TOXICOLOGY
HANDBOOK

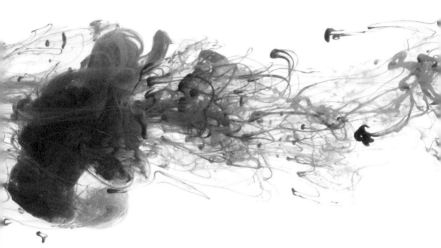

TOXICOLOGY HANDBOOK

4TH EDITION

Jason Armstrong
Ovidiu Pascu

ELSEVIER

Elsevier

Elsevier Australia. ACN 001 002 357
(a division of Reed International Books Australia Pty Ltd)
Tower 1, 475 Victoria Avenue, Chatswood, NSW 2067

Notice

Knowledge and best practice in this field are constantly changing. As new research and
experience broaden our understanding, changes in research methods, professional practices
or medical treatment may become necessary.

Practitioners and researchers must always rely on their own experience and knowledge in
evaluating and using any information, methods, compounds or experiments described herein.
In using such information or methods they should be mindful of their own safety and the safety
of others, including parties for whom they have a professional responsibility.

With respect to any drug or pharmaceutical products identified, readers are advised to check
the most current information provided (i) on procedures featured or (ii) by the manufacturer of
each product to be administered, to verify the recommended dose or formula, the method and
duration of administration and contraindications. It is the responsibility of practitioners, relying
on their own experience and knowledge of their patients, to make diagnoses, to determine
dosages and the best treatment for each individual patient and to take all appropriate safety
precautions.

To the fullest extent of the law, neither the Publisher nor the authors, contributors or editors,
assume any liability for any injury and/or damage to persons or property as a matter of product
liability, negligence or otherwise, or from any use or operation of any methods, products,
instructions or ideas contained in the material herein.

National Library of Australia Cataloguing-in-Publication entry

Jason Armstrong, Ovidiu Pascu authors.
    Toxicology handbook, 4th edition / Jason Armstrong, Ovidiu Pascu.
    4th edition.
    978-0-7295-4436-8 (paperback)
    Includes index.
    Armstrong, Jason
    Pascu, Ovidiu.

Content Strategist: Larissa Norrie
Content Project Manager: Shivani Pal
Edited by Katie Millar
Index by SPI
Typeset by Aptara
Cover and internal design by Gopalakrishnan Venkatraman

Printed in Singapore
Last digit is the print number: 9 8 7 6 5 4 3 2 1

CONTENTS

CHAPTER 6 ANTIVENOMS

APPENDICES

It gives me great personal pleasure to welcome the arrival of the
4th Edition of the Toxicology Handbook. This text was originally
produced by an enthusiastic group of Western Australian Emergency
Physicians trying to establish the sub-speciality of Clinical Toxicology.
Its aim was to provide a concise bedside text to assist the clinician
charged with treating the acutely poisoned patient. The point of
difference was that it did not just provide factual information. It also
encouraged the user to adopt a rigorous and structured risk assessment-
based approach to decision making in the context of Clinical Toxicology.
The Handbook's success in disseminating this approach, and its utility at
the bedside, are attested to by the well-thumbed editions found in
Emergency Departments across Australasia.

This updated edition of the Handbook incorporates necessary and
important modifications to reflect an evolving evidence base and
pharmaco-epidemiology. As such, its appearance is welcome and timely.
Reassuringly, the newest edition continues to be soundly based on the
same structured approach to assessment and management of the acutely
poisoned patient. As such, it will continue to serve the Emergency
Medicine community and their poisoned patients as a trusted pragmatic
source of clinical toxicology guidance.

I congratulate the editors of the fourth edition of the Toxicology
Handbook.

Lindsay Murray MBBS FACEM
Co-Director, Emergency Medicine
Lismore Base Hospital, Northern NSW Local Health District

PREFACE TO 4TH EDITION

It is a great honour for us to have been involved with the Toxicology Handbook since its inception, and now to take over from Lindsay Murray as primary authors of the 4th edition. The Handbook has become a standard reference for medical practitioners and health-care professionals, ranging from the pre-hospital environment to the intensive care unit. The strength of the book is its role as a concise, practical bedside text, providing the clinician with the confidence to make safe, well-informed management decisions in treating the poisoned patient.

The structured approach to assessment and management represents the distillation of many years of clinical experience and expertise. The R RSI DEAD framework is a simple, easily-remembered and elegant approach which forms the basis of care for all toxicology patients. We continue in this 4th edition with the same essential emphasis on the risk assessment and have significantly updated the content based on new research and guidelines, to cover the wide variety of presentations encountered in Clinical Toxicology. Additional chapters have been added to discuss newer agents that are seen with increasing frequency in poisoned patients.

Treatment recommendations for cardiotoxicity and dysrhythmias, particularly resulting from drug-induced conduction abnormalities (QRS and QT prolongation), have been simplified and standardised throughout the Handbook to improve the approach to patient management. In addition, we have expanded the sections on Controversies for a number of important topics, to highlight and address the dilemmas faced by clinicians as they make management decisions at the bedside.

We feel great satisfaction to visit other Emergency Departments and find a well-used version of the Handbook lying on the desk - we hope that this reflects the relevant, useful and enlightening information it provides.

We dedicate this edition to Lindsay Murray, our teacher and mentor, whose clear and compassionate approach to Clinical Toxicology and to patient care in general has influenced us throughout our careers.

Jason Armstrong
Ovidiu Pascu

EDITORS

Jason Armstrong MD FACEM
Consultant Emergency Physician and Clinical Toxicologist, Sir
Charles Gairdner Hospital, Perth, WA
Medical Director, WA Poisons Information Centre
Clinical Senior Lecturer in Emergency Medicine, University of
Western Australia, Australia
Ovidiu Pascu MD FACEM
Consultant Emergency Physician and Clinical Toxicologist, Sir
Charles Gairdner Hospital, Perth, WA
Clinical Toxicologist, WA Poisons Information Centre

CONTRIBUTORS

Alan Gault, MBChB FACEM
Consultant Emergency Physician and Clinical Toxicologist
Sir Charles Gairdner Hospital, Perth, WA;
Clinical Toxicologist, WA Poisons Information Centre
Candice Hanson, BMedSci MBBS(Hons) FACEM
Consultant Emergency Physician and Clinical Toxicology Fellow,
Sir Charles Gairdner Hospital, Perth, WA
Jeremy Mason, MBBS
Toxicology Registrar, Sir Charles Gairdner Hospital, Perth, WA
Nick Merwood, BSc MPharm
Poisons Information Specialist, WA Poisons Information Centre, Sir
Charles Gairdner Hospital, Perth, WA
Gareth Wahl, MBBS FACEM
Consultant Emergency Physician and Clinical Toxicologist, Sir
Charles Gairdner Hospital, Perth, WA; Clinical Toxicologist, WA
Poisons Information Centre

CHAPTER 1
APPROACH TO THE POISONED PATIENT

1.1 OVERVIEW

Acute poisoning is a common emergency medicine presentation. Between 150 and 400 acute poisoning presentations annually can be expected for each 100 000 population served by an emergency department. Acute poisoning is a dynamic medical illness that frequently represents a potentially life-threatening exacerbation of a chronic psychosocial disorder. However, this is a highly heterogeneous patient population: deliberate self-poisoning, recreational drug abuse, occupational poisoning and envenoming challenge with myriad potential presentations. The clinician needs a robust and simple clinical approach that can address this heterogeneity but that allows the development of a management plan tailored to the individual patient at that particular presentation at that particular medical facility.

Risk assessment is pivotal to that robust approach. It is a distinct cognitive process through which the clinician attempts to predict the likely clinical course and potential complications for the individual at that particular presentation. Risk assessment should wherever possible be quantitative and take into account the agent, dose and time of ingestion, clinical features and progress, and individual patient factors (e.g. weight and co-morbidities).

Toxicology management guidelines frequently focus on the agent involved. This makes adaptation of treatment recommendations to an individual patient in a particular location difficult. A risk-assessment-based approach ensures the clinician addresses potentially time-critical management priorities in an appropriate order but avoids unnecessary investigations or interventions.

Risk assessment is secondary only to resuscitation in the management of acute poisoning. It allows subsequent management decisions regarding supportive care and monitoring, investigations, decontamination, use of enhanced elimination techniques, antidotes and disposition to be made in a sensible structured manner.

Ideally, this risk-assessment-based approach is supported by a healthcare system designed to address both the medical and the psychological needs of the poisoned patient. Where the medical needs of a patient exceed local resources, a risk-assessment-based management approach ensures that this is identified early and disposition planning and communication occur in a proactive manner within that organised system.

In this handbook, the authors offer a systematic risk-assessment-based approach to the management of acute poisoning as it presents to the emergency department (see **Table 1.1.1**). Separate chapters cover the pharmaceutical, chemical and natural toxins of most importance to the

TABLE 1.1.1   Risk-assessment-based approach to poisoning (R RSI DEAD)

Resuscitation
   Airway
   Breathing
   Circulation
   Detect and correct
   — Hypoglycaemia
   — Seizures
   — Hyper-/hypothermia
   Emergency antidote administration
Risk assessment
   Agent(s)
   Dose(s)
   Time since ingestion
   Clinical features and course
   Patient factors
Supportive care and monitoring
Investigations
   Screening—12-lead ECG, paracetamol, blood glucose level (BGL)
   Specific
Decontamination
Enhanced elimination
Antidotes
Disposition

practitioner in emergency departments in Australia and New Zealand. It will also be of use to ambulance and emergency paramedic personnel and staff of general intensive care units. The approach to acute poisoning presented in this book is honed at the bedside and on the telephone. The authors collectively have directly cared for many thousands of patients in the Western Australian Toxicology Service and offered consultation in thousands more acute poisonings across Australia and overseas via the Western Australian, New South Wales, Victorian and Queensland Poisons Information Centres (PICs). The agents covered are carefully selected to cover all common poisonings, rare but life-threatening poisonings and poisonings where particular interventions make a difference to outcome or which result in frequent consultations with clinical toxicologists through the PIC network. Chapters are also offered on the important antidotes and antivenoms with practical information on administration, dose and adverse effects. All chapters highlight the important features of the risk assessment. All chapters have special sections on 'pitfalls' and 'handy tips'. These are not for show! They are designed to respond to the real questions and mistakes that regularly occur in clinical practice across Australasia.

Clinical toxicology has rightly become an area of expertise of the emergency doctor but the infinite variation in presentation constantly confounds and surprises all of us. We hope that the information in this book, when combined with a structured approach, will improve the care delivered to the poisoned patient.

Poisoning is most frequently the presentation of an individual suffering from exacerbation of very significant underlying psychiatric, social or drug and alcohol problems. Excellence in care of the poisoning delivered in a compassionate manner offers the best opportunity to intervene and produce a positive outcome for this vulnerable group of patients.

References

Daly FFS, Little M, Murray L. A risk assessment based approach to the management of acute poisoning. Emergency Medicine Journal 2006; 23(5):396–399. doi:10.1136/emj.2005.030312.

Erickson TB, Thompson TM. The approach to the patient with an unknown overdose. Emergency Medicine Clinics of North America 2007; 25(2):249–281.

1.2 RESUSCITATION

INTRODUCTION

Poisoning is a leading cause of death in patients under the age of 40 years and is a leading differential diagnosis when cardiac arrest occurs in a young adult.

Unlike cardiac arrest in the older population, resuscitation following acute poisoning may be associated with good neurological outcomes even after prolonged periods (hours) of cardiopulmonary resuscitation (CPR). Therefore, when poisoning is considered part of the differential diagnosis in a patient with cardiac arrest, resuscitation should continue until expert advice can be obtained. Extracorporeal membrane oxygenation therapy (ECMO) may provide life-saving bridging therapy in selected cases of severe refractory shock or adult respiratory distress syndrome.

Attempts at decontamination of the skin or gastrointestinal tract almost never take priority over resuscitation and institution of supportive care measures.

AIRWAY, BREATHING AND CIRCULATION

Acute poisoning is a dynamic medical illness and patients may deteriorate within a few minutes or hours of presentation. Altered conscious state, loss of airway protective reflexes, hypoventilation and hypotension are immediate life-threats in the poisoned patient.

As in all life-threatening emergencies, attention to airway, breathing and circulation are paramount. These priorities are usually managed along conventional lines. Basic resuscitative and supportive care measures ensure the survival of the vast majority of patients (see **Table 1.2.1**).

TABLE 1.2.1	Resuscitation

Airway
Breathing
Circulation
Detect and correct:
    Seizures
        Always generalised when due to toxicological causes
        Benzodiazepines are first-line therapy
    Hypoglycaemia
        Check bedside blood glucose level (BGL) in all patients with altered
            mental status
        Treat if BGL <4.0 mmol/L
    Hyper-/hypothermia
        Temp >38.5°C prompts urgent intervention
Emergency antidote administration

Although commonly used to describe a patient's mental status, clinical scores such as the Glasgow Coma Scale (GCS) or Alert–Verbal–Pain–Unresponsive (AVPU) system have never been systematically validated across all poisonings. A patient's ability to guard their airway is not well correlated to GCS. An increased risk of aspiration has been noted with GCS less than 15. Moreover, a patient's ability to guard the airway and ventilate effectively may change within a short period of time.

In some specific situations, standard resuscitation algorithms do not apply (see **Table 1.2.2**).

DETECT AND CORRECT SEIZURES

Toxic seizures are generalised and can usually be controlled with intravenous benzodiazepines (e.g. midazolam or diazepam). The most common causes of seizures in poisoned patients in Australia are agents with stimulant properties such as amphetamines, tramadol and venlafaxine. Seizures related to ethanol or benzodiazepine withdrawal are also common.

The presence of focal or partial seizures indicates a focal neurological disorder that is either a complication of poisoning or due to a non-toxicological cause, and prompts further investigation.

Barbiturates are recommended as second-line therapy for refractory seizures in acute poisoning. Pyridoxine is indicated in the extremely rare presentation of recurrent seizures secondary to isoniazid poisoning.

Phenytoin is contraindicated in the management of seizures related to acute poisoning because of poor efficacy and the potential to exacerbate sodium channel blockade, which may be a causative mechanism. Other anticonvulsant agents such as levetiracetam have a limited role in the management of acute toxicological seizures.

TABLE 1.2.2 Specific resuscitation situations in toxicology where conventional algorithms or approaches may not apply

Life-threat	Mechanism	Agent(s)	Comments
AIRWAY			
Airway compromise	Corrosive injury to oropharynx	• Alkalis • Acids • Glyphosate • Paraquat	• Stridor, dysphagia and dysphonia indicate airway injury and potential for imminent airway compromise • Early endotracheal intubation or surgical airway often required
BREATHING			
Acidosis Acidaemia	Various	• Ethylene glycol • Methanol • Salicylates	• Until late in the clinical course there is usually prominent respiratory compensation • Intubation and ventilation at standard settings worsens acidaemia and may precipitate rapid clinical deterioration • Maintain hyperventilation and consider bolus IV sodium bicarbonate 1–2 mmol/kg to prevent worsening of acidaemia
Hypoventilation	Opioid mu receptor stimulation	• Opioids	• Prompt administration of naloxone may obviate need for intubation and ventilation
Respiratory failure	Cholinergic crisis	• Carbamates • Nerve agents • Organophosphates	• Rapid administration of atropine to achieve drying of respiratory secretions may improve oxygenation
Hypoxaemia	Oxygen free-radical-mediated pulmonary injury	• Paraquat	• Avoid supplemental oxygen; if hypoxia occurs, titrate supplemental oxygen to maintain oxygen saturation of ~90% or PaO_2 60 mmHg

TABLE 1.2.2 Specific resuscitation situations in toxicology where conventional algorithms or approaches may not apply—cont'd

Life-threat	Mechanism	Agent(s)	Comments
CIRCULATION			
Torsades de pointes (polymorphic ventricular tachycardia)	QT prolongation	• Amisulpride • Antipsychotics • Chloroquine/ hydroxychloroquine • Citalopram/ escitalopram • Methadone • Sotalol	• Electrical cardioversion may be required for persistent episodes • Magnesium, isoprenaline or overdrive electrical pacing are recommended treatment options • Ensure that all QT-dependent electrolytes are at the upper limit of normal (potassium, calcium, magnesium)
Ventricular dysrhythmias	Fast sodium channel blockade	• Chloroquine/ hydroxychloroquine • Cocaine • Flecainide • Local anaesthetic agents • Procainamide • Propranolol • Quinine • Tricyclic antidepressants	• Cardioversion or defibrillation unlikely to be efficacious • Urgently intubate and hyperventilate • Bolus IV sodium bicarbonate 1–2 mmol/kg repeated every 1–2 minutes until restoration of perfusing rhythm and pH established at 7.5–7.55 • Lidocaine is third-line therapy once therapeutic pH is established • Amiodarone is not a recommended agent
Ventricular ectopy/ ventricular tachycardia	Toxin-induced myocardial sensitisation to catecholamines	• Chloral hydrate • Hydrocarbons • Organochlorines	• Cardioversion or defibrillation unlikely to be efficacious • IV beta-blockers indicated

Continued

TABLE 1.2.2 Specific resuscitation situations in toxicology where conventional algorithms or approaches may not apply—cont'd

Life-threat	Mechanism	Agent(s)	Comments
CIRCULATION cont'd			
Cardiovascular collapse/ arrest	Fast sodium channel blockade	• Local anaesthetic agents	• Consider intravenous lipid emulsion in addition to standard resuscitation protocols
Cardiogenic shock	Various	• Diltiazem and verapamil • Beta-blockers • Acute stress-induced (sympathomimetic) cardiotoxicity	• High-dose insulin therapy
Tachycardia	Central and peripheral sympathomimetic response	• Amphetamines • Cocaine	• Beta-blockers contraindicated • Administer IV benzodiazepines, titrated to response
Supraventricular tachycardia	Adenosine antagonism	• Theophylline	• Adenosine ineffective • Beta-blockers titrated to effect • Urgent haemodialysis indicated

Hypertension	Central and peripheral sympathomimetic response	• Amphetamines
		• Cocaine
			• Beta-blockers contraindicated
			• Administer IV benzodiazepines, titrated to response
			• If further therapy necessary, use agents that can be given by titratable intravenous infusion
			  — Glyceryl trinitrate (GTN)
			  — Phentolamine
			  — Sodium nitroprusside

TABLE 1.2.2 Specific resuscitation situations in toxicology where conventional algorithms or approaches may not apply—cont'd

Life-threat	Mechanism	Agent(s)	Comments
CIRCULATION cont'd			
Cardiac dysrhythmias	Na⁺-K⁺-ATPase pump inhibition	• Digoxin	• Usual resuscitation interventions futile • Digoxin-specific antibodies (Fab)
Acute coronary syndrome	Central and peripheral sympathomimetic response	• Amphetamines • Cocaine	• Beta-blockers contraindicated • Benzodiazepines • GTN • Antiplatelet and anticoagulation therapy if no contraindication • Reperfusion therapy along conventional lines
OTHER			
Hyperkalaemia	Na⁺-K⁺-ATPase pump inhibition	• Digoxin	• Digoxin-specific antibodies (Fab)
Hypoglycaemia	Hyperinsulinaemia	• Sulfonylureas	• Difficult to maintain euglycaemia with glucose supplementation alone • Octreotide
Seizures	Inhibition of GABA production	• Isoniazid	• IV pyridoxine 1 g per gram of isoniazid ingested, up to 5 g
Seizures	Adenosine antagonism	• Theophylline	• Urgent haemodialysis indicated

DETECT AND CORRECT HYPOGLYCAEMIA

Hypoglycaemia is an easily detectable and correctable cause of significant neurological features. Bedside blood glucose level (BGL) estimation should be performed as soon as possible in all patients with altered mental status.

If the blood glucose is less than 4.0 mmol/L, 50 mL of 50% glucose should be given intravenously (2–5 mL/kg 10% glucose in children) to urgently correct hypoglycaemia.

Hypoglycaemia in acute poisoning is associated with numerous agents including insulin, sulfonylureas, beta-blockers, quinine, chloroquine, salicylates and valproic acid.

DETECT AND CORRECT HYPER-/HYPOTHERMIA

Hyperthermia is associated with a number of life-threatening acute poisonings and is associated with poor outcome.

A temperature greater than 38.5°C during the resuscitation phase of management is an indication for continuous core-temperature monitoring.

A temperature greater than 39.5°C is an emergency that requires prompt management to prevent multiple organ failure and neurological injury. Neuromuscular paralysis with intubation and ventilation leads to a cessation of muscle-generated heat production and a rapid reduction of temperature.

Profound hypothermia (core temperature <29°C) may mimic or cause cardiac arrest. Clinical manifestations include coma, fixed and dilated pupils, bradycardia (usually atrial fibrillation) and hypotension. Vital signs may be difficult to elicit and the cardiac rhythm may degenerate to ventricular fibrillation or asystole. In the patient with undetectable vital signs, immediate exogenous rewarming is indicated while CPR continues. Cardiopulmonary bypass or extracorporeal membrane oxygenation (ECMO), if available, are the most effective means.

EMERGENCY ANTIDOTE ADMINISTRATION

Administration of antidotes is sometimes indicated during the resuscitation phase of management. As with all drugs, antidotes have indications, adverse effects and contraindications. The decision to administer an antidote during resuscitation will depend on the perceived benefit compared to possible adverse effects.

Examples where early administration of an antidote is necessary to ensure a successful resuscitation include intravenous sodium bicarbonate in tricyclic antidepressant poisoning, naloxone in severe opioid poisoning, atropine in severe organophosphorus agent poisoning and digoxin-specific antibodies for patients with digoxin poisoning and cardiovascular compromise.

References

Albertson TE, Dawson AH, de Latorre F et al. TOX-ACLS: toxicologic-oriented advanced cardiac life support. Annals of Emergency Medicine 2001; 37:S78–S90.

Australian Resuscitation Council. Adult advanced life support: Australian Resuscitation Council guidelines 2006: Guideline 11.6. Emergency Medicine Australasia 2006; 18:337–356.

De Lange DW, Sikma MA, Meulenbelt J. Extracorporeal membrane oxygenation in the treatment of poisoned patients. Clinical Toxicology 2013; 51:385–393.

Gunja N, Graudins A. Management of cardiac arrest following poisoning. Emergency Medicine Australasia 2011; 23:16–22.

Isbister GK, Downes F, Sibbritt D et al. Aspiration pneumonitis in an overdose population: frequency, predictors, and outcomes. Critical Care Medicine 2004; 32:88–93.

Kopec KT, Brent J, Banner W et al. Management of cardiac dysrhythmias following hydrocarbon abuse: clinical toxicology case from NACCT acute and intensive care symposium. Clinical Toxicology 2014; 52:141–145.

Vanden Hoek TL, Morrison LJ, Shuster M et al. Part 12: Cardiac arrest in special situations: 2010 American Heart Association guidelines for cardiopulmonary and emergency cardiovascular care. Circulation 2010; 122:S829–S861.

1.3 RISK ASSESSMENT

Risk assessment should occur as soon as possible in the management of the poisoned patient. Only resuscitation is a greater priority. Risk assessment is a distinct quantitative cognitive step through which the clinician attempts to predict the likely clinical course and potential complications for the individual patient at that particular presentation.

The five key components of the history and examination required to formulate a risk assessment are listed in **Table 1.3.1**.

Risk assessment is pivotal as it allows the clinician to identify potential problems and make specific balanced decisions about all subsequent management steps (supportive care and monitoring, screening and specialised testing, decontamination, enhanced elimination, antidotes and disposition).

Provided their mental status is normal, patients with deliberate self-poisoning are generally both willing and able to give a good history from which an accurate risk assessment can be constructed. Doctors ignore the patient's history at their peril.

TABLE 1.3.1 Information required to formulate a risk assessment
1 Agent(s)
2 Dose(s)
3 Time since ingestion
4 Clinical features and progress
5 Patient factors (weight and co-morbidities)

If altered mental status precludes obtaining a direct history, back-up strategies are employed to gather the necessary information. These include:

1 asking ambulance officers or family to search for agents
2 counting missing tablets
3 checking medical records for previous prescriptions
4 questioning relatives about agents potentially available to the patient.

Under these circumstances, the risk assessment is less accurate and is often based on a 'worst-case scenario'. This is commonly the case with small children where ingestions are rarely witnessed. As the clinical course progresses, the risk assessment and management plan may be refined.

In unknown ingestions, the patient's clinical status is correlated with the clinician's knowledge of the agents commonly available in that geographical area. For example, central nervous system (CNS) and respiratory depression associated with miotic pupils indicates opioid intoxication in a young adult male in urban Australia but is more likely to indicate organophosphate intoxication in rural Sri Lanka.

The agent, dose and time since ingestion should correlate with the patient's current clinical status. If they do not, the risk assessment needs to be reviewed and revised.

Acute poisoning is a dynamic process and important decisions can often be made at particular time points. For example, following tricyclic antidepressant self-poisoning, life-threatening events occur within 6 hours (and usually within the first 2 hours) of ingestion. Therefore, low-risk patients can be identified on clinical grounds at 6 hours post ingestion. In contrast, following deliberate self-poisoning with sustained-release calcium channel blockers, patients may not exhibit clinical features of poisoning during the first few hours. A properly performed risk assessment anticipates the development of severe cardiovascular toxicity and allows appropriate preparation of staff, equipment and resources.

In the majority of cases, the risk assessment allows early recognition of medically trivial poisonings. This reassures attending staff, family and patient and permits the avoidance of unnecessary investigations, interventions and prolonged observation or admission. Early psychosocial assessment and discharge planning may commence, which shortens hospital length of stay.

Less commonly, but very importantly, risk assessment allows early identification of potentially serious poisoning and the implementation of a tailored proactive management plan. Informed decisions about the requirement for gastrointestinal decontamination can be made and appropriate investigations selected. If a specialised procedure or antidote might be required in the next few hours, early communication and disposition planning may begin.

ROLE OF THE POISONS INFORMATION CENTRE

The clinician's ability to construct an accurate risk assessment relies on knowledge and experience of the toxic agents concerned. Although this is straightforward for many exposures, new or unusual agents are frequently encountered. A variety of sources of information may be used to obtain the information necessary to formulate a risk assessment. Textbooks and databases may be difficult to evaluate emergently and apply to the individual patient. When faced with a time-critical poisoning emergency, a call to the poisons information centre is the most rapid mechanism to obtain accurate information and individualised risk assessment.

The Australian Poisons Information Centre network comprises centres located in Sydney, Perth, Brisbane and Melbourne that can be accessed nationwide by calling 131126. The New Zealand Poisons Information Centre located in Dunedin is accessed by calling 0800 764 766 (0800-POISON). Trained poisons information specialists with a background in pharmacy or medical science are familiar with accessing information from computerised databases and other information sources. They can assist in the identification of commercial products and their constituents and in the formulation of a risk assessment, provided the clinician is able to provide appropriate information. Where necessary, medical callers treating an acute poisoning case are referred to an on-call clinical toxicologist who is able to offer more detailed individualised risk assessment and management advice.

Reference
Daly FF, Little M, Murray L. A risk assessment based approach to the management of acute poisoning. Emergency Medicine Journal 2006; 23:396–399.

1.4 SUPPORTIVE CARE AND MONITORING

Following resuscitation and risk assessment, supportive care and disposition planning can begin.

Poisoning morbidity and mortality usually result from the acute effects of the toxin on the cardiovascular, central nervous or respiratory systems. Support of these and other systems for the duration of the intoxication will ensure a good outcome for the vast majority of acute poisonings. Monitoring is essential to detect the progress of the intoxication and the timing of institution, escalation and withdrawal of supportive care and other measures.

An initial period of close observation in the emergency department is usually appropriate. During this time, the patient's clinical status is monitored closely to ensure that it correlates with the previous risk assessment. If early complications are expected (e.g. decreased level of consciousness requiring intubation in the following 2 hours), preparations can be made to secure the airway as soon as the intoxication declares itself and before the patient is moved elsewhere. If unexpected deterioration occurs at any time, the clinician's priorities revert to resuscitation prior to revising the risk assessment.

The duration of observation depends on the agent(s) ingested, the formulations involved (e.g. sustained-release preparations) and potential complications. For example, patients with significant beta-blocker and tricyclic antidepressant deliberate self-poisoning develop symptoms and signs of major intoxication within 2–4 hours of ingestion. In contrast, patients with sustained-release calcium channel blocker or valproic acid deliberate self-poisoning may take 6–12 hours to develop signs of major toxicity.

Disposition from the emergency department depends on the current and expected clinical status of the patient. If specific complications are anticipated, the chosen inpatient clinical area must be resourced to detect and manage them.

The accuracy and skill of the initial management and risk assessment are wasted if the subsequent plan of management is not documented and communicated to the treating team. Good practice includes the documentation of a comprehensive management plan that informs the team looking after the patient of:

1   expected clinical course
2   potential complications according to the individual risk assessment
3   type of observation and monitoring required
4   end points that must trigger notification of the treating doctor or further consultation
5   management plans for agitation or delirium
6   criteria for changing management
7   provisional psychosocial risk assessment with contingency plan should the patient attempt to abscond prior to formal psychosocial assessment.

The needs of the vast majority of patients can be met in the emergency department, emergency observation unit or intensive care unit. The emergency observation unit is appropriate for the ongoing management of most acute poisonings, where the general supportive measures outlined in **Table 1.4.1** can be provided.

Criteria for admission to an emergency observation unit following acute poisoning include:

1   clinical deterioration not anticipated
2   adequate sedation achieved.

TABLE 1.4.1 Supportive care measures

Airway
  Intubation
Breathing
  Supplemental oxygen
  Ventilation
Circulation
  Intravenous fluids
  Inotropes
  Control of hypertension
  Extracorporeal membrane oxygenation
Sedation
  Titrated IV benzodiazepines
Seizure control/prophylaxis
  IV benzodiazepines
Metabolic
  Ensuring normoglycaemia
  Control of pH
Fluids and electrolytes
Renal function
  Adequate hydration
  Haemodialysis
General
  Nutrition
  Respiratory toilet
  Bladder care (serial bladder scans and indwelling catheter as indicated)
  Prevention of pressure areas
  Thromboembolism prophylaxis
  Mobilisation as mental status changes resolve

Criteria for admission to an intensive care unit following acute poisoning include requirements for:

1 airway control
2 ventilation
3 prolonged or invasive haemodynamic monitoring or support
4 haemodialysis.

1.5 INVESTIGATIONS

Investigations in acute poisoning are employed either as screening tests or for specific purposes.

Screening refers to the performance of a medical evaluation and/or diagnostic test in asymptomatic persons in the hope that early diagnosis may lead to improved outcome. In the acutely poisoned patient, screening tests aim to identify occult toxic ingestions for which early specific treatment is indicated.

TABLE 1.5.1 Screening tests
12-lead ECG
Rate
Rhythm
PR interval
QRS interval
QT interval
Dominant R wave in aVR
Bedside BGL
Serum paracetamol level

The recommended screening tests for acute poisoning are a 12-lead electrocardiogram (ECG), a bedside blood glucose level (BGL) and a serum paracetamol level (see **Table 1.5.1**).

The ECG is a readily available non-invasive tool that assists in the identification of occult but potentially lethal cardiac conduction abnormalities, such as those in tricyclic antidepressant cardiotoxicity.

The bedside BGL is used to detect hypoglycaemia that may be missed, particularly in the patient with altered mental status due to other drug effects. It is performed during the initial resuscitation and assessment phase of any poisoned patient with altered mental status.

Paracetamol is a ubiquitous analgesic in the western world. Deliberate self-poisoning with paracetamol is common, comprising up to 15% of adult poisoning presentations in Australasia. Life-threatening paracetamol poisoning may be occult in the early stages, but progression to fulminant hepatic failure and death can be prevented by timely administration of N-acetylcysteine. Although a thorough cost–benefit analysis has never been performed, it is postulated that the cost of several thousand serum paracetamol measurements is offset by the detection of one potentially preventable paracetamol-related death or liver transplant. For this reason, it is advisable to screen for paracetamol in all cases of known or suspected acute deliberate self-poisoning. Screening is particularly important where altered mental status precludes obtaining an ingestion history directly from the patient.

The screening paracetamol level may be performed at presentation and does not need to be delayed until 4 hours after ingestion. A non-detectable paracetamol level more than 1 hour after ingestion excludes significant paracetamol ingestion and further paracetamol levels are not required.

If paracetamol poisoning is suspected after the initial risk assessment, then a screening paracetamol level is not the appropriate test. Instead, a timed paracetamol level should be performed 4 hours post ingestion (or as soon as possible after 4 hours) as part of the toxicological evaluation.

Serum salicylate and tricyclic antidepressant assays have been advocated as routine screening tests. Salicylate poisoning is now relatively uncommon in Australasia. Significant acute intoxication is associated with a recognisable pattern of symptoms and acid–base disturbances and is rarely occult. Therefore, routine screening for salicylate in patients without symptoms or signs of salicylism does not comply with the rationale for screening and should not be performed. Serum tricyclic antidepressant levels correlate with complications and outcome following acute poisoning. However, the major complications of tricyclic antidepressant poisoning usually occur within 2–4 hours of ingestion. The 12-lead ECG, correlated to the patient's clinical status, reflects target organ effects more accurately and is the preferred screening test.

Many poisoned patients are young and have few medical co-morbidities. After appropriate risk assessment and the institution of supportive care, they may require no further investigation beyond the screening ECG, bedside BGL and serum paracetamol measurement. In a young and otherwise healthy patient presenting with normal mental status and vital signs, additional tests such as electrolytes, full blood picture, liver function tests and coagulation studies are not routinely indicated.

Other investigations are ordered selectively where it is anticipated that the results will assist risk assessment or management. Potential indications for specific tests in the acute poisoning patient are shown in **Table 1.5.2**.

For most patients and poisonings, the risk assessment and subsequent clinical course dictate management decisions. Drug concentrations do not usually assist decision making. Some of the few agents where serum levels assist in risk assessment or management decisions are shown in **Table 1.5.3**.

Qualitative urine screens for drugs of abuse (e.g. opioids, benzodiazepines, amphetamines, cocaine, barbiturates and cannabinoids) rarely alter the management of the acutely poisoned patient and are not

---

TABLE 1.5.2   Indications for other investigations
Refine risk assessment or prognosis
Exclude or confirm an important differential diagnosis
Exclude or confirm an important specific poisoning
Exclude or confirm a complication that requires specific management
Establish an indication for antidote administration
Establish an indication for institution of enhanced elimination
Monitor response to therapy or define an end point for a therapeutic intervention

TABLE 1.5.3	Useful drug levels that may assist risk assessment or management in specific settings	
Carbamazepine	Lithium	Salicylate
Digoxin	Methanol	Theophylline
Ethanol	Methotrexate	Valproic acid
Ethylene glycol	Paracetamol	
Iron	Phenobarbitone	

routinely indicated. Patients with acute intoxication with one or more of these agents may be managed according to their clinical presentation. On occasion, a urine drug screen can be indicated to provide evidence of illicit or recreational drug use if the history is not evident or forthcoming.

References

Ashbourne JF, Olson KR, Khayam-Bashi H. Value of rapid screening for acetaminophen in all patients with intentional drug overdose. Annals of Emergency Medicine 1989; 18(10):1035–1038.

Chiew AL, Reith DM, Pomerleau AC et al. Updated guidelines for the management of paracetamol poisoning in Australia and New Zealand. Medical Journal of Australia 2019; 212(4):175–183.

Sporer KA, Khayam-Bashi H. Acetaminophen and salicylate serum levels in patients with suicidal ingestion or altered mental status. American Journal of Emergency Medicine 1996; 14(5):443–446.

1.6 GASTROINTESTINAL DECONTAMINATION

Doctors have long directed great effort into attempts at gastrointestinal decontamination following ingestion of toxic substances. They have employed a variety of methods (see **Table 1.6.1**) in the reasonable expectation that, by reducing the dose absorbed, they will also reduce the subsequent severity and duration of clinical toxicity. Unfortunately, the tendency has been to overestimate the potential benefits while underestimating the potential hazards of gastrointestinal decontamination procedures. These procedures do not provide significant benefit when applied to unselected deliberate self-poisoned patients and are no longer considered routine.

TABLE 1.6.1 Methods of gastrointestinal decontamination
● Activated charcoal
● Whole bowel irrigation
No longer recommended:
● Induced emesis (syrup of ipecac)
● Gastric lavage

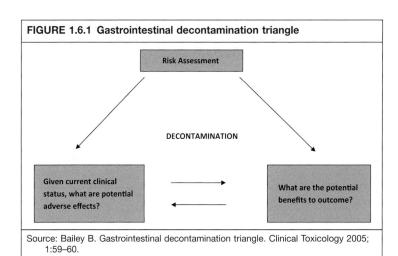

FIGURE 1.6.1 Gastrointestinal decontamination triangle

Source: Bailey B. Gastrointestinal decontamination triangle. Clinical Toxicology 2005; 1:59–60.

The theoretical benefits of gastrointestinal decontamination have not been definitively evaluated in controlled studies for all poisonings. The decision to decontaminate is one of clinical judgement in which the potential benefits are weighed against the potential risks and the resources required to perform the procedure (see **Figure 1.6.1** and **Table 1.6.2**).

Employing this rationale, gastrointestinal decontamination is reserved for cases where the risk assessment predicts severe or life-threatening toxicity and where supportive care or antidote treatment alone is insufficient to ensure a satisfactory outcome. There should be reasonable grounds to believe that a significant amount of agent remains unabsorbed and is amenable to removal by the selected procedure. This requires

TABLE 1.6.2 Gastrointestinal decontamination: risk–benefit analysis

Potential benefits	Potential risks
<ul><li>Improved clinical outcome (morbidity and mortality)</li><li>More benign clinical course requiring lower level of supportive care</li><li>Reduced need for other potentially hazardous interventions or expensive antidotes</li><li>Reduced hospital length of stay</li></ul>	<ul><li>Pulmonary aspiration</li><li>Gastrointestinal complications<ul><li>— Bowel obstruction</li><li>— Perforation</li></ul></li><li>Distraction of staff from resuscitation and supportive care priorities</li><li>Diversion of departmental resources for performance of procedure</li></ul>

knowledge of the absorption kinetics of the agent(s) involved. For most ingested agents, absorption is virtually complete within 1 hour.

Gastrointestinal decontamination is never performed to the detriment of basic resuscitation or supportive care. To avoid pulmonary aspiration, the procedure is not performed without first securing the airway in a patient with a depressed level of consciousness or in whom the risk assessment indicates the potential for imminent seizures or decline in conscious state.

SINGLE-DOSE ACTIVATED CHARCOAL

Activated charcoal (AC) is produced by the super-heating of distilled wood pulp. The resulting fine porous particles are suspended in water or sorbitol prior to oral or nasogastric administration. Most commonly ingested agents are bound (adsorbed) by electrostatic and other intermolecular forces to the extensive surface area provided by these particles, preventing further absorption from the gastrointestinal tract (see **Table 1.6.3** for a list of agents that do not bind to activated charcoal).

Oral AC is the preferred method of gastrointestinal decontamination. However, it does not improve clinical outcome in all patients with self-poisoning and should not be regarded as routine. It is most likely to benefit a subgroup of patients with severe poisoning by reducing the length of hospital stay, level of supportive care required or requirement for use of enhanced elimination techniques or antidote administration.

AC is indicated where it is likely that toxin remains in the gastrointestinal tract (particularly if given within the first 1–2 hours after ingestion for most agents) and where the potential benefits outweigh the potential risks. The main concern is pulmonary aspiration of charcoal, due to vomiting or loss of airway reflexes associated with impaired level of consciousness or seizures. It is recommended to routinely administer AC via a nasogastric tube to unconscious patients who have ingested pharmaceutical agents once the airway is protected by intubation, as the risk–benefit analysis is almost always in favour of administration. Administration of AC to an uncooperative patient either orally or by insertion of a nasogastric tube is not safe or practical and should not be attempted. The one possible exception is following ingestion of colchicine, where administration of AC can be considered a justified life-saving intervention.

There are several important presentations where administration of AC is indicated even many hours after ingestion, including for salicylates, massive ingestions (particularly paracetamol) or slow-release formulations of diltiazem or verapamil.

There are no data supporting the preferential use of AC in sorbitol or other cathartic agents over AC in water.

TABLE 1.6.3 Agents poorly bound to activated charcoal		
Hydrocarbons and alcohols	**Metals**	**Corrosives**
Ethanol Isopropyl alcohol Ethylene glycol Methanol	Lithium Iron Potassium Lead Arsenic Mercury	Acids Alkalis

Potential complications

- Increased risk of vomiting
- Pulmonary aspiration of AC
- Direct administration into lung via misplaced nasogastric tube (potentially fatal)
- Impaired absorption of subsequently administered oral antidotes or other therapeutic agents
- Corneal abrasions
- Distraction of attending staff from resuscitation and supportive care priorities

Contraindications

- Non-toxic ingestion
- Uncooperative patient
- Decreased level of consciousness or risk of seizures (unless airway protected by endotracheal intubation)
- Agent not bound to AC (see **Table 1.6.3**)
- Corrosive ingestion

Technique

- Give 50 g (adults) or 1 g/kg (children) as a single oral dose.
- Mixing with ice cream improves palatability for children.
- In the intubated patient, AC may be given via orogastric or nasogastric tube after tube placement is confirmed on chest X-ray.

Note: Insertion of a nasogastric tube in children in order to administer AC can result in significant complications and is not recommended.

WHOLE BOWEL IRRIGATION

This labour-intensive method of gastrointestinal decontamination attempts to empty the entire gastrointestinal tract by administering large volumes of osmotically balanced polyethylene glycol electrolyte lavage solution

(PEG-ELS). It is not routinely performed because the risk–benefit analysis reserves this intervention for life-threatening ingestions of sustained-release or enteric-coated preparations, or agents that do not bind to charcoal and where good clinical outcome is not expected with supportive care and antidote administration, and the patient presents before established severe toxicity (see **Table 1.6.4**).

Large volumes of PEG-ELS (up to 2 L/hour in adults) are recommended by some authorities in order to perform whole bowel irrigation effectively, and patients are often unable to tolerate the procedure. Smaller volumes may be better tolerated and still result in a beneficial effect on patient outcome. Whole bowel irrigation has been attempted on ventilated patients but is usually unable to be completed because even with the airway protected by an endotracheal tube, there is a significant risk of pulmonary aspiration.

Potential complications

- Nausea, vomiting and abdominal bloating
- Pulmonary aspiration
- Distraction from resuscitation and supportive care priorities
- Delayed retrieval to a hospital offering definitive care

Contraindications

- Uncooperative patient
- Uncontrolled vomiting
- Decreased level of consciousness or risk of seizures
- Ileus or intestinal obstruction
- Intubated and ventilated patient (relative contraindication)

Technique

- One-to-one nursing is recommended to ensure close supervision during the procedure.
- Consider placement of a nasogastric tube and confirm position on chest X-ray.
- Give activated charcoal 50 g (children 1 g/kg) unless agent does not bind to AC.

TABLE 1.6.4 Potential indications for whole bowel irrigation
• Iron overdose >60 mg/kg
• Slow-release potassium chloride ingestion >2.5 mmol/kg
• Life-threatening slow-release verapamil or diltiazem ingestions
• Symptomatic arsenic trioxide ingestion
• Lead ingestion
• 'Body packers' (see **Chapter 2.14: Body packers and stuffers**)

- Administer PEG-ELS solution as tolerated up to a maximum of 2 L/hour (children up to 25 mL/kg/hour).
- Consider metoclopramide to minimise vomiting and enhance gastric emptying.
- Consider use of a bedside commode to manage explosive diarrhoea.
- Continue irrigation until the effluent is clear. This may take several hours.
- Cease whole bowel irrigation if abdominal distension or loss of bowel sounds is noted.
- Abdominal X-ray may be useful to assess effectiveness of decontamination of radio-opaque substances such as iron and potassium salts or other metallic substances.

NO LONGER RECOMMENDED

Induced Emesis (Syrup of Ipecac)

Emptying the stomach by inducing emesis was historically the main method of oral decontamination for toxic ingestions. Administration of syrup of ipecac, a preparation containing a potent plant-derived emetic, reliably induces vomiting via central and peripheral mechanisms with a mean time to onset of 18 minutes. For many years, it was routinely recommended for home use following accidental paediatric ingestions with the intention of reducing the requirement for hospital management. Available evidence indicates that the amount of toxin removed is unreliable and decreases rapidly with time to the point that it is negligible by 1 hour. Ipecac-induced vomiting can be prolonged and render subsequent administration of activated charcoal more difficult. The potential benefit of syrup of ipecac to improve outcome is now considered so unlikely that it is no longer used either in the home or in emergency departments.

Gastric Lavage

This invasive technique attempts to remove toxic substances from the stomach by the sequential administration and drainage of small volumes of fluid via a large-bore orogastric tube. Historically, this procedure was commonly performed in emergency departments, but has now been all but abandoned because of the lack of proven benefit and risk of considerable adverse effects including pulmonary complications (aspiration and hypoxia) and mechanical injury to the gastrointestinal tract.

References

American Academy of Clinical Toxicology and the European Association of Poison Centres and Clinical Toxicologists. Position paper: whole bowel irrigation. Clinical Toxicology 2004; 42:843–854.

American Academy of Clinical Toxicology and the European Association of Poison Centres and Clinical Toxicologists. Position paper: single-dose activated charcoal. Clinical Toxicology 2005; 43:61–87.

Bailey B. Gastrointestinal decontamination triangle. Clinical Toxicology 2005; 1:59–60.

Benson BE, Hoppu K, Troutman WG et al. Position paper update: gastric lavage for gastrointestinal decontamination. Clinical Toxicology 2013; 51:140–146.

Hojer J, Troutman WG, Hoppu K et al. Position paper update: ipecac syrup for gastrointestinal decontamination. Clinical Toxicology 2013; 51:134–139.

Isbister GK, Pavan Kumar VV. Indications for single dose activated charcoal administration. Current Opinion in Critical Care 2011; 17:351–357.

Juurlink DN. Activated charcoal for acute overdose: a reappraisal. British Journal of Clinical Pharmacology 2016; 81(3):482–487. doi:10.1111/bcp.12793.

1.7 ENHANCED ELIMINATION

Techniques of enhanced elimination (see **Table 1.7.1**) are employed to increase the rate of removal of an agent from the body with the aim of reducing the severity and duration of clinical intoxication.

These interventions are only indicated if it is thought they will reduce mortality, length of stay, complications or the need for other more invasive interventions. In practice, these techniques are useful in the treatment of poisoning by only a few agents that are characterised by:

- severe toxicity
- poor outcome despite good supportive care/antidote administration
- slow endogenous rates of elimination
- suitable pharmacokinetic properties.

Accurate risk assessment allows early identification of those patients who may benefit from enhanced elimination and institution of the intervention before severe life-threatening intoxication develops.

TABLE 1.7.1	Techniques of enhanced elimination and potential indications
Multiple-dose activated charcoal	**Haemodialysis and haemofiltration**
Carbamazepine	Carbamazepine
Dapsone	Lithium
Phenobarbitone	Metformin lactic acidosis
Quinine	Potassium
Theophylline	Salicylate
Urinary alkalinisation	Theophylline
Salicylate	Toxic alcohols
Herbicides	Valproic acid
Methotrexate	**Charcoal haemoperfusion**
Phenobarbitone	Theophylline

Some of these techniques require specialised equipment and staff, and early identification of candidates facilitates the timely communication, planning and transport necessary to ensure a good outcome.

The final decision as to whether to initiate a technique of enhanced elimination depends on a risk–benefit analysis in which the expected benefits of the procedure are balanced against the resource utilisation and risks associated with the procedure.

Techniques of enhanced elimination are never carried out to the detriment of resuscitation, good supportive care, decontamination and antidote treatment.

Once the decision to initiate a technique of enhanced elimination is made, it is important to establish pre-defined clinical or laboratory end points for therapy.

MULTIPLE-DOSE ACTIVATED CHARCOAL (MDAC)

Rationale

Repeated administration of oral AC progressively fills the entire gut lumen with charcoal. This has the potential to enhance drug elimination in two ways:

1 Interruption of enterohepatic circulation
   — A number of drugs are excreted in the bile and then reabsorbed from the distal ileum. Charcoal in the small intestine binds drug and prevents reabsorption, thus enhancing elimination.
   — This is only significant if a drug not only undergoes enterohepatic circulation but also has a relatively small volume of distribution.
2 Gastrointestinal dialysis
   — Drug passes across the gut mucosa from a relatively high concentration in the intravascular compartment to a low concentration in the gut lumen, which is maintained by continuing adsorption to charcoal.
   — This is only effective if the drug is a relatively small molecule, lipid soluble, has a small volume of distribution and low protein binding.

Indications

Enhanced elimination by this technique has been proposed as clinically useful in the following scenarios:

- Carbamazepine coma
  — Most common indication for MDAC
  — Used in the expectation that enhanced elimination will reduce duration of ventilation and length of stay in intensive care

- Phenobarbitone coma
  — Rare
  — Used in the expectation that enhanced elimination will reduce duration of ventilation and length of stay in intensive care
- Dapsone overdose with methaemoglobinaemia
  — Very rare
  — MDAC may enhance elimination of dapsone and reduce the duration of severe prolonged methaemoglobinaemia
- Quinine overdose
  — MDAC may enhance drug elimination and limit the severity of toxicity (especially retinal injury)
- Theophylline overdose
  — Attempts at enhanced elimination with MDAC should never delay more effective elimination techniques (haemodialysis) following life-threatening overdose.

Contraindications

- Decreased level of consciousness or anticipated decreased level of consciousness without prior airway protection
- Bowel obstruction

Potential complications

Although rare in carefully selected patients, they may include:

- Vomiting (30%)
- Aspiration of charcoal, especially if there is a decreased level of consciousness or seizures
- Constipation
- Charcoal bezoar formation, bowel obstruction, bowel perforation (rare)
- Corneal abrasion
- Distraction of attending staff from resuscitation and supportive care priorities.

Technique

- Give an initial dose of AC 50 g (adults) or 1 g/kg (children) PO.
- Give repeat doses of 25 g (0.5 g/kg in children) every 2 hours.
- In the intubated patient, AC is given via orogastric or nasogastric tube after tube placement has been confirmed on chest X-ray.
- Check for bowel sounds and high nasogastric aspirates prior to administration of each dose.
- Cease further administration if bowel sounds are inaudible or nasogastric aspirates of high volume.
- Reconsider the indications and clinical end points for therapy every 6 hours. MDAC should rarely be required beyond 6 hours.

URINARY ALKALINISATION

Rationale

The production of an alkaline urine pH promotes the ionisation of acidic drugs and prevents reabsorption across the renal tubular epithelium, thus promoting excretion in the urine. For this method to be effective, the drug must be filtered at the glomerulus, have a small volume of distribution and be a weak acid.

Indications

- Salicylate poisoning
    - Salicylates are normally eliminated by hepatic metabolism and are not readily excreted in acidic urine. In overdose, metabolism is saturated and elimination half-life greatly prolonged.
    - Urinary alkalinisation greatly enhances elimination and is indicated in any symptomatic patient in an effort to reduce the duration and severity of symptoms or to avoid progression to severe poisoning and the need for haemodialysis.
    - Severe established salicylate toxicity is an indication for immediate haemodialysis in addition to urinary alkalinisation.
- Urinary alkalinisation is considered in poisoning from other agents including methotrexate, phenobarbitone and some herbicides (see relevant chapters).

Contraindications

- Fluid overload

Complications

- Alkalaemia (usually well-tolerated)
- Fluid overload
- Hypokalaemia
- Hypocalcaemia (not usually clinically significant)

Technique

- Correct hypokalaemia if present (it is difficult to alkalinise the urine in the presence of systemic hypokalaemia).
- Give 1–2 mmol/kg sodium bicarbonate IV bolus.
- Commence infusion of 150 mmol sodium bicarbonate in 850 mL 5% glucose at 250 mL/hour.
- 20 mmol of potassium chloride may be added to the infusion to maintain normokalaemia.
- Monitor serum bicarbonate and potassium at least every 4 hours.
- Regularly dipstick urine and aim for urinary pH >7.5.
- Continue until clinical and laboratory evidence of toxicity is resolving.

EXTRACORPOREAL TECHNIQUES OF ELIMINATION

A number of such techniques have been used to enhance elimination of toxins including:

- haemodialysis
  - intermittent
  - continuous
- haemofiltration
- haemoperfusion
- plasmapheresis
- exchange transfusion.

All of the above techniques are invasive and require specialised staff, equipment and monitoring, and may be associated with significant complications. For these reasons, they are reserved for life-threatening poisonings where a good outcome cannot be achieved by other means, including good supportive care and antidote administration.

Haemodialysis effectively enhances elimination of any drug that is a small molecule and has a small volume of distribution, rapid redistribution from tissues and plasma and slow endogenous elimination. Clinical situations that involve life-threatening poisoning with agents fulfilling these criteria include:

- toxic alcohol poisoning
  - methanol
  - ethylene glycol
- theophylline poisoning
- severe salicylate intoxication
  - acute overdose with established severe toxicity
  - chronic intoxication with altered mental status
- severe lithium toxicity with significant neurological features and/or renal impairment
- phenobarbitone coma
- metformin lactic acidosis
- massive valproate overdose
- massive carbamazepine overdose
- potassium salt overdose with life-threatening hyperkalaemia.

Precise clinical indications for extracorporeal elimination in each of these important poisonings are discussed in the relevant sections of **Chapter 3**. The decision to institute extracorporeal elimination should be made early as soon as the risk assessment indicates potential lethality. In general, intermittent dialysis achieves greater clearance rates than continuous haemodialysis or haemofiltration techniques and is preferred where available. Facilities for charcoal haemoperfusion are not available in most centres.

References

American Academy of Clinical Toxicology, European Association of Poisons Centres and Clinical Toxicologists. Position statement and practice guidelines on the use of multi-dose activated charcoal in the treatment of acute poisoning. Journal of Toxicology–Clinical Toxicology 1999; 37(6):731–751. doi:10.1081/clt-100102451.

Dorrington CL, Johnson DW, Brant R. The frequency of complications associated with the use of multiple-dose activated charcoal. Annals of Emergency Medicine 2003; 41(3):370–377.

Ouellet GI, Bouchard J, Ghannoum M et al. Available extracorporeal treatments for poisoning: overview and limitations. Seminars in Dialysis 2014; 27(4):342–349.

Pond SM, Olson KR, Osterloh JD et al. Randomised study of the treatment of phenobarbital overdose with repeated doses of activated charcoal. Journal of the American Medical Association 1984; 251:3104–3108.

Proudfoot AT, Krenzelok EP, Vale JA. Position paper on urine alkalinization. Journal of Toxicology–Clinical Toxicology 2004; 42:1–26.

1.8 ANTIDOTES

Antidotes are drugs that correct the effects of poisoning. Only a few antidotes exist and many are used only rarely. Specific antidotes likely to be used in clinical practice are discussed in **Chapter 4** of this book.

Like all pharmaceuticals, antidotes have specific indications, contraindications, optimal administration methods, monitoring requirements, appropriate therapeutic end points and adverse effect profiles.

The decision to administer an antidote to an individual patient is based upon a risk–benefit analysis. An antidote is administered when the potential therapeutic benefit is judged to exceed the potential adverse effects, cost and resource requirements. An accurate risk assessment combined with pharmaceutical knowledge of the antidote is essential to clinical decision making.

Many antidotes are rarely prescribed, expensive and not widely stocked. Planning of stocking, storage, access, monitoring, training and protocol development are essential components of rational antidote use. It is often appropriate for stocking to be coordinated on a regional basis in association with regional policies concerning the treatment of poisoned patients. It is frequently cheaper and safer to transport an antidote to a patient rather than vice versa.

References

Daly FFS, Little M, Murray L. A risk assessment based approach to the management of acute poisoning. Emergency Medicine Journal 2006; 23(5):396–399. doi:10.1136/emj.2005.030312.

Dart RC, Borrow SW, Caravati EM et al. Expert consensus guidelines for stocking of antidotes in hospitals that provide emergency care. Annals of Emergency Medicine 2009; 54:386–394.

1.9 DISPOSITION

A medical disposition is required for all patients who present with poisoning or potential exposure to a toxic substance. Those who have deliberately self-poisoned also require psychiatric and social review. A risk-assessment-based approach to the management of acute poisoning allows early planning for appropriate medical and psychosocial disposition. Patients must be admitted to an environment capable of providing an adequate level of monitoring and supportive care and, if appropriate, where staff and resources are available to undertake decontamination, enhanced elimination techniques or administration of antidotes.

Early risk assessment in the pre-hospital setting, usually by poisons information centre staff, often allows non-intentional exposures to be observed outside of the hospital environment. For those that present to hospital, it minimises the duration and intensity of monitoring. Frequently, patients can be 'cleared' for medical discharge directly from the emergency department immediately following assessment or following a few hours of observation. No arrangements for admission to hospital need to be made unless unexpected signs or symptoms of toxicity develop.

At other times, the risk assessment will indicate the need for ongoing observation, supportive care or the need for specific enhanced elimination techniques or antidote administration. Under these circumstances, the patient must be admitted to an environment capable of providing a level of care appropriate for the anticipated clinical course. In many hospitals, this is now the emergency observation unit rather than the general medical ward. Where ongoing airway control, ventilation or advanced haemodynamic support is required, admission to an intensive care unit is appropriate.

EMERGENCY OBSERVATION UNITS

Emergency observation units (EOUs) have been established in many emergency departments in Australasia and elsewhere. These units vary in capacity, design and staffing. Ideally, they are located adjacent to emergency departments, staffed by emergency doctors and provide short-term, focused, goal-oriented care. They have been remarkably successful in:

- streamlining treatment in suitable conditions
- reducing total bed days
- increasing patient satisfaction
- reducing inappropriate discharges and litigation.

TOXICOLOGY PATIENTS IN THE EMERGENCY OBSERVATION UNIT

In most hospitals where EOUs are established, the units appear to provide an ideal environment for the management of acute poisoning beyond the initial assessment and monitoring phase. Advantages of using the EOU to admit toxicology patients include the ready availability of appropriate resources, staff and training; 24-hour availability of experienced medical staff; an open-plan environment that facilitates observation; and an emergency department ethos that is geared towards rapid assessment and disposition. Adequate resources must be dedicated to the EOU, particularly medical, nursing, psychiatric and social services.

Ideal design features and staffing that facilitate the management of toxicology patients in the EOU include:

- central nursing stations with clear vision of all areas
- an environment that protects from self-harm
- secure entrances
- dedicated areas for private interviews
- dedicated social work, drug and alcohol, plus outpatient liaison services
- appropriate monitors ± telemetry
- dedicated resuscitation equipment
- duress alarms
- appropriate staff, skills and equipment
- appropriate 24/7/365 senior staff coverage
- dedicated psychiatric services
- nurse–patient ratios appropriate for the acuity of patients (e.g. 1 : 4 for monitored 'step-down' patients; 1 : 8 for non-monitored general patients).

Criteria need to be developed for admission to the EOU following acute poisoning. Such criteria might include:

- cardiac monitoring not required (but this can be provided in some EOUs)
- adequate sedation in cases of delirium
- deterioration not anticipated (based on accurate risk assessment and initial period of observation in the emergency department).

Admission of toxicology patients to the EOU helps counter several of the difficulties encountered when poisoned patients are admitted to other areas of the hospital:

- admissions scattered all over the hospital
- less experienced nursing staff
- poor availability of medical staff
- frequent security incidents/absconding patients
- most clinicians managing patients on general medical wards are junior and have no formal training in clinical toxicology
- longer admissions.

RETRIEVAL OF THE POISONED PATIENT

Usually, the initial receiving hospital is adequately resourced to provide an acceptable level of supportive care, monitoring and therapy for the poisoned patient. If this is not the case, transfer is necessary. Risk assessment ensures that the need to transfer is recognised early so that appropriate planning and consultation takes place in an effort to ensure as smooth a retrieval as possible (see **Table 1.9.1**). Poisoning is unusual in that transfer frequently takes place during the most severe phase of the illness.

Resuscitation

The need to retrieve a patient to another centre should not distract attending staff from resuscitation and supportive care priorities. Attention to airway, breathing and circulation ensure an optimum outcome in the majority of cases. Whenever possible, the patient should be stabilised before retrieval begins. Interventions such as intubation, ventilation, initial resuscitation of hypotension, cessation of seizures, assessment of blood glucose and management of hyperthermia are completed before a patient is placed in the transport vehicle, where further assessment and

---

TABLE 1.9.1   Principles of retrieval of the poisoned patient
• Risk assessment is vital
• Identify patients who may need retrieval to another hospital as soon as possible
• Patients should only be retrieved for specific clinical indications
• Recognise that transport may occur during the worst phase of the intoxication
• Consider bringing expertise and resources to the patient, rather than vice versa
• Assess, manage and stabilise potential resuscitation and supportive care priorities prior to transfer
• Ensure that transport does not lead to an interval of lower level of care
• Transport to a centre capable of definitive care

detailed management are often impossible. If the referring team does not possess the necessary skills or resources to complete these resuscitation and stabilisation tasks adequately, this should be communicated to the receiving and retrieval teams so that these resources can be brought to the patient.

Transport

As transport usually occurs during the most severe phase of the poisoning, the patient should never be subjected to an interval of a lower level of care during the transfer. Consideration of the mode and staffing of transport takes this into account.

Planning

Planning is required to ensure that any potential complications are identified and managed in a proactive fashion. Thus, if coma requiring intubation and ventilation is anticipated in the next few hours (e.g. controlled-release carbamazepine), early intubation and ventilation should occur prior to transfer. Similarly, if significant hypotension is expected (e.g. calcium channel blockers), appropriate monitoring, intravenous access and resuscitation resources should be ready prior to transfer.

Communication

Communication is vital. Retrieval is always to a higher level of care. Thus, transport must occur to a facility with appropriate resources to manage the potential complications identified by the risk assessment. For example, if haemodialysis may be required (e.g. theophylline or salicylate poisoning), the patient must be transported to a facility capable of instituting this intervention at short notice. Ideally, communication should include the team of clinicians who will ultimately manage the patient. Consultations with other specialist teams (e.g. paediatricians, intensivists or clinical toxicologists) may also occur to assist the process. This improves continuity of care and decreases the inefficiencies and errors that may be associated with multiple handovers.

Antidotes

If an antidote is likely to definitively treat the patient and render them stable (e.g. N-acetylcysteine, digoxin-specific antibodies), it is preferable to transfer the antidote to the patient, start treatment, then move the patient only if necessary.

Psychosocial assessment

Most episodes of acute poisoning represent an exacerbation of an underlying psychosocial disorder and the final disposition of the patient is made in this context. All patients with deliberate self-poisoning should undergo psychosocial assessment prior to discharge. Ideally, this process begins before the medical treatment of the poisoning is complete so that final disposition is facilitated.

References

Daly FFS, Little M, Murray L A risk assessment based approach to the management of acute poisoning. Emergency Medicine Journal 2006; 23(5):396–399. doi: 10.1136/emj.2005.030312.

Isoardi KZ, Armitage MC, Harris K et al. Establishing a dedicated toxicology unit reduces length of stay of poisoned patients and saves hospital bed days. Emergency Medicine Australasia 2017; 29(3):310–314. doi.org/10.1111/1742-6723.12755.

Parish S, Carter A, Liu YH, et al. The impact of the introduction of a toxicology service on the intensive care unit. Clinical Toxicology 2019;57(9):778–783. doi:10.1080/15563650.2019.1566553.

Ross MA, Graff LG. Principles of observation medicine. Emergency Medicine Clinics of North America 2001; 19(1):1–17.

Warren J, Fromm RE, Orr RA et al. Guidelines for the inter- and intrahospital transport of critically ill patients. Critical Care Medicine 2004; 32:256–262.

CHAPTER 2
SPECIFIC CONSIDERATIONS

Coma describes a clinical state of impaired responsiveness where the patient cannot be roused. It is a common manifestation of poisoning by many agents (see **Table 2.1.1**).

In a poisoned patient, coma may be the result of:

- direct toxic effect on the CNS
- secondary effect of poisoning on the CNS – hypoxaemia, hypoglycaemia, hyponatraemia, hypotension or cerebral oedema
- co-existing non-toxicological causes: metabolic encephalopathy, neurotrauma, space occupying lesion or CNS infections.

Coma presents an immediate threat to life, irrespective of the underlying cause. Assessment and management is a core emergency competency. Most agents that cause toxic coma produce a temporary alteration in mental status that has a good prognosis with good supportive care.

MANAGEMENT

Resuscitation

Poisoning is a dynamic illness. The patient's ability to maintain an airway and ventilate effectively may change in a short period of time. Early risk assessment allows the clinician to anticipate the development of coma and prepare to manage it effectively. Maintaining a patent airway and adequate ventilation are the immediate priorities using standard airway techniques. Definitive control of the airway is achieved as soon as practical by rapid sequence intubation according to the individual risk assessment.

A common pitfall in poisoning is failure of the risk assessment to anticipate the likely duration of coma and to leave the airway unprotected for a prolonged period of time. This increases the risk of hypoxaemia, hypoventilation and pulmonary aspiration. A patient's ability to guard their airway is poorly correlated to the Glasgow Coma Scale (GCS). Conventionally, a GCS of 8 or less has been considered an indication for intubation. However, in poisoned patients, the risk of pulmonary aspiration increases with any drop in GCS below 15, especially where there has been a delay to hospital presentation.

Once neuromuscular paralysis and intubation is achieved, it is vital to ventilate the patient at an appropriate minute volume. Several poisonings (e.g. methanol, ethylene glycol, salicylate) are associated with severe metabolic acidosis and it is essential to maintain appropriate compensatory hyperventilation to prevent rapid clinical deterioration and possibly death.

TABLE 2.1.1 Toxicological causes of coma

PRIMARY NEUROLOGICAL EFFECT

Alcohols
  Ethanol
  Ethylene glycol
  Isopropyl alcohol
  Methanol
Antipsychotic agents
  Amisulpride
  Chlorpromazine
  Clozapine
  Olanzapine
  Quetiapine
Anticonvulsant agents
  Carbamazepine
  Lamotrigine
  Valproic acid
Antidepressants
  Selective serotonin reuptake
    inhibitors
  Tricyclic antidepressants
Antihistamines
  Diphenhydramine
  Promethazine
Antimalarial agents
  Chloroquine
  Hydroxychloroquine
  Quinine
Baclofen
Beta-adrenergic blockers
  Propranolol
Centrally acting alpha-2-agonists
  Clonidine
  Oxymetazoline

Cholinergic agents
  Acetylcholinesterase inhibitors
    (e.g. donepezil)
  Carbamates
  Nicotine
  Organophosphates
Hydrocarbons
  Essential oils
  Toluene
Local anaesthetics
  Bupivacaine
  Cocaine
  Lidocaine
  Ropivacaine
Mushrooms
  Gyromitra species
**Non-steroidal anti-inflammatory
  agents**
  Ibuprofen
  Mefenamic acid
Opioids
  Codeine
  Heroin
  Morphine
  Methadone
Sedative-hypnotic agents
  Barbiturates
  Benzodiazepines
  Chloral hydrate
  Gamma-hydroxybutyrate
  Non-benzodiazepine agents
    (zolpidem, zopiclone)

SECONDARY EFFECT

Cerebral oedema
  Salicylates
  Valproic acid
Hypoglycaemia
  Insulin
  Sulfonylurea agents
  Beta-blockers
  Chloroquine
  Venlafaxine, desvenlafaxine
Hypotension
  Cardiotoxic agents
Hypoxaemia (systemic or cellular)
  Agents causing
    methaemoglobinaemia
  Carbon monoxide
  Cyanide
  Hydrogen sulfide

Neuroleptic malignant syndrome
  Antipsychotic agents
Seizures
  Bupropion
  Isoniazid
  Tramadol
  Venlafaxine
Serotonin toxicity
  Monoamine oxidase inhibitors
  Selective serotonin reuptake
    inhibitors
  Serotonin and noradrenaline
    reuptake inhibitors (e.g.
    venlafaxine)

Risk assessment

The risk assessment can usually predict the development of coma if the agent and dose are known. If coma is unexpected, the risk assessment must subsequently be reviewed to consider ingestion of alternative agents, ingestion of a larger dose than suspected or a non-toxicological cause for coma.

Where the patient presents with coma of unknown origin and there is no definite history of ingestion, the clinician must rigorously evaluate the historical, clinical and laboratory features of the case in order to:

- identify alternative non-toxicological causes of coma
- recognise important complications of coma
- identify poisonings where specific interventions are required to ensure a good outcome.

Toxic agents usually act on the CNS in a global and symmetrical fashion and any focal or unilateral neurological sign is suggestive of an alternative cause.

Patients may have been comatose for a prolonged period of time prior to arrival in hospital. These patients are at risk of a number of secondary complications, which may have greater impact on their morbidity and mortality than the intoxication itself. These complications must be specifically sought and managed in any patient presenting with coma. They include:

- pulmonary aspiration
- hypoxic brain injury
- rhabdomyolysis
- acute renal failure
- compartment syndromes
- pressure areas.

Supportive care, monitoring and disposition

In order to minimise the complications of coma, close attention to the following supportive care measures is imperative:

- monitoring of conscious state and airway
- respiratory toilet and prophylaxis (mobilisation and/or physiotherapy)
- fluid monitoring and management
- bladder care (serial bladder scans and indwelling catheter as indicated)
- prevention of pressure areas
- thromboembolism prophylaxis
- mobilisation as mental status changes resolve.

Investigations

- **Screening (12-lead ECG, BGL and serum paracetamol level):**
  — These tests are particularly important in the comatose patient where no ingestion history is available.
  — A measurable paracetamol level mandates empiric treatment with N-acetylcysteine if the time of ingestion cannot be determined.
- **To detect toxic ingestions for which specific interventions are required:**
  — blood gases, anion gap and lactate
  — osmolar gap
  — specific drug levels: carbamazepine, ethanol, ethylene glycol or methanol (when available), salicylate, valproic acid.
- **To detect and assess complications:**
  — blood gases, anion gap and lactate
  — electrolytes, urea and creatinine (EUC)
  — liver function tests
  — CK
  — chest X-ray.
- **To exclude or confirm important differential diagnoses:**
  — blood gases, anion gap and lactate
  — electrolytes, urea and creatinine (EUC)
  — liver function tests
  — head CT scan
  — lumbar puncture
  — blood and urine cultures
  — EEG.

Decontamination

Administration of activated charcoal (AC) is contraindicated in poisoned patients who present with coma and have an unprotected airway. Activated charcoal via nasogastric tube (NGT) is recommended in all comatose poisoned patients once the airway is secured by rapid sequence intubation and the appropriate position of the NGT has been confirmed radiologically.

Enhanced elimination techniques and antidote administration

The vast majority of patients presenting with or developing toxic coma are assured of a good outcome with timely institution of supportive care. There are a small number of agents where specific interventions are indicated (see **Table 2.1.2**). Details of management of these agents are found in the relevant drug and antidote chapters. Poisoning with carbamazepine, valproic acid or phenobarbitone is excluded by obtaining a negative specific drug level in any comatose patient with access to

TABLE 2.1.2	Agents causing coma that may require specific intervention

Carbamazepine
   Multi-dose activated charcoal
   Haemodialysis
Isoniazid
   Pyridoxine
Opioids
   Naloxone
Organophosphates
   Atropine
   Pralidoxime
Phenobarbitone
   Multi-dose activated charcoal
   Haemodialysis
	Salicylate
	   Urinary alkalinisation
	   Haemodialysis
	Sulfonylureas
	   Glucose
	   Octreotide
	Toxic alcohols (ethylene glycol, methanol)
	   Ethanol
	   Fomepizole
	   Haemodialysis
	Valproic acid
	   Haemodialysis

these anticonvulsant agents. Toxic alcohol and salicylate poisoning must be excluded in any comatose patient with metabolic acidosis.

References

Daly FFS, Little M, Murray L. A risk assessment approach to the management of acute poisoning. Emergency Medicine Journal 2006; 23:396–399.

International Liaison Committee on Resuscitation. 2005 American Heart Association Guidelines for Cardiopulmonary and Emergency Cardiovascular Care – Part 10.2: Toxicology in ECC. Circulation 2005; 112(24 Supplement I):IV126–IV132.

Isbister GK, Downes F, Sibbritt D et al. Aspiration pneumonitis in an overdose population: frequency, predictors and outcomes. Critical Care Medicine 2004; 32:88–93.

2.2 HYPOTENSION

Hypotension is common in poisoned patients. It is usually mild, secondary to peripheral vasodilatation and responsive to intravenous fluids. Hypotension refractory to basic fluid resuscitation is associated with increased morbidity. Poisoning secondary to medications with direct cardiotoxic effects is frequently associated with refractory hypotension of multi-factorial origin and mortality is higher.

Every attempt should be made to determine the cause of hypotension. The main differentiation in this evaluation is between vasodilatory and cardiogenic aetiologies.

Vasodilatory shock is the more common cause of hypotension. The usual mechanism is peripheral vasodilatation, which can occur via numerous pathophysiological processes. The classes of drugs most frequently involved include:

- α_1-adrenergic receptor blockers
- calcium channel blockers (CCB) – predominantly dihydropyridines (see **Chapter 3.21: Calcium channel blockers**)
- renin–angiotensin system inhibitors: angiotensin-converting enzyme inhibitors (ACEIs) or angiotensin receptor blockers (ARBs).

Cardiogenic shock occurs via multiple aetiologies, resulting in a decrease in cardiac contractility and cardiac output. Agents and mechanisms include:

- calcium channel blockers (CCB) – predominantly diltiazem and verapamil (see **Chapter 3.21: Calcium channel blockers**)
- beta-blockers
- acute stress-induced (sympathomimetic) cardiotoxicity:
  — amphetamines and amphetamine-like substances
  — serotonin and noradrenaline reuptake inhibitors (SNRIs)
  — cocaine
  — envenomings
    – Irukandji jellyfish
    – funnel-web spiders
- ischaemia from various causes including:
  — myocardial infarction from coronary thrombosis or vascular dissection (e.g. amphetamines, cocaine)
  — cellular hypoxia (e.g. carbon monoxide, cyanide, methaemoglobinaemia).

Echocardiography is the most useful initial investigation to determine the cause of hypotension due to its ready availability compared to invasive cardiac output monitoring. In the absence of these modalities, the clinical features provide an indication of the likely aetiology.

In a hypotensive patient, following attention to airway and breathing a thorough and sequential step-wise assessment is required to guide appropriate management interventions:

1 Check cardiac rhythm and review a current 12-lead ECG. Commence continuous ECG monitoring while the risk assessment is performed.
2 Correct cardiac dysrhythmias. Under certain circumstances, standard resuscitation guidelines may be ineffective and the administration of specific antidotes is a priority (see **Chapter 1.2: Resuscitation**).
3 Give 10–20 mL/kg of IV crystalloid to ensure euvolaemia. Further fluid administration may be indicated but depends on the clinical evaluation of intravascular volume status and the individual risk assessment.
4 Commence appropriate inotropic and/or vasopressor agents. The choice depends on the aetiology of hypotension.

5 Consider early administration of high-dose insulin therapy in the setting of cardiogenic shock from toxicological causes (see **Chapter 4.14: Insulin (high-dose)**).

6 Consider interventions such as extracorporeal membrane oxygenation (ECMO), cardiopulmonary bypass or intra-aortic balloon pump:

— Acute cardiovascular toxicity is frequently reversible once the poisoning has resolved. Supportive bridging therapy with mechanical assist devices is therefore warranted in the appropriate setting.

References

Vanden Hoek TL, Morrison LJ, Shuster M et al. Part 12: Cardiac arrest in special situations: 2010 American Heart Association guidelines for cardiopulmonary and emergency cardiovascular care. Circulation 2010; 122:S829–S861.

Weiner L, Mazzeffi MA, Hines EQ et al. Clinical utility of venoarterial-extracorporeal membrane oxygenation (VA-ECMO) in patients with drug-induced cardiogenic shock: a retrospective study of the Extracorporeal Life Support Organizations' ECMO case registry. Clinical Toxicology 2010; 58(7):705–710. doi:10.1080/1556 3650.2019.1676896.

2.3 SEIZURES

Toxic seizures are characteristically generalised and self-limiting and usually respond to the administration of benzodiazepines. The most common causes of toxic seizures in Australia are tramadol, venlafaxine, antidepressants and amphetamines (see **Table 2.3.1** for a summary of causes). Toxic seizures may be delayed in onset as a result of extended-release formulations of several of these agents.

Seizures are also a prominent manifestation of a number of withdrawal syndromes, in particular those associated with ethanol and benzodiazepines.

In certain poisonings, seizures herald severe intoxication and a grave prognosis unless definitive care is rapidly instituted (e.g. chloroquine, propranolol, salicylates, theophylline, tricyclic antidepressants).

The presence of focal or partial seizures indicates a focal neurological disorder that is either a complication of poisoning or non-toxicological in origin. In either case, further investigation and targeted management is required.

Seizures of any cause are treated as a matter of priority. Prolonged seizure activity is associated with irreversible CNS injury. Secondary hypoxia and acidosis increase the susceptibility for dysrhythmias and multi-organ failure. Secondary hyperpyrexia and rhabdomyolysis may lead to dehydration, hyperkalaemia and renal failure.

There are multiple complex mechanisms responsible for the promotion of toxicological seizures. The most common causes are a decrease in

TABLE 2.3.1 Toxicological causes of seizures

Anticonvulsants	**Local anaesthetic agents**
Carbamazepine	Bupivacaine
Topiramate	Lidocaine
Antidepressants	Ropivacaine
Bupropion	**Nicotine**
Citalopram	**Non-steroidal anti-inflammatory**
Escitalopram	**agents**
Venlafaxine	Mefenamic acid
Antidysrhythmic agents	**Opioids**
Quinidine	Dextropropoxyphene
Antihistamines	Pethidine
Antimalarial agents	Tramadol
Chloroquine	**Propranolol**
Hydroxychloroquine	**Salicylates**
Quinine	**Sympathomimetic agents**
Antipsychotic agents	Amphetamines and
Atypical antipsychotics	amphetamine-like
Butyrophenones	substances
Olanzapine	Cocaine
Phenothiazines	Synthetic cannabinoids and
Quetiapine	cathinones
Baclofen	**Theophylline**
Hypoglycaemic agents	**Tricyclic antidepressants**
Insulin	**Withdrawal syndromes**
Sulfonylureas	Alcohol
Isoniazid	Barbiturates
	Benzodiazepines
	Non-benzodiazepine sedative-
	hypnotic agents (e.g.
	gamma-hydroxybutyrate,
	zopiclone, zolpidem)

activity of the neuro-inhibitory pathways (primarily gamma aminobutyric acid (GABA) receptors) or an increase in excitatory pathways (glutamate and N-methyl-D-aspartate (NMDA) receptors). Other neurotransmitter pathways involved include noradrenaline, dopamine, serotonin, acetylcholine, histamine and adenosine. Secondary hypoxia, hypotension and metabolic disturbances can also lead to the development of seizures.

The first-line treatment for toxicological seizures is benzodiazepines, preferably by the intravenous route. Midazolam and diazepam are the agents most commonly used. If intravenous access is not established, intramuscular midazolam is an effective alternative route of administration.

Barbiturates are recommended as second-line therapy for refractory seizures in acute poisoning. Intubation and ventilation are indicated in this setting due to the risk of significant respiratory depression with barbiturate administration.

Propofol is another option for treatment of refractory seizures based on limited published data. As for the use of barbiturates, management in an intensive care environment is required.

Phenytoin is not indicated in the management of seizures from acute poisoning or withdrawal syndromes as it does not reverse the generalised lowering of seizure threshold or suppress the increase in neuronal excitability. It is used for epileptic seizures, where it blocks voltage-dependent sodium channels located at the epileptic focus and inhibits the propagation of seizure activity.

There are currently limited data to support a beneficial role for other anticonvulsants such as levetiracetam in the management of toxicological seizures.

MANAGEMENT

See **Chapter 1.2: Resuscitation**.

1 Attention to airway, breathing and circulation is paramount and proceeds along standard lines. Consider the requirement for rapid-sequence intubation and ventilation if the conscious state does not recover promptly.

2 Check bedside blood glucose level and correct hypoglycaemia if present.

3 Give intravenous benzodiazepine (e.g. midazolam or diazepam 5–10 mg; children 0.1–0.3 mg/kg over 3–5 minutes). If intravenous access is not established, intramuscular midazolam at a similar dose is an alternative route of administration.

4 Consider barbiturates as second-line therapy for refractory seizures in acute poisoning – options include phenobarbitone 100–300 mg slow IV (no faster than 1 mg/kg/min), repeated as required to a dose of 20 mg/kg or a maximum of 2 g (children 10–20 mg/kg slow IV), or thiopentone 3–5 mg/kg IV. Intubation and ventilation are indicated in this setting due to the risk of significant respiratory depression with barbiturate administration.

5 Consider propofol as an alternative second-line agent (see above).

6 Pyridoxine is the agent indicated in intractable seizures secondary to isoniazid and other hydrazines (gram for gram dose to match suspected isoniazid dose, up to 5 g IV; children 70 mg/kg not exceeding 5 g).

References

Chen HY, Albertson TE, Olson KR. Treatment of drug-induced seizures. British Journal of Clinical Pharmacology 2016; 81(3):412–419. doi:10.1111/bcp.12720.

Kunisaki TA, Augenstein WL. Drug- and toxin-induced seizures. Emergency Medical Clinics of North America 1994; 12(4):1027–1056.

Reichert C, Reichert P, Monnet-Tschudi F et al. Seizures after single-agent overdose with pharmaceutical drugs: analysis of cases reported to a poison center. Clinical Toxicology 2014; 52(6):629–634.

Shah ASV, Eddleston M. Should phenytoin or barbiturates be used as second-line anticonvulsant therapy for toxicological seizures? Clinical Toxicology 2010; 48:800–805.

2.4 APPROACH TO DELIRIUM

Delirium is a disorder of impaired attention and awareness. The key diagnostic features are shown in **Table 2.4.1**.

The pathophysiology of delirium is poorly understood and in the poisoned patient it is likely to be multi-factorial with alterations of the neurotransmitter and humoral mechanisms playing a key role. Intoxication with or withdrawal from a variety of agents may present with delirium (**Table 2.4.2**). Toxicological delirium usually has an acute onset, is transient and improves as intoxication resolves over hours to days.

Patients with delirium may be disruptive and present an immediate threat to themselves and others. These presentations are challenging emergencies in which the clinician must, concomitantly, control the patient's agitation, resuscitate the patient and perform an accurate risk assessment.

DUTY OF CARE

Patients with delirium lack capacity – the cognitive ability to understand the consequences of their decisions or actions. The clinician has a duty of care to protect the patient from serious harm or death. Similarly, the clinician has a duty of care to others (staff and the community at large) to protect them from potential harm resulting from the actions of the delirious patient.

In this setting, failure to control the situation (allowing the patient to abscond or injure themselves) represents an act of omission. In contrast,

---

TABLE 2.4.1 Diagnostic features of delirium (based on DSM-V criteria)

A. A disturbance in attention (i.e. reduced ability to direct, focus, sustain and shift attention) and awareness (reduced orientation to the environment)

B. The disturbance develops over a short period of time (usually hours to a few days), represents a change from baseline attention and awareness and tends to fluctuate in severity during the course of a day

C. An additional disturbance in cognition (e.g. memory deficit, disorientation, language, visuospatial ability or perception)

D. The disturbances in criteria A and B are not better explained by another pre-existing, established or evolving neurocognitive disorder and do not occur in the context of a severely reduced level of arousal, such as coma

E. There is evidence from the history, physical examination or laboratory findings that the disturbance is a direct physiological consequence of another medical condition, substance intoxication or withdrawal (i.e. due to a drug of abuse or to a medication), or exposure to a toxin, or is due to multiple aetiologies

TABLE 2.4.2 Toxicological causes of delirium
Alcohol
Anticholinergic toxicity
Antidepressants
Bupropion
Monoamine oxidase inhibitors
Venlafaxine
Atypical antipsychotic agents
Clozapine
Olanzapine
Quetiapine
Baclofen
Benzodiazepines and other sedative-hypnotic agents (e.g. zolpidem)
Cannabis
Hallucinogenic agents
Dimethyltryptamine (DMT)
Ketamine
Phencyclidine
2,5-Dimethoxy-4-iodophenethylamine (2C-I)
Neuroleptic malignant syndrome (NMS)
Nicotine
Salicylates
Serotonin toxicity
Sympathomimetic toxicity
Amphetamine and amphetamine-like substances
Cocaine
Synthetic cannabinoids
Theophylline
Withdrawal syndromes

while the delirium lasts, temporary physical restraint, pharmacological sedation and ongoing medical management, perhaps against the patient's wishes at the time, is appropriate under this duty of care.

MANAGEMENT

Resuscitation

Assess and manage airway, breathing and circulation as appropriate.

Delirium may occur due to seizures (post-ictal state) or represent non-convulsive status epilepticus. Manage seizures with benzodiazepines as first-line therapy or specific anti-convulsants as indicated (see **Chapter 2.3: Seizures**).

Check bedside serum glucose as soon as possible in all patients with altered mental status to exclude hypoglycaemia. If the serum glucose is <4.0 mmol/L, 50 mL of 50% glucose should be given intravenously immediately (5 mL/kg 10% glucose in children) to correct hypoglycaemia. If hypoglycaemia is detected, the underlying cause must be considered and managed.

All patients manifesting delirium and agitation should have frequent temperature measurements as part of their monitoring. A temperature greater than 38.5°C is an indication for continuous core-temperature monitoring. A temperature greater than 39.5°C is an emergency that requires prompt management to prevent multiple-organ failure and neurological injury. Neuromuscular paralysis, intubation and ventilation will decrease muscle-generated heat production and can lead to rapid improvement in hyperthermia.

Risk assessment

A detailed risk assessment is essential, as for any poisoned patient, so that a specific management plan can be tailored for the patient.

Where the patient presents with delirium but no definite history of ingestion, the clinician must rigorously evaluate the historical, clinical and laboratory features of the case in order to diagnose:

- alternative (non-toxicological) causes (see **Table 2.4.3**)
- toxicities or syndromes where specific interventions (enhanced elimination techniques or antidotes) are necessary to ensure a good outcome (see **Table 2.4.4**)
- important complications of delirium (see **Table 2.4.5**).

Supportive care and monitoring

Manage the patient in a calm environment to minimise external distractions and stimulation. Reassure the patient, explain their circumstances (including the medical team's duty of care) and outline the plan of management. One-to-one nursing is usually necessary to allow close observation and management during the initial stages.

TABLE 2.4.3   Other conditions mimicking or contributing to delirium

Acid–base disturbance
Behavioural disturbance
CNS infection (e.g. encephalitis)
Dementia
Electrolyte disturbance (e.g. hyponatraemia)
Endocrine emergency (e.g. thyrotoxicosis)
Head injury
Hypoglycaemia
Hypoxia
Organ failure (e.g. hepatic encephalopathy)
Psychosis
Seizures (e.g. non-convulsive status epilepticus, post-ictal)
Stroke
Trauma (e.g. subdural haemorrhage)
Withdrawal (e.g. alcohol or sedative-hypnotic agents)

TABLE 2.4.4 Agents or syndromes associated with delirium that may require specific interventions

Agent	Possible interventions
Anticholinergic agents	Physostigmine (see **Chapter 4.21: Physostigmine**)
Neuroleptic malignant syndrome	Bromocriptine
Salicylates	Urinary alkalinisation Haemodialysis
Serotonin toxicity	Cyproheptadine (see **Chapter 4.3: Cyproheptadine**) Neuromuscular paralysis, intubation and ventilation
Theophylline	Multi-dose activated charcoal Haemodialysis

If initial reassurance does not improve the behavioural disturbance, and the patient remains a threat to themselves or others, temporary physical restraint may be required. Physical restraint should be achieved quickly by broad-based control of the arms and legs. Physical restraint must never threaten the patient's airway or respiratory efforts, and should only ever be used until appropriate pharmacological sedation can be achieved.

The ideal pharmacological agent used for sedation has a rapid onset of action, predictable dose response and minimal side effects. The agents best matching these characteristics are antipsychotics, benzodiazepines and ketamine. The choice of agent is dictated by the individual risk assessment and how quickly sedation is required to be achieved. Local guidelines and protocols for sedation should be available to indicate the preferred agents for use at an individual institution.

In mild cases of delirium, oral or sublingual dosing is appropriate. Lorazepam, olanzapine and risperidone (in elderly patients) are the agents of choice.

TABLE 2.4.5 Complications of delirium in the poisoned patient

Aspiration pneumonitis
Deep vein thrombosis and pulmonary embolism
Fluid, electrolyte and acid–base disturbances, most commonly dehydration
Hypoventilation, hypoxia
Hyperthermia
Physical injury to the patient or others
Rhabdomyolysis
Urinary retention

In severe cases, or in any case requiring physical restraint, intravenous or intramuscular dosing is required. Droperidol, midazolam and ketamine are the agents of choice:

- Droperidol monotherapy is a safe and effective sedation agent for the undifferentiated patient with delirium, either by the IM or IV route. Droperidol has the potential to cause QT prolongation and in the United States, the FDA has given the drug a 'black box' warning. However, the risk of torsades de pointes in the acute setting is rare. An upper dose limit of 20 mg within a 24-hour period is recommended in published series.
- Midazolam as a sole agent has an increased risk of respiratory depression, particularly with rapidly escalating doses, and can also cause paradoxical agitation.
- The combination of droperidol and midazolam achieves more rapid sedation then either drug alone.
- Ketamine is an appropriate choice for immediate control of the severely agitated patient due to its rapid onset of action and good safety profile. As a third-line agent there is an additive risk of airway complications, and doses should be titrated carefully.

On occasion, intubation and ventilation is indicated to control severe delirium or behavioural disturbance that does not respond to parenteral sedation, thereby minimising the risk of secondary complications such as physical injury or pulmonary aspiration.

Once agitation is adequately controlled, the patient is managed in an area capable of providing appropriate supervision and monitoring, and where further sedation can be administered if required. Delirium may persist for days, depending on the cause. Patients with anticholinergic delirium frequently develop urinary retention and attempts to achieve adequate sedation will not be effective until this is relieved by placement of an indwelling urinary catheter.

General supportive care, as detailed in **Chapter 1.4: Supportive care and monitoring**, includes:

- monitoring of conscious state and airway
- respiratory toilet and prophylaxis (mobilisation and/or chest physiotherapy)
- fluid monitoring and management
- bladder care (indwelling urinary catheter)
- prevention of pressure areas
- thromboembolism prophylaxis
- mobilisation as mental status changes resolve.

Investigations

Investigations in acute poisoning are used either as screening tests or for specific purposes. Specific investigations in the patient with delirium should be ordered selectively where it is anticipated that the results will refine risk assessment, exclude significant complications or exclude potential non-toxicological diagnoses.

Enhanced elimination techniques and antidote administration

There are relatively few instances where these interventions are required in the management of delirium (see **Table 2.4.4**). For the use of physostigmine in anticholinergic delirium, see **Chapter 2.6: Anticholinergic toxicity** and **Chapter 4.21: Physostigmine**.

References

Calver L, Page CB, Downes MA et al. The safety and effectiveness of droperidol for sedation of acute behavioral disturbance in the emergency department. Annals of Emergency Medicine 2015; 66(3):230–238.e1. doi:10.1016/j.annemergmed. 2015.03.016.

Chan EW, Taylor DM, Knott JC. Intravenous droperidol or olanzapine as an adjunct to midazolam for the acutely agitated patient; a multicenter, randomized, double-blind, placebo-controlled clinical trial. Annals of Emergency Medicine 2013; 61:72–81.

Horowitz BZ, Bizovi K, Moreno R. Droperidol – behind the black box warning. Academic Emergency Medicine 2002; 9(6):615–618.

Isbister GK, Calver LA, Page CB et al. Randomised controlled trial of intramuscular droperidol versus midazolam for violence and acute behavioral disturbance: the DORM study. Annals of Emergency Medicine 2010; 56(4):392–401.e1. doi:10.1016/j.annemergmed.2010.05.037.

Korczak V, Kirby A, Gunja N. Chemical agents for the sedation of agitated patients in the ED: a systematic review. American Journal of Emergency Medicine 2016; 34(12):2426–2431. doi:10.1016/j.ajem.2016.09.025.

2.5 SEROTONIN TOXICITY

Serotonin toxicity is the clinical manifestation of increased stimulation of serotonin receptors in the CNS. This occurs when excess serotonin (5-hydroxytryptamine) accumulates in the CNS, secondary to a number of pharmacological mechanisms: inhibition of serotonin metabolism (monoamine oxidase inhibitors), prevention of serotonin reuptake in nerve terminals (serotonin reuptake inhibitors), increased serotonin release (amphetamine-like substances) or increased intake of serotonin precursors (tryptophan).

CLINICAL FEATURES

Serotonin toxicity manifests as a constellation of signs and symptoms reflecting the triad of clinical features: mental status changes, autonomic stimulation and neuromuscular excitation (see **Table 2.5.1**).

TABLE 2.5.1 Clinical features of serotonin toxicity		
Mental status changes	**Autonomic stimulation**	**Neuromuscular excitation**
Apprehension Anxiety Agitation, psychomotor acceleration and delirium Confusion	Diarrhoea Flushing Hypertension Hyperthermia Mydriasis Sweating Tachycardia	Clonus (esp. ocular and ankle) Hyperreflexia Increased tone (lower limbs > upper limbs) Myoclonus Rigidity Tremor

There is a spectrum of severity ranging from mild symptoms in ambulatory patients to fulminant life-threatening toxicity characterised by severe generalised rigidity, hyperthermia, marked mental state changes and autonomic instability. Without prompt intervention, severe toxicity progresses to multi-organ failure, disseminated intravascular coagulation (DIC) and death.

Symptoms are usually of rapid onset and may occur within hours of changes in medication or overdose. The toxicity usually resolves over 24 hours following discontinuation of the causative agent(s) and appropriate treatment. More severe toxicity may require several days of intensive care management.

DIAGNOSIS

Serotonin toxicity is a clinical diagnosis and requires the history of ingestion of one or more serotonergic agents (or a change in their dose) and the presence of characteristic clinical features. Some symptoms are more significantly associated with the diagnosis (see **Table 2.5.1**) and diagnostic algorithms have been developed (see **Figure 2.5.1**).

Clinical settings in which serotonin toxicity may develop include:

- introduction or increase in dose of a single serotonergic drug
- change in therapy from one serotonergic drug to another without an adequate intervening 'washout' period
- drug interaction between two serotonergic agents
- interaction between a serotonergic drug and an illicit drug or herbal preparation
- deliberate self-poisoning with serotonergic agent(s).

Numerous agents are implicated in the development of serotonin toxicity, of which the most important ones are listed in **Table 2.5.2**.

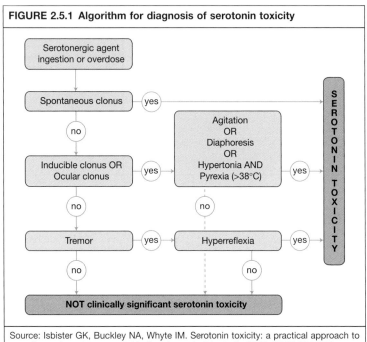

FIGURE 2.5.1 Algorithm for diagnosis of serotonin toxicity

Source: Isbister GK, Buckley NA, Whyte IM. Serotonin toxicity: a practical approach to diagnosis and treatment. Medical Journal of Australia 2007; 187(6):361–365.

TABLE 2.5.2 Agents implicated in development of serotonin toxicity

Analgesics and antitussives
  Dextromethorphan
  Fentanyl
  Pethidine
  Tramadol
Herbal preparations
  Spirulina
  St John's wort (*Hypericum perforatum*)
Ilicit drugs
  Amphetamines
  Methylenedioxymethamphetamine
    (MDMA; ecstasy)
Lamotrigine
Lithium
Monoamine oxidase inhibitors (MAOIs)
  Moclobemide
  Phenelzine
  Tranylcypromine

Selective serotonin reuptake inhibitors (SSRIs)
  Citalopram
  Escitalopram
  Fluoxetine
  Fluvoxamine
  Paroxetine
  Sertraline
Serotonin and noradrenaline reuptake inhibitors (SNRIs)
  Desvenlafaxine
  Duloxetine
  Reboxetine
  Venlafaxine
Tricyclic antidepressants
Tryptophan

Severe serotonin toxicity can occur following overdose with irreversible monoamine oxidase inhibitors (phenelzine and tranylcypromine) in isolation. More commonly, it occurs following deliberate self-poisoning with multiple serotonergic agents. Life-threatening serotonin toxicity does not develop after ingestion of single SSRIs.

DIFFERENTIAL DIAGNOSIS

Careful consideration of drug history, clinical features and clinical course is essential to distinguish serotonin toxicity from neuroleptic malignant syndrome, anticholinergic toxicity and malignant hyperthermia (see **Table 2.5.3**). Other differential diagnoses include CNS infections, withdrawal syndromes (alcohol, benzodiazepines) and sympathomimetic intoxication.

MANAGEMENT

Severe serotonin toxicity is potentially life-threatening if not recognised and treated promptly. It should be anticipated following deliberate self-poisoning with multiple serotonergic medications.

Mild serotonin toxicity, with normal mental status and vital signs, is a self-limiting condition and will resolve with minimal intervention.

- Attention to airway, breathing and circulation is paramount. Immediate life threats include:
  — severe rigidity compromising ventilation
  — hyperthermia
  — altered mental status.
- Rapid sequence intubation, ventilation and neuromuscular paralysis is indicated for patients with established severe toxicity or if there is no immediate response to intravenous benzodiazepines and fluids.
  - Give titrated doses of intravenous benzodiazepines (midazolam or diazepam 2.5–10 mg IV). Further doses may be required to achieve improvement in agitation and neuromuscular activity.
  - Give appropriate intravenous fluids.
  - A temperature >38.5°C is an indication for continuous core-temperature monitoring. A temperature >39.5°C is an emergency and requires prompt intervention with intubation, neuromuscular paralysis and active cooling to prevent further muscle-generated heat production and severe hyperthermia leading to multi-organ failure, neurological injury and death.
  - Tachycardia and hypertension usually respond to appropriate intravenous benzodiazepines. If there is no improvement, intubation and paralysis may be required.

TABLE 2.5.3 Differential diagnosis of serotonin toxicity

Condition	Drug history	Cadence	Vital signs	Pupils	Skin	Bowel sounds	Neuromuscular tone	Reflexes	Mental status
Serotonin toxicity	$5HT_{2A}$ or $5HT_{1A}$ agonist	<12 hours	↑HR, BP, RR and Temp	Mydriasis	Sweaty	Hyperactive	Increased, esp. lower limbs	Hyperreflexia and clonus	Agitation progressing to coma
Neuroleptic malignant syndrome	Dopamine antagonist	Days	↑HR, BP, RR and Temp	Mydriasis or normal	Sweaty but pale	Normal	Lead-pipe rigidity	Bradyreflexia	Mutism, staring, bradykinesia, coma
Anticholinergic toxicity	Anticholinergic agent	<12 hours	↑HR, BP, RR and Temp	Mydriasis	Hot, red and dry	Decreased or absent	Normal	Normal	Agitated delirium
Malignant hyperthermia	Inhalational anaesthetic	Minutes–24 hours	↑HR, BP, RR and Temp	Normal	Sweaty and mottled	Decreased	Generalised rigidity	Hyporeflexia	Agitation

Adapted from Boyer EW, Shannon M. The serotonin syndrome. New England Journal of Medicine 2005; 352(11):1112–1120.

Antidote therapy: specific serotonin antagonists

A number of serotonin antagonists have been used to treat serotonin toxicity although their efficacy has not been established in controlled trials. Cyproheptadine, an antihistamine with anti-serotonergic effects (see **Chapter 4.3: Cyproheptadine**), can be given orally or via a nasogastric tube. The initial dose is 12 mg, and further doses of 8 mg can be given 8 hourly. Alternative agents – particularly indicated if agitation is a prominent feature – are olanzapine 5–10 mg SL or PO, or chlorpromazine (25–100 mg given in 100 mL of normal saline IV over 30–60 minutes). Adverse effects are common with chlorpromazine and include significant sedation, orthostatic hypotension and anticholinergic side effects.

Serotonin antagonists are not indicated for severe serotonin toxicity where a good outcome can only be achieved with timely institution of good supportive care including intravenous benzodiazepines, cooling measures, endotracheal intubation, ventilation and neuromuscular paralysis.

Disposition

The patient with mild serotonin toxicity related to therapeutic drug administration may be discharged once the causative agent is ceased.

Patients at risk of developing serotonin toxicity following deliberate self-poisoning should be observed for this complication for at least 6 hours (12 hours if a slow-release preparation is ingested).

Any patient with abnormal mental status or vital signs requires admission for observation and management. The duration of admission will usually be less than 24 hours.

Patients who develop severe serotonin toxicity requiring neuromuscular paralysis, intubation and ventilation are managed in an intensive care unit.

References

Boyer EW, Shannon M. The serotonin syndrome. New England Journal of Medicine 2005; 352(11):1112–1120.

Dunkley EJ, Isbister GK, Sibbritt D et al. The Hunter Serotonin Toxicity Criteria: simple and accurate diagnostic decision rules for serotonin toxicity. Quarterly Journal of Medicine 2003; 96:635–642.

Isbister GK, Buckley NA, Whyte IM. Serotonin toxicity: a practical approach to diagnosis and treatment. Medical Journal of Australia 2007; 187(6):361–365.

2.6 ANTICHOLINERGIC TOXICITY

Anticholinergic (antimuscarinic) toxicity is caused by competitive inhibition of central and peripheral acetylcholine muscarinic receptors and can result in significant morbidity if not managed appropriately.

CLINICAL FEATURES

Anticholinergic toxicity is best characterised as an agitated delirium associated with variable signs of peripheral muscarinic blockade (see **Table 2.6.1**).

The diagnosis of anticholinergic toxicity is clinical, usually based on the characteristic appearance of the delirium, the presence of peripheral signs and a history of ingestion of a known anticholinergic agent (see **Table 2.6.2**). Signs and symptoms are variable and no particular pattern of central or peripheral signs reliably diagnoses the syndrome.

Many anticholinergic pharmaceuticals and plants have other toxic effects including coma, which may obscure the anticholinergic features of their clinical presentation following poisoning. If a clear history of ingestion is not forthcoming, a differential diagnosis should be considered (see **Table 2.6.3**). Focal neurological signs do not occur as part of the syndrome and their presence prompts immediate investigation for an alternative diagnosis.

When inadequately managed, patients with anticholinergic toxicity are at risk of a number of complications that significantly affect their clinical course. These include:

- injury to themselves or others
- dehydration
- hyperthermia
- rhabdomyolysis
- urinary retention and bladder stretch injury
- pulmonary aspiration and atelectasis.

In the patient who presents late to medical care, some or all of these complications may already be present.

TABLE 2.6.1 Clinical features of anticholinergic toxicity	
Central	**Peripheral**
Agitated delirium characterised by: • fluctuating mental status • confusion • restlessness • fidgeting • visual hallucinations • picking at objects in the air • mumbling slurred speech • disruptive behaviour Tremor Myoclonus Coma Seizures (rare)	Mydriasis Tachycardia Dry mouth Dry skin Flushing Hyperthermia Sparse or absent bowel sounds Urinary retention

TABLE 2.6.2 Anticholinergic agents	

Antiparkinsonian drugs
  Amantadine
  Benztropine
Antihistamines
  Brompheniramine
  Chlorpheniramine
  Cyproheptadine
  Dexchlorpheniramine
  Dimenhydrinate
  Diphenhydramine
  Doxylamine
  Pheniramine
  Promethazine
  Trimeprazine
Antitussives
  Dextromethorphan
Antidepressants
  Tricyclic antidepressants
Antipsychotic agents
  (butyrophenones and
  phenothiazines)
  Chlorpromazine
  Droperidol
  Fluphenazine
  Haloperidol
  Thioridazine
  Trifluoperazine
	Atypical antipsychotic agents
	  Olanzapine
	  Quetiapine
	Anticonvulsant agents
	  Carbamazepine
	Motion sickness agents
	  Hyoscine or scoploamine
	  Meclizine
	Antimuscarinic agents
	  Atropine
	  Hyoscine
	  Glycopyrrolate
	Topical ophthalmological agents
	  Cyclopentolate
	  Homatropine
	  Tropicamide
	Urinary antispasmodic agents
	  Oxybutynin
	Muscle relaxants
	  Cyclobenzaprine
	  Orphenadrine
	Plants and herbal remedies
	  Selected mushrooms
	  Datura species
	  Numerous other plant-derived
	    compounds

MANAGEMENT

Resuscitation

- Attention to airway, breathing and circulation.
- Detect and correct seizures (give benzodiazepines).
- Detect and correct hypoglycaemia.
- Detect and correct hyperthermia.

Risk assessment

The development of anticholinergic toxicity is anticipated following deliberate self-poisoning with potent anticholinergic agents. It usually

TABLE 2.6.3 Differential diagnosis of anticholinergic toxicity	
Encephalitis Hypoglycaemia Hyponatraemia Post-ictal Neuroleptic malignant syndrome	Neurotrauma Sepsis Serotonin toxicity Subarachnoid haemorrhage Wernicke's encephalopathy

manifests within the first few hours of ingestion. Once established, it is difficult to predict the duration of delirium but it may persist for up to 5 days in some circumstances, such as deliberate self-poisoning with benztropine or carbamazepine.

Supportive care
- Manage in a quiet but well-lit area.
- Reassure the patient.
- Intravenous fluids to maintain hydration.
- Insert an indwelling urinary catheter as urinary retention is almost universal.
- Treat agitation with titrated doses of intravenous benzodiazepines until the patient is resting quietly but able to be roused easily. Repeat doses are often required. Droperidol is another treatment option for agitation as it has relatively minor anticholinergic effects at therapeutic dosing.
- One-to-one nursing is frequently necessary to ensure adequate levels of supervision, reassurance and appropriate sedation.
- Avoid using drugs with potent anticholinergic effects.
- Patients with severe agitation may require intubation and ventilation for definitive management. Patients who develop coma following administration of sedative agents may require intubation and ventilation to protect their airway.

Investigations
- Screening tests in deliberate poisoning
  - 12-lead ECG, BGL and paracetamol level
- Specific testing as indicated to identify and treat alternative diagnoses or complications

Decontamination
Patients who present with established anticholinergic toxicity should only receive activated charcoal if they are intubated.

Enhanced elimination
Not clinically indicated for the majority of anticholinergic agents.

Antidotes
Physostigmine is a centrally acting acetylcholinesterase inhibitor that may be used to reverse anticholinergic delirium in selected patients, particularly where it proves difficult to manage them with titrated benzodiazepines. It is also useful to confirm the diagnosis of anticholinergic delirium and avoid the need for further investigation to exclude alternative diagnoses. For further details on this antidote, see **Chapter 4.21: Physostigmine**.

References

Liang HK. Clinical evaluation of the poisoned patient and toxic syndromes. Clinical Chemistry 1996; 42(8):1350–1355.

Patel RJ, Saylor T, Williams SR et al. Prevalence of autonomic signs and symptoms in antimuscarinic drug poisonings. Journal of Emergency Medicine 2004; 26(1): 89–94.

2.7 CHOLINERGIC TOXICITY

Cholinergic toxicity is the result of increased acetylcholine activity at central and peripheral muscarinic and nicotinic receptors and is potentially lethal. Acetylcholine is the neurotransmitter at pre- and post-ganglionic parasympathetic, pre-ganglionic sympathetic and somatic nerves. It is also an important neurotransmitter in the CNS. Cholinergic toxicity arises from either acetylcholinesterase enzyme inhibition or direct agonist action at muscarinic or nicotinic receptors.

Most cases of clinically significant toxicity are due to poisoning from organophosphate or carbamate pesticides. A comprehensive list of causative agents is shown in **Table 2.7.1**.

TABLE 2.7.1 Cholinergic toxicity: causative agents

ACETYLCHOLINESTERASE INHIBITORS	

Organophosphate insecticides
  Chlorpyrifos
  Coumafos
  Diazinon
  Dimethoate
  Fenthion
  Malathion
Carbamate insecticides
  Aldicarb
  Arasan
  Cycloate
  Terbucarb
  Thiram
	Chemical warfare nerve agents
	  Tabun (GA)
	  Sarin (GB)
	  Soman (GD)
	  VX
	Agents used in dementia
	  Donepezil
	  Galantamine
	  Rivastigmine
	  Tacrine
	Agents used in myasthenia gravis
	  Edrophonium
	  Neostigmine
	  Physostigmine
	  Pyridostigmine

ACETYLCHOLINE AGONISTS	

Muscarinic agents
  Acetylcholine
  Bethanechol
  Carbachol
  Pilocarpine
	Nicotinic agents
	  Nicotine (tobacco, gums,
	    patches)
	Mushrooms

CLINICAL FEATURES

Excessive stimulation of cholinoreceptors produces a constellation of CNS, autonomic and neuromuscular effects (see **Table 2.7.2**). Classically, the patient in cholinergic crisis has copious secretions, vomiting, diarrhoea and altered mental status. Fasciculation and muscle weakness may be prominent. Death is secondary to respiratory failure from excessive respiratory secretions and weakness of ventilatory muscles.

Signs and symptoms are variable. Although bradycardia secondary to increased vagal tone is expected, tachycardia is very common secondary to hypoxia, peripheral vasodilatation and the effects of nicotinic stimulation (see **Chapter 3.59: Organophosphorus agents (organophosphates and carbamates)**).

The diagnosis is clinical and based on the characteristic features and progress, usually supported by an exposure history. Miosis appears to be a consistent feature of chemical warfare nerve agent poisoning. Laboratory testing is useful to exclude other diagnoses (see **Risk assessment** below and **Table 2.7.3**) or complications. Complications may include:

- rapid onset of respiratory failure
- seizures
- medium- and long-term neurological sequelae of organophosphate intoxication.

MANAGEMENT
Resuscitation

In the setting of organophosphate poisoning, efforts to decontaminate the patient or use sophisticated personal protective equipment should not delay resuscitation efforts.

TABLE 2.7.2	Clinical features of cholinergic toxicity		
Central nervous system	Neuromuscular	Parasympathetic muscarinic effects	Sympathetic nicotinic effects

Agitation
Central
    respiratory
    depression
Coma
Confusion
Lethargy
Seizures
	Fasciculation
	Muscle
	    weakness
		Abdominal cramping
		Bradycardia
		Bronchoconstriction
		Bronchorrhoea
		Diarrhoea
		Lacrimation
		Miosis
		Salivation
		Urinary incontinence
		Vomiting
			Hypertension
			Mydriasis
			Sweating
			Tachycardia

TABLE 2.7.3 Differential diagnosis of cholinergic toxicity
Causes of weakness (neurotoxic snakebite, Guillain–Barré syndrome, myasthenia gravis, botulism)
Cardiotropic intoxication resulting in bradycardia and vomiting (digoxin, oleander, beta-adrenergic blockers, calcium channel blockers)
Gastroenteritis and abdominal emergencies
Ictal phenomena
Mushroom ingestion
Respiratory disorders (asthma, congestive cardiac failure)
Salicylate intoxication
Serotonin toxicity
Sympathomimetic toxicity
Theophylline intoxication

- Attention to airway, breathing and circulation is paramount. Early control of pulmonary secretions and administration of oxygen is the key to survival.
- Give supplemental oxygen.
- Administer atropine if there are any objective signs of muscarinic excess, such as cough, dyspnoea, respiratory failure, vomiting, diarrhoea, salivation, lacrimation or bradycardia. Repeated escalating doses are given (see **Chapter 4.1: Atropine**) until drying of respiratory secretions is achieved.
- Control seizures with benzodiazepines.
- If adequate oxygenation and ventilation are not rapidly achieved with oxygen and atropine, proceed immediately to intubation and ventilation.

Risk assessment

Deliberate self-poisoning with any organophosphate agent is expected to lead to a life-threatening cholinergic crisis. Any ingestion of an organophosphate agent by a child is also regarded as potentially life-threatening. The need for large doses of atropine should be anticipated. If a clear history of ingestion is not forthcoming, a differential diagnosis should be considered (see **Table 2.7.3**).

Supportive care

- In organophosphate poisoning, staff should manage the patient in a well-ventilated room using standard precautions. Sophisticated personal protective equipment is not required.
- Reassure the patient.
- Commence fluid resuscitation. Patients may already be dehydrated at presentation and require intravenous fluid resuscitation. Increased

insensible fluid losses are likely and often patients cannot drink, so ongoing intravenous fluid management is frequently required.

- Insert an indwelling catheter. Monitor fluid balance until the patient is drinking normally.

Investigations

- Screening tests (12-lead ECG, BGL and serum paracetamol level) indicated if deliberate self-poisoning is suspected
- Specific testing as dictated by the individual agent (e.g. cholinesterase levels)
- Chest X-ray
- Blood gases
- Electrolytes and renal function

Decontamination

The need for gastrointestinal decontamination is determined by a risk–benefit analysis that incorporates the risk assessment. In the setting of organophosphate poisoning, efforts to decontaminate the patient or use sophisticated personal protective equipment should not delay resuscitation efforts.

Enhanced elimination

The need for enhanced elimination will be determined by a risk–benefit analysis that incorporates the risk assessment.

Antidotes

Atropine (see **Chapter 4.1: Atropine**).
The utility of pralidoxime (see **Chapter 4.22: Pralidoxime**) for organophosphate or nerve agent intoxication is controversial.

References

Eddleston M, Dawson A, Karalliedde L et al. Early management after self-poisoning with an organophosphorus or carbamate insecticide: a treatment protocol for junior doctors. Critical Care 2004; 8(6):R391–R397.

Liang HK. Clinical evaluation of the poisoned patient and toxic syndromes. Clinical Chemistry 1996; 42(8):1350–1355.

Little M, Murray L. Consensus statement: risk of nosocomial organophosphate poisoning in emergency departments. Emergency Medicine Australasia 2004; 16:456–458.

2.8 NEUROLEPTIC MALIGNANT SYNDROME

Neuroleptic malignant syndrome (NMS) is a rare but potentially lethal syndrome complicating the use of neuroleptic medications. It is characterised by neuromuscular rigidity, altered mental status and autonomic instability.

The aetiology of NMS remains controversial. Although a central deficiency of dopaminergic neurotransmission at nigrostriatal, mesolimbic and hypothalamic–pituitary pathways appears pivotal, peripheral mechanisms involving altered skeletal muscle mitochondrial function may also be involved. The syndrome develops in 0.02–2.5% of patients taking neuroleptic medication and this incidence does not appear to have changed significantly with the introduction of atypical antipsychotics into clinical practice.

CLINICAL FEATURES

The syndrome is characterised by altered mental status, autonomic instability and neuromuscular dysfunction (see **Table 2.8.1**). The onset of NMS typically occurs over 24–72 hours and recovery may take days or weeks.

DIAGNOSTIC CRITERIA

The diagnosis is clinical, based on a high index of suspicion, presence of characteristic signs and symptoms, and the history of ingestion of one or more neuroleptic agents. Neuroleptic malignant syndrome is a clinical diagnosis made after other medical conditions have been considered and excluded as necessary.

The diagnostic criteria detailed in **Table 2.8.2** are present in the majority of patients.

Leucocytosis, ranging up to $40\,000 \times 10^9$ cells per litre, is common. The creatine kinase (CK) can be significantly elevated (>100 000 IU), particularly if severe rigidity is present. Decreased serum iron is commonly seen but is not specific for the diagnosis. Other biochemical features include metabolic acidosis, abnormalities of hepatic and renal function, hypocalcaemia and hypomagnesaemia. Head CT and MRI are typically normal in NMS, although cerebral oedema has been reported in

TABLE 2.8.1   Clinical features of neuroleptic malignant syndrome

Central nervous system	Autonomic instability	Neuromuscular
Confusion Delirium Stupor Coma	Hyperthermia Tachycardia Hypertension Tachypnoea Cardiac dysrhythmias Diaphoresis Urinary incontinence or retention	'Lead-pipe' rigidity Generalised bradykinesia or akinesia Mutism and staring Dysarthria Dystonia and abnormal postures Abnormal involuntary movements

---

TABLE 2.8.2   Criteria for diagnosis of NMS

- Recent exposure to dopamine antagonist, or dopamine agonist withdrawal
- Hyperthermia
- Rigidity
- Mental status alteration
- CK elevation (at least 4 times upper limit of normal)
- Sympathetic nervous system lability, defined as at least two of the following:
  - blood pressure elevation (systolic or diastolic >25% above baseline)
  - blood pressure fluctuation (>20 mmHg diastolic change or >25 mmHg systolic change within 24 hours)
  - diaphoresis
  - urinary incontinence
- Tachycardia plus tachypnoea
- Negative work-up for infectious, toxic, metabolic and neurological causes

Adapted from Gurrera RJ, Caroff SN, Cohen A et al. An international consensus study of neuroleptic malignant syndrome diagnostic criteria using the Delphi method. Journal of Clinical Psychiatry 2011; 72:1222–1228.

---

isolated, severe cases. Lumbar puncture, usually performed to exclude encephalitis, may show elevated CSF protein in over 30% of cases. Generalised slow wave activity, consistent with a metabolic encephalopathy, is seen on electroencephalogram (EEG).

The following risk factors for NMS have been suggested:

- high doses of neuroleptic agent
- increased dose of neuroleptic agent within the previous 5 days
- large magnitude dosage increase
- parenteral administration
- simultaneous use of two or more neuroleptic agents
- use of haloperidol or depot fluphenazine
- young age
- male sex
- psychiatric co-morbidity
- genetic factors
- pre-existing organic brain disorders (infectious encephalitis, AIDS, tumours)
- dehydration
- high CK levels during episodes of psychosis not associated with NMS
- intercurrent illness.

DIFFERENTIAL DIAGNOSIS

Neuroleptic malignant syndrome is a diagnosis of exclusion and important alternative diagnoses that share some features with NMS must be considered:

- acute lethal (malignant) catatonia
- malignant hyperthermia
- serotonin toxicity (see **Chapter 2.5: Serotonin toxicity**)
- anticholinergic toxicity (see **Chapter 2.6: Anticholinergic toxicity**)
- sympathomimetic toxicity
- encephalitis
- metabolic encephalopathies.

Acute lethal (malignant) catatonia is clinically very similar to NMS. The diagnostic criteria are nearly identical but NMS is distinguished by a history of recent antipsychotic medication use. Neuroleptic malignant syndrome is usually characterised by bradykinesia and mutism, whereas acute lethal catatonia may be characterised by abnormal posturing and waxy flexibility.

COMPLICATIONS

- Respiratory failure
- Dehydration
- Renal failure
- Multiple-organ failure
- Thromboembolism
- Residual catatonia and parkinsonian symptoms
- Recurrence after rechallenge with an antipsychotic agent may occur

MANAGEMENT

Resuscitation

- Attention to airway, breathing and circulation is paramount. If there is coma, hyperthermia >39.5°C or severe rigidity compromising ventilation, proceed to rapid-sequence intubation and ventilation.
- Detect and correct hypoglycaemia.
- Detect and correct hyperthermia. A temperature >38.5°C is an indication for continuous core-temperature monitoring. A temperature >39.5°C is an emergency and requires prompt intervention with neuromuscular paralysis, intubation and ventilation to prevent further muscle-generated heat production, and severe hyperthermia leading to multiple-organ failure, neurological injury and death.
- Avoid any agent with dopamine antagonist effects.
- Intravenous benzodiazepines are frequently used in the management of NMS to achieve muscle relaxation and control of delirium.

- Haemodynamic instability requires close physiological monitoring.
- Bromocriptine (see below) is indicated if there is significant autonomic instability.

Investigations

Based on clinical assessment, investigations are required to exclude alternative diagnoses and detect significant complications:

- chest X-ray
- 12-lead ECG
- full blood count
- renal function and electrolytes
- creatine kinase
- serum calcium and magnesium
- liver function tests
- blood gases
- blood and urine cultures
- head CT
- lumbar puncture
- MRI brain
- electroencephalogram.

Supportive care

- Cease causative agent(s).
- Reassure the patient.
- Administer intravenous fluids and institute fluid balance monitoring.
- Monitor temperature.
- Thromboembolism prophylaxis.

Antidote therapy

The roles of bromocriptine, dantrolene and electroconvulsive therapy (ECT) have not been defined by prospective trials. It is not known whether they increase survival or shorten the clinical course when compared with good supportive care alone.

Bromocriptine is a dopamine agonist that may be given orally or via a nasogastric tube. It is indicated in moderate and severe cases. Dosing commences at 2.5 mg every 8 hours, increasing to 5 mg every 4 hours (30 mg/day). Adverse effects include postural hypotension, headache, nausea, vomiting, dyskinesia and erythromelalgia (painful erythematous extremities). Autonomic instability and fever usually improve within 24 hours of commencing bromocriptine therapy but neuromuscular changes and delirium may take longer to resolve (1–2 days and several days, respectively). If bromocriptine is used, it should be continued for 1–2 weeks before tapering the dose.

Dantrolene is indicated if there is severe muscle rigidity and fever. It is administered intravenously 2–3 mg/kg/day up to a total dose of 10 mg/kg/day. Once oral treatment can be tolerated, it may be given in an oral dose of 100–400 mg/day in divided doses for 10 days, or the patient may be switched to bromocriptine.

Electroconvulsive therapy (ECT) has been reported to significantly improve clinical features of NMS, particularly in severe cases. It is thought to act by increasing central dopaminergic activity. Improvement may be seen after the third or fourth treatment. It has been advocated for:

- severe NMS refractory to supportive care and antidote treatment
- severe NMS that is difficult to differentiate from acute lethal catatonia
- treatment of residual catatonic symptoms after NMS
- when the psychiatric disorder underlying severe NMS is psychotic depression or catatonia.

Disposition and follow-up

Patients with NMS are admitted for observation and management until full recovery has occurred. Recurrence of NMS after reinstitution of an antipsychotic agent occurs in a significant percentage of patients.

References

Bhanushali MJ, Tuite PJ. The evaluation and management of patients with neuroleptic malignant syndrome. Neurology Clinics of North America 2004; 22:389–411.

Gurrera RJ, Caroff SN, Cohen A et al. An international consensus study of neuroleptic malignant syndrome diagnostic criteria using the Delphi method. Journal of Clinical Psychiatry 2011; 72:1222–1228.

Rosebush P, Stewart T. A prospective analysis of 24 episodes of neuroleptic malignant syndrome. American Journal of Psychiatry 1989; 146(6):717–725.

Rusyniak DE, Sprague JE. Toxin-induced hyperthermic syndromes. Medical Clinics of North America 2005; 89:1277–1296.

Trollor JN, Chen X, Sachdev PS. Neuroleptic malignant syndrome associated with atypical antipsychotic drugs. CNS Drugs 2009; 23(6):477–492.

2.9 ALCOHOL USE DISORDER

Alcohol abuse and dependence is formally defined as alcohol use disorder (AUD) (see **Box 2.9.1**). Alcohol withdrawal is a potentially life-threatening medical condition.

More harm occurs in the community as a result of the acute health and social effects of alcohol use than from the consequences of long-term alcohol dependence (see **Table 2.9.1**). Upwards of 30% of all emergency department presentations are alcohol-related. The incidence of alcohol-related problems is even higher in the population that presents

---

BOX 2.9.1   Psychiatric definition of alcohol use disorder (DSM-V)

- Alcohol is often taken in larger amounts or over a longer period than was intended.
- There is a persistent desire or unsuccessful efforts to cut down or control alcohol use.
- A great deal of time is spent in activities necessary to obtain alcohol, use alcohol or recover from its effects.
- Craving or a strong desire or urge to use alcohol occurs.
- Recurrent alcohol use results in a failure to fulfil major role obligations at work, school or home.
- Alcohol use continues despite having persistent or recurrent social or interpersonal problems caused or exacerbated by the effects of alcohol.
- Important social, occupational or recreational activities are given up or reduced because of alcohol use.
- Recurrent alcohol use occurs in situations in which it is physically hazardous.
- Alcohol use is continued despite knowledge of having a persistent or recurrent physical or psychological problem that is likely to have been caused or exacerbated by alcohol.
- Tolerance occurs, as defined by either of the following:
  - a need for markedly increased amounts of alcohol to achieve intoxication or desired effect
  - a markedly diminished effect with continued use of the same amount of alcohol.
- Withdrawal occurs, as manifested by either of the following:
  - the characteristic withdrawal syndrome for alcohol
  - alcohol (or a closely related substance, such as a benzodiazepine) is taken to relieve or avoid withdrawal symptoms.

The presence of at least 2 of these symptoms indicates an alcohol use disorder (AUD).

The severity of AUD is defined as:

- mild: the presence of 2 to 3 symptoms
- moderate: the presence of 4 to 5 symptoms
- severe: the presence of 6 or more symptoms.

Adapted from Diagnostic and Statistical Manual of Mental Disorders. 5th edn. Arlington, Virginia: American Psychiatric Association; 2013.

---

to emergency departments with deliberate self-poisoning with either self-harm or recreational intent.

SCREENING AND BRIEF INTERVENTION STRATEGIES

Presentation to the emergency department, particularly with acute poisoning, provides an ideal opportunity to identify individuals with alcohol-related problems and provide brief intervention with the aim of improving long-term outcomes.

In most settings, doctors identify fewer than 50% of patients with alcohol-related problems. Factors associated with failure to identify these individuals include:

TABLE 2.9.1   Medical complications of chronic alcohol abuse

Cardiovascular	**Malignancy**
Atrial fibrillation	Breast
Cardiomyopathy	Colorectal
Electrolytes	Hepatic
Hypocalcaemia	Larynx
Hypokalaemia	Oesophagus
Hypomagnesaemia	Oropharynx
Hypophosphataemia	**Malnutrition**
Endocrine	Folate deficiency
Hypoglycaemia	Niacin deficiency (pellagra)
Hypogonadism	Stomatitis
Osteoporosis	Vitamin C deficiency (scurvy)
Steatosis	**Neurological**
Haematological	Dementia
Anaemia	Cerebellar degeneration
Coagulopathy	Korsakoff's syndrome
Leucopenia	Peripheral neuropathy
Macrocytosis	Wernicke's encephalopathy
Thrombocytopenia	**Psychiatric**
Gastrointestinal	Alcoholic hallucinosis
Alcoholic hepatitis	Depression and suicide
Cirrhosis	Delusions
Gastritis	
Malabsorption	
Oesophageal varices and	
gastrointestinal haemorrhage	
Pancreatitis	

Adapted from Sivilotti ML. Ethanol, isopropanol and methanol. In: Dart RC, ed. Medical Toxicology. 3rd edn. Philadelphia: Lippincott Williams & Wilkins; 2003.

- inadequate training about substance abuse
- negative attitudes towards patients with substance abuse
- scepticism about effectiveness of treatments
- belief that alcohol problems are not in the realm of the generalist clinician
- excessive time required to perform formal screening procedures.

A number of tools have been developed to assist identification of potentially hazardous alcohol consumption and are suitable for application in the emergency department. The Alcohol Use Disorders Identification Test (AUDIT) identifies patients with at-risk, hazardous or harmful drinking with a sensitivity of 51–97% and a specificity of 78–96% (see **Box 2.9.2**). The 'CAGE' questions detect alcohol abuse and dependence with a sensitivity of 43–94% and specificity of 70–97% (see **Box 2.9.3**).

BOX 2.9.2 The Alcohol Use Disorders Identification Test (AUDIT) Score (WHO 1992)

Questions pertain to behaviour in the last year

Score	0	1	2	3	4
How often do you have a drink containing alcohol?	Never	Monthly or less	Two to four times per month	Two to three times per week	Four or more times per week
How many drinks containing alcohol do you have on a typical day when you are drinking?	1 or 2	3 or 4	5, 6 or 7	8 or 9	10 or more
How often do you have 6 or more drinks on one occasion?	Never	Less than monthly	Monthly	Weekly	Daily or almost daily
How often during the last year have you found that you were not able to stop drinking once you had started?	Never	Less than monthly	Monthly	Weekly	Daily or almost daily
How often during the last year have you failed to do what was normally expected from you because of drinking?	Never	Less than monthly	Monthly	Weekly	Daily or almost daily
How often during the last year have you needed a first drink in the morning to get yourself going after a heavy drinking session?	Never	Less than monthly	Monthly	Weekly	Daily or almost daily

BOX 2.9.2 The Alcohol Use Disorders Identification Test (AUDIT) Score (WHO 1992)—cont'd

Questions pertain to behaviour in the last year

Score	0	1	2	3	4
How often during the last year have you had a feeling of guilt or remorse after drinking?	Never	Less than monthly	Monthly	Weekly	Daily or almost daily
How often during the last year have you been unable to remember what happened the night before because you had been drinking?	Never	Less than monthly	Monthly	Weekly	Daily or almost daily
Have you or someone else been injured as a result of your drinking?	No		Yes, but not in the last year		Yes, during the last year
Has a relative or friend or doctor or other health worker been concerned about your drinking or suggested you cut down?	No		Yes, but not in the last year		Yes, during the last year
Score >20	Hazardous alcohol usage. Help required				
Score 16–19	Hazardous alcohol usage. Help urged				
Score 8–15	Drinking exceeding safe levels				
Score 0–7	Normal usage				

BOX 2.9.3 'CAGE' questions

Two or more positive responses identify patients with lifetime risk of alcohol problems.

Cut down: Have you ever tried to cut down your drinking?

Annoyed: Have you ever been annoyed by criticism of your drinking?

Guilty: Do you feel guilty about your drinking?

Eye-opener: Do you need an eye-opener when you get up in the morning?

The following single question when administered to trauma patients, using a cut-off of three drinks, correlates well with the AUDIT score: 'On a typical day when you are drinking, how many drinks do you have?' Abbreviated screening tools such as this consume minimal time and do not require detailed training.

Early detection of alcohol problems allows implementation of brief intervention strategies such as 'FRAMES', which has been shown to decrease alcohol consumption in non-dependent patients (see **Box 2.9.4**).

BOX 2.9.4 'FRAMES' acronym

Feedback: review problems caused by alcohol with the patient.

Responsibility: point out that changing behaviour is the patient's responsibility.

Advice: advise the patient to cut down or abstain from alcohol.

Menu: provide options to assist the patient to change behaviour.

Empathy: use an empathetic approach.

Self-efficacy: encourage optimism that the patient can change behaviour.

ALCOHOL WITHDRAWAL

The alcohol withdrawal syndrome usually develops within 6–24 hours of cessation or reduction in alcohol consumption in dependent individuals. It commonly develops in patients admitted to hospital for other conditions.

Pathophysiology

Prolonged alcohol use leads to the development of tolerance and physical dependence due to down-regulation of inhibitory gamma-aminobutyric acid ($GABA_A$) receptors and increased expression of excitatory N-methyl-D-aspartate (NMDA) receptors, which enhance glutamate neurotransmission.

Abrupt cessation of chronic alcohol consumption unmasks these changes, with increased glutamate-mediated CNS excitation and a reduction in inhibitory $GABA_A$ receptors, resulting in the clinical features of autonomic overactivity, delirium and seizures. Increased dopaminergic and noradrenergic neurotransmission also occur.

Clinical features

Alcohol withdrawal manifests as a constellation of clinical autonomic and neurological features with a wide spectrum of severity and a typical time course.

Autonomic excitation

- Occurs within hours of cessation and peaks at 24–48 hours:
    — tremor
    — anxiety and agitation
    — sweating
    — tachycardia
    — hypertension
    — nausea and vomiting
    — hyperthermia.

Neuro-excitation

- Occurs within 12–48 hours of cessation:
    — hyperreflexia
    — nightmares
    — hallucinations (visual, tactile and occasionally auditory)
    — generalised tonic–clonic seizures

Delirium tremens

- Severe form with mortality approaching 8%.
- Up to 20% of patients admitted to urban hospitals with alcohol withdrawal.
- Associated with medical co-morbidities and delayed presentation:
    — hallucinations
    — confusion, disorientation and clouding of consciousness
    — autonomic hyperactivity
    — respiratory and cardiovascular collapse
    — death.

Co-morbidities

A number of important co-morbidities should be considered, detected and managed in all patients with high or regular alcohol intake:

- Wernicke's encephalopathy (see **Table 2.9.2**)
- dehydration
- hypoglycaemia
- electrolyte abnormalities
- coagulation disorders/thrombocytopenia
- anaemia, usually macrocytic

TABLE 2.9.2   Signs of Wernicke's encephalopathy
Acute confusion
Reduced level of consciousness
Coma
Memory disturbance
Ataxia
Ophthalmoplegia
Nystagmus
Unexplained hypotension
Hypothermia

- alcoholic gastritis and gastrointestinal bleeding
- pancreatitis
- alcoholic liver disease and hepatic encephalopathy
- subdural haemorrhage
- alcoholic ketoacidosis.

Management

There is a spectrum of severity for presentations of alcohol withdrawal. The mainstay of treatment for significant withdrawal symptoms is appropriate administration of benzodiazepines, in either a fixed-dose or a weaning regimen, or by symptom-triggered dosing based on an alcohol withdrawal score (AWS). Numerous scoring systems are proposed, of varying complexity, and every institution should have a formal protocol to guide management.

Alcohol withdrawal scores are not specific for the diagnosis of withdrawal as other medical or psychiatric conditions can cause similar clinical features. Excessive dosing of benzodiazepines based on the AWS can lead to significant side effects (e.g. over-sedation or worsened delirium). It is recommended that an upper limit of daily benzodiazepine dosing is incorporated into a withdrawal protocol to ensure appropriate review of the clinical management.

Mild forms of alcohol withdrawal can be managed with appropriate medication and supportive care in an outpatient setting. Symptoms typically settle in 2–7 days. Relapse is common without implementation of adequate psychosocial support.

Withdrawal in a residential setting with professional supervision is more appropriate in the following circumstances:

- history of severe alcohol withdrawal
- poor social support
- failure of unsupervised outpatient withdrawal.

Inpatient alcohol withdrawal is indicated for the minority of patients in whom there is a significant risk of delirium tremens, seizures or significant co-morbidities:

- presentation with severe alcohol withdrawal
    - abnormal vital signs after initial treatment
    - hallucinations
    - altered conscious state
    - seizures
- presence of medical complications or co-morbidities (see above)
- presence of significant psychiatric co-morbidities.

Management approach to severe alcohol withdrawal in the hospital setting

Resuscitation, supportive care and monitoring

- Florid delirium tremens constitutes a medical emergency and is managed in an area fully equipped for resuscitation and monitoring with the following priorities:
    - immediate attention to airway, breathing and circulation
    - establishment of IV access
    - control of seizures and delirium by administration of repeated doses of IV diazepam 5–10 mg until seizures and agitation are controlled
    - detection and treatment of hypoglycaemia.
- Alcohol withdrawal onset, severity, progress and response to therapy is best monitored with an alcohol withdrawal chart incorporating an alcohol withdrawal score (AWS) (see **Appendix 4: Alcohol Withdrawal Score** for a validated example).
- Institute monitoring for alcohol withdrawal in any patient judged to be at risk of developing alcohol withdrawal, not solely patients who present in established withdrawal.
- Give regular oral diazepam or lorazepam as guided by the AWS to maintain adequate control of withdrawal.
- Give thiamine 100–300 mg IV tds for the first 24 hours and then review. This should be continued for 3 days if there is altered mental status and even higher doses should be given if Wernicke's encephalopathy is strongly suspected (see **Table 2.9.2**).
- Ensure adequate hydration, electrolyte balance and nutrition.
- Detect and treat co-morbidities.
- Notes:
    - Phenytoin is not indicated for the treatment or prevention of alcohol-related seizures.
    - Lorazepam is the preferred benzodiazepine for alcohol withdrawal in patients with severe liver disease because its shorter half-life minimises the risk of worsening hepatic encephalopathy.

— Low-dose baclofen is associated with reduced use of high-dose benzodiazepines in some patients and may be considered as adjunctive therapy in severe withdrawal (see **References**).

Investigations as indicated
EUC, FBE, LFTs, coagulation profile, serum lipase

Disposition and follow-up
- Medical admission is indicated if:
  — Large doses of diazepam are required to control withdrawal.
  — Medical co-morbidities require care.
- Referral to residential or home detoxification and rehabilitation services for assessment and psychosocial support is considered once acute withdrawal is controlled or resolving.

References

Friedman PD. Alcohol use in adults. The New England Journal of Medicine 2013; 368:365–373.

Hall W, Zador D. The alcohol withdrawal syndrome. Lancet 1997; 349:1897–1900.

Holmwood C. Alcohol related problems in Australia: is there a role for general practice? Medical Journal of Australia 2002; 177:102–103.

Jesse S, Bråthen G, Ferrara M et al. Alcohol withdrawal syndrome: mechanisms, manifestations, and management. Acta Neurologica Scandinavica 2017; 135(1): 4–16. doi:10.1111/ane.12671.

Lieber CS. Medical disorders of alcoholism. New England Journal of Medicine 1995; 333(16):1058–1065.

Lyon JE, Khan RA, Gessert CE et al. Treating alcohol withdrawal with oral baclofen: a randomized, double-blind, placebo-controlled trial. Journal of Hospital Medicine 2011; 6(8):469–474.

Reed DN, Saxe A, Montanez M et al. Use of a single question to screen trauma patients for alcohol dependence. Journal of Trauma 2005; 59:619–623.

Sechi GP, Serra A. Wernicke's encephalopathy: new clinical settings and recent advances in diagnosis and management. Lancet Neurology 2007; 6:442–455.

Sullivan JT, Sykora K, Schneiderman J et al. Assessment of alcohol withdrawal: the revised clinical institute withdrawal assessment for alcohol scale (CIWA-Ar). British Journal of Addiction 1989; 84(11):1353–1357. doi:10.1111/j.1360-0443.1989.tb00737.x.

Tjipto AC, McD Taylor D, Liew H. Alcohol use among young adults presenting to the emergency department. Emergency Medicine Australasia 2006; 18(2):125–130.

2.10 AMPHETAMINE USE DISORDER

Amphetamine use disorder is defined by DSM-V along the lines of substance use disorder in general as outlined for alcohol (see **Box 2.9.1**). Lifetime prevalence of stimulant use disorder is estimated at 3.3% and peaks in 16–29 year-olds. Amphetamine and other stimulant-related presentations represent a significant burden on emergency departments,

TABLE 2.10.1 Effects of long-term amphetamine abuse
Medical
Poor dentition
Weight loss
Skin excoriations
Cardiomyopathy (rare)
Psychiatric
Confusion
Emotional lability
Insomnia
Memory loss
Paranoid psychosis
Social
Damage to social relationships
Neglect of social, interpersonal and occupational responsibilities

accounting for over 1% of all presentations. Most of these presentations relate to medical, social and psychiatric sequelae of acute amphetamine intoxication. The management of these presentations together with the clinical toxicology of amphetamines is dealt with in **Chapter 3.7: Amphetamines and amphetamine-like substances**.

Long-term amphetamine abuse is associated with medical, psychiatric and social sequelae (see **Table 2.10.1**). These sequelae may result directly in hospital presentation or complicate the management of intercurrent illness. Amphetamines, particularly methamphetamine, are highly addictive and patients may also present in withdrawal or develop withdrawal during admission for other reasons.

No pharmacological agent has been demonstrated to be effective in the treatment of amphetamine withdrawal, dependence or abuse. Management relies on counselling and social support.

AMPHETAMINE WITHDRAWAL

Prolonged or heavy use of amphetamines results in tachyphylaxis (reduced response to repeated doses). This phenomenon is thought to be due to depleted concentrations of neurotransmitters. The symptoms are largely psychiatric and mood-related, and include depression, fatigue, insomnia, increased appetite and cognitive impairment. Symptoms usually peak 2–4 days following cessation of use but may continue for 7–14 days. Amphetamine withdrawal in itself is rarely severe enough to warrant specific medical treatment or admission. Management consists of referral for appropriate psychosocial support.

References

Romanelli F, Smith KM. Clinical effects and management of amphetamines. Pharmacotherapy 2006; 26(8):1148–1156.

Sara GE, Burgess PM, Harris MG et al. Stimulant use and stimulant use disorders in Australia: findings from the national survey of mental health and wellbeing. Medical Journal of Australia 2011; 195:607–610.

Shoptaw SJ, Kao U, Heinzerling K et al. Treatment for amphetamine withdrawal. Cochrane Database of Systematic Reviews 2009; 2:C0003021.

Srisurapanont M, Jarusuraisin N, Krittirattanapaiboon P. Treatment for amphetamine dependence and abuse. Cochrane Database of Systematic Reviews 2001; 4: C0003022.

2.11 OPIOID USE DISORDER

Opioid use disorder is defined by DSM-V along the lines of substance use disorder in general as outlined for alcohol (see **Box 2.9.1**). Opioid-related presentations represent an increasing burden on the health system. In particular, there has been a doubling of hospital admissions and deaths related to prescription opioids in the past decade in Australia and the United Kingdom. The management of these presentations together with the clinical toxicology of opioids is dealt with in **Chapter 3.57: Opioids**.

OPIOID WITHDRAWAL

Opioid withdrawal syndrome is the physiological response that develops when there is abrupt cessation or rapid reduction in opioid dose in a dependent individual or when that individual is administered an opioid antagonist or partial agonist.

Pathophysiology

Opioids exert their analgesic and euphoric effects by agonist activity at CNS mu receptors, leading to decreased intracellular cAMP via the membrane-bound G-proteins. Prolonged opioid use leads to a process of cellular adaptation and down-regulation through multiple mechanisms. When opioids are ceased, a withdrawal syndrome develops.

Clinical features

Although unpleasant, uncomplicated opioid withdrawal is not life-threatening. This is in contrast to withdrawal from alcohol or sedative-hypnotics. The symptoms usually prompt concerted efforts to obtain opioids by the individual concerned.

The timing of onset of symptoms depends on the elimination kinetics of the specific opioid, the usual dose ingested and the degree of dependence. Symptoms may begin within 6 hours of the last heroin dose, peak at 36–48 hours and resolve within 1 week. In contrast, onset of symptoms may be delayed 2–3 days after cessation of methadone, peak at several days and last for up to 2 weeks. Patients may present with withdrawal symptoms associated with cessation of more than one agent.

The clinical manifestations of opioid withdrawal include intense craving, dysphoria, autonomic hyperactivity and gastrointestinal distress. More specifically, symptoms include:

- anxiety, restlessness and dysphoria
- insomnia
- intense craving
- yawning
- lacrimation
- salivation
- rhinorrhoea
- anorexia, nausea and vomiting
- abdominal cramps and diarrhoea
- mydriasis
- piloerection
- diaphoresis
- flushing
- myalgia and arthralgia
- hypertension and tachycardia in severe cases.

Altered mental status, delirium, hyperthermia and seizures are not direct features of opioid withdrawal. Their presence should alert the clinician to an alternative diagnosis or complication.

Co-morbidities

Co-morbidities that should be considered in patients with opioid withdrawal include:

- alcohol or sedative-hypnotic withdrawal syndrome
- dehydration
- electrolyte abnormalities
- infective complications of intravenous drug abuse
- psychiatric morbidities.

Management

Administration of opioids in sufficient dose will abolish all physiological manifestations of the withdrawal syndrome. Administration of opioids to control withdrawal may be the appropriate course of action, particularly where the management of co-morbidities demands attention.

Managed withdrawal (detoxification) is a necessary step towards drug-free treatment. The aims of early management of drug detoxification are safe cessation or dose reduction, management of symptoms and medical complications and retention of the patient in a treatment program.

Most patients with opioid withdrawal can be managed in an outpatient setting. Information and reassurance provided in a non-judgemental way are vital to engage the patient in a realistic withdrawal treatment program.

Admission to hospital may be required in the following circumstances:

- severe withdrawal syndrome (e.g. following administration of antagonist)
- significant complications (e.g. severe dehydration)
- significant intercurrent illness (e.g. sepsis)
- psychiatric co-morbidity.

Pharmacological treatment of opioid withdrawal is categorised into three types: opioid replacement therapy (e.g. methadone, buprenorphine), antagonist detoxification (e.g. naltrexone) and symptomatic treatment.

Opioid replacement therapy

Methadone is used in opioid withdrawal and for maintenance in abstinence programs. Methadone maintenance treatment achieves significant reduction in heroin use and reduces mortality from heroin overdose but does not produce an overall reduction in mortality when compared with drug-free maintenance.

To commence methadone, patients should be referred for evaluation and ongoing management by a specialist drug and alcohol service. Methadone doses typically start at 20–40 mg/day and are tapered over many weeks (e.g. by 3–5% each week).

Buprenorphine is a high-affinity partial mu-opioid agonist used as an alternative to methadone. Doses start at 2–16 mg/day and are tapered over many weeks. Buprenorphine treatment is as effective as methadone in maintenance treatment of heroin dependence but less effective in achieving treatment retention, particularly with low-dose or flexible-dose regimens.

Buprenorphine is administered orally or sublingually, frequently as a co-formulation with naloxone to prevent illicit diversion for intravenous misuse.

Detoxification

Rapid detoxification using naltrexone, buprenorphine and clonidine in various combinations, or by rapid tapering of methadone, has been successful in selected patients. Efficacy depends on patient selection and close clinical supervision by a team experienced in specialised drug and alcohol treatment. Ultra-rapid detoxification is an invasive procedure involving the precipitation of severe opioid withdrawal using naltrexone, occasionally under general anaesthesia. This technique does not improve abstinence rates and carries a high risk of serious adverse events including death.

TABLE 2.11.1 Symptomatic treatment of opioid withdrawal

Dehydration
  Fluid resuscitation
Nausea and vomiting
  Metoclopramide 10 mg or prochlorperazine 5 mg or ondansetron 4 mg
    PO, 6 hourly as required
Abdominal cramps and diarrhoea
  Hyoscine 20 mg PO every 6 hours or atropine–diphenoxylate
    (25 micrograms–2.5 mg) two tablets PO every 6–8 hours
Myalgia and arthralgia
  Paracetamol (1 g every 6 hours) or ibuprofen (400 mg every 6 hours)
Anxiety, dysphoria and insomnia
  Diazepam 5–10 mg PO every 6–8 hours for 2–3 days
  Clonidine
    Centrally acting alpha-2-adrenergic receptor agonist used to
      attenuate the physical and psychological symptoms of opioid
      withdrawal
    Adverse effect is postural hypotension, especially in patients with
      dehydration and bradycardia
    Give a test dose of 75 micrograms PO, followed by lying and
      standing blood pressure monitoring for 1 hour
    If symptomatic postural hypotension does not occur, commence
      50 micrograms PO three times a day. The dose may be
      increased if tolerated (e.g. up to 200–300 micrograms three
      times daily) before tapering over the subsequent 5 days

Supportive care

Patients should be reassured and assessed for potential co-morbidities and complications. Fluid resuscitation for dehydration may be required. The presence of altered mental status, fever or seizures prompts further investigation for an alternative cause. Several medications are of value in providing symptomatic relief (see **Table 2.11.1**).

Presentation with drug-related problems provides an opportunity for patient counselling regarding the risks of drug abuse and dependence and engagement in strategies to change behaviour.

References

Anonymous. Deaths and severe adverse events associated with anesthesia-assisted rapid opioid detoxification – New York City, 2012. Morbidity and Mortality Weekly Report 2013; 38:777–780.

Kosten TR, O'Connor PG. Management of drug and alcohol withdrawal. New England Journal of Medicine 2003; 348:1786–1795.

Mattick RP, Breen C, Kimber J et al. Methadone maintenance therapy versus no opioid replacement therapy for opioid dependence. Cochrane Database of Systematic Reviews 2009; 3:CD002209.

Mattick RP, Breen C, Kimber J et al. Buprenorphine maintenance versus placebo or methadone maintenance for opioid dependence. Cochrane Database of Systematic Reviews 2014; 2:C0002207.

Olmedo R, Hoffman RS. Withdrawal syndromes. Emergency Medicine Clinics of North America 2000; 18(2):273–288.

Roxburgh A, Bruno R, Larance B et al. Prescription of opioid analgesics and related harms in Australia. Medical Journal of Australia 2011; 195:280–284.

Tetrault JM, O'Connor PG. Substance abuse and withdrawal in the critical care setting. Critical Care Clinics 2008; 24:767–788.

2.12 SEDATIVE-HYPNOTIC USE DISORDER

Sedative-hypnotic use disorder is defined by DSM-V along the lines of substance use disorder in general as outlined for alcohol (see **Box 2.9.1**). Sedative-hypnotics include benzodiazepines, barbiturates, non-benzodiazepine agents (zolpidem, zopiclone), baclofen, gamma-hydroxybutyrate, chloral hydrate and paraldehyde. Deliberate self-poisoning with these agents is extremely common and the management of these presentations together with the clinical toxicology of the specific sedative-hypnotics is dealt with in **Chapter 3.14: Baclofen, Chapter 3.15: Barbiturates, Chapter 3.16: Benzodiazepines, Chapter 3.26: Chloral hydrate** and **Chapter 3.37: Gamma-hydroxybutyrate (GHB)**.

SEDATIVE-HYPNOTIC WITHDRAWAL

Abrupt cessation or reduction in dose of a sedative-hypnotic agent can produce a characteristic withdrawal syndrome in a dependent individual similar to that of alcohol withdrawal. Withdrawal syndromes are described for:

- benzodiazepines
- barbiturates
- non-benzodiazepine sedative-hypnotic agents (zolpidem, zopiclone)
- baclofen
- gamma-hydroxybutyrate (GHB)
- chloral hydrate.

Pathophysiology

The sedative-hypnotic agents cause down-regulation of inhibitory gamma-aminobutyric acid ($GABA_A$) receptors, and increased expression of excitatory N-methyl-D-aspartate (NMDA) receptors which enhance glutamate neurotransmission.

Abrupt cessation of these agents unmasks these changes, with increased glutamate-mediated CNS excitation and a reduction in inhibitory $GABA_A$ receptors resulting in the clinical features of autonomic overactivity, delirium and seizures.

Clinical features

There is a high degree of inter-individual difference in the rate of onset, type and severity of withdrawal symptoms. Variability is determined by dose and duration of therapy, rapidity of withdrawal, elimination kinetics of the agent and patient factors. Onset of symptoms generally occurs within 2–10 days of abrupt cessation, although withdrawal of short-acting agents (e.g. GHB) or agents administered by the intrathecal route (e.g. baclofen) may produce symptoms within hours. The clinical presentation may reflect withdrawal from more than one class of agent.

Rarely, a severe and potentially lethal syndrome similar to delirium tremens can occur. This is in contrast to opioid or cannabis withdrawal, which does not cause delirium, autonomic instability or seizures (see **Chapter 2.11: Opioid use disorder** and **Chapter 3.22: Cannabinoids (and synthetic cannabinoid receptor agonists (SCRAs))**.

The commonly observed clinical features resemble those of alcohol withdrawal (see **Chapter 2.9: Alcohol use disorder**), although psychomotor and autonomic nervous system signs may be more prominent:

- irritability and agitation
- anorexia
- inattention
- memory disturbances
- insomnia
- palpitations
- perceptual disturbances, including photophobia and hyperacusis
- hallucinations
- increased spasticity (baclofen).

Co-morbidities

Co-morbidities that should be considered in patients with sedative-hypnotic withdrawal include:

- alcohol withdrawal syndrome
- dehydration
- electrolyte abnormalities
- psychiatric morbidities.

Management

Where withdrawal develops as a result of an interruption in regular benzodiazepine (or other sedative-hypnotic agent) use due to an intercurrent medical illness, it is best to reverse the withdrawal syndrome by reinstitution of the responsible agent until the precipitating illness is treated.

Where the aim is to achieve permanent safe withdrawal or dose reduction, alternative management strategies are adopted. The usual strategy is to substitute a longer acting benzodiazepine for the agent being ceased and then to slowly taper the dose. Tapering is titrated to individual patient symptoms. If withdrawal symptoms increase, the dose may be increased transiently or tapering attempted more slowly. Typically, withdrawal takes weeks to complete with dosage decreases of 10–15% per week.

Management of severe sedative-hypnotic withdrawal with delirium or seizures is similar to alcohol withdrawal syndrome (see **Chapter 2.9: Alcohol use disorder**).

Several scores have been used to assess the severity of the benzodiazepine withdrawal syndrome in order to guide admission decisions and benzodiazepine dosing. However, most scores have not been prospectively validated and should be used with caution.

Disposition

In most patients, sedative-hypnotic withdrawal is mild and management in an outpatient setting is appropriate. Presentation with drug-related problems provides an opportunity for patient counselling regarding the risks of drug abuse and dependence and engagement in strategies to change behaviour.

Withdrawal in a residential setting, with supervision by specialised staff with training in drug and alcohol issues, is appropriate in selected circumstances:

- history of severe withdrawal
- poor social support
- failure of unsupervised outpatient withdrawal.

Inpatient sedative-hypnotic withdrawal is appropriate for a minority of patients in whom there is a significant risk of delirium or seizures:

- presentation in severe withdrawal
- abnormal vital signs after initial treatment
- hallucinations
- altered conscious state
- seizures
- presence of medical complications or co-morbidities
- presence of significant psychiatric co-morbidities.

References

Kosten TR, O'Connor PG. Management of drug and alcohol withdrawal. New England Journal of Medicine 2003; 348:1786–1795.

Leo RJ, Baer D. Delirium associated with baclofen withdrawal: a review of common presentations and management strategies. Psychosomatics 2005; 46:503–507.

McDonough M, Kennedy N, Glasper A et al. Clinical features of gamma-hydroxybutyrate (GHB) withdrawal: a review. Drug and Alcohol Dependence 2004; 75:3–9.

Olmedo R, Hoffman RS. Withdrawal syndromes. Emergency Medicine Clinics of North America 2000; 18(2):273–288.

2.13 SOLVENT ABUSE

A solvent is defined as a liquid that has the ability to dissolve, suspend or extract another material without chemical change to either the material or solvent. Organic solvents are found in numerous household and industrial products, including glues, household cleaners, degreasers, thinners, paints, pharmaceuticals, cosmetics and pesticides. The group includes aliphatic, cyclical, aromatic and halogenated hydrocarbons, ethers, esters, glycols, ketones, aldehydes and amines (see **Table 2.13.1**). Common solvents include isopropanol, toluene and xylene. Other volatile hydrocarbons more commonly used as fuels, such as petrol, kerosene and butane (used as lighter fuel), have similar physicochemical properties, clinical effects and abuse potential.

TABLE 2.13.1 Chemicals used for inhalational abuse	

Aliphatic hydrocarbons
    Acetylene
    n-Butane
    Cyclopropane
    Isobutane
    n-Hexane
    Propane
Aromatic hydrocarbons
    Toluene
    Xylene
Mixed hydrocarbons
    Petrol
    Kerosene
Halogenated hydrocarbons
    Bromochlorodifluoromethane
    Carbon tetrachloride
    Chlorodifluoromethane
    Chloroform
    Dichlorodifluoromethane
    Dichloromethane (methylene
        chloride)
    1,2-Dichloropropane
    Enflurane
    Ethyl chloride
    Halothane
    Isoflurane
    Methoxyflurane
    Tetrachloroethylene
    1,1,1-Trichloroethane
    Trichloroethylene
    Trichlorofluoromethane
	Nitrites
	    Amyl nitrite
	    Butyl nitrite
	    Cyclohexyl nitrite
	Oxygenated compounds
	    Acetone
	    Butanone
	    Diethyl ether
	    Dimethyl ether
	    Ethyl acetate
	    Methyl acetate
	    Methyl isobutyl ketone
	    Nitrous oxide

Adapted from Flanagan RJ, Ruprah M, Meredith TJ et al. An introduction to the clinical toxicology of volatile substances. Drug Safety 1990; 5:359–383.

The recreational abuse of solvents involves inhalation of these volatile substances for the purpose of achieving an alteration in mental status, principally euphoria. Inhalational organic solvent abuse is a major public health problem particularly afflicting adolescents and Indigenous communities. The agent with the highest potential for abuse is toluene, found primarily in glues, spray paints and lacquers.

PHYSICOCHEMICAL PROPERTIES

The organic solvents are all volatile liquids and well absorbed via the inhalational route. Peak blood concentrations are achieved within 15–30 minutes of inhalation. These agents are highly lipid soluble and following absorption are preferentially distributed to lipid-rich organs notably the CNS and liver. After inhalation stops, excretion by the lungs takes place. Solvents are also metabolised by the liver with elimination half-lives in the order of 15–72 hours.

MECHANISM OF TOXICITY

While agents vary in their end-organ specificity, acute solvent toxicity generally correlates with the volatility of an agent. They are lipophilic and potent CNS depressants. High volatility is associated with a greater risk of micro-aspiration and pneumonitis. Myelin toxicity is thought to be the cause of the neuropsychiatric consequences associated with long-term inhalational abuse and occupational exposure. Myocardial sensitisation to catecholamines may be associated with cardiac dysrhythmias and sudden death.

MODES OF ABUSE

Solvent abusers always employ the inhalational route with the following methods described:

- 'Huffing': the liquid solvent is poured into a bag or piece of cloth such as a sock and the liquid-soaked material is then held up to the face as the abuser inhales deeply.
- 'Bagging': the liquid is poured into a bag and the bag held over the head.
- 'Sniffing' or 'snorting': liquid is inhaled directly from the container.

CLINICAL FEATURES

The solvent abuser may present with acute solvent neurotoxicity or with the CNS, metabolic, behavioural and social complications associated with chronic abuse.

Acute inhalational exposure

Acute inhalation predominantly affects the CNS, causing altered cognition that resembles ethanol intoxication. There is general impairment of psychomotor function, as measured by reaction time, manual dexterity, coordination and body balance. Patients are euphoric, disinhibited, lethargic and ataxic with slurred speech and inappropriate affect. More severe intoxication is characterised by confusion, depressed level of consciousness, seizures and coma.

Inhalational exposure to solvents also causes intense irritation to the mucous membranes of the eye, nose, throat and lower airways. Inadvertent aspiration can induce chemical pneumonitis.

Sudden death, particularly associated with butane and propane, may occur during acute exposure. Possible mechanisms are asphyxiation or cardiac dysrhythmias induced by sensitisation of the myocardium to endogenous circulating catecholamines.

Chronic inhalational abuse

There is strong evidence to suggest that long-term toluene exposure leads to persistent neurotoxicity characterised by structural and functional brain abnormalities, as well as neuropsychological impairment. Neuro-imaging studies suggest injury preferentially affects white matter structures (lipid-rich myelinated structures), a pattern which could be explained by the lipid-dependent distribution to myelinated areas of the brain.

Persistent neurotoxicity is characterised by impaired cognition and poor performance on most neuropsychological tests, including those testing working memory and executive cognitive function. Although the individuals engaging in chronic toluene abuse are likely to come from a background of psychomotor, emotional and social deprivation, it does appear that the abuse itself is associated with adverse effects in cognitive and intellectual abilities. These effects further exacerbate the pre-existing problems and complicate efforts to achieve detoxification, long-term abstinence and rehabilitation.

It remains controversial as to whether long-term abstinence is associated with significant improvement in neuropsychological function.

Chronic toluene abuse is also associated with a normal anion gap metabolic acidosis largely due to distal renal tubular acidosis. Acidaemia, hyperchloraemia and hypokalaemia may be profound (25% of chronic abusers have serum K^+ <2 mmol/L).

MANAGEMENT

The solvent abuser who presents with acute solvent neurotoxicity requires standard resuscitative measures for management of coma and seizures. Behavioural disorders frequently necessitate early sedation with titrated doses of intravenous benzodiazepine or droperidol (see **Chapter 2.4: Approach to delirium**). Management of secondary complications such as hypoxia, hypoglycaemia, electrolyte disturbances and seizures usually ensures survival.

Cardiac dysrhythmias, while a cause of early sudden death, are rarely observed after arrival at hospital. Management along advanced cardiac life support (ACLS) guidelines with consideration of early use of beta-blocking agents for tachydysrhythmias is appropriate.

Acid–base and electrolyte status should be checked early in the patient suspected of chronic solvent abuse. Acidaemia may be prominent even in a relatively asymptomatic patient. Patients may present with life-threatening acidaemia requiring intensive care management to correct acid–base disturbances and profound hypokalaemia.

DISPOSITION

A period of observation lasting hours to days may be required until the acute CNS and metabolic disorders resolve. This may occur in the emergency department or intensive care unit, but continuous and adequate supervision is essential to prevent injury to the patient and staff.

After resolution of acute toxicity, the issues associated with chronic solvent abuse must be addressed. Management is challenging and as much socio-political as medical or psychological. Achieving sustained abstinence in the setting of ongoing social deprivation is difficult. Many of the neuropsychiatric effects associated with chronic abuse are likely to be irreversible and further complicate management.

SOLVENT WITHDRAWAL

Physical withdrawal from solvents is generally mild with lethargy, headaches, anxiety or depressed mood. It may last from several days to a few weeks and does not require any specific treatment.

SOLVENT ABUSE DURING PREGNANCY AND LACTATION

Most solvents, including toluene, are highly lipid soluble and cross the placenta easily. A fetal solvent syndrome similar to fetal alcohol syndrome is described, as is a withdrawal syndrome in the neonate in the postpartum period.

References

Carlisle EJF, Donnelly SM, Vasuvattakul S et al. Glue-sniffing and distal renal tubular acidosis: sticking to the facts. Journal of the American Society of Nephrology 1991; 1:1019–1027.

Dick FD. Solvent neurotoxicity. Occupational and Environmental Medicine 2006; 63:221–226.

Flanagan RJ, Ruprah M, Meredith TJ et al. An introduction to the clinical toxicology of volatile substances. Drug Safety 1990; 5:359–383.

Kopec KT, Brent J, Banner W et al. Management of cardiac dysrhythmias following hydrocarbon abuse: clinical toxicology teaching case from NAACT acute and intensive care symposium. Clinical Toxicology 2014; 52:141–145.

Maruff P, Burns CB, Tyler P et al. Neurological and cognitive abnormalities associated with chronic petrol sniffing. Brain 1998; 121:1903–1917.

Rosenberg NL, Grigsby J, Driesbach J et al. Neuropsychological impairment and MRI abnormalities associated with chronic solvent abuse. Clinical Toxicology 2002; 40(1):21–24.

Yucel M, Takagi M, Walterfang M et al. Toluene misuse and long-term harms: a systematic review of the neuropsychological and neuroimaging literature. Neuroscience and Biobehavioural Reviews 2008; 32:910–926.

2.14 BODY PACKERS AND STUFFERS

Body packing refers to the internal concealment of illicit drugs (usually in large quantities) for transportation across international borders. The drug is usually of a single type and meticulously packaged in plastic, latex, condoms or balloons. Many hours have usually elapsed before presentation to the emergency department, so most packets have already entered the small or large intestine. The vagina and rectum are not usually used for body packing as the drugs are more likely to be discovered on physical examination. Cocaine, heroin, amphetamine, 3-4-methylenedioxymethamphetamine (MDMA, 'ecstasy'), cannabis and hashish have all been reported to have been transported by body packing. Up to 1 kg of drug, divided into more than 100 packets, may be transported by a single individual. Body packers (often referred to as 'mules' or 'swallowers') use constipating agents such as atropine-diphenoxylate to slow gastrointestinal transit such that it may take from days to weeks for all packages to pass.

Body stuffing refers to the hasty internal concealment of illicit drugs immediately prior to apprehension by authorities. The packages are more likely to contain multiple different drugs, are usually prepared in a rushed manner and much more likely to leak. They may consist simply of a small plastic bag or foil pouch. The delay from ingestion to presentation to the emergency department is much shorter and the ingested packets are frequently still within the stomach. The vagina and rectum are alternative sites for drug concealment in body stuffing.

The management of body packers and body stuffers poses multiple challenges:

- Many times the lethal dose of illicit drug may have been ingested.
- Patients may not provide an accurate history, making risk assessment problematic.
- The treating clinician may be asked by law enforcement officers to conduct procedures for which the patient has not consented.
- There are few prospective studies to guide management.

The medico-legal issues in cases of body packing can be complex and require senior medical decision making. An essential factor to consider is whether the patient is under arrest and will remain in custody – a decision requiring formal legal oversight.

Even if the patient is under arrest, they can refuse medical assessment, including examination and radiological imaging, and it is important that medical or nursing staff do not feel compelled to ignore the patient's right to autonomy. However, if there is evidence of medical complications from body packing (e.g. drug intoxication; bowel obstruction or perforation), a clinician's duty of care to the patient allows appropriate investigations and management to be performed. If the patient is not under arrest, they can decline management advice or treatment provided they have capacity. Clear documentation of the assessment and decision making is an essential medico-legal requirement.

CLINICAL PRESENTATION

Body packers present in three settings:

- acute drug intoxication or fear of impending rupture and intoxication
- request by authorities for medical assessment following arrest
- development of surgical complications, usually bowel obstruction but bowel perforation, oesophageal obstruction and oesophageal rupture are also reported.

MANAGEMENT OF BODY STUFFERS

Patients are initially observed in a monitored environment with intravenous access. If the patient presents within 1 hour and is cooperative, a single dose of 50 g oral activated charcoal is indicated.

Depending on the history and patient consent, body cavities may be examined. CT scanning is unreliable in the setting of body stuffing and cannot be used to confirm or exclude the presence of packets or drugs. The duration of observation required to ensure that significant toxicity does not occur is not well established. Available data from retrospective studies suggest that most body stuffers will develop symptoms within 6 hours. Therefore, it is reasonable to consider a patient safe for discharge once observed for 6–12 hours and they remain asymptomatic, particularly if the history suggests ingestion of a small number of packets. However, patients who will remain under arrest are often kept for medical supervision up to 24 hours before discharge due to concerns about access to medical and nursing care while in custody.

Although it is likely that a 6–12-hour observation period is adequate for body stuffers, it is essential that the clinician responsible for the patient appreciates that available evidence does not guarantee that the patient will remain asymptomatic once discharged from medical care. Patients with clinical features of intoxication are managed until resolution of symptoms.

MANAGEMENT OF BODY PACKERS

Resuscitation, supportive care and monitoring

Body packers should be given high triage priority and are initially managed in an area equipped for cardiopulmonary monitoring and resuscitation. Immediate resuscitation priorities are attended to as outlined in **Chapter 1.2: Resuscitation**.

Risk assessment

Body packers transport many times the lethal dose of cocaine, heroin or amphetamines. The onset of signs of drug intoxication may herald imminent catastrophic deterioration.

It is important to obtain a detailed history from the patient, if possible. The type of drug, number and construction of packages and time of ingestion are vital components of the history. In those patients admitting (or proven) to have swallowed drug packets, there is good correlation between the number of packets self-reported and the total number of packets retrieved. The physical examination should look for any evidence of drug intoxication and surgical complications (e.g. bowel obstruction or perforation).

Supportive care and disposition

The patient should be admitted to a clinical area equipped and staffed to manage the potentially rapid onset of drug intoxication. In most settings, this will be an intensive care unit or emergency observation ward. Staff are briefed on the potential symptoms of intoxication that will prompt urgent review and appropriate management. Senior medical staff must be available 24 hours a day. Intravenous access is maintained until discharge. Continuous ECG and pulse oximetry monitoring are kept in place when the patient is not ambulating, and especially when asleep. Asymptomatic patients may eat a normal diet. Ambulation around the ward is encouraged as bed rest appears to be a risk factor for bowel obstruction. Patients are observed until the expected numbers of packets are passed and repeat abdominal CT scanning (if indicated) is negative. The mean time to pass all packages is approximately 5 days.

Investigations

Patients may refuse to undergo investigations, even when under arrest. In this scenario, the decision for a patient to remain in custody under medical supervision is determined by an appropriate legal authority.

Abdominal X-ray is able to detect internal drug concealment in a significant percentage of body packers and delivers a low dose of radiation. Abdominal CT scanning is a more sensitive investigation and is considered the investigation of choice, but delivers a higher dose of radiation and does not have 100% sensitivity. Packet counts on CT are most accurate when <15 packets exist. However, for higher numbers of packets, correlation between packets counted on CT and total number passed is poor. Once all expected packets have been retrieved, repeat abdominal CT scan can be performed in an attempt to exclude additional retained packets. However, it may be reasonable to confirm the tally of packages with a reliable history from the patient to avoid repeated CT scanning and additional irradiation.

Urine toxicology screening has low clinical utility. A positive test suggests the need for further investigation and observation but a negative test does not exclude body packing or indicate that the patient is safe for discharge.

Decontamination

Cooperative asymptomatic patients may be administered 50 g activated charcoal in case of package leakage or rupture.

Asymptomatic patients, even those transporting cocaine, may be treated conservatively and observed until all packages are retrieved. The incidence of serious complications such as late-onset drug intoxication, bowel obstruction, urgent laparotomy or death is less than 5% with conservative management. A light or liquid diet plus laxatives are often ordered in an effort to speed passage of packages.

The role of whole bowel irrigation to achieve more rapid and complete decontamination is controversial. There are unproven concerns that it may increase the risk of bowel obstruction or package leakage. Judicious administration can be considered under appropriate supervision (see **Chapter 1.6: Gastrointestinal decontamination**). The requirement for use of this technique for heroin body packers may be less compelling, where a good outcome can be expected with supportive care and antidote administration, even in the event of package rupture.

Endoscopy may be considered to retrieve packages from the stomach that are too large to pass the pylorus. Colonoscopy may be considered to retrieve packages retained in either of the colonic flexures. These procedures may be technically difficult to perform and carry a risk of package rupture.

Patients with severe cocaine or other stimulant toxicity requiring resuscitation are considered for urgent laparotomy. Similarly, patients who develop signs of bowel obstruction or perforation should have their packages surgically removed.

Antidotes

Naloxone is indicated for the management of opioid intoxication. In body packers, large initial doses may be required (e.g. 2–10 mg) followed by an intravenous infusion (see **Chapter 4.18: Naloxone**). The management of cocaine and amphetamine intoxication is described in **Chapter 3.29: Cocaine** and **Chapter 3.7: Amphetamines and amphetamine-like substances**.

References

Asha SE, Higham M, Child P. Sensitivity and specificity of CT scanning for determining the number of internally concealed packages in 'body-packers'. Emergency Medicine Journal 2015; 32(5):387–391.

Beckley I, Ansari NA, Khwaja HA et al. Clinical management of cocaine body packers: the Hillingdon experience. Canadian Journal of Surgery 2009; 52(5):417–421.

Das D, Ali B, Mackway-Jones K. Conservative management of asymptomatic cocaine body packers. Emergency Medicine Journal 2003; 20:172–174.

De Bakker JK, Nanayakkara PWB, Geeraedts LMG et al. Body packers: a plea for conservative management. Langenbecks Archives of Surgery 2012; 397:125–130.

Hergan K, Kofler K, Oser W. Drug smuggling by body packing: what radiologists should know about it. European Radiology 2004; 14(4):736–742.

Moreira M, Buchanan J, Heard K. Validation of a 6-hour observation period for cocaine body stuffers. The American Journal of Emergency Medicine 2011; 29(3):299–303. https://doi.org/10.1016/j.ajem.2009.11.022.

Traub SJ, Hoffman RS, Nelson LS. Body packing – the internal concealment of illicit drugs. New England Journal of Medicine 2003; 349:2519–2526.

West PL, McKeown NJ, Hendrickson RG. Methamphetamine body stuffers: an observational case series. Annals of Emergency Medicine 2010; 55(2):190–197. https://doi.org/10.1016/j.annemergmed.2009.08.005.

Yamamoto T, Malavasi E, Archer JR et al. Management of body stuffers presenting to the emergency department. European Journal of Emergency Medicine 2016; 23(6):425–429.

2.15 OSMOLAR GAP

The osmolar gap is a calculated value that assists in the diagnosis of toxic alcohol poisoning. It is particularly useful when laboratory estimation of serum methanol and ethylene glycol levels are not readily available.

Osmolality (see **Table 2.15.1**) of a solution is measured by an osmometer in a laboratory, usually by freezing point depression.

Osmolarity of a solution is calculated from a formula that represents the solutes, which under ordinary circumstances contribute nearly all of the osmolality of the sample. The most widely used formula is:

$$\text{Osmolarity (mOsmol/L)} = [2 \times \text{sodium mmol/L}]$$
$$+ \text{urea (mmol/L)} + \text{glucose (mmol/L)}$$

TABLE 2.15.1 Definitions
Osmole: the amount of a substance that yields, in ideal solution, that number of particles that would depress the freezing point of the solvent by 1.86°K
Osmolality: the number of osmoles of solute per kilogram of solvent
Osmolarity: the number of osmoles of solute per litre of solution

In clinical toxicology, ethanol is so ubiquitous that it is routinely included in the calculation. The ethanol level in mmol/L is multiplied by 1.25, because ethanol has an osmotic coefficient that is higher than expected:

Osmolarity (mOsmol/L) = [2 × sodium (mmol/L)] + urea (mmol/L) + glucose (mmol/L) + [ethanol (mmol/L) × 1.25]

Osmolar gap is the difference between the osmolality (as measured in the laboratory) and the osmolarity (as calculated from measured solute concentrations):

Osmolar gap = measured osmolality - calculated osmolarity

Notes:

1 All solute concentrations must be in mmol/L (SI units). If ethanol is reported in non-SI units, it is converted to mmol/L as follows: ethanol mg/dL/4.6 or ethanol mg/dL × 0.217; or ethanol % × 217.

2 The units of osmolarity and osmolality are different so the osmolar gap is expressed as a number without units.

A normal osmolar gap is <10. A small gap exists because the calculation does not take into account the osmotic effects of potassium, sulfate, phosphate, calcium, magnesium, lactate, ammonia, serum proteins and lipids.

To safely interpret an elevated osmolar gap, the following principles apply:

- An elevated osmolar gap suggests the presence of high concentrations of unmeasured (and potentially toxic) osmotically active compounds (see **Table 2.15.2**).
- A number of non-toxicological conditions also cause an elevated osmolar gap (see **Table 2.15.3**).

TABLE 2.15.2   Exogenous agents associated with elevated osmolar gap
Acetone
Ethanol
Ethylene glycol
Glycerol
Glycine
Isopropyl alcohol
Mannitol
Methanol
Propylene glycol (diluent in several medications e.g. diazepam, phenytoin)

Adapted from Dart RC, ed. Medical Toxicology. 3rd edn (text). Philadelphia: Lippincott Williams & Wilkins; 2004.

TABLE 2.15.3   Non-toxicological conditions associated with elevated osmolar gap

Alcoholic ketoacidosis
Chronic renal failure
Diabetic ketoacidosis
Hyperlipidaemia
Hyperproteinaemia
Severe lactic acidosis
Shock
Trauma and burns

Adapted from Dart RC, ed. Medical Toxicology. 3rd edn (text). Philadelphia: Lippincott Williams & Wilkins; 2004.

- In suspected toxic alcohol ingestion (due to history of ingestion or presence of anion gap metabolic acidosis), an elevated osmolar gap supports the diagnosis.
  — In confirmed significant toxic alcohol ingestion, the osmolar gap is frequently very elevated (>50).
- A normal osmolar gap does not exclude potentially life-threatening toxic alcohol ingestion for the following reasons:
  — Small concentrations of toxic alcohols not detected by this surrogate measure may still cause significant intoxication.
  — Late in the clinical course, the parent compounds (alcohols) are already metabolised to non-osmotically active compounds.

The serum concentration of a particular alcohol suspected to be present can be estimated from the osmolar gap. Multiply the osmolar gap by the conversion factors (the molecular weight of the alcohol divided by 10) listed in **Table 2.15.4** to estimate the alcohol concentration in conventional units (mg/dL).

For further detail on the assessment and management of toxic alcohol poisoning, see the relevant chapters **(Chapter 3.1: Alcohol: Ethanol,**

TABLE 2.15.4   Estimated alcohol levels based on osmolar gap

To calculate the serum alcohol level in mg/dL multiply the osmolar gap by the conversion factor

Alcohol	Conversion factor
Ethanol	4.6
Ethylene glycol	6.2
Isopropyl alcohol	6.0
Methanol	3.2
Propylene glycol	7.2

Adapted from Olsen KR. Poisoning and drug overdose. 2nd edn. Norwalk, CT: Appleton and Lange; 1994.

Chapter 3.2: Alcohol: Ethylene glycol, Chapter 3.3: Alcohol: Isopropanol (isopropyl alcohol) and Chapter 3.4: Alcohol: Methanol (methyl alcohol).

References
Koga Y, Purssell RA, Lynd LD. The irrationality of the present use of the osmole gap: applicable physical chemistry principles and recommendations to improve the validity of current practices. Toxicological Reviews 2004; 23(3):203–211.

Krasowski MD. A retrospective analysis of glycol and toxic alcohol ingestion: utility of anion and osmolal gaps. BMC Clinical Pathology 2012; 12:1.

Purssell RA, Lynd LD, Koga Y. The use of the osmole gap as a screening test for the presence of exogenous substances. Toxicological Reviews 2004; 23(3):189–202.

Purssell RA, Pudek M, Brubacher J et al. Derivation and validation of a formula to calculate the contribution of ethanol to the osmolal gap. Annals of Emergency Medicine 2001; 38(6):653–659.

2.16 ACID–BASE DISORDERS

The assessment of acid–base abnormalities is a core competency in critical care and clinical toxicology. These disorders are manifestations of underlying disease processes and not diagnoses in themselves. Several potentially lethal poisonings produce characteristic acid–base abnormalities. The detection of any acid–base disorder during assessment of the poisoned or potentially poisoned patient mandates careful characterisation to produce a differential diagnosis as the initial step to definitive diagnosis and management.

Assessment and characterisation of an acid–base disturbance requires information derived from the history, physical examination and basic investigations including electrolytes, creatinine, blood glucose and blood gases.

In the history and physical examination, particular attention is paid to:

- past medical history
  — diabetes
  — renal failure
- current medications
  — metformin
  — salicylates
- potential chemical or pharmaceutical ingestions
- diarrhoea or vomiting
- level of consciousness
- respiratory rate
- hydration and urine output.

This information can be evaluated in a systematic fashion using the five-step approach proposed by Whittier and Rutecki:

Step 1: Determine primary acid–base disturbance by assessing pH.
   Acidaemia exists if pH <7.36.
   Alkalaemia exists if pH >7.44.

Note: The body always compensates for an acid–base disturbance but this compensation is never complete (the pH cannot return to normal). Therefore, if a single acid–base disturbance exists, the primary process can be identified by the serum pH. If there is significant abnormality of HCO_3^- and $PaCO_2$ with normal pH, there must be at least two counteracting pathologies.

Step 2: Determine whether the primary process is respiratory, metabolic or both by assessing $PaCO_2$ and HCO_3^-.

Respiratory acidosis exists if $PaCO_2$ >44 mmHg.
Respiratory alkalosis exists if $PaCO_2$ <40 mmHg.
Metabolic acidosis exists if HCO_3^- <25 mmol/L.
Metabolic alkalosis exists if HCO_3^- >25 mmol/L.

Step 3: Calculate the anion gap.

The anion gap represents the concentration of all unmeasured anions in the plasma. It is calculated from the following formula:

$$Anion\ gap = Na^+ - (Cl^- + HCO_3^-)$$

Notes:

1 The normal anion gap ranges from 8 to 16 mmol/L.

2 Addition of K^+ to the anion gap calculation is not required.

3 Correct for hypoalbuminaemia (albumin is an anion) if present. For every 10 g/L below normal, add 2.5 to the anion gap.

4 Acid anions produced during a metabolic acidosis are not measured as part of the usual laboratory biochemical profile. The H^+ ions produced are buffered by HCO_3^-, leading to a reduction in measured anions (HCO_3^-) to accompany the increase in unmeasured acid anions, and so the calculated anion gap increases.

5 Minor degrees of acidosis and elevation of anion gap are common in clinical practice. An idiopathic minor abnormality prompts supportive care and re-evaluation in 4 hours. In most cases, the abnormality will be improving.

An anion gap that is rising or >20 at any time prompts immediate investigation (see **Table 2.16.1**). Two-thirds of patients with an anion gap in the range of 20–29 mmol/L will be found to have a metabolic acidosis. If the anion gap is >30, metabolic acidosis is invariably present.

Step 4: Assess the degree of compensation.

Metabolic acidosis: expected $PaCO_2$ in mmHg is $1.5 \times HCO_3^- + 8$ (range: ± 2).

Metabolic alkalosis: expected $PaCO_2$ in mmHg is $0.7 \times HCO_3^- + 20$ (range: ± 2).

TABLE 2.16.1 Causes of anion-gap acidosis (mnemonic 'CAT MUDPILES')

C	Carbon monoxide, cyanide
A	Alcohol, alcoholic ketoacidosis
T	Toluene
M	Metformin, methanol
U	Uraemia
D	Diabetic ketoacidosis
P	Paracetamol, propylene glycol, paraldehyde
I	Iron, isoniazid (INH)
L	Lactic acidosis (numerous causes)
E	Ethylene glycol
S	Salicylates, starvation ketoacidosis

TABLE 2.16.2 Causes of a low anion gap (<6)

Increased unmeasured cations	**Artefactual hyperchloraemia**
Hypercalcaemia	Bromism
Hypermagnesaemia	Iodism
Lithium intoxication	Hypertriglyceridaemia
Multiple myeloma and other 'gammopathies'	
Decreased unmeasured anions	
Dilution	
Hypoalbuminaemia	

TABLE 2.16.3 Causes of non-anion-gap metabolic acidosis

Abnormal bicarbonate loss or chloride retention	Mnemonic 'USED CARP'
Drugs	
Acetazolamide (+ others with carbonic anhydrase activity, e.g. topiramate)	**U** Ureterostomy
	S Small bowel fistula
	E Extra Cl$^-$
Acidifying agents (e.g. ammonium chloride)	**D** Diarrhoea
	C Carbonic anhydrase inhibitors
Cholestyramine	**A** Adrenal insufficiency
Gastrointestinal bicarbonate loss	**R** Renal tubular acidosis
Diarrhoea	**P** Pancreatic fistula
Pancreatic fistula	
Rapid hydration with normal saline (increased chloride)	
Renal bicarbonate loss	
Renal tubular acidosis	
Uretoenterostomy	

TABLE 2.16.4   Causes of metabolic alkalosis

Administration of bases	**Urinary acid loss**
Antacids	Adrenogenital syndrome
Dialysis	Bartter's syndrome
Milk–alkali syndrome	Cushing's syndrome
Gastrointestinal acid loss	Diuretics
Protracted vomiting or	Licorice (glycyrrhizic acid)
nasogastric suction	Primary hyperaldosteronism
(chloride loss)	**Volume contraction**
Renal bicarbonate retention	
Chronic hypercapnia	
Hypochloraemia	
Hypokalaemia	

TABLE 2.16.5   Causes of respiratory acidosis

Acute	**Chronic**
Airway obstruction	Kyphoscoliosis
Aspiration	Lung diseases
Bronchospasm	Neuromuscular disorders
Drug-induced CNS depression	Obesity
Hypoventilation of CNS or muscular origin	
Pulmonary disease	

TABLE 2.16.6   Causes of respiratory alkalosis

CNS-mediated hyperventilation	**Pulmonary**
Increased intracranial pressure	Congestive cardiac failure
Cerebrovascular accidents	Mechanical hyperventilation
Psychogenic	Pneumonia
Hypoxia-mediated hyperventilation	Pulmonary emboli
Altitude	**Sepsis**
Anaemia	**Toxin-induced hyperventilation**
V/Q mismatch	Nicotine
	Salicylate
	Xanthines

Respiratory acidosis: HCO_3 should increase by 1 mmol/L (acute) or 4 mmol/L (chronic) for every 10 mmHg increase in $PaCO_2$.

Respiratory alkalosis: HCO_3^- should decrease by 2 mmol/L (acute) or 5 mmol/L (chronic) for every 10 mmHg decrease in $PaCO_2$.

TABLE 2.16.7   Causes of hyperlactataemia

Type A: Imbalance between oxygen demand and supply	Type B: Metabolic derangements
Carbon monoxide poisoning Cyanide Excessive oxygen demand-seizure, hyperpyrexia, shivering, exercise Shock Severe anaemia Severe hypoxia Psychogenic hyperventilation	Beta-2-agonists Cancer Ethanol (increased hepatic NADH and decreased conversion of lactate to pyruvate) Hepatic failure Inborn errors of metabolism Ketoacidosis Metformin Sepsis Vitamin deficiency (thiamine, biotin)

TABLE 2.16.8   Interpretation of delta ratio

Delta ratio	Interpretation
<0.4	Hyperchloraemic normal anion gap acidosis
0.4–0.8	Consider combined high anion gap and low anion gap acidosis but ratio of <1 is also associated with renal failure
1–2	Usual for high anion gap acidosis Average value for lactic acidosis is 1.6 Diabetic ketoacidosis usually close to 1 due to ketone loss
>2	Pre-existing elevated HCO_3^- likely – consider concurrent metabolic acidosis or pre-existing compensated respiratory acidosis
http://www.anaesthesiamcq.com/AcidBaseBook	

Step 5: Determine if there is a 1 : 1 relationship between anions in the blood (delta ratio).

Assuming all buffering in metabolic acidosis is by HCO_3^-, the increase in the anion gap should be equal to the decrease in HCO_3^- concentration and the ratio between these two changes ('delta ratio') should be equal to one.

The delta ratio can be useful in the assessment of metabolic acid–base disorders (see **Table 2.16.8**), but one should always be wary of over-interpretation and always look for other evidence to support the diagnosis.

References

Brandis K. Acid–base physiology. Available at: http://www.anaesthesiamcq.com/AcidBaseBook.

Gabow PA, Kaehny WD, Fennessey PV et al. Diagnostic importance of an increased serum anion gap. New England Journal of Medicine 1980; 303(15):854–858.

Whittier WL, Rutecki GW. Primer on clinical acid–base problem solving. Disease Monitoring 2004; 50:117–162.

2.17 THE 12-LEAD ECG IN TOXICOLOGY

The 12-lead ECG is a non-invasive, inexpensive and readily available tool that identifies occult but potentially lethal cardiac conduction abnormalities, such as those seen in tricyclic antidepressant cardiotoxicity. For these reasons, it is recommended as a screening test in all patients who present following deliberate self-poisoning. The 12-lead ECG provides valuable real-time prognostic information that reflects toxic effects at the target organ, often not available from clinical evaluation or serum drug assays. Serial ECGs allow monitoring of the progression or regression of cardiotoxicity during the clinical course. They inform decision making with regard to the level of care and monitoring required and appropriate disposition planning.

ELECTROPATHOPHYSIOLOGY

The changes in rate, rhythm and intervals detected on the 12-lead ECG in acute poisoning reflect a variety of toxic effects on the cardiac conducting system (see **Figure 2.17.1**). Normal intervals are shown in **Figure 2.17.2**. Pathophysiological mechanisms include:

Fast sodium channel blockade (agents listed in Table 2.17.1)
- Slowed sodium influx during phase 0 of the cardiac action potential manifesting as:
  — widened QRS
  — right axis deviation of the terminal QRS (see **Figure 2.17.3**)
  — bradycardia (although tachycardia secondary to other factors is more commonly observed)
  — ventricular tachycardia and ventricular fibrillation.

Blockade of potassium efflux during cardiac repolarisation (agents listed in Table 2.17.2)
- Prolongation of the QT interval
- Torsades de pointes

FIGURE 2.17.1 The myocardial action potential and corresponding ECG trace

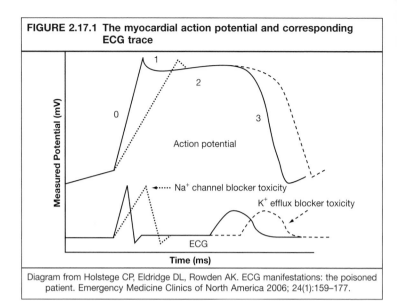

Diagram from Holstege CP, Eldridge DL, Rowden AK. ECG manifestations: the poisoned patient. Emergency Medicine Clinics of North America 2006; 24(1):159–177.

FIGURE 2.17.2 Normal ECG parameters

Rate 60–100/minute
PR interval: <200 ms (5 small squares)
QRS duration: <100 ms (2.5 small squares)
QT interval: <450 ms
$QTc = QT/\sqrt{R-R}$

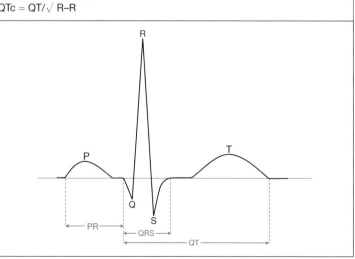

TABLE 2.17.1	Agents associated with fast sodium channel blockade (QRS widening)

Tricyclic antidepressants	Local anaesthetics
Amitriptyline	Bupivacaine
Clomipramine	Cocaine
Dothiepin	Lidocaine
Doxepin	Ropivacaine
Imipramine	**Phenothiazines**
Nortriptyline	Thioridazine
Class 1A antidysrhythmic agents	**Carbamazepine**
Disopyramide	**Diphenhydramine**
Procainamide	**Hydroxychloroquine/chloroquine**
Quinidine	**Lamotrigine**
Class 1C antidysrhythmic agents	**Propoxyphene/dextropropoxyphene**
Flecainide	**Propranolol**
	Quinine
	Venlafaxine

FIGURE 2.17.3	ECG changes in tricyclic antidepressant (or other fast Na channel blocker) toxicity

Features consistent with fast sodium channel blockade:
- QRS >100 ms in lead II
- Right axis deviation of terminal QRS
  - Terminal R wave >3 mm in aVR
  - R/S ratio >0.7 in aVR

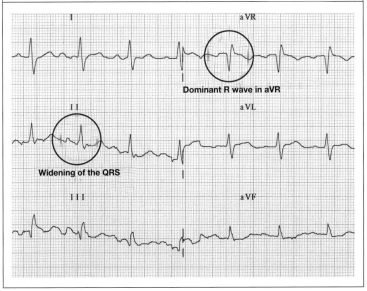

TABLE 2.17.2 Agents associated with blockade of potassium efflux (QT prolongation)

Antipsychotic agents
    Amisulpride
    Chlorpromazine
    Droperidol
    Haloperidol
    Olanzapine
    Quetiapine
    Thioridazine
    Ziprasidone
Class 1A antidysrhythmic agents
    Quinidine
    Disopyramide
    Procainamide
Class 1C antidysrhythmic agents
    Flecainide
Class III antidysrhythmic agents
    Sotalol
Tricyclic antidepressants
    Amitriptyline
    Desimipramine
    Doxepin
    Imipramine
    Nortriptyline
	Other antidepressants
	    Bupropion
	    Citalopram
	    Escitalopram
	    Mianserin
	    Moclobemide
	Antihistamines
	    Diphenhydramine
	    Doxylamine
	    Loratadine
	    Promethazine
	    Terfenadine
	Chloroquine
	Hydroxychloroquine
	Quinine
	Fluoroquinolones
	    Moxifloxacin
	Macrolides
	    Azithromycin
	    Erythromycin
	Methadone

Na^+–K^+-ATPase pump blockade (cardiac glycosides)

- Increased automaticity
  - Atrial or ventricular ectopic beats
  - Accelerated supraventricular or junctional tachycardias with or without AV block
  - Ventricular tachycardia
- Decreased AV node conduction
  - 1st-degree heart block (prolonged PR interval)
  - 2nd-degree heart block
  - 3rd-degree (complete) heart block

Calcium channel blockade

- Sinus bradycardia
- Decreased AV node conduction
  - 1st-degree heart block (prolonged PR interval)
  - 2nd-degree heart block
  - 3rd-degree (complete) heart block
- Intraventricular conduction defects

Beta-adrenergic receptor blockade

- Bradycardia
- Decreased AV node conduction

— 1st-degree heart block (prolonged PR interval)
— 2nd-degree heart block
— 3rd-degree (complete) heart block

Myocardial ischaemia
- ST-segment depression or elevation
- Conduction abnormalities

Hyperkalaemia
- Peaked T waves
- QRS prolongation

Hypocalcaemia, hypokalaemia, hypomagnesaemia
- QT prolongation.

TRICYCLIC ANTIDEPRESSANTS (TCAs)

The toxicological significance of QRS widening is best studied in the setting of TCA poisoning. A QRS duration >100 ms indicates blockade of cardiac fast sodium channels, and in combination with right axis deviation of the terminal QRS, it is virtually pathognomonic (see **Figure 2.17.3** and **Chapter 3.78: Tricyclic antidepressants (TCAs)**). Most studies examining ECG changes in TCA intoxication are small or retrospective. However, the following features are associated with major toxicity:

- QRS >100 ms (2.5 small squares) is associated with seizures.
- QRS >160 ms (4 small squares) is associated with ventricular dysrhythmias
- Right axis deviation of the terminal QRS as defined by
  — terminal R wave >3 mm in aVR
  — R/S ratio >0.7 in aVR.

SYSTEMATIC ANALYSIS OF THE 12-LEAD ECG OF A POISONED PATIENT

1 Determine rate and rhythm.
2 Determine PR interval.
3 Determine QRS duration in multiple leads. Studies examining the prognostic significance of QRS duration in tricyclic antidepressant poisoning use manual measurements, particularly in limb lead II. In general, the manually measured QRS corresponds well with the duration calculated by automated ECG machine algorithms, but it is always preferable to check the intervals manually. Serial ECGs are useful to determine whether QRS prolongation is dynamic (due to acute poisoning) or static (due to pre-existing conduction delays e.g. bundle-branch blocks).

4   Check for right axis deviation of the QRS. A large terminal R wave in aVR or increased R/S ratio indicates slow rightward conduction and is characteristic of fast sodium channel blockade. If not pathological, it will remains static in appearance throughout the course of the poisoning. Comparison with pre-poisoning ECGs is useful.

5   Determine QT interval. A prolonged QT interval predisposes to the development of torsades de pointes, a polymorphic ventricular tachycardia. Torsades de pointes may be self-limiting but can degenerate into ventricular fibrillation. Torsades de pointes is more likely to occur where there is co-existing bradycardia. The risk for developing dysrhythmia related to drug-induced QT prolongation is best predicted by the QT nomogram, which plots QT versus heart rate (see **Figure 2.17.4**) and is more reliable than derived calculations such as the QTc (see **References**).

6   Check for evidence of increased cardiac ectopy or automaticity related to digoxin or other cardiac glycoside toxicity.

7   Check for evidence of hyperkalaemia.

8   Check for evidence of myocardial ischaemia.

FIGURE 2.17.4 QT interval nomogram for determining 'at risk' QT-HR pairs from a single 12-lead ECG

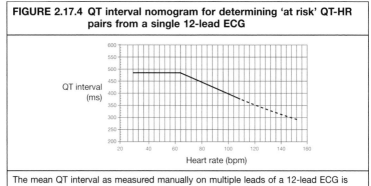

The mean QT interval as measured manually on multiple leads of a 12-lead ECG is plotted against the heart rate (HR) measured on the ECG. If the point is above the line, the QT-HR is regarded 'at risk' for the development of torsades de pointes.

Chan A, Isbister GK, Kirkpatrick CMJ et al. Drug-induced QT prolongation and torsades de pointes: evaluation of a QT nomogram. Quarterly Journal of Medicine 2007; 100:609–615.

MANAGEMENT OF ACUTE CONDUCTION ABNORMALITIES FOLLOWING POISONING

QRS WIDENING DUE TO SODIUM CHANNEL BLOCKADE

Sodium channel blockade resulting from acute poisoning causes dynamic widening of the QRS and is associated with development of ventricular dysrhythmias and seizures. Treatment is best described for poisoning caused by tricyclic antidepressants (TCAs) but can be extrapolated to other agents causing similar electrophysiological effects.

If QRS widening is associated with altered mental state or haemodynamic instability (seizures, coma, hypotension or cardiac dysrhythmias), the mainstays of treatment for both cardiovascular and CNS toxicity are administration of IV sodium bicarbonate, intubation and hyperventilation.

- Administer sodium bicarbonate 1–2 mmol/kg IV boluses repeated every 1–2 minutes until:
  — restoration of perfusing rhythm
  — improvement in QRS widening
  — pH established at 7.5–7.55.
- Intubation and hyperventilation to control the airway and maintain a therapeutic end point of pH 7.5–7.55.

The majority of TCA poisonings will respond to these interventions with a dynamic improvement in QRS widening and clinical status. Other agents, particularly propranolol, are also likely to show improvement, particularly if the presentation is associated with significant metabolic and/ or respiratory acidosis.

However, a number of agents (including lamotrigine and venlafaxine) may not show a clear improvement in QRS duration or haemodynamic status following these interventions, and attempts to improve QRS widening by ongoing administration of IV sodium bicarbonate boluses once the pH has reached 7.5–7.55 carries the risk of worsening outcome (see **Chapter 1.2: Resuscitation**).

QT PROLONGATION

A number of agents cause drug-mediated QT prolongation due to effects on cardiac potassium channels, which are encoded by the human ether-a-go-go-related gene (hERG). Drug-induced QT prolongation can occur either in acute poisoning or during therapeutic use and predisposes to the development of torsades de pointes. The risk of torsades is greater at slower heart rates and is thought to result from ectopic beats (early afterdepolarisations – EADs) occurring during cardiac repolarisation ('R on T' phenomenon).

Treatment interventions attempt to decrease the incidence of early afterdepolarisations (administration of magnesium and potassium) or increase the resting heart rate to decrease the absolute R-R interval, thereby limiting the opportunity for ventricular depolarisation (R wave) to occur during repolarisation (the preceding T wave). Management of asymptomatic QT prolongation differs from management of established torsades de pointes.

FIGURE 2.17.5 Torsades de pointes secondary to QT prolongation

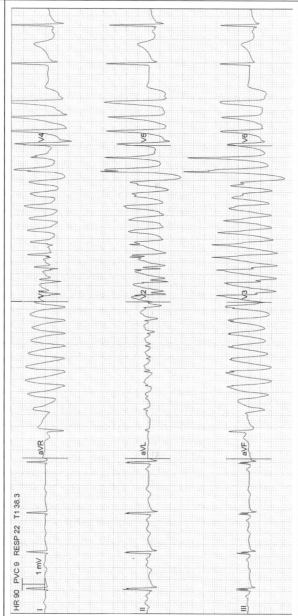

- Treatment of asymptomatic QT prolongation
  - Ensure that all QT-dependent electrolytes are at the upper limit of normal (potassium, calcium, magnesium).
  - Prophylactic treatment with an IV bolus of magnesium, or use of isoprenaline or overdrive electrical pacing to increase heart rate, are not proven to decrease the incidence of torsades de pointes and are not routinely recommended.

- Treatment of torsades de pointes
  - Electrical cardioversion may be required for persistent episodes that result in altered mental state or haemodynamic instability.
  - Magnesium 10 mmol IV bolus (0.05 mmol/kg in children) over 1–2 minutes, repeated once if torsades de pointes recurs.
  - Isoprenaline or overdrive electrical pacing are other treatment options to increase the resting heart rate to a target of >100 beats/min.

In all cases, continue ECG monitoring until abnormalities of the QT interval (as defined by the QT nomogram) have resolved.

References

Boehnert MT, Lovejoy FH. Value of the QRS duration versus the serum drug level in predicting seizures and ventricular arrhythmias after an acute overdose of tricyclic antidepressants. New England Journal of Medicine 1985; 313:474–479.

Chan A, Isbister GK, Kirkpatrick CMJ et al. Drug-induced QT prolongation and torsades de pointes: evaluation of a QT nomogram. Quarterly Journal of Medicine 2007; 100:609–615.

Holstege CP, Eldridge DL, Rowden AK. ECG manifestations: the poisoned patient. Emergency Medicine Clinics of North America 2006; 24(1):159–177.

Liebelt EL, Francis D, Woolf AD. ECG lead aVR versus QRS interval in predicting seizures and arrhythmias in acute tricyclic antidepressant toxicity. Annals of Emergency Medicine 1995; 26:195–201.

Niemann JT, Bessen HA, Rothstein RJ et al. Electrocardiographic criteria for tricyclic antidepressant cardiotoxicity. American Journal of Cardiology 1986; 57: 1154–1159.

Wolfe TR, Caravati EM, Rollins DE. Terminal 40-ms frontal plane QRS axis as a marker for tricyclic antidepressant overdose. Annals of Emergency Medicine 1989; 18:348–351.

2.18 APPROACH TO MUSHROOM POISONING

Poisoning from ingestion of mushrooms occurs worldwide usually when wild mushrooms containing toxins are misidentified as edible species. Multiple individuals may be poisoned simultaneously. The most common presentation is a benign self-limited gastrointestinal disturbance but a number of other important toxic syndromes, including potentially lethal hepatotoxicity, are recognised. Assessment and management is based on the recognition of the principal clinical syndromes that may develop following ingestion of toxic mushrooms. To complicate the assessment, poisoned patients may present with overlapping clinical features after ingestion of different mushroom species.

RISK ASSESSMENT

- The vast majority of mushroom poisoning cases in Australasia manifest with acute gastrointestinal toxicity. A rapid resolution of symptoms and good outcome with supportive care is anticipated.
- A variety of other toxic syndromes may develop and a favourable outcome can usually be anticipated with good supportive care.
- Worldwide, cyclopeptide hepatotoxic poisoning, particularly from *Amanita phalloides*, accounts for the majority of mushroom-related deaths. This form of poisoning is reported but extremely rare within Australasia.
  - Within Australia, almost all cases of cyclopeptide hepatotoxic poisoning have occurred in the Australian Capital Territory. *Amanita phalloides* is thought to have been imported along with oak trees and is now naturalised particularly in the older suburbs of Canberra. *Amanita phalloides* has also been reported in Melbourne, Adelaide and the surrounding rural areas.
- Cyclopeptide hepatotoxic poisoning must be considered whenever gastrointestinal symptoms develop more than 6 hours after ingestion of mushrooms and with a high degree of suspicion if the mushrooms were growing wild in the regions mentioned above.
- **Children:** accidental ingestion of wild mushrooms by children is usually benign.

CLINICAL SYNDROMES

There are hundreds of thousands of mushroom species and reliable mushroom identification, even by expert mycologists, is difficult. In the clinical setting, identification is frequently impossible because the mushrooms are unavailable, decomposing, partly digested or cooked. A variety of clinical syndromes may develop following ingestion of toxic mushrooms. They are diagnosed on the basis of the clinical features and the timing of the onset and duration in relation to mushroom ingestion (see **Table 2.18.1**). Laboratory abnormalities are important in the diagnosis of some syndromes, especially hepatotoxicity. Identification of the mushroom species by a mycologist may provide important supportive evidence if available. Conventional food poisoning should be considered in the differential diagnosis for

TABLE 2.18.1 Clinical syndromes of mushroom poisoning

Syndrome	Clinical features	Clinical course	Toxin (mushroom species)
EARLY ONSET (WITHIN 6 HOURS)			
Gastrointestinal*	Malaise, abdominal pain, nausea, vomiting, diarrhoea	Onset 30 min–3 hours Resolution 6–24 hours	Toxins not fully identified Multiple mushroom species
Cholinergic*	Vomiting, diarrhoea, lacrimation, salivation, urinary incontinence, bronchorrhoea, bronchospasm, miosis	Onset 30 min–2 hours Resolution 12–24 hours	Muscarine (*Clitocybe*, *Inocybe* and *Boletus* species)
Hallucinogenic*	Ataxia, anxiety, mydriasis, tachycardia, dyskinesias, delirium and hallucinations	Onset 30 min–2 hours Resolution 4–6 hours	Psilocybin (*Psilocybe* species) Toxin resembles lysergic acid diethylamide (LSD)
Disulfiram-like*	Nausea, vomiting, tachycardia, facial flushing, sweating, chest pain	Onset 30 min–2 hours following ethanol consumption (may occur up to 7 days after mushroom ingestion) Resolution within 6 hours	Coprine (*Coprinus* species)
Glutaminergic*	Drowsiness, delirium, dysphoria, hallucinations, myoclonus, hyperreflexia, seizures	Onset 30 min–2 hours Resolution 6–24 hours	Ibotenic acid Muscimol (*Amanita muscaria* and *pantherina*)

Continued

TABLE 2.18.1 Clinical syndromes of mushroom poisoning—cont'd

Syndrome	Clinical features	Clinical course	Toxin (mushroom species)
Seizures Delayed onset: Gastroenteritis Hepatotoxicity Haemolysis Methaemoglobinaemia	Headache, tremor, ataxia, nystagmus, vertigo, seizures Nausea, vomiting, diarrhoea	Onset of symptoms up to 24 hours	Gyromitrin (*Gyromitra* species) Activated to monomethylhydrazine – similar action to isoniazid to inhibit pyridoxine-dependent synthesis of GABA
	Delayed hepatotoxicity with raised transaminases (rare)	Onset 2–3 days	
	Delayed haemolysis and methaemoglobinaemia (rare)	Onset 1–3 days after hepatic injury	
Immune-mediated haemolytic anaemia	Haemolytic anaemia, haemoglobinuria, immune-complex nephritis and acute renal failure	Onset 2–3 days	*Paxillus* species Antibodies develop following repeated ingestion
Allergic bronchoalveolitis	Nausea, vomiting and rhinitis	Onset within 6 hours	Inhalation of dried *Lycoperdonosis* spores
	Acute bronchopneumonia	Within days	

TABLE 2.18.1 Clinical syndromes of mushroom poisoning—cont'd

Syndrome	Clinical features	Clinical course	Toxin (mushroom species)
DELAYED ONSET (6–24 HOURS)			
Hepatotoxic*	Asymptomatic	6–24 hours	Three classes of cyclopeptide: • Amatoxins • Phallotoxins • Virotoxins (*Amanita, Galerina* and *Lepiota* species)
	Nausea, vomiting, abdominal cramps and diarrhoea	Onset 6–24 hours	
	Transient clinical improvement during asymptomatic increase in hepatic transaminases	18–36 hours	
	Progressive hepatic failure, kidney injury, coagulopathy with progression to multisystem organ failure and up to 30% mortality	1–7 days	
	Recovery in survivors	>7 days	

Continued

SPECIFIC CONSIDERATIONS

TABLE 2.18.1 Clinical syndromes of mushroom poisoning—cont'd

Syndrome	Clinical features	Clinical course	Toxin (mushroom species)
Erythromelalgia	Burning pain, redness and oedema of the hands and feet, exacerbated by heat and relieved by cold	Onset 24–72 hours Resolution days to months	Acromelic acids (*Clitocybe acromelalga*)
GREATLY DELAYED ONSET (>24 HOURS)			
Nephrotoxic	Anorexia, headache, nausea, vomiting, abdominal pain and flank pain Interstitial nephritis and acute renal failure	Initial GI symptoms may be mild Renal failure develops over 3–20 days	Orellanine (*Cortinarius* and *A. smithiana* species)
Rhabdomyolysis	Myalgias, muscle weakness and myocarditis (very rare)	Onset 24–72 hours	(*Tricholoma* and *Russula* species)

*Denotes syndromes described in Australia.

any patient who presents with gastrointestinal symptoms following ingestion of mushrooms.

Numerous toxins are identified and are usually species-specific (see **Table 2.18.1**).

The most clinically significant poisoning syndrome is delayed hepatotoxicity, primarily due to *Amanita phalloides*. Amatoxins (chiefly α-amanitin) are highly lethal and cause fulminant hepatic failure, as well as gastrointestinal and renal toxicity. The toxins are actively transported into hepatic cells and bind irreversibly to RNA polymerase II, leading to the death of rapidly dividing cells.

MANAGEMENT

Resuscitation and supportive care

Patients may present with altered conscious state, seizures or significant hypovolaemia secondary to gastrointestinal fluid losses. These priorities are managed along conventional lines as outlined in **Chapter 1.2: Resuscitation, Chapter 2.3: Seizures** and **Chapter 2.4: Approach to delirium**.

Decontamination

Administration of activated charcoal 50 g (1 g/kg in a child) is indicated if onset of gastrointestinal symptoms is delayed beyond 6 hours after ingestion.

Investigations

Examination of any available mushrooms by a mycologist is useful, particularly in cases where ingestion of species containing cyclopeptide hepatotoxins is considered.

FBC and EUC are performed to exclude haematological or biochemical derangements. Liver function tests and venous blood gases should be monitored for 24–48 hours where ingestion of mushrooms containing cyclopeptide hepatotoxins is suspected.

Enhanced elimination

Methods of enhanced elimination are frequently considered in patients with potential cyclopeptide hepatotoxic mushroom poisoning but their effect on outcome has not been studied in controlled trials. If cyclopeptide hepatotoxic mushroom poisoning is suspected, multiple-dose activated charcoal (see **Chapter 1.7: Enhanced elimination**) is indicated because amatoxin undergoes enterohepatic circulation.

Antidotes

Multiple therapies have been advocated in patients with cyclopeptide hepatotoxic mushroom poisoning but their effect on outcomes has not been well evaluated in controlled trials. They include silibinin, rifampicin and high-dose benzyl penicillin (penicillin G), all of which act to limit amatoxin uptake into hepatic cells by blocking the organic anion transporting polypeptide (OATP) co-transporter located in hepatocyte membranes. If delayed onset of gastrointestinal symptoms or rising hepatic transaminases raises suspicion of cyclopeptide hepatotoxic mushroom poisoning, commence:

- N-acetylcysteine at the standard dosing recommended for paracetamol hepatotoxicity (see **Chapter 4.17: N-acetylcysteine**)
- silibinin (if available) 5 mg/kg by intravenous infusion over 1 hour followed by a continuous infusion of 20 mg/kg/day for up to 5 days
- rifampicin 600 mg IV daily (15 mg/kg in children) over 1–2 hours if silibinin is not available
- benzylpenicillin 3 g IV (60 mg/kg, maximum 2.4 g in children) 4 hourly may be given if IV silibinin or IV rifampicin are not available. The risk of toxicity from such large doses of IV penicillin may outweigh any possible benefit.

Intravenous therapies are recommended in amatoxin poisoning because the concurrent use of oral activated charcoal will limit efficacy of orally administered agents. For this reason, PO rifampicin or silymarin are not likely to be useful.

Atropine may be considered in patients with peripheral cholinergic signs and symptoms (see **Chapter 4.1: Atropine**).

Management of seizures secondary to monomethylhydrazine poisoning from ingestion of *Gyromitra* mushrooms is similar to the management of isoniazid poisoning and includes administration of pyridoxine (see **Chapter 4.23: Pyridoxine**).

Disposition and follow-up

- Asymptomatic paediatric patients may be observed at home following suspected ingestion of wild mushrooms.
- Patients with early onset gastrointestinal illness are managed supportively in a ward environment. They may be discharged when clinically well. Patients with significant symptoms lasting more than 6 hours should have liver function tests and renal function checked prior to discharge. Abnormal liver or renal function prompts further inpatient management.
- Cyclopeptide hepatotoxic mushroom poisoning is extremely rare and most clinicians have very limited clinical experience. If this syndrome is suspected due to delayed onset gastrointestinal symptoms or rising hepatic transaminases, early consultation with a hepatologist and clinical toxicologist is recommended. In severe

cases, hepatic transplantation has been attempted but prognosis remains poor.

References

Diaz JH. Syndromic diagnosis and management of confirmed mushroom poisonings. Critical Care Medicine 2006; 33:427–436.

Enjalbert F, Rapior S, Nouguier-Soulé J et al. Treatment of amatoxin poisoning: 20-year retrospective analysis. Journal of Toxicology–Clinical Toxicology 2002; 40(6):715–757.

Persson H. Mushrooms. Medicine 2012; 40(3):135–138.

Roberts DM, Hall MJ, Falkland MM et al. Amanita phalloides poisoning and treatment with silibinin in the Australian Capital Territory and New South Wales. Medical Journal of Australia 2013; 198:43–47.

2.19 APPROACH TO PLANT POISONING

Numerous pharmacologically active substances are produced by plants and many pharmaceutical agents and recreational drugs are of plant origin. Serious human poisoning from plant exposures is, however, extremely rare.

Exposure to toxic plants may occur unintentionally when they are mistakenly identified as edible plants or when young children ingest parts of plants, usually berries or seeds. Intentional exposure to toxic plants occurs with recreational or medicinal intent or, less commonly, as an attempt at deliberate self-harm. It often involves the ingestion of teas made from the plant. Non-intentional cutaneous and ocular exposures may also cause symptoms.

Assessment of plant exposures is difficult even when the plant is positively identified because it is virtually impossible to quantify dose; there is enormous variation in toxin concentrations between species, plant part, location and season.

RISK ASSESSMENT

- Most plant exposures are asymptomatic or cause minor irritative symptoms only.
- Plants containing calcium oxalate crystals may cause more severe irritation to exposed mucous membranes.
- A few plants or parts of plants are capable of causing severe poisoning when ingested in sufficient quantity.
- Accurate plant identification usually allows refinement of the risk assessment.
- In the absence of accurate plant identification, risk assessment relies on knowledge of local plants and observation of clinical features and progress.

- **Children:** significant plant poisoning is extremely rare. Ingestion of yellow oleander or castor bean seeds can theoretically cause significant poisoning but hospital assessment is not indicated unless symptoms develop.

IMPORTANT PLANT TOXINS

Calcium oxalate

Some plants contain needle-like calcium oxalate crystals packaged into bundles that can cause mechanical injury to mucosal membranes when ingested. The plants most commonly associated with this type of injury are *Dieffenbachia* spp. and *Philodendron* spp.

Toxins capable of causing severe poisoning

A number of plant toxins are known to have caused significant human poisoning or death following ingestion of fresh plant material. Important examples are listed in **Table 2.19.1** and discussed here.

Aconite (*Aconitum* spp. and *Delphinium* spp.) is found in some Asian herbal medicines. It binds to voltage-dependent sodium channels leading to permanent activation of cardiac muscle and voltage-dependent nervous tissue receptors. Dose-dependent toxicity develops rapidly after ingestion and manifests with CNS, cardiovascular and gastrointestinal effects. Bradycardia and hypotension may progress to tachydysrhythmias and cardiac arrest; paraesthesias may progress to CNS depression, respiratory depression, paralysis and seizures; and nausea and vomiting may progress to diarrhoea and abdominal cramping.

Belladonna alkaloids (atropine, scopolamine, hyoscyamine) are found in numerous plant species. Those most commonly associated with human poisoning are belladonna (*Atropa* spp.), angel's trumpet (*Datura* spp.) and henbane (*Hyoscyamus* spp.). These alkaloids cause competitive blockade of central and peripheral acetylcholine muscarinic receptors leading to the anticholinergic syndrome (see **Chapter 2.6: Anticholinergic toxicity**).

Cardiac glycosides of various types are found in all parts of several plants, including foxglove (*Digitalis purpurea*), pink and white oleander (*Nerium* spp.) and yellow oleander (*Thevetia* spp.). These all have digoxin-like effects on cardiac conduction and Na^+–K^+-ATPase (see **Chapter 3.33: Digoxin: Acute overdose**).

The antimitotic agent, colchicine, is found in all parts of the autumn crocus (*Colchicum autumnale*) and glory lily (*Gloriosa superba*), and human colchicine poisoning (see **Chapter 3.30: Colchicine**) is reported after ingestion of bulbs and leaves.

TABLE 2.19.1 Plant toxins with potential to cause serious toxicity or death following a single acute ingestion

Toxin(s)	Plant(s)	Clinical features
Aconite	*Aconitum* spp. *Delphinium* spp.	Severe cardiovascular, neurological and gastrointestinal toxicity High mortality from ventricular dysrhythmias and cardiovascular collapse
Belladonna alkaloids	*Datura* spp. (jimsonweed, angel's trumpet) *Atropa belladonna* *Hyoscyamus niger* (henbane)	Anticholinergic poisoning: tachycardia, delirium, agitation, ileus, urinary retention
Cardiac glycosides	*Digitalis* spp. (foxglove) *Nerium* spp. (pink or white oleander) *Thevetia* spp. (yellow oleander)	Bradycardia, dysrhythmias, GI disturbance, hyperkalaemia
Colchicine	*Colchicum autumnale* (autumn crocus) *Gloriosa superba* (glory lily)	GI disturbance, bone marrow depression, multi-system organ failure
Coniine	*Conium maculatum* (poison hemlock)	Bradycardia, tachycardia, GI disturbance, ascending paralysis, rhabdomyolysis, renal failure
Cyanogenic glycosides	*Prunus* spp. seed kernels (apricot, plum, pear, cherry, almond)	Tachycardia, bradycardia, coma, acidosis, multi-system organ failure
Hypoglycin	*Blighia sapida* (ackee)	Hypoglycaemia, acidaemia, vomiting, seizures
Nicotine	*Nicotiana* spp. (tobacco)	Tachycardia, hypotension, tremor, sweating, GI symptoms, seizures
Psychotropic alkaloids	*Ipomea* spp. (morning glory) seeds *Lophophora williamsii* (peyote cactus)	Acute psychosis, visual hallucinations
Ricin	*Ricinus communis* (castor beans)	GI disturbance, multi-system organ failure
Taxine	*Taxus* spp. (yew)	Bradycardia, dysrhythmias, GI disturbance

Coniine is an alkaloid found in poison hemlock (*Conium maculatum*). It is structurally related to nicotine and produces both nicotinic effects and neuromuscular blockade with potential for respiratory failure.

Amygdalin is a cyanogenic glycoside found in the seeds or pits of apricots, almonds, apples, peaches and wild cherries (*Prunus* spp.). Laetrile, derived from amygdalin from apricot pits, is sometimes marketed as a health food. After ingestion, amygdalin is hydrolysed to produce cyanide (see **Chapter 3.32: Cyanide**).

Hypoglycin A is found in the unripe fruit and seeds of the ackee tree (*Blighia sapida*). It interferes with fatty acid metabolism and causes hypoglycaemia. It also causes vomiting, CNS depression and seizures.

Nicotine is found in the tobacco plant (*Nicotiana tabacum*). Excessive ingestion, inhalation or transdermal exposure leads to overstimulation of nicotinic receptors. This manifests with GI symptoms, sweating, mydriasis, tachycardia, hypertension and seizures.

Psychotropic alkaloids include lysergic acid and mescaline. They act as direct serotonin agonists and can produce vivid visual hallucinations. Lysergic acid is found in morning glory seeds (*Ipomea* spp.) and mescaline in the peyote cactus (*Lophophora williamsii*).

Ricin, a lectin, is found in the castor bean plant (*Ricinus communis*). The highest concentration is in the seeds. An intracellular toxin, it inhibits protein synthesis, leading to a severe gastrointestinal disturbance together with cardiac, haematological, hepatic and renal toxicity.

Taxine is a mixture of alkaloids found in yew trees (*Taxus* spp.), which inhibit both sodium and calcium currents. Ingestion of seeds has produced gastrointestinal symptoms, paraesthesias, mental status changes, bradycardia, conduction blocks, ventricular dysrhythmias and cardiac arrest.

CLINICAL FEATURES

The vast majority of plant exposures remain asymptomatic. Minor transient gastrointestinal symptoms may be observed.

The clinical features of oxalate crystal ingestion are immediate onset of pain and swelling usually affecting the lips, tongue, oral cavity and pharynx. Rarely, severe exposures may produce dysphagia, profuse salivation and upper airways obstruction. It may take days for symptoms to subside.

Potentially serious exposures manifest onset of signs and symptoms suggestive of the toxic mechanism. As detailed above, the clinical syndromes that may develop include cardiovascular collapse, anticholinergic syndrome, nicotinic poisoning, cardiac glycoside poisoning, colchicine or cyanide poisoning.

MANAGEMENT

Resuscitation

Immediate resuscitation is unlikely to be required except in the patient with delayed presentation after severe poisoning. An important exception is aconite poisoning in which death from ventricular dysrhythmias or respiratory paralysis may occur within hours of ingestion. Resuscitation follows standard ACLS protocols, including the use of anti-arrhythmics such as amiodarone, lidocaine or flecainide. Successful outcome from cardiac arrest from aconite poisoning using cardiopulmonary bypass is reported.

Supportive care and monitoring

The management of most plant poisonings entails supportive care and monitoring along the standard lines described in **Chapter 1.4: Supportive care and monitoring**. Particular attention to fluid and electrolyte status is required with colchicine (see **Chapter 3.30: Colchicine**), aconite and ricin poisoning. Maintenance of euglycaemia with glucose infusion is required in ackee fruit poisoning. Management of seizures and delirium requires administration of titrated doses of benzodiazepines as outlined in **Chapter 2.3: Seizures** and **Chapter 2.4: Approach to delirium**.

Investigations

Investigations are performed as dictated by clinical signs and symptoms. Serum digoxin levels do not accurately reflect toxicity from cardiac glycoside poisoning of plant origin.

Decontamination

Administration of oral activated charcoal 50 g (1 g/kg in a child) is indicated where the risk assessment suggests the possibility of life-threatening toxicity. Where there is any potential for imminent depression in the level of consciousness or seizures, the airway must be secured prior to administration of activated charcoal.

Skin exposure requires thorough washing of the exposed skin and eye exposure requires thorough irrigation of the affected eye.

Antidotes

Physostigmine is useful in reversing severe anticholinergic poisoning (see **Chapter 4.21: Physostigmine**). Cyanide antidotes may be useful in treating cyanogenic glycoside poisoning (see **Chapter 4.13: Hydroxocobalamin** and **Chapter 4.26: Sodium thiosulfate**). Digoxin immune Fab in relatively high doses has been used successfully to reverse cardiotoxicity from oleander poisoning (see **Chapter 4.5: Digoxin immune Fab**).

Enhanced elimination

Not useful in plant poisoning.

Disposition

Hospital assessment or observation is not required if the patient is asymptomatic or has minor gastrointestinal symptoms only and the plant is identified as not having potential for serious toxicity. This is the case for the vast majority of plant exposure cases.

Hospital assessment and observation is necessary if there has been significant ingestion of plant material containing potentially life-threatening toxins. Any patient with symptoms beyond minor gastrointestinal ones should also be assessed in hospital. The period of observation continues until all risk of serious toxicity has elapsed. Where significant toxicity develops, the level of care and length of stay will be determined by the clinical course.

Dermal, mucosal and ophthalmic plant exposures

A wide variety of plants are able to cause either primary or allergic contact dermatitis. Some plants such as nettles have a specialist stinging apparatus that acts like a hypodermic syringe to deliver irritant chemical to the skin. Contact dermatitis is frequently associated with exposure to the sap of certain plants such as the mango tree. It is rarely serious. Allergic contact dermatitis results from type IV hypersensitivity response to plant exposures. Certain plants have a greater propensity to cause allergic contact dermatitis.

References

Challoner KR, McCarron MM. Castor bean intoxication. Annals of Emergency Medicine 1990; 19:1177–1183.

Chan TY. Aconite poisoning. Clinical Toxicology 2009; 47(4):279–285.

Eddleston M, Ariaratnam CA, Sjostrom L et al. Acute yellow oleander (Thevetia peruviana) poisoning: cardiac arrhythmias, electrolyte disturbances, and serum cardiac glycoside concentrations on presentation to hospital. Heart 2000; 83:301–306.

Eddleston M, Rajapakse S, Rajakanthan K et al. Anti-digoxin Fab fragments in cardiotoxicity induced by ingestion of yellow oleander: a randomised controlled trial. Lancet 2000; 355:967–972.

Froberg B, Ibrahim D, Furbee RB. Plant poisoning. Emergency Clinics of North America 2007; 25:375–433.

Rajapakse S. Management of yellow oleander poisoning. Clinical Toxicology 2009; 47(3):206–212.

Schep LJ, Slaughter RJ, Beasley DM. Nicotinic plant poisoning. Clinical Toxicology 2009; 47(8):771–781.

Suchard JR, Wallace KL, Gerkin RD. Acute cyanide toxicity caused by apricot kernel ingestion. Annals of Emergency Medicine 1998; 32:742–744.

2.20 POISONING DURING PREGNANCY AND LACTATION

Management decisions regarding poisoning or envenoming in the pregnant or lactating patient take into consideration the risks to the fetus or infant of the poisoning or its treatment.

Pregnancy-induced physiological changes affect drug pharmacokinetics and pharmacodynamics in the following ways:

1 Absorption – delayed gastric emptying and intestinal transit time slow drug absorption and may prolong the period where decontamination is of potential benefit.
2 Distribution – increased blood volume (45–50%) increases volume of distribution and potentially decreases plasma levels; dilution of plasma proteins increases free drug levels.
3 Elimination – hepatic enzyme systems are altered by circulating hormones; renal blood flow and glomerular filtration rate increase.

Most drugs cross the placenta by diffusion and maternal blood levels are the most significant determinant of fetal exposure. Maternal blood levels are usually greater than those of the fetus, although for some agents they are the same and for others fetal levels exceed maternal levels (e.g. valproic acid and diazepam).

On a practical level, acute management of overdose in the pregnant patient rarely differs from that of the non-pregnant patient. In particular, paracetamol and iron overdose, which are relatively common in this group, are managed along standard lines.

Excellence in supportive care of the poisoned mother ensures the best physiological conditions to minimise fetal compromise. Early detection and correction of hypoxia, hypotension, hypoglycaemia and seizures in the mother ensure the best outcome for the fetus. Fetal monitoring may be useful in detecting fetal compromise and the response to treatment.

Greater circulating volumes, increased respiratory rate and physiological resting tachycardia in the pregnant patient disguise hypovolaemia and respiratory compromise until later stages.

Oral activated charcoal and whole bowel irrigation do not pose any special risks to pregnant patients and these forms of decontamination are implemented whenever indicated as for non-pregnant patients.

Poisoning with a limited number of agents poses a potentially greater risk to the fetus than the mother and the threshold for treatment is lowered. These include:

● carbon monoxide
● methaemoglobin-inducing agents

- lead
- salicylates.

Consideration of the need to emergently deliver near-term infants in poisoned mothers is a complicated issue that should be managed with toxicology and obstetric expertise.

In general, if the fetus survives a maternal intentional ingestion, the risk of teratogenicity is low. The teratogenic risk is theoretically greater when the exposure occurs during the first trimester. It is important that the pregnant patient be counselled regarding these risks once she has recovered. Assistance in providing such advice can be obtained by contacting the drug information services at tertiary women's hospitals. Australian drug risk classifications for pregnancy are available for all therapeutic agents. Paracetamol overdose treated with N-acetylcysteine does not appear to be associated with fetal abnormality even when the exposure occurs during the first trimester.

The decision to continue breastfeeding during acute poisoning involves a risk–benefit analysis. Most drugs are excreted in breast milk. The percentage of maternal dose likely to be received by an infant is very low (<2–3%) and usually does not pose a poisoning risk. Nonetheless, it is usually best to interrupt breastfeeding until the mother recovers, provided this can be done without compromising infant nutrition.

References

Anderson GD. Pregnancy-induced changes in pharmacokinetics: a mechanistic-based approach. Clinical Pharmacokinetics 2005; 44(10):989–1008.

McElhatton PR, Sullivan FM, Volans GN. Paracetamol overdose in pregnancy: analysis of the outcomes of 200 cases referred to the teratology information service. Reproductive Toxicology 1997; 10:85–94.

Syme MR, Paxton JW, Keelan JA. Drug transfer and metabolism by the human placenta. Clinical Pharmacokinetics 2004; 43(8):487–514.

Wiles JM, Clark LE, Herrera JL. Acetaminophen overdose in pregnancy. Southern Medical Journal 2005; 98(11):1118–1122.

2.21 POISONING IN CHILDREN

Unintentional paediatric exposures generate over 80 000 calls to Australian poisons information centres (PICs) each year. Many children are also brought directly to emergency departments without initial PIC consultation. The following information refers to unintentional exposures in children under the age of 6 years. Older children and adolescents may present with deliberate self-poisoning and these cases are assessed and managed according to the principles outlined for adults.

MANAGEMENT

Resuscitation

Paediatric resuscitation in poisoning follows the principles outlined in **Chapter 1.2: Resuscitation**. Attention to airway, breathing and circulation are paramount and ensure survival in the vast majority of patients.

Risk assessment

The principles of risk assessment in acute paediatric poisoning are the same as outlined for adults in **Chapter 1.3: Risk assessment**. However, the process is influenced by the difficulty in obtaining an accurate history regarding dose and agent, and the different range of agents ingested by small children.

Paediatric unintentional exposures occur most frequently with children in the 12–36 months age group. It is normal behaviour at that age to ingest small items found in the immediate environment. Not surprisingly, the range of agents ingested differs substantially from that ingested by adolescents or adults who deliberately self-poison (see **Table 2.21.1**). The ingested agent is more likely to be non-pharmaceutical and often virtually non-toxic when ingested in the readily available dose (see **Table 2.21.2**).

The toxic effects exerted by most agents on a mg/kg basis are the same for children as for adults. Small children rarely ingest more than 2–3 tablets or a mouthful of most agents, which equates to doses well below those ingested by adults or adolescents intending self-harm. However, some pharmaceutical agents, particularly large-dose controlled-release preparations, have the potential to cause serious toxicity if ingested by a 10-kg toddler in one, two or three dose units (see **Table 2.21.3**). Some non-pharmaceutical agents are also potentially lethal to children in small doses (see **Table 2.21.4**). In envenoming cases, the dose of venom is determined by the venomous creature, not

TABLE 2.21.1 Agents involved in accidental paediatric exposures	
Agent	**Percentage**
Pharmaceuticals	40%
Household cleaning products	14%
Plants	13%
Cosmetics	10%
Pesticides	6%

TABLE 2.21.2 Non-toxic household exposures	
Antacids	Inks
Antibiotics	Laxatives
Bath oil	Lipstick
Candles (wax)	Matches (red phosphorus)
Chalk	Newsprint
Colognes and perfumes	Oral contraceptives
Corticosteroids	Paint
Cosmetics	Shampoo
Deodorants	Shaving cream
Detergents (sips)	Shoe polish
Fertilisers	Silica
Glues	Soap
Hair products	Suntan lotions
Hand lotions	Thermometer mercury
Incense	Vaseline (petroleum jelly)

the victim, and children receive a larger venom dose on a microgram/kg basis.

Agents that do not cause significant toxicity when ingested in one, two or three dose units by small children include paracetamol (more than four 500-mg tablets, or more than 42 mL of 240 mg/5 mL solution required to exceed 200 mg/kg), iron (six or more tablets containing 105 mg elemental iron required to exceed 60 mg/kg), colchicine (10 or more 0.5-mg tablets required to exceed 0.5 mg/kg), digoxin (16 or more 250-microgram tablets required to exceed 4 mg) and anticoagulant rodenticides (less than one packet is generally considered non-toxic following a single unintentional ingestion).

Unfortunately, accurate estimation of dose and time is frequently challenging because of the inability to obtain an accurate dosing history. Risk assessment and subsequent management decisions are always based on a 'worst-case scenario' determined as follows:

1 The time of ingestion is assumed to be the latest possible time (except paracetamol).
2 Assume all missing or unaccounted agent(s) have been ingested.
3 Do not attempt to account for spillage, which is difficult to estimate.
4 If more than one child is involved, it is assumed that each child ingested all the missing or unaccounted agent(s).

This approach means that many children are assessed and observed in hospital but do not go on to develop toxicity.

Ingestion of a few unidentified tablets, often found in a public space, presents a difficult scenario around which to construct a risk assessment. If a tablet remains available for inspection, a PIC may be consulted to assist with identification. If this cannot be done with complete accuracy,

TABLE 2.21.3 Pharmaceuticals with potential for severe toxicity if 1 or 2 tablets ingested by a 10-kg toddler

Agent	Features of severe toxicity
Amphetamines Amphetamine Methamphetamine MDMA (ecstasy)	Agitation, confusion, hypertension, hyperthermia
Baclofen 25 mg	Coma
Calcium channel blockers Diltiazem CD 180, 240 or 360 mg Verapamil SR 160, 180 or 240 mg	Delayed onset of bradycardia, hypotension, conduction defects, refractory shock
Carbamazepine 400 mg	Coma
Chloroquine 155 mg **Hydroxychloroquine** 200 mg	Rapid onset of coma, seizures and cardiovascular collapse
Clozapine 100 or 200 mg	Coma
Dextropropoxyphene 100 mg	Ventricular tachycardia
Opioids Oxycodone 5 mg, 10 mg, 20 mg, 40 mg, 80 mg Hydromorphone 2 mg, 4 mg, 8 mg Methadone 10 mg Morphine sulfate 5, 10, 15, 30, 60, 100, 200 mg (controlled release) Diphenoxylate 2.5 mg/atropine 25 microgram	Coma, respiratory arrest Note: Onset of toxicity may be delayed with diphenoxylate/atropine and controlled-release morphine
Propranolol 160 mg	Coma, seizures, ventricular tachycardia, hypoglycaemia
Sulfonylureas Glibenclamide 5 mg Glibenclamide/metformin 1.25/250 mg, 2.5/500 mg, 5/500 mg Gliclazide 80 mg Gliclazide modified-release 30 mg Glimepiride 1, 2, 3, 4 mg Glipizide 5 mg	Hypoglycaemia; onset may be delayed up to 8 hours
Theophylline SR 200, 250, 300 mg	Seizures, supraventricular tachycardia, vomiting
Tricyclic antidepressants Dothiepin 75 mg	Coma, seizures, hypotension, ventricular tachycardia
Venlafaxine XR 150 mg	Seizures

Adapted from McCoubrie D, Murray L, Daly FFS et al. Ingestion of two unidentified tablets by a toddler. Emergency Medicine Journal 2006; 23:718–720.

TABLE 2.21.4 Non-pharmaceuticals with potential for severe toxicity if sip or mouthful ingested by a 10-kg toddler

Agent	Features of severe toxicity
Organophosphate and carbamate insecticides	Cholinergic symptoms Seizures Depressed level of consciousness
Paraquat/diquat	Oropharyngeal burns Multiple-organ failure Pulmonary fibrosis
Hydrocarbons Solvents Eucalyptus oil Kerosene	Rapid depressed level of consciousness Seizures Aspiration pneumonia
Camphor	Rapid depressed level of consciousness Seizures Hypotension
Corrosives Sodium hydroxide Strong acids	Gastro-oesophageal injury including perforation
Naphthalene (one mothball) NB: Most mothballs contain paradichlorobenzene, which is non-toxic after a single unintentional ingestion	Methaemoglobinaemia Haemolysis
Strychnine	Rapid onset of generalised muscle spasm Death by respiratory failure

the risk assessment assumes that the ingested tablets are one of the potentially lethal agents (see **Table 2.21.3**). A management plan based on this risk assessment is shown in **Table 2.21.5**.

Supportive care and disposition

Most ingestions are benign and do not need referral to hospital or gastrointestinal decontamination (see **Table 2.21.2**). For those ingestions that require management in a hospital setting, risk assessment based on the 'worst-case scenario' guides a defined period of focused observation.

Investigations

The screening tests performed on all adolescents and adults who deliberately self-poison are not indicated in the context of unintentional

TABLE 2.21.5	Management of a toddler who ingests unidentified tablets

- Admit for a minimum 12-hour observation period
- Ensure healthcare facility has appropriate resources to observe, resuscitate and treat patient if evidence of poisoning occurs
- IV access can be deferred until early evidence of toxicity is apparent
- Check bedside glucose level at presentation, if there is clinical evidence of hypoglycaemia, and at discharge
- Brief staff regarding clinical features for which the patient is being observed (see **Table 2.21.3**)
- Monitor level of consciousness, vital signs (pulse, blood pressure and respiratory rate) and early clinical features of hypoglycaemia
- Cardiac monitoring may be instituted if there is any abnormality of conscious state or vital signs
- Discharge patient only during daylight hours

paediatric poisoning. Investigations are performed only for specific purposes and are usually not necessary. Early measurement of drug levels, such as paracetamol, digoxin or theophylline, may be useful to exclude ingestion and obviate the need for prolonged observation, further investigation or transfer between facilities.

Decontamination

Gastrointestinal decontamination following unintentional paediatric ingestion is not routine. It is unusual that even the risk assessment based on a 'worst-case scenario' implies potential benefits that outweigh the risk associated with gastrointestinal decontamination procedures in children. Where activated charcoal is indicated, mixing with ice cream improves its palatability and the ease of administration. Administration of activated charcoal via a nasogastric tube inadvertently placed in the bronchial tree has resulted in paediatric death. Decontamination should be reserved for severe or life-threatening poisoning where the risk assessment suggests that supportive care or antidote treatment alone may not be adequate to ensure a satisfactory outcome.

Enhanced elimination and antidotes

Antidotes and enhanced elimination techniques have specific indications, contraindications, methods of administration, monitoring requirements, appropriate therapeutic end points and adverse effect profiles. The risk–benefit analysis is rarely in favour of these interventions following paediatric exposures. Doses of antidotes, where indicated, are usually the same as for adults on a mg/kg basis. However, antivenom doses are the same as for adults in absolute terms.

DISPOSITION AND FOLLOW-UP

The vast majority of paediatric exposures are benign and do not require referral to hospital for assessment or observation. This decision based on risk assessment is often made by a PIC when contacted by parents, carers or medical professionals working outside of hospital; in less than 7% of such cases is the child referred to hospital by the PIC. Most children referred or presenting to hospital can be discharged home if clinical evidence of toxicity does not develop within a short period of observation. Those who develop toxicity require admission to a facility able to provide an appropriate level of care.

Following any unintentional paediatric exposure, the circumstances of exposure are evaluated and parents or carers advised on safe storage of medicines and chemicals in the home if indicated. Unusually severe intoxication suggesting large, repeated or unusual exposure prompts consideration of non-accidental injury (NAI). This diagnosis is also considered if poisoning is diagnosed in an infant under 12 months of age. Children in this age group are not normally capable of self-administering tablets or other foreign materials. They may be administered toxins by adult carers with malicious intent, or by older siblings.

References

Bar-Oz B, Levichek Z, Koren G. Medications that can be fatal for a toddler with one tablet or teaspoonful. Pediatric Drugs 2004; 6:123–126.

Calello DP, Henretig FM. Pediatric toxicology: specialized approach to the poisoned child. Emergency Clinics of North America 2014; 32:29–52.

McCoubrie D, Murray L, Daly FFS et al. Ingestion of two unidentified tablets by a toddler. Emergency Medicine Journal 2006; 23:718–720.

Mofenson HC, Greensher J, Carraccio TR. Ingestions considered non-toxic. Emergency Medicine Clinics of North America 1984; 2(1):159–174.

2.22 POISONING IN THE ELDERLY

The assessment and management of the poisoned elderly patient is challenging.

The co-existence of limited physiological reserves, deteriorating cognition, multiple medical problems and their multiple prescribed medications provides the basis for exaggerated and unpredictable responses to any toxicological insult. The risk assessment for an overdose in the elderly patient predicts a more severe clinical course for the same agent taken in the same dose by a healthy young adult. Higher levels of vigilance, supportive care and monitoring are necessary. The clinical course of overdose or chronic poisoning is likely to be more severe and also have a higher complication rate. Age is highly correlated with case fatality rate and it is estimated that each 10-year increase in age is associated with a 36% increase in the odds ratio for death as an outcome following poisoning. Elderly patients are more likely to require hospital care as a result of accidental exposures and adverse drug effects.

Pharmacokinetic changes with ageing include delayed gastrointestinal absorption, decreased protein binding with resultant increased free drug levels and reduced hepatic metabolic function and glomerular filtration rate with resultant impaired elimination. Acute renal failure secondary to intercurrent medical problems or prescribed medications commonly leads to poisoning syndromes in the elderly, such as chronic lithium or digoxin toxicity.

Pharmacodynamic differences in the elderly are a result of drug actions on physiologically impaired organs. This is particularly seen with cardiovascular, respiratory and CNS depressant agents. An elderly patient's ability to respond to cardiovascular compromise with usual mechanisms such as peripheral vasoconstriction and increased cardiac output varies greatly. Clinical assessment of volume status in order to optimise renal and cardiac function is often unreliable and a lower threshold for invasive monitoring is required in these patients.

Most elderly patients will have a relatively delayed recovery from serious poisoning. The complications of immobility and hospital admission are observed more frequently in the elderly. These include atelectasis, pneumonia, pulmonary embolism, catheter-induced sepsis, muscle wasting and acute confusional states.

Reference
Roger JJ, Heard K. Does age matter? Comparing case fatality rates for selected poisonings reported to U.S. poison centers. Clinical Toxicology 2007; 45:705–708.

CHAPTER 3
SPECIFIC TOXINS

3.1 ALCOHOL: ETHANOL

See also Chapter 2.9: Alcohol use disorder.

Ethanol causes the rapid onset of dose-related CNS depression and is commonly ingested during deliberate self-poisoning. There is a high degree of inter-individual variability and care is essentially supportive.

RISK ASSESSMENT
- There is no clearly defined dose/kg threshold for toxicity that applies to all patients.
- The dose ingested may be estimated if the number of standard drinks consumed is known:
  - Standard drinks containing approximately 10 g ethanol:
    - 375-mL can of mid-strength beer (3.5%)
    - 100-mL glass of wine
    - 30-mL shot of spirit.
- Co-ingestion of other CNS depressants (e.g. sedative-hypnotic agents, antidepressants, opioids) increases the risk of respiratory depression.
- Seizures may occur in the setting of ethanol intoxication or withdrawal.
- **Children:** ingestion of even small amounts of ethanol can result in significant hypoglycaemia and CNS depression.

Toxic mechanism
The CNS depressant effects of ethanol are primarily mediated by stimulation of inhibitory $GABA_A$ receptors, but multiple other neurotransmitters are also affected, including glutamate, N-methyl-D-aspartate (NMDA) and serotonin ($5-HT_3$). Metabolic effects include hypoglycaemia and ketoacidosis, resulting from impaired gluconeogenesis and fatty acid oxidation. Hyperlactataemia occurs due to impaired conversion of lactate to pyruvate following an increase in the $NADH:NAD^+$ ratio. Ethanol causes direct, dose-dependent cardiovascular depression and vasodilatation. Tolerance and withdrawal phenomena result from adaptation of inhibitory and excitatory receptors in the setting of chronic ethanol use.

Toxicokinetics
Ethanol is rapidly absorbed following oral administration. It distributes readily across total body water (volume of distribution 0.6–0.7 L/kg). Ethanol is oxidised by cytosolic and microsomal alcohol dehydrogenases to form acetaldehyde, which in turn is metabolised by aldehyde dehydrogenase to acetate (see **Appendix 5: Alcohol pathways**). Both cytosolic steps involve the reduction of NAD to NADH. Above a serum ethanol concentration of 4 mmol/L (20 mg/dL), metabolism changes to zero order kinetics, so a constant amount of ethanol is metabolised per unit time. In most patients, serum ethanol levels decrease by approximately 4 mmol/L/hour (20 mg/dL/hour; 0.02%/hour).

CLINICAL FEATURES
Clinical features are progressive with increasing degrees of intoxication (see **Table 3.1.1**).
- Disinhibition, emotional lability and euphoria
- Nystagmus, ataxia, slurred speech
- Agitation, aggression and disorientation
- Nausea, vomiting
- Tachycardia, hypotension, hypothermia

TABLE 3.1.1 Guide to dose-related serum ethanol concentrations and clinical features

| Ethanol dose (g/kg) | Serum ethanol concentration | | | Clinical features |
| | SI units (mmol/L) | Conventional units | | |
		mg/dL	g/dL (%)	
0.5	11	50	0.05	Disinhibition and euphoria
1	22	100	0.10	Slurred speech. Impaired judgement and coordination. Significant CNS depression in non-tolerant individuals, especially children
2	43	200	0.20	Potential for coma, although ethanol-dependent individuals are usually ambulant
>5	>87	>400	>0.40	Coma, respiratory depression, hypotension, except in patients with marked tolerance

Note: To convert SI units to mg/dL, multiply by 4.61. To convert mg/dL to SI units, multiply by 0.217.

- Coma with loss of airway protective reflexes and respiratory depression.

Improvement in conscious state is usually seen within 2–4 hours, but 6–12 hours may elapse before patients are ambulant.

INVESTIGATIONS
Screening tests in deliberate self-poisoning
- 12-lead ECG, BGL and paracetamol level

Specific investigations
- Serum, blood or breath alcohol levels.
- Ethanol levels assist risk assessment in patients with CNS depression. However, elevated serum blood ethanol concentrations should not be assumed to be the sole contributor to CNS depression and appropriate evaluation for other causes is required.
- The serum ethanol concentration is not the same as the whole blood ethanol level, which defines legal driving limits. Whole blood concentrations are approximately 10% lower than corresponding serum concentrations.

- Breath ethanol estimation provides a convenient bedside estimation of blood ethanol concentration but the result is influenced by minute ventilation.

MANAGEMENT
Resuscitation, supportive care and monitoring
- Attention to airway, breathing and circulation is paramount. These priorities are managed along conventional lines as outlined in **Chapter 1.2: Resuscitation**.
- Basic resuscitative measures ensure the survival of the vast majority of patients.
- General supportive care measures are indicated, as outlined in **Chapter 1.4: Supportive care and monitoring**.
- Give thiamine 100–300 mg PO or IV tds to patients with potential thiamine deficiency.
- Close clinical and physiological monitoring is indicated.
- Monitor for urinary retention and place an indwelling urinary catheter as required.

Decontamination
- Activated charcoal does not bind ethanol and is not indicated.

Enhanced elimination
- Elimination of ethanol is enhanced by haemodialysis. However, this intervention is not routinely indicated because good supportive care generally ensures a favourable outcome.

Antidotes
- None available.

DISPOSITION AND FOLLOW-UP
- Patients with mild CNS depression are managed supportively in a ward environment. The patient is fit for medical discharge when clinically well and able to ambulate safely.
- Patients with significant CNS depression may require intubation and admission to an intensive care unit.
- Where appropriate, patients are counselled regarding ethanol misuse prior to discharge, as discussed in **Chapter 2.9: Alcohol use disorder**.

HANDY TIPS
- A blood ethanol concentration confirms the diagnosis of ethanol intoxication but does not exclude other causes of CNS depression (e.g. co-ingestions, trauma, metabolic disorder).
- Anticipate alcohol withdrawal during the observation period in patients with alcohol dependence.

PITFALLS
- Failure to regard ethanol intoxication as potentially life-threatening.
- Failure to detect and manage co-existing intoxications or other medical conditions in the ethanol intoxicated patient.

- Discharge of ethanol intoxicated patients before they are competent to make decisions about their own welfare and ensure their own safety.

Presentations

Ethanol is found in varying concentrations in a large number of beverages and domestic and commercial products:

beers: 2.8–12.0%
wines: 9–14%
spirits: 35–50%
methylated spirits: 95%
hand sanitisers
mouth wash, food extracts and flavourings (e.g. vanilla extract 35% ethanol), cough and cold syrups, perfumes and cosmetics.

References

Baselt RC. Disposition of toxic drugs and chemicals in man 5th edn Foster City, California: Chemical Toxicology Institute;2000.

Lieber CS. Medical disorders of alcoholism. New England Journal of Medicine 1995; 333(16):1058–1065.

O'Connor PG, Schottenfeld RS. Patients with alcohol problems. New England Journal of Medicine 1998; 338(9):592–602.

Tjipto AC, Taylor DMcD, Liew H. Alcohol use among young adults presenting to the emergency department. Emergency Medicine Australasia 2006; 18(2):125–130.

3.2 ALCOHOL: ETHYLENE GLYCOL

Ethylene glycol is a toxic alcohol and poisoning is potentially lethal. Ethanol, fomepizole and haemodialysis are treatment options for the management of patients with significant poisoning.

RISK ASSESSMENT

- Ingestion of >1 mL/kg of 100% ethylene glycol is potentially lethal.
- All deliberate self-poisonings are assumed to be potentially lethal.
- Co-ingestion of ethanol complicates risk assessment because the onset of clinical features will be delayed (see **Investigations** below).
- Dermal and inhalation exposure does not lead to ethylene glycol intoxication.
- **Children:** an accidental lick or taste does not require hospital evaluation unless symptoms develop.

Toxic mechanism

Ethylene glycol causes initial CNS effects similar to those of ethanol. The more significant toxic effects are due to accumulation of glycolic and oxalic acid metabolites, resulting in a severe, progressive high anion-gap metabolic acidosis (HAGMA). Hyperlactataemia is caused by impaired conversion of lactate to pyruvate following an increase in the NADH:NAD$^+$ ratio. Acute oliguric renal failure occurs secondary to calcium oxalate crystal deposition in renal tubules and the nephrotoxic effects of glycolic acid. Calcium oxalate deposition can also occur in other tissues (myocardium, brain and skeletal muscle), resulting in hypocalcaemia with a risk of cardiac dysrhythmias and seizures.

Toxicokinetics

Ethylene glycol is rapidly absorbed following ingestion and peak concentrations occur within 2 hours. It is distributed across total body water with rapid CNS penetration. Ethylene glycol is metabolised sequentially by alcohol dehydrogenase (ADH) and aldehyde dehydrogenase (ALDH) to glycoaldehyde and glycolic acid, which in turn is converted to glyoxylic acid and oxalic acid (see **Appendix 5: Alcohol pathways**). The elimination half-life of ethylene glycol is 3–9 hours with inter-individual variability, but this increases to approximately 20 hours in the presence of ethanol or fomepizole, which competitively inhibit ADH. In this setting, ethylene glycol is slowly eliminated by the renal route.

CLINICAL FEATURES

- Initial clinical features develop within the first 2 hours and are similar to those of ethanol intoxication:
  - euphoria, nystagmus, drowsiness, nausea and vomiting.
- Progressively severe features develop over the subsequent 4–12 hours:
  - dyspnoea, tachypnoea, tachycardia and decreased conscious level progressing to hypotension, seizures, coma and death.
- Flank pain and oliguria indicate acute renal failure.
- Persistent coma or neurocognitive deficits may result from cerebral oedema or ischaemic encephalopathy.
- Multiple cranial and peripheral neuropathies may become evident during recovery.

INVESTIGATIONS

Screening tests in deliberate self-poisoning
- 12-lead ECG, BGL and paracetamol level

Specific investigations
Calculation of osmolar and anion gaps:
- Calculated serum osmolarity (EUC, blood gas, blood glucose, serum ethanol level)
- Measured serum osmolality (laboratory assay measuring freezing point depression)
- Calculated or measured anion gap (EUC, blood gas)
  - Ingestion of ethylene glycol results in initial elevation of the osmolar gap.
  - As ethylene glycol is metabolised, the osmolar gap decreases, and a high anion-gap metabolic acidosis (HAGMA) develops.
  - Reliable calculation and measurement of osmolar and anion gaps requires simultaneous sampling of the relevant biochemical markers.
  - Interpretation of the osmolar and anion gaps is dependent on the time course of the poisoning and is related to the time since ingestion and the presence or absence of ADH blockade (see **Chapter 2.15: Osmolar gap** and **Chapter 2.16: Acid–base disorders** for discussion regarding osmolar and anion gaps and interpretation of acid–base disturbances).
- Progressive decrease in the pH and venous bicarbonate concentration indicate worsening acidosis, but these are late signs of toxicity.
  - Note: Some blood gas analysers incorrectly measure glycol metabolites as lactate, and a falsely elevated serum lactate may be a useful early indicator of ethylene glycol poisoning.

- Breath or serum ethanol level
  - Confirm or exclude co-ingestion of ethanol.
  - Monitor antidotal treatment with ethanol.
    - Note: Ethylene glycol is not detected by breath or serum ethanol assays.
- Serum ethylene glycol level
  - Not usually available in a clinically relevant time frame.
  - Significant metabolism may have occurred by the time of collection.
  - Serial levels (if available) guide cessation of antidote therapy and haemodialysis, in combination with other clinical and biochemical markers.
- Urine microscopy
  - Presence of calcium oxalate crystals in the urine is pathognomonic of ethylene glycol intoxication but their absence does not exclude the diagnosis.
- CT or MRI brain
  - May demonstrate characteristic ischaemic or haemorrhagic injury to the basal ganglia.

MANAGEMENT
Resuscitation, supportive care and monitoring
- Severe ethylene glycol poisoning is a life-threatening emergency managed in an area equipped for cardiorespiratory monitoring and resuscitation.
- Patients may present with established toxicity, characterised by severe metabolic acidosis and a degree of respiratory compensation:
  - Attention to airway and breathing is paramount. In patients maintaining effective ventilation, intubation is to be avoided as even a brief period of apnoea during standard rapid sequence intubation can lead to cardiac arrest.
  - If intubation and ventilation is required for coma or ineffective ventilation, it is imperative to maintain adequate hyperventilation to maximise respiratory alkalosis.
- Sodium bicarbonate is an immediate priority in patients with severe metabolic acidosis awaiting haemodialysis:
  - Administer IV sodium bicarbonate boluses 1–2 mmol/kg guided by serial blood gases and clinical response.
  - Maintain hyperventilation and consider further bolus IV sodium bicarbonate to prevent worsening acidaemia pending haemodialysis.
- Patients who present early after ingestion, or who have co-ingested ethanol, may not yet have developed metabolic acidosis:
  - Calculation and assessment of the osmolar and anion gaps is vital to guide management decisions (see **Investigations**).
- Administration of ethanol (or fomepizole if available) is indicated prior to definitive blood results if ethylene glycol poisoning is considered a likely diagnosis.
- Treat seizures with IV benzodiazepines as discussed in **Chapter 2.3: Seizures**.
- Detect and correct hypoglycaemia, hyperkalaemia, hypocalcaemia and hypomagnesaemia.

- General supportive care measures are indicated, as outlined in **Chapter 1.4: Supportive care and monitoring**.
- Monitor fluid balance and urine output.
- Cofactor therapy: pyridoxine 50 mg IV 6 hourly and thiamine 100–300 mg IV or PO 6 hourly are indicated to enhance metabolism of glyoxylic acid.

Decontamination
- Activated charcoal does not adsorb ethylene glycol and is not indicated.

Enhanced elimination
- Haemodialysis is definitive management of ethylene glycol poisoning, as it removes ethylene glycol and corrects acidosis.
- Lactate-free dialysate with added bicarbonate is indicated in the setting of significant acidaemia.
- The threshold for haemodialysis is not clearly defined for all cases, and discussion with a clinical toxicologist or Poisons Information Centre is indicated. Reasonable indications include:
  — ingestion of ethylene glycol with an elevated osmolar gap >20
  — acidaemia with pH <7.3 or bicarbonate <20 mmol/L
  — renal impairment
  — worsening clinical status or progressive acidosis despite supportive care
  — ethylene glycol level >8 mmol/L (50 mg/dL) if available.
- End points for haemodialysis
  — Correction of acidosis
  — Correction of osmolar gap
  — Ethylene glycol level <3.2 mmol/L (20 mg/dL) if available.
- Acid–base status and electrolytes are repeated every 4 hours for 12 hours following cessation of haemodialysis to confirm that further dialysis is not required.

Antidotes
- Ethanol (see **Chapter 4.8: Ethanol**) and fomepizole (see **Chapter 4.11: Fomepizole**) are used in the treatment of suspected or confirmed ethylene glycol poisoning.
- Ethanol at a serum concentration of 22 mmol/L (100 mg/dL; 0.1%) competitively inhibits ADH so that ethylene glycol is not metabolised.
- Fomepizole is a more potent competitive inhibitor of ADH but is not readily available in most centres in Australia.
- Fomepizole is the preferred antidotal therapy for paediatric poisoning with ethylene glycol, due to the risk of serious adverse effects from ethanol administration and the logistical difficulties inherent in instituting haemodialysis in paediatric patients.

DISPOSITION AND FOLLOW-UP
- Children and adult patients who remain clinically well following accidental ingestion and have a normal venous bicarbonate level (≥20 mEq/L) 4 hours after serum or breath ethanol level is demonstrated to be undetectable are fit for medical discharge.

- All symptomatic patients, and those with deliberate ingestion, are assumed to have potentially lethal ethylene glycol intoxication and are admitted to hospital for further evaluation and definitive management if required.
- If established renal failure develops, ongoing dialysis may be required for several weeks, but renal function usually returns to normal.
- Patients who survive severe intoxication are followed up to exclude the development of cranial or peripheral neuropathies.

HANDY TIPS
- Co-ingestion of ethanol delays the onset of clinical features of ethylene glycol intoxication.
- Plan for transfer to a facility with haemodialysis as soon as the provisional diagnosis of ethylene glycol intoxication is made.
- Serum bicarbonate levels provide a surrogate marker of glycolic and oxalic acid production, and may be useful to exclude significant ingestion in the absence of formal osmolar calculations, particularly in the setting of accidental ingestions.
- Anion gap acidosis with elevated lactate (± elevated osmolar gap) associated with hypocalcaemia and rising creatinine is pathognomonic of ethylene glycol intoxication.

PITFALLS
- Absence of symptoms on presentation does not exclude a significant ingestion.
- Normal osmolar gap (<10) does not exclude significant poisoning.
- Failure to recognise the concurrent presence of ethanol as a confounding factor in the risk assessment for ethylene glycol poisoning.

CONTROVERSIES
- Haemodialysis is an effective treatment for significant ethylene glycol poisoning but is an invasive intervention.
- ADH blockade with ethanol or fomepizole (if available) may allow native renal elimination of ethylene glycol to occur in an acceptable time frame (<48 hours) that justifies prolonged intoxication (ethanol) or expensive antidote (fomepizole).
- Paediatric poisoning with ethylene glycol is a clear indication for antidotal therapy with fomepizole if it is available.

Sources
Radiator coolants and antifreeze in concentrations 20–98%
De-icing solutions
Solvents
Brake fluids

References
Brent J. Current management of ethylene glycol poisoning. Drugs 2001; 61(7):979–988.
Caravati EM, Erdman AR, Christianson G et al. Ethylene glycol exposure: an evidence based consensus guideline for out-of-hospital management. Clinical Toxicology 2005; 43:327–345.

Jolliff HA, Dart RC, Bogdan GM et al. Can the diagnosis of ethylene glycol (EG) toxicity be made without serum EG levels and osmolality values (abstract)? Journal of Toxicology–Clinical Toxicology 2000; 38(5):539–540.

Levine M, Curry SC, Ruha AM et al. Ethylene glycol elimination kinetics and outcomes in patients managed without hemodialysis. Annals of Emergency Medicine 2012; 59(6):527–531.

McMartin K, Jacobsen D, Hovda KE. Antidotes for poisoning by alcohols that form toxic metabolites. British Journal of Clinical Pharmacology 2015; 81(2):505–515.

Miller H, Barceloux DG, Krenzelok EP et al. American Academy of Clinical Toxicology practice guidelines on the treatment of ethylene glycol poisoning. Clinical Toxicology 1999; 37(5):537–560.

3.3 ALCOHOL: ISOPROPANOL (ISOPROPYL ALCOHOL)

Isopropanol produces a CNS intoxication syndrome similar to that of ethanol. In addition, gastrointestinal irritation and ketosis are prominent features, but significant acidosis does not occur. Management is essentially supportive.

RISK ASSESSMENT

- Isopropanol causes dose-related CNS depression following ingestion, although there is a high degree of inter-individual variability.
- As little as 1 mL/kg of a 70% solution causes symptoms of inebriation, and more than 4 mL/kg may cause coma and respiratory depression.
- Co-ingestion of other CNS depressants (e.g. sedative-hypnotic agents, opioids, ethanol) increases the risk of respiratory depression.
- **Children:** minor ingestions such as a taste or lick do not require hospital evaluation unless symptoms develop. Significant isopropanol toxicity is reported from dermal absorption following application of 'rubbing alcohol' to small children as an antipyretic.

Toxic mechanism

Isopropanol causes CNS effects similar to those of ethanol (see **Chapter 3.1: Alcohol: Ethanol**). Ketonaemia without acidosis is the characteristic feature of isopropanol intoxication – unlike ethylene glycol or methanol, isopropanol does not cause a severe, progressive high anion-gap metabolic acidosis (HAGMA) because acetone is either eliminated unchanged or metabolised to carbon dioxide and water. Isopropanol is a gastrointestinal irritant and also causes dose-dependent cardiovascular depression.

Toxicokinetics

Isopropanol is rapidly absorbed following ingestion, dermal contact or inhalation. It distributes across the total body water with a volume of distribution around 0.5 L/kg. Up to 80% is metabolised by hepatic alcohol dehydrogenase (ADH) to acetone and the remainder is excreted unchanged by renal and pulmonary routes (see **Appendix 5: Alcohol pathways**). The metabolism of isopropanol is effectively blocked in the presence of ethanol and the elimination half-life is correspondingly prolonged. Acetone is mostly excreted unchanged (also via the kidneys and lungs) or metabolised to carbon dioxide and water, with a half-life greater than 16 hours.

CLINICAL FEATURES

- An intoxication syndrome similar to ethanol develops rapidly following ingestion (see **Chapter 3.1: Alcohol: Ethanol**).

- A sweet, fruity odour on the breath indicates the presence of acetone and may be a prominent clinical feature.

INVESTIGATIONS
Screening tests in deliberate self-poisoning
- 12-lead ECG, BGL and paracetamol level

Specific investigations
Isopropanol and acetone will cause an increase in the serum osmolarity, but unlike ethylene glycol or methanol, a severe HAGMA will not occur.
- Calculation of osmolar and anion gaps is warranted to ensure that no other toxic alcohols are present if there is any doubt about the agent ingested (see **Chapter 2.15: Osmolar gap, Chapter 2.16: Acid–base disorders, Chapter 3.2: Alcohol: Ethylene glycol** and **Chapter 3.4: Alcohol: Methanol** for discussion regarding osmolar and anion gaps and interpretation of acid–base disturbances).
- Breath or serum ethanol level
  - Confirm or exclude co-ingestion of ethanol.
    - Note: Isopropanol is not detected by breath or serum ethanol assays.
- Serum and urine ketones
  - Note: Some point-of-care ketone analysers may not reliably detect acetone.
- Isopropanol levels are not routinely available and do not assist acute management.

MANAGEMENT
Resuscitation, supportive care and monitoring
- Attention to airway, breathing and circulation are paramount. These priorities are managed along conventional lines, as outlined in **Chapter 1.2: Resuscitation**.
- Basic resuscitative measures ensure the survival of the vast majority of patients.
- General supportive care measures are indicated, as outlined in **Chapter 1.4: Supportive care and monitoring**.
- Give thiamine 100–300 mg PO or IV tds to patients with potential thiamine deficiency.
- Close clinical and physiological monitoring is indicated.

Decontamination
- Activated charcoal does not adsorb isopropanol and is not indicated.

Enhanced elimination
- Haemodialysis is highly effective at removing isopropanol but is rarely indicated as a good outcome can be anticipated with supportive care.

Antidotes
- Ethanol and fomepizole are contraindicated as they inhibit metabolism of isopropanol to acetone, prolonging isopropanol half-life. Isopropanol as the parent alcohol is the primary cause of toxicity.

DISPOSITION AND FOLLOW-UP

- Patients with mild CNS depression are managed supportively and discharged when clinically well.
- Patients who are clinically well after confirmed isopropanol ingestion and have a normal venous bicarbonate level (≥20 mEq/L) 4 hours after serum or breath ethanol level is demonstrated to be undetectable are fit for medical discharge.

HANDY TIPS

- Isopropanol intoxication mimics ethanol intoxication.
- A patient presenting with a prominent fruity or sweet odour on the breath, with ketonaemia or ketonuria, an elevated osmolar gap and no evident or developing acidosis, is highly suggestive of isopropanol intoxication.
- Acetone can cause false elevation of the creatinine concentration when measured by colorimetric methods, and an elevated serum creatinine should be confirmed with formal laboratory testing using enzymatic assays.

Sources

Isopropanol (50–70% concentration) is found in hand sanitisers, disinfectants, solvents, window cleaners and perfumes.

References

Slaughter RJ, Mason RW, Beasley DMG et al. Isopropanol poisoning. Clinical Toxicology 2014; 52(5):470–478.

Stremski E, Hennes H. Accidental isopropanol ingestion in children. Pediatric Emergency Care 2000; 16(4):238–240.

Zaman F, Pervez A, Abreu K. Isopropyl alcohol intoxication: a diagnostic challenge. American Journal of Kidney Diseases 2002; 40(3):E12.

3.4 ALCOHOL: METHANOL (METHYL ALCOHOL)

Methanol is a toxic alcohol. Poisoning frequently occurs following ingestion of home-made distilled spirits 'homebrew/moonshine/ bootleg liquor' or adulterated commercially available drinks, particularly from countries with poor regulatory environments. Ethanol, fomepizole and haemodialysis are treatment options for the management of patients with significant poisoning.

RISK ASSESSMENT

- Ingestion of >0.5 mL/kg of 100% methanol is potentially lethal.
- Deliberate self-poisonings are assumed to be potentially lethal.
- Co-ingestion of ethanol complicates risk assessment because the onset of clinical features will be delayed (see **Investigations** below).
- Inhalational or dermal absorption is less likely to lead to significant methanol intoxication, although toxicity has been reported with prolonged exposure or misuse.
- **Children:** all exposures in children require medical assessment. Ingestion of >0.15 mL/kg (1.5 mL in a 10-kg toddler) of 100% methanol can lead to significant toxicity.

Toxic mechanism

Methanol causes initial CNS effects similar to those of ethanol. The more significant toxic effects are due to accumulation of the metabolite formic acid, resulting in a severe, progressive high anion-gap metabolic acidosis (HAGMA). Hyperlactataemia is secondary to inhibition of mitochondrial cytochrome oxidase and impaired conversion of lactate to pyruvate following an increase in the NADH:NAD$^+$ ratio. Direct toxic effects on the retina and optic nerve lead to blindness. In the brain, characteristic features of methanol encephalopathy include subcortical white matter haemorrhages and symmetrical necrosis of highly metabolically active structures such as the basal ganglia and thalamus.

Toxicokinetics

Methanol is rapidly absorbed after ingestion with peak levels occurring within 60 minutes. Systemic and ocular toxicity have been reported after prolonged inhalational exposure. It is rapidly distributed across total body water with a volume of distribution of 0.6–0.7 L/kg. Methanol is metabolised in the liver by alcohol dehydrogenase (ADH) to formaldehyde, which in turn is metabolised by aldehyde dehydrogenase (ALDH) to formic acid (see **Appendix 5: Alcohol pathways**). The elimination half-life of methanol has been reported between 2.5 and 12 hours, with significant inter-individual variability. This increases to greater than 48 hours in the presence of ethanol or fomepizole, which competitively inhibit ADH. In this setting, methanol is very slowly eliminated by respiratory or renal routes.

CLINICAL FEATURES

- Mild CNS depression similar to that of ethanol intoxication is evident within 1 hour of ingestion. Nausea, vomiting and abdominal pain may occur.
- Progressively severe features occur over the subsequent 12 hours as metabolic acidosis develops:
  - Malaise, dyspnoea, tachypnoea, tachycardia and decreased conscious level, progressing to hypotension, seizures, coma and death.
  - Retinal toxicity is characteristic, ranging from mydriasis and blurred vision to visual field defects and blindness. Papillo-oedema may be evident on fundoscopy.
- Persistent coma or neurocognitive deficits may result from cerebral oedema or ischaemic encephalopathy.
- Patients who survive severe poisoning may have permanent blindness and extrapyramidal movement disorders.

INVESTIGATIONS

Screening tests in deliberate self-poisoning
- 12-lead ECG, BGL and paracetamol level

Specific investigations
Calculation of osmolar and anion gaps:
- Calculated serum osmolarity (EUC, blood gas, blood glucose, serum ethanol level)
- Measured serum osmolality (laboratory assay measuring freezing point depression)
- Calculated or measured anion gap (EUC, blood gas)
  - Ingestion of methanol results in initial elevation of the osmolar gap.
  - As methanol is metabolised, the osmolar gap decreases, and a HAGMA develops.

- Reliable calculation and measurement of osmolar and anion gaps requires simultaneous sampling of the relevant biochemical markers.
- Interpretation of the osmolar and anion gaps is dependent on the time course of the poisoning and is related to the time since ingestion and the presence or absence of ADH blockade (see **Chapter 2.15: Osmolar gap** and **Chapter 2.16: Acid–base disorders** for discussion regarding osmolar and anion gaps and interpretation of acid–base disturbances).
- Progressive decrease in the pH and venous bicarbonate concentration indicate worsening acidosis, but these are late signs of toxicity.
- Breath or serum ethanol level
  - Confirm or exclude co-ingestion of ethanol.
  - Monitor antidotal treatment with ethanol.
    - Note: methanol is not detected by breath or serum ethanol assays.
- Serum methanol level
  - Not usually available in a clinically relevant time-frame
  - Significant metabolism may have occurred by the time of collection
  - Serial levels (if available) guide cessation of antidote therapy and haemodialysis, in combination with other clinical and biochemical markers.
- CT or MRI brain
  - May demonstrate characteristic ischaemic or haemorrhagic injury to the basal ganglia.

MANAGEMENT
Resuscitation, supportive care and monitoring
Severe methanol poisoning is a life-threatening emergency managed in an area equipped for cardiorespiratory monitoring and resuscitation.
- Patients may present with established toxicity, characterised by severe metabolic acidosis and a degree of respiratory compensation:
  - Attention to airway and breathing is paramount. In patients maintaining effective ventilation, intubation is to be avoided as even a brief period of apnoea during standard rapid sequence intubation can lead to cardiac arrest.
  - If intubation and ventilation is required for coma or ineffective ventilation, it is imperative to maintain adequate hyperventilation to maximise respiratory alkalosis.
- Sodium bicarbonate is an immediate priority in patients with severe metabolic acidosis, as systemic acidosis enhances formic acid inhibition of cytochrome oxidase:
  - Administer IV sodium bicarbonate boluses 1–2 mmol/kg guided by serial blood gases and clinical response.
  - Maintain hyperventilation and consider further bolus IV sodium bicarbonate to prevent worsening acidaemia pending haemodialysis.
- Patients who present early after ingestion, or who have co-ingested ethanol, may not yet have developed metabolic acidosis:
  - Calculation and assessment of the osmolar and anion gaps is vital to guide management decisions (see **Investigations**).

- Administration of ethanol (or fomepizole if available) is indicated prior to definitive blood results if methanol poisoning is considered a likely diagnosis.
- Treat seizures with IV benzodiazepines, as discussed in **Chapter 2.3: Seizures**.
- Detect and correct hypoglycaemia.
- General supportive care measures are indicated, as outlined in **Chapter 1.4: Supportive care and monitoring**.
- Cofactor therapy: folinic acid or folic acid 50 mg IV 6 hourly is indicated to enhance metabolism of formic acid to non-toxic metabolites (see **Chapter 4.10: Folinic acid**).

Decontamination
- Activated charcoal does not adsorb methanol and is not indicated.

Enhanced elimination
- Haemodialysis is definitive management of methanol poisoning, as it removes both methanol and formic acid and corrects acidosis.
- Lactate-free dialysate with added bicarbonate is indicated in the setting of significant acidaemia.
- The threshold for haemodialysis is not clearly defined for all cases, and discussion with a clinical toxicologist or Poisons Information Centre is indicated. Reasonable indications include:
  — ingestion of methanol with an elevated osmolar gap >20
  — acidaemia with pH <7.3 or bicarbonate <20 mmol/L
  — visual symptoms
  — worsening clinical status or progressive acidosis despite supportive care
  — methanol level >16 mmol/L (50 mg/dL) if available.
- End points for haemodialysis
  — Correction of acidosis
  — Correction of osmolar gap
  — Methanol level <6 mmol/L (20 mg/dL) if available.
- Acid–base status and electrolytes are repeated every 4 hours for 12 hours following cessation of haemodialysis to confirm that further dialysis is not required.

Antidotes
- Ethanol (see **Chapter 4.8: Ethanol**) and fomepizole (see **Chapter 4.11: Fomepizole**) are used in the treatment of suspected or confirmed methanol poisoning.
- Ethanol at a serum concentration of 22 mmol/L (100 mg/dL; 0.1%) competitively inhibits ADH so that methanol cannot be metabolised to formaldehyde.
- Fomepizole is a more potent competitive inhibitor of ADH, but is not readily available in most centres in Australia.
- Fomepizole is the preferred antidotal therapy for paediatric poisoning with methanol due to the risk of serious adverse effects from ethanol administration and the logistical difficulties inherent in instituting haemodialysis in paediatric patients.

DISPOSITION AND FOLLOW-UP

- Children and adult patients who remain clinically well after suspected accidental ingestion and have a normal venous bicarbonate level (≥20 mEq/L) at 8 or more hours post ingestion may be discharged.
- Adult patients who remain clinically well following accidental ingestion and have a normal venous bicarbonate level (≥20 mEq/L) 8 hours after serum or breath ethanol level is demonstrated to be undetectable are fit for medical discharge.
- All symptomatic patients and those with deliberate ingestion are assumed to have potentially lethal methanol intoxication and are admitted to hospital for further evaluation and management.

HANDY TIPS

- Most commercial products available in Australia labelled as 'methylated spirits' do not contain methanol, but it is essential to confirm the constituents.
- Co-ingestion of ethanol delays the onset of clinical features of methanol intoxication.
- Plan for transfer to a facility with haemodialysis as soon as the provisional diagnosis of methanol intoxication is made.
- Serum bicarbonate levels provide a surrogate marker of formic acid production and are useful to exclude significant ingestion in the absence of formal osmolar calculations, particularly in the setting of accidental ingestions.
- Methanol motor-racing fuels may also contain nitromethane, an additive used to improve engine performance. Nitromethane causes false elevation of the creatinine concentration when measured by colorimetric methods, and an elevated serum creatinine should be confirmed with formal laboratory testing using enzymatic assays.

PITFALLS

- Absence of symptoms on presentation does not exclude a significant ingestion.
- Normal osmolar gap (<10) does not exclude significant poisoning.
- Failure to recognise the concurrent presence of ethanol as a confounding factor in the risk assessment for methanol poisoning.

CONTROVERSIES

- Haemodialysis is an effective treatment for significant methanol poisoning but is an invasive intervention.
- Native elimination of methanol by respiratory or renal routes is so slow (unlike for ethylene glycol) that the prolonged duration of intoxication (ethanol) or administration of expensive antidote (fomepizole) required for definitive management may not be justified in adults.
- Paediatric poisoning with methanol is a clear indication for antidotal therapy with fomepizole if it is available.

Sources

Automotive cleaning fluid
Chemical applications in industry and science
Solvent in thinners, varnishes, paints and enamels
Model aeroplane and car fuel

Fuel additive
Dyes and stains
Racing car fuel
Home-made or adulterated distilled spirits
Wood alcohol, wood spirits

References

Barceloux DG, Bond R, Krenzelok EP et al. American Academy of Clinical Toxicology practice guidelines on the treatment of methanol poisoning. Journal of Toxicology–Clinical Toxicology 2002; 40(4):415–446.

Hassanian-Moghaddam H, Zamani N, Roberts DM et al. Consensus statements on the approach to patients in a methanol poisoning outbreak. Clinical Toxicology 2019; 57(12):1129–1136.

Kostic MA, Dart RC. Rethinking the toxic methanol level. Journal of Toxicology–Clinical Toxicology 2003; 41(6):793–800.

McMartin K, Jacobsen D, Hovda KE. Antidotes for poisoning by alcohols that form toxic metabolites. British Journal of Clinical Pharmacology 2016; 81(3):505–515.

Roberts DM, Yates C, Mégarbane B et al. EXTRIP workgroup: recommendations for the role of extracorporeal treatments in the management of acute methanol poisoning: a systematic review and consensus statement. Critical Care Medicine 2015; 43(2):461–472.

3.5 ALCOHOL: OTHER TOXIC ALCOHOLS

Diethylene glycol, Dipropylene glycol, Ethylene glycol monobutyl ether (EGBE), Ethylene glycol monoethyl ether (EGME), Propylene glycol, Triethylene glycol

These alcohols are found in a variety of automotive products, solvents and pharmaceuticals. Diethylene glycol poisoning can occur as epidemics, related to illicit use as a solvent in pharmaceutical preparations. Deliberate self-poisoning is potentially lethal.

RISK ASSESSMENT

- Deliberate self-poisonings are assumed to be potentially lethal.
- Ingestion of >1 mL/kg of 100% diethylene glycol is potentially lethal.
- There are limited data on the toxicity of glycol ethers (EGBE or EGME), but intentional, large-volume ingestions should be considered potentially lethal.
- Co-ingestion of ethanol complicates risk assessment because the onset of clinical features will be delayed (see **Investigations** below).
- The toxic effects of propylene glycol as a pharmaceutical product are a function of dose and rate of administration.
- Inhalational or dermal absorption is unlikely to lead to significant intoxication, although toxicity has been reported with prolonged exposure or misuse.
- **Children:** minor ingestions such as a taste or lick do not require hospital evaluation unless symptoms develop.

Toxic mechanism

These alcohols cause CNS effects similar to those of ethanol. More significant toxicity is a consequence of accumulation of metabolites. Diethylene glycol consists of two ethylene glycol molecules linked by a stable ether bond, and free ethylene glycol is not liberated. It is sequentially metabolised by alcohol dehydrogenase (ADH) and aldehyde dehydrogenase (ALDH) to the metabolites 2-hydroxyethoxyacetic acid (HEAA) and diglycolic acid (DGA), which cause renal and neurological toxicity.

EGBE and EGME also have stable ether linkages, preventing the formation of ethylene glycol – there are few case reports of poisoning from these agents, but toxicity is likely due to acid metabolites.

The cardiovascular and CNS effects of propylene glycol appear to be a direct toxic action, and metabolism of the molecule results in production of lactic acid.

Toxicokinetics
These alcohols are rapidly absorbed following ingestion and peak levels occur within 1 hour. They are distributed across total body water with volumes of distribution of 0.6 L/kg. They are metabolised sequentially by hepatic alcohol dehydrogenase (ADH) to pyruvate and lactate (propylene glycol), and aldehyde dehydrogenase (ALDH) to various alkoxy acetic acid products.

CLINICAL FEATURES
- Initial clinical features develop within the first 1–2 hours and are similar to those of ethanol intoxication: euphoria, nystagmus, drowsiness, nausea and vomiting.
- Progressively severe features develop over subsequent hours as metabolism progresses and acidosis worsens.
- Severe effects include coma, seizures, refractory shock and renal failure.
- Diethylene glycol is associated with early gastrointestinal features and metabolic acidosis:
  - Progressive renal and hepatic injury develop over 1–3 days, and renal failure may occur.
  - Multiple cranial and peripheral neuropathies may become evident during recovery.
  - Persistent coma or neurocognitive deficits may result from toxic encephalopathy.
- Onset of severe toxicity may be delayed up to 48 hours following ingestion of glycol ethers (EGBE, EGME).
- Over-rapid intravenous administration of excessive propylene glycol (administration of large quantities of drug with propylene glycol as a diluent) is associated with hypotension, bradycardia and sudden cardiovascular collapse.

INVESTIGATIONS
Screening tests in deliberate self-poisoning
- 12-lead ECG, BGL and paracetamol level

Specific investigations
Detection of toxic alcohols in the serum requires calculation of osmolar and anion gaps:
- Calculated serum osmolarity (EUC, blood gas, blood glucose, serum ethanol level)
- Measured serum osmolality (laboratory assay measuring freezing point depression)
- Calculated or measured anion gap (EUC, blood gas):
  - Ingestion of toxic alcohols results in initial elevation of the osmolar gap.

- As toxic alcohols are metabolised, the osmolar gap decreases and a high anion-gap metabolic acidosis (HAGMA) develops.
- Reliable calculation and measurement of osmolar and anion gaps requires simultaneous sampling of the relevant biochemical markers.
- Interpretation of the osmolar and anion gaps is dependent on the time course of the poisoning and is related to the time since ingestion and the presence or absence of ADH blockade (see **Chapter 2.15: Osmolar gap** and **Chapter 2.16: Acid–base disorders** for discussion regarding osmolar and anion gaps and interpretation of acid–base disturbances).
- Progressive decrease in the pH and venous bicarbonate concentration indicate worsening acidosis, but these are late signs of toxicity.
- Breath or serum ethanol level
  - Confirm or exclude co-ingestion of ethanol.
  - Monitor antidotal treatment with ethanol.
    - Note: Toxic alcohols are not detected by breath or serum ethanol assays.
- Serum toxic alcohol levels
  - Not readily available in a clinically useful time frame.

MANAGEMENT
Resuscitation, supportive care and monitoring
Severe toxic alcohol poisoning is a life-threatening emergency managed in an area equipped for cardiorespiratory monitoring and resuscitation.

- Patients may present with established toxicity, characterised by severe metabolic acidosis and a degree of respiratory compensation:
  - Attention to airway and breathing is paramount. In patients maintaining effective ventilation, intubation is to be avoided as even a brief period of apnoea during standard rapid sequence intubation can lead to cardiac arrest.
  - If intubation and ventilation is required for coma or ineffective ventilation, it is imperative to maintain adequate hyperventilation to maximise respiratory alkalosis.
- Sodium bicarbonate is an immediate priority in patients with severe metabolic acidosis awaiting haemodialysis:
  - Administer IV sodium bicarbonate boluses 1–2 mmol/kg guided by serial blood gases and clinical response.
  - Maintain hyperventilation and consider further bolus IV sodium bicarbonate to prevent worsening acidaemia pending haemodialysis.
- Patients who present early after ingestion, or who have co-ingested ethanol, may not yet have developed metabolic acidosis:
  - Calculation and assessment of the osmolar and anion gaps is vital to guide management decisions (see **Investigations**).
- Administration of ethanol (or fomepizole if available) is indicated prior to definitive blood results if significant toxic alcohol poisoning is considered a likely diagnosis.

Decontamination

- Activated charcoal does not adsorb toxic alcohols and is not indicated.

Enhanced elimination

- Haemodialysis is effective at removing toxic alcohols and correcting acidosis. The threshold for haemodialysis is less clearly defined for these toxic alcohols compared to ethylene glycol or methanol. Discussion with a clinical toxicologist or Poisons Information Centre is indicated. Reasonable indications include:
  - ingestion of toxic alcohol with an elevated osmolar gap >20
  - acidaemia with pH <7.3 or bicarbonate <20 mmol/L
  - renal impairment
  - worsening clinical status despite supportive care.

Antidotes

- Ethanol (see **Chapter 4.8: Ethanol**) and fomepizole (see **Chapter 4.11: Fomepizole**) are used in the treatment of diethylene glycol and glycol ether (EGBE, EGME) poisoning in the same way as they are for ethylene glycol poisoning.
- Ethanol at a serum concentration of 22 mmol/L (100 mg/dL; 0.1%) competitively inhibits ADH so that toxic alcohols are not metabolised.
- Fomepizole is a more potent competitive inhibitor of ADH, but is not readily available in most centres in Australia.
- Fomepizole is the preferred antidotal therapy for paediatric poisoning with toxic alcohols due to the risk of serious adverse effects from ethanol administration and the logistical difficulties inherent in instituting haemodialysis in paediatric patients.

DISPOSITION AND FOLLOW-UP

- Children and adult patients who remain clinically well after suspected accidental ingestion and have a normal venous bicarbonate level (≥20 mEq/L) at 8 or more hours post ingestion may be discharged.
- Adult patients who remain clinically well following accidental ingestion and have a normal venous bicarbonate level (≥20 mEq/L) 8 hours after serum or breath ethanol level is demonstrated to be undetectable are fit for medical discharge.
- All symptomatic patients and those with deliberate ingestion are assumed to have potentially lethal intoxication and are admitted to hospital for further evaluation and management.

HANDY TIPS

- Co-ingestion of ethanol delays the onset of clinical features of toxic alcohol poisoning.
- Plan for transfer to a facility with haemodialysis as soon as the provisional diagnosis of toxic alcohol poisoning is made.
- Serum bicarbonate and pH provide surrogate markers of toxic acid production and are useful to exclude significant ingestion in the absence of formal osmolar calculations, particularly in the setting of accidental ingestions.

PITFALLS
- Absence of symptoms on presentation does not exclude a significant ingestion.
- Normal osmolar gap (<10) does not exclude significant poisoning.
- Failure to recognise the concurrent presence of ethanol as a confounding factor in the risk assessment for toxic alcohol poisoning.
- Failure to recognise the potential for delay in development of toxicity in glycol ether and diethylene glycol ingestions.

CONTROVERSIES
- The indications for haemodialysis and antidote therapy in the management of these toxic alcohols is not well defined.
- The requirement for prolonged observation and monitoring following ingestion of complex glycol ethers (EGBE, EGME) to exclude the possibility of delayed onset (>24 hours) metabolic acidosis.

Sources

Diethylene glycol: hydraulic fluids, solvents
Glycol ethers (ethylene glycol monoethyl ether (EGME), ethylene glycol monobutyl ether (EGBE)): brake fluids, cleaning products, many solvents
Propylene glycol: solvents, many parenteral drug formulations
Benzyl alcohol: bacteriostatic agent frequently found in parenteral drug formulations

References

Kraut JA, Mullins ME. Toxic alcohols. The New England Journal of Medicine 2018; 378:270–280.
McMartin K, Jacobsen D, Hovda KE. Antidotes for poisoning by alcohols that form toxic metabolites. British Journal of Clinical Pharmacology 2016; 81(3):505–515.
Mégarbane B, Borron SW, Baud FJ. Current recommendations for treatment of severe toxic alcohol poisonings. Intensive Care Medicine 2005; 31(2):189–195.
Schep LJ, Slaughter RJ, Temple WA et al. Diethylene glycol poisoning. Clinical Toxicology 2009; 47(6):525–535.
Zar T, Graeber C, Perazella MA. Recognition, treatment, and prevention of propylene glycol toxicity. Seminars in Dialysis 2007; 20(3):217–219.

3.6 AMISULPRIDE

Amisulpride overdose is associated with QT prolongation and torsades de pointes. Patients ingesting >4 g should be monitored for at least 16 hours and until all ECG intervals are normal.

RISK ASSESSMENT
- Small overdoses (<4 g) are generally benign; however, QT prolongation and torsades de pointes have been reported.
- Larger ingestions (>4 g) pose an increasing risk of severe toxicity (see **Table 3.6.1**):
- **Children:** all accidental ingestions require assessment in hospital.

TABLE 3.6.1	Dose-related risk assessment: amisulpride
Dose	Risks
<4 g	QT prolongation and torsades de pointes have been reported in this dose range, especially in the presence of electrolyte abnormalities
>4 g	Cardiotoxicity including bradycardia, hypotension, QT prolongation, torsades de pointes and rate-dependent bundle branch blocks Seizures and coma with large ingestions

Toxic mechanism

Amisulpride is an atypical antipsychotic (benzamide derivative). It is a highly selective dopamine antagonist (binds to D_2 and D_3 receptors) with minimal affinity for other receptors.

Toxicokinetics

Amisulpride has an oral bioavailability of 50%. Peak serum concentrations are reached by 4 hours but may occur later than this in overdose. It has a large volume of distribution and limited metabolism to inactive metabolites. Most drug is excreted unchanged via faecal and renal routes, with an elimination half-life of 12 hours following therapeutic doses.

CLINICAL FEATURES

Patients may appear only mildly symptomatic for some hours, although QT prolongation may be evident on early 12-lead ECGs.

- Onset of sedation, bradycardia, hypotension and torsades de pointes is usually delayed some hours. The time to first episode of torsades de pointes is from 5 to 20 hours following ingestion. The latest reported occurrence of torsades de pointes is 32 hours following ingestion.
- Seizures and coma are rare but reported with large ingestions.

INVESTIGATIONS
Screening tests in deliberate self-poisoning
- 12-lead ECG, BGL and paracetamol level

Specific investigations
- Serial ECGs
  - The key investigation is the ECG. Any prolongation of the QT is significant and mandates continuous cardiac monitoring until it resolves (see **Chapter 2.17: The 12-lead ECG in toxicology**).
- EUC
  - Potassium, calcium and magnesium (QT dependent electrolytes).

MANAGEMENT
Resuscitation, supportive care and monitoring
- Amisulpride overdose is a potentially life-threatening emergency and is managed in a resuscitation area.
- Clinical features that require immediate intervention include:

- Hypotension
  - Volume resuscitation as appropriate.
- Torsades de pointes
  - Electrical cardioversion may be required for persistent episodes that result in altered mental state or haemodynamic instability.
  - Magnesium 10 mmol IV bolus (0.05 mmol/kg in children) over 1–2 minutes, repeated once if torsades de pointes recurs.
  - Isoprenaline or overdrive electrical pacing are other treatment options to increase the resting heart rate to a target of >100 beats/min.
  - Ensure that all QT-dependent electrolytes (potassium, calcium, magnesium) are at the upper limit of normal (see **Chapter 2.17: The 12-lead ECG in toxicology**).
- Seizures and coma: prompt intubation and ventilation is indicated in the presence of a depressed conscious state.
- Rate-related bundle branch blockade can occur, but sodium channel blockade similar to tricyclic antidepressant toxicity is not a feature of amisulpride poisoning.
  - Intravenous bolus sodium bicarbonate is not expected to improve QRS widening and is avoided due to the risk of exacerbating hypokalaemia and QT prolongation and promoting development of torsades de pointes (see **Chapter 4.24: Sodium bicarbonate**).
- Continuous cardiac and haemodynamic monitoring with serial 12-lead ECGs for a minimum of 16 hours is required if the ingested dose exceeds 4 g.

Decontamination
- Oral activated charcoal is appropriate following ingestion of >4 g within the previous 4 hours.

Enhanced elimination
- Not clinically useful.

Antidotes
- None available.

DISPOSITION AND FOLLOW-UP
- Patients who ingest <4 g, are clinically well and have a normal ECG and QT interval 6 hours post ingestion have a relatively low risk of clinical deterioration and may not require ongoing medical observation and cardiac monitoring.
- Patients who ingest >4 g are at higher risk of cardiotoxicity. If they are asymptomatic and have a normal ECG and QT interval at 16 hours post ingestion they do not require further medical management.
- The presence of any symptoms or QT prolongation mandates continued cardiac monitoring until these abnormalities resolve. Cardiac monitoring may be required for greater than 24 hours.

HANDY TIPS
- Following large ingestions, patients may demonstrate only mild symptoms for several hours prior to sudden deterioration.

- Bradycardia occurs in up to 25% of cases and is strongly associated with a higher risk of torsades de pointes.
- The magnitude of QT prolongation is a strong predictor of torsades de pointes.

PITFALL
- Failure to identify ECG abnormalities as risk factors for clinical deterioration.

CONTROVERSIES
- The threshold dose for risk of amisulpride-related QT prolongation and torsades de pointes. These features can occur at therapeutic doses.
- The duration of cardiac monitoring required for patients who remain asymptomatic with normal QT intervals, particularly for ingestions <4 g.

References
Isbister GK, Balit CR, MacLeod D et al. Amisulpride overdose is frequently associated with QT prolongation and torsades de pointes. Journal of Clinical Pharmacology 2010; 30(4):391–395.

Isbister GK, Murray L, John S et al. Amisulpride deliberate self poisoning causing severe cardiac toxicity including QT prolongation and torsades de pointes. Medical Journal of Australia 2006; 184:354–356.

Joy JP, Coulter CV, SB Duffull SB et al. Prediction of torsade de pointes from the QT interval: analysis of a case series of amisulpride overdoses. Clinical Pharmacology and Therapeutics 2011; 90(2):243–245.

3.7 AMPHETAMINES AND AMPHETAMINE-LIKE SUBSTANCES

Pharmaceutical agents: **Dexamphetamine, Lisdexamfetamine, Methylphenidate, Phentermine.**

Illicit agents: **Methamphetamine, 3,4-methylenedioxyamphetamine (MDA), 3,4 methylenedioxymethamphetamine (MDMA, ecstasy), Paramethoxyamphetamine (PMA), Cathinones, Phenylethylamines, Piperazines.**

See also Chapter 2.10: Amphetamine use disorder.

Amphetamines and amphetamine-like substances produce prominent central and peripheral sympathomimetic effects. Lethal complications include severe hyperthermia, acute coronary syndrome, cardiac dysrhythmias, aortic dissection, cardiomyopathy and intracranial haemorrhage. Repeated use leads to long-term neuropsychiatric sequelae.

Many emerging analogues have prominent hallucinogenic and serotonergic effects in addition to sympathomimetic properties. The principles of management – most importantly benzodiazepines and supportive care – are the same.

RISK ASSESSMENT
- Small doses of illicit agents may result in severe toxicity.
- Ingestion of pharmaceutical agents is less likely to cause life-threatening effects.
- The presence of hyperthermia, headache, impaired level of consciousness, focal neurological signs, chest pain or hypotension herald potentially life-threatening complications and warrant immediate management and investigation.
- Seizures are a feature of amphetamine emergency presentations.
- **Children:** one illicit amphetamine-derivative pill may lead to life-threatening sympathomimetic toxicity. Accidental ingestion of pharmaceutical sympathomimetic agents carries less risk of severe toxicity, but it is safest for all patients to be assessed in hospital.

Toxic mechanism
Amphetamine is structurally related to ephedrine (a phenylethylamine). Substitutions on the basic structure yield numerous derivatives with varying clinical effects. Amphetamines enhance the release of multiple neurotransmitters and block their reuptake. Inhibition of monoamine oxidase also occurs, leading to enhanced central and peripheral noradrenergic, dopaminergic and serotonergic stimulation. Sympathomimetic features are prominent in the clinical presentation. Long-term CNS effects occur due to neurotransmitter and receptor adaptation, as well as permanent destruction of dopaminergic neuropathways. MDMA at recreational doses can induce the syndrome of inappropriate antidiuretic hormone secretion (SIADH), leading to profound hyponatraemia, seizures and coma.

Toxicokinetics
Amphetamines and their analogues are well absorbed following ingestion and inhalation, and are also commonly injected intravenously. They are lipid-soluble weak bases and have large volumes of distribution (methamphetamine 3.5 L/kg). Most amphetamines undergo hepatic metabolism to form metabolites that are excreted in the urine. Elimination half-life varies from 8 to 30 hours.

CLINICAL FEATURES
Patients may present with symptoms of acute intoxication, medical complications of abuse or psychiatric sequelae. The most frequent presentation is agitation with sweating, tachycardia and hypertension. Acute clinical features may persist for more than 24 hours and include:
- Central nervous system
  - Euphoria
  - Anxiety, dysphoria, agitation and aggression
  - Hyperthermia, rigidity and myoclonic movements
  - Seizures
- Cardiovascular
  - Tachydysrhythmias
  - Hypertension
  - Hypotension
  - Acute coronary syndrome
  - Acute cardiomyopathy
  - Acute pulmonary oedema

- Peripheral sympathomimetic
  - Mydriasis, sweating and tremor
- Clinical features associated with medical complications
  - Rhabdomyolysis, dehydration and renal failure
  - Hyponatraemia and cerebral oedema (particularly following MDMA ingestion)
  - Aortic and carotid artery dissection
  - Intracerebral haemorrhage
  - Subarachnoid haemorrhage can occur and may arise from pre-existing cerebral aneurysms.
- Psychiatric
  - Paranoid psychosis with visual and tactile hallucinations.
  - Paranoid ideation commonly occurs in acute intoxication and may persist as part of a post-amphetamine psychosis when other features of acute intoxication have resolved.

INVESTIGATIONS

Screening tests in deliberate self-poisoning
- 12-lead ECG, BGL and paracetamol level

Specific investigations
- Blood gas, EUC and creatine kinase
  - Detect hyponatraemia, metabolic acidosis, rhabdomyolysis and renal failure.
- ECG and troponin
  - Detect acute coronary syndrome.
- CT head/neck/chest
  - Detect intracranial haemorrhage or vascular dissection.
- Echocardiogram
  - Assess cardiac function.
- Serum or urine amphetamine levels rarely assist acute management. They may be useful to confirm use, particularly during forensic or psychiatric evaluation.

MANAGEMENT

Resuscitation, supportive care and monitoring
- Amphetamine intoxication is a potentially life-threatening emergency and patients are managed in an area capable of cardiorespiratory monitoring and resuscitation.
- Attention to airway, breathing and circulation are paramount. These priorities are managed along conventional lines, as outlined in **Chapter 1.2: Resuscitation**.
- Early life-threats that require immediate intervention include:
  - tachydysrhythmias
  - hypertension
  - hypotension
  - acute coronary syndrome
  - seizures and agitated delirium
  - hyperthermia
  - hyponatraemia.

- Treat tachycardia and hypertension initially with titrated parenteral benzodiazepines. If haemodynamic toxicity is refractory to benzodiazepine sedation, consider:
  - titrated vasodilator infusion (glyceryl trinitrate, sodium nitroprusside)
  - labetalol 10–20 mg IV repeated every 10 minutes to a maximum of 300 mg (or as an infusion)
  - clonidine 50–100 microgram IV tds
- Acute coronary syndrome is largely managed according to standard protocols with the following caveats:
  - Pure beta-blockers are relatively contraindicated – labetalol may be preferable because of its combined alpha- and beta-blocking effects (see **Controversies**).
  - Thrombolysis may not be appropriate as the pathophysiology is frequently vasospasm or dissection.
- Persistent hypotension is a significant feature that suggests cardiogenic shock from acute stress-induced (sympathomimetic) cardiomyopathy. Immediate resuscitation and investigations are indicated to guide ongoing management, including decisions regarding inotropic support (see **Chapter 2.2: Hypotension**).
- Seizures are managed with IV benzodiazepines (see **Chapter 2.3: Seizures**).
- Agitation is managed with titrated doses of benzodiazepines. Oral diazepam may be considered in mild cases (10–20 mg diazepam PO repeated as necessary) but IV therapy should be instituted early where agitation is moderate or severe.
  - Give midazolam or diazepam 2.5–10 mg IV titrated to effect. Further doses may be required.
  - Additional or alternative agents include droperidol 5–10 mg IM or IV, or olanzapine 5–10 mg SL, IM or IV (see **Chapter 2.4: Approach to delirium**).
- Hyperthermia:
  - Temperature >38.5°C is an indication for continuous core-temperature monitoring, benzodiazepine sedation and fluid resuscitation.
  - Temperature >39.5°C requires rapid external cooling to prevent multiple organ failure and neurological injury. Paralysis, intubation and ventilation may be required.
- Hyponatraemia:
  - Immediate correction with hypertonic saline is indicated if the serum sodium is <120 mmol/L and is associated with altered mental status or seizures. Give hypertonic saline (3% sodium chloride) 3 mL/kg over 30 minutes, aiming for an increase in serum sodium of 4–6 mmol/L and improvement in clinical features. Resolution of SIADH manifests by diuresis and correction of hyponatraemia, usually within 24 hours.

Decontamination
- Amphetamines ingested orally are rapidly absorbed, and activated charcoal is not recommended.

Enhanced elimination
- Not clinically useful.

Antidotes
- None available.

DISPOSITION AND FOLLOW-UP
- Children with accidental ingestions should be observed in hospital for 4 hours following immediate-release and 12 hours following controlled-release preparations. If they do not develop symptoms during that period, they may be safely discharged.
- Patients whose intoxication is adequately controlled with benzodiazepine sedation and have normal vital signs and 12-lead ECG may be managed supportively in a ward environment. They may be discharged when clinically well.
- Patients with significant alteration of conscious state, ongoing chest pain or hyperthermia are managed in a critical care area.

HANDY TIPS
- Early control of agitation with adequate doses of IV benzodiazepines calms the patient and improves tachycardia, hypertension and hyperthermia.
- Abnormal mental status or focal neurological signs prompt exclusion of hyponatraemia, hypoglycaemia, aortic dissection or intracranial haemorrhage.
- Phentolamine 1–5 mg IV (repeated as necessary up to 15 mg) is an effective treatment for hypertension, but it is not readily available.
- Beta-blockers and verapamil may cause significant haemodynamic deterioration due to negative inotropic effects if cardiomyopathy is present.
- Amphetamine-induced movement disorder can result from excessive dopaminergic stimulation. It is characterised by choreoathetoid movements and dysphoria and must be differentiated from acute dystonic reactions. It responds to antipsychotic (antidopaminergic) medication such as droperidol or olanzapine if benzodiazepines are not effective.

PITFALLS
- Failure to adequately sedate the agitated or hyper-adrenergic patient.
- Failure to recognise the significance of persistent hypotension as a marker of acute cardiomyopathy, and institute therapy appropriately.
- Failure to detect and treat hyperthermia promptly.
- Failure to detect and treat hyponatraemia in a patient presenting with altered mental status or seizures.

CONTROVERSIES
- Administration of beta-adrenergic blockers in the acute management of amphetamine intoxication. They are relatively contraindicated as unopposed alpha-adrenergic stimulation may cause severe vasoconstriction. However, emerging data suggest that titrated dosing may be used. Labetalol is a theoretically

preferable agent due to combined alpha- and beta-blocking effects.
— Note: Both beta-blockers and verapamil may cause significant haemodynamic deterioration due to negative inotropic effects in the presence of catecholamine-induced cardiomyopathy.

Presentations

Prescription medications
Dexamphetamine 5 mg tablets (100)
Methylphenidate 10 mg tablets (100)
Methylphenidate 20 mg, 30 mg, 40 mg capsules (30)
Methylphenidate 18 mg, 27 mg, 36 mg, 54 mg extended-release tablets (30)
Phentermine

Illicit amphetamine-derivative pills
Methamphetamine: ice, speed, P
3,4-methylenedioxymethamphetamine (MDMA): ecstasy, XTC
3,4-methylenedioxyamphetamine (MDA): love drug

Cathinones
Khat (*Catha edulis*)
Mephedrone (4-methylmethcathinone): Bath salts, Plant food

Phenylethylamines

Piperazines

References
Downes M, Whyte I. Amphetamine-induced movement disorder. Emergency Medicine Australasia 2005; 17:277–280.
Richards JR, Albertson TE, Derleta RW et al. Treatment of toxicity from amphetamines, related derivatives, and analogues: a systematic clinical review. Drug and Alcohol Dependence 2015. http://dx.doi.org/10.1016/j.drugalcdep.2015.01.040.
Rietjens SJ, Hondebrink L, Jorna T et al. Methylphenidate poisoning: relatively mild symptoms even after high dose exposure. Clinical Toxicology 2017; 55(8):941–942.

SPECIFIC TOXINS

163

TOXICOLOGY HANDBOOK

3.8 ANGIOTENSIN-CONVERTING ENZYME INHIBITORS (ACEIs) AND ANGIOTENSIN II RECEPTOR BLOCKERS (ARBs)

ACEIs: Captopril, Enalapril, Fosinopril, Lisinopril, Perindopril, Quinapril, Ramipril, Trandolapril.

ARBs: Candesartan, Eprosartan, Irbesartan, Losartan, Olmesartan, Telmisartan, Valsartan.

Overdose with angiotensin-converting enzyme inhibitors (ACEIs) or angiotensin II receptor blockers (ARBs) is relatively benign. The principal toxic effect is mild-to-moderate hypotension usually responsive to fluid therapy.

RISK ASSESSMENT
- Overdose with these agents usually causes only mild hypotension, irrespective of the dose ingested.
- Hypotension is apparent within 4 hours of ingestion and is managed primarily with intravenous fluid administration.
- Co-ingestion with other vasodilating agents (e.g. dihydropyridine calcium channel blockers, alpha-blockers) can cause more

profound and resistant hypotension requiring haemodynamic support.
- **Children:** accidental paediatric ingestion of ACEIs or ARBs only requires hospital evaluation if symptoms develop.

Toxic mechanism
ACE inhibitors reversibly inhibit angiotensin-converting enzyme, preventing conversion of angiotensin I to angiotensin II, a potent vasoconstrictor. Angiotensin II has endocrine effects and its inhibition leads to a reduction in circulating aldosterone, which can result in hyperkalaemia. Angiotensin II receptor blockers cause similar clinical effects by their action at vascular and tissue receptors.

Toxicokinetics
All these agents are rapidly absorbed with peak levels occurring within 1–2 hours. Many agents are prodrugs requiring hepatic conversion to active metabolites. Elimination is by hepatic and renal pathways.

CLINICAL FEATURES
Patients are usually asymptomatic. The principal clinical feature is mild hypotension, which occurs within 4 hours of the ingestion and may last several hours.

INVESTIGATIONS
Screening tests in deliberate self-poisoning
- 12-lead ECG, BGL and paracetamol level

Specific investigations
- EUC
    - Detect hyperkalaemia or renal impairment.

MANAGEMENT
Resuscitation, supportive care and monitoring
- Resuscitation is rarely required and management is supportive.
- Patients presenting with significant hypotension usually respond to a fluid bolus of 10–20 mL/kg of intravenous fluid.
- Vasopressor therapy may be required if hypotension persists despite appropriate volume resuscitation.
- Non-invasive haemodynamic monitoring is usually sufficient.

Decontamination
- Oral activated charcoal may be given to the patient who presents within 1 hour of ingestion.

Enhanced elimination
- Not clinically useful.

Antidotes
- None available.

DISPOSITION AND FOLLOW-UP
- The patient who remains asymptomatic with normal vital signs at 4 hours following ingestion does not require further medical management.
- The symptomatic or hypotensive patient is admitted for ongoing supportive care until clinical features of poisoning resolve.

Presentations
Captopril 12.5 mg, 25 mg, 50 mg tablets (90)
Captopril 50 mg tablets (90)
Enalapril maleate 5 mg, 10 mg, 20 mg tablets (30)
Enalapril maleate 20 mg/hydrochlorothiazide 6 mg tablets (30)
Fosinopril sodium 10 mg, 20 mg tablets (30)
Fosinopril sodium 10 mg/hydrochlorothiazide 12.5 mg tablets (30)
Fosinopril sodium 20 mg/hydrochlorothiazide 12.5 mg tablets (30)
Lisinopril dihydrate 5 mg, 10 mg, 20 mg tablets (30)
Perindopril erbumine 2 mg, 4 mg, 8 mg tablets (30)
Perindopril erbumine 4 mg/indapamide hemihydrate 1.25 mg tablets (30)
Quinapril hydrochloride 5 mg, 10 mg, 20 mg tablets (30)
Ramipril 1.25 mg, 2.5 mg, 5 mg, 10 mg tablets (30)
Trandolapril 0.5 mg, 1 mg, 2 mg, 4 mg tablets (28)
Trandolapril 2 mg/verapamil hydrochloride 180 mg sustained-release tablets (28)
Trandolapril 4 mg/verapamil hydrochloride 240 mg sustained-release tablets (28)

References

Balit CR, Gilmore SP, Isbister GK. Unintentional paediatric ingestions of angiotensin converting enzyme inhibitors and angiotensin II receptor antagonists. Journal of Paediatrics and Child Health 2007; 43(10):686–688.

Christie GA, Lucas C, Bateman DN et al. Redefining the ACE-inhibitor dose–response relationship: substantial blood pressure lowering after massive doses. European Journal of Clinical Pharmacology 2006; 62(12):989–993.

Huang J, Buckley NA, Isoardi KZ et al. Angiotensin axis antagonists increase the incidence of haemodynamic instability in dihydropyridine calcium channel blocker poisoning. Clinical Toxicology 2021; 59(6):464–471.

Prasa D, Hoffmann-Walbeck P, Barth S et al. Angiotensin II antagonists – an assessment of their acute toxicity. Clinical Toxicology 2013; 51(5):429–434.

3.9 ANTICOAGULANT RODENTICIDES

Brodifacoum, Bromadiolone, Chlorophacinone, Difenacoum, Diphacinone, Flocoumafen

Long-acting anticoagulant rodenticides or 'superwarfarins' were developed to counter rodent resistance to warfarin. Single unintentional paediatric ingestions are non-toxic. In contrast, massive or repeated dosing leads to profound and prolonged (weeks to months) anticoagulation. Warfarin is discussed in Chapter 3.81: Warfarin.

RISK ASSESSMENT

- Single accidental ingestion does not cause significant anticoagulation.
- Massive single ingestion of >0.1 mg/kg of brodifacoum will cause anticoagulation but this equates to 2 g/kg of 0.005% bait or 3 × 50-g pellet packs in a 75-kg adult.
- Anticoagulation is usually associated with repeated ingestion. In this scenario, severe, prolonged (weeks to months) anticoagulation requiring massive doses of vitamin K is anticipated.
- **Children:** it is estimated that a young child needs to ingest >30 g of a 0.005% preparation as a single dose to cause significant anticoagulation. This has never been reported.

Toxic mechanism

These agents inhibit hepatic vitamin K-dependent production of clotting factors II, VII, IX and X in the same way as warfarin. Several mechanisms confer increased potency and prolonged duration of action: greater affinity for vitamin K_1 2,3-epoxide reductase, disruption of vitamin K cycle at several sites and hepatic accumulation. These agents have prolonged elimination half-lives.

Toxicokinetics

These agents are completely absorbed following oral administration. They are highly lipid soluble and have large volumes of distribution. They are concentrated in the liver. Superwarfarins undergo hepatic metabolism and enterohepatic recirculation and have very prolonged elimination phases of weeks to months.

CLINICAL FEATURES

- Patients are usually asymptomatic.
- Severe coagulopathy manifests as bruising, petechial or purpuric rashes, gingival bleeding, epistaxis or haematuria.
- Following acute single ingestions, coagulopathy may not be evident for 12 hours, and is frequently delayed 24–48 hours. Peak effects occur at 72–96 hours.

INVESTIGATIONS
Screening tests in deliberate self-poisoning
- 12-lead ECG, BGL and paracetamol level

Specific investigations
- INR
  - In patients who are not anticoagulated, INR will be normal during the first 6–12 hours after deliberate overdose. Following massive overdose, perform serial INRs every 12 hours for 48 hours to rule out toxicity. Vitamin K should be withheld until anticoagulation is documented. Normal INR at 48 hours excludes toxic ingestion.
  - Following repeated ingestion over several days, INR is abnormal at presentation. Vitamin K therapy may commence immediately. Outpatient INR estimations are required to monitor therapy.
- Superwarfarin levels
  - Not widely available.
  - Useful to confirm diagnosis in cases where paediatric non-accidental injury or occult poisoning is suspected.
  - Useful to determine when vitamin K therapy can safely be stopped.

MANAGEMENT
Resuscitation, supportive care and monitoring
- In patients with evidence of haemorrhage, attention to airway, breathing and circulation are paramount. These priorities can usually be managed along conventional lines, as outlined in **Chapter 1.2: Resuscitation**.
- If there is active uncontrolled bleeding, administer prothrombin complex concentrate (PCC; 25–50 IU/kg as an initial dose). It is likely that this will provide rapid and adequate immediate reversal of the coagulopathy in most situations (see **Controversies** below).
  - Three-factor PCC contains factors II, IX and X, but only low levels of factor VII.

- — Four-factor PCC has higher levels of factor VII but is not currently available in Australia.
- Fresh frozen plasma (150–300 mL as an initial dose) provides additional coagulation factors (particularly factor VII). It is recommended in addition to PCC or if the severity of bleeding is such that all available reversal agents are required.
- If PCC is not available, a higher initial dose of FFP is recommended (10–15 mL/kg).
- Vitamin K 5–10 mg IV is given after consideration of the requirement for ongoing anticoagulation with warfarin (see **Antidotes** below). If alternative agents will be used for ongoing therapeutic anticoagulation, full reversal with large doses of vitamin K is appropriate.
- In the absence of active bleeding, the decision to give reversal therapy is determined by the INR level and the presence of high-risk factors for clinically significant bleeding (see **Chapter 3.81: Warfarin**).
- General supportive care measures are indicated, as outlined in **Chapter 1.4: Supportive care and monitoring**.

Decontamination
- Activated charcoal is not indicated following accidental ingestions.
- Following massive single acute deliberate self-poisoning, administer 50 g activated charcoal to cooperative patients who present within 12 hours of ingestion.

Enhanced elimination
- Not clinically useful.

Antidotes
- Vitamin K (phytomenadione) is indicated where there is documented anticoagulation from repeated deliberate ingestion or following acute deliberate self-poisoning. Prophylactic vitamin K is not indicated. In patients with proven anticoagulation, vitamin K is titrated to achieve safe INR levels. Very large daily doses of oral vitamin K may be required for weeks or months. Initial daily dose is variable and requires close medical supervision with repeated INR measurements until stable dosing is determined. See antidote **Chapter 4.27: Vitamin K** for details.

DISPOSITION AND FOLLOW-UP
- Minor accidental ingestions by adults or children do not require hospital observation or investigation.
- Referral for an INR is indicated where there is acute deliberate self-poisoning, suspicion of repeated ingestion or abnormal bleeding. A normal INR 48 hours after the last ingestion excludes toxicity.
- Following massive single ingestions, INR is monitored for 48 hours. A normal INR at 48 hours excludes toxicity and the patient does not require further medical monitoring.
- Established anticoagulation requires hospital admission for stabilisation on high-dose oral vitamin K. Prolonged supervision of INRs and compliance with vitamin K therapy is essential and arranged prior to discharge in consultation with mental health services.

PITFALL

- Prophylactic vitamin K therapy following an acute ingestion delays diagnosis of subsequent toxicity and prolongs the need for medical supervision.

Presentations

Pellets, wax blocks, paste and liquid concentrate. Often coloured blue, green or red and may contain a bittering agent.
Typical concentration is 0.005% (5 mg/100 g).
Pellet packs are typically 50 g (i.e. contain 2.5 mg brodifacoum).
Concentrates may be up to 0.25% (250 mg/100 g).

References

Gunja N, Coggins A, Bidny S. Management of intentional superwarfarin poisoning with long-term vitamin K and brodifacoum levels. Clinical Toxicology 2011; 49:385–390.

Ingels M, Lai C, Tai W et al. A prospective study of acute, unintentional, pediatric superwarfarin ingestions managed without decontamination. Annals of Emergency Medicine 2002; 40(1):73–78.

Shepherd G, Klein-Schwartz W, Anderson BD. Acute unintentional pediatric brodifacoum ingestions. Pediatric Emergency Care 2002; 18(3):174–178.

Watt BE, Proudfoot AT, Bradberry SM et al. Anticoagulant rodenticides. Toxicological Reviews 2005; 24(4):259–269.

3.10 ANTICONVULSANTS: NEWER AGENTS

Gabapentin, Levetiracetam, Oxcarbazepine, Tiagabine, Topiramate, Vigabatrin

The newer anticonvulsants are generally much less toxic in overdose than the older agents – phenobarbitone (see Chapter 3.15: Barbiturates), carbamazepine (see Chapter 3.23: Carbamazepine), phenytoin (see Chapter 3.65: Phenytoin) and valproic acid (see Chapter 3.79: Valproic acid). Sedation and non-specific neurological symptoms may occur. Treatment is supportive and a favourable outcome can be anticipated.

RISK ASSESSMENT

- Most overdoses with these agents produce mild and transient CNS symptoms only.
- Symptoms usually appear within 2 hours and resolve within 24 hours.
- Coma and seizures can occur but are rare.
- **Children:** accidental paediatric ingestion is unlikely to cause significant toxicity. Referral to hospital is indicated if neurological features occur.

Toxic mechanism

These agents exert anticonvulsant effect by inhibiting excitatory neurotransmission or enhancing GABA activity. Additional mechanisms of toxicity in overdose are not clearly defined. Gabapentin is a structural analogue of GABA but exerts its effect by blockade of voltage-gated calcium channels in the CNS. Topiramate has multiple pharmacological effects, including inhibition of carbonic anhydrase enzymes. Oxcarbazepine, although structurally similar to carbamazepine, is much less toxic in overdose.

Toxicokinetics

Most agents are well absorbed orally, with linear kinetics, and undergo hepatic metabolism to inactive metabolites that are excreted renally. Topiramate is primarily excreted unchanged in the urine. Absorption of gabapentin from the GI tract is saturable at higher doses and this limits toxicity following overdose.

CLINICAL FEATURES

- Gabapentin overdose
  - Nausea, vomiting mild sedation and tachycardia
- Levetiracetam overdose
  - Sedation and respiratory depression
- Oxcarbazepine overdose
  - Sedation, usually mild even after massive overdose
- Tiagabine overdose
  - Sedation, coma, respiratory depression and seizures
- Topiramate overdose
  - Ataxia, sedation, coma and seizures
  - Non-anion gap metabolic acidosis secondary to carbonic anhydrase inhibition can occur, and resolves over several days. It is of little clinical significance.
- Vigabatrin overdose
  - Drowsiness and delirium

INVESTIGATIONS
Screening tests in deliberate self-poisoning
- 12-lead ECG, BGL and paracetamol level

Specific investigations
- EUC and venous blood gas for topiramate overdose.
- Specific drug levels are neither readily available nor clinically useful.

MANAGEMENT
Resuscitation, supportive care and monitoring
- Attention to airway, breathing and circulation are paramount. These priorities are managed along conventional lines, as outlined in **Chapter 1.2: Resuscitation**.
- Clinical features that require immediate intervention include:
  - Respiratory depression or coma are indications for intubation and ventilation.
  - Seizures are managed with titrated doses of benzodiazepines as described in **Chapter 2.3: Seizures**.
- General supportive care measures are indicated, as outlined in **Chapter 1.4: Supportive care and monitoring**.

Decontamination
- Routine gastrointestinal decontamination is not indicated for these agents, due to rapid absorption and relatively mild toxicity.
- A dose of activated charcoal 50 g (1 g/kg in children) may be given via a nasogastric tube to the patient with coma or seizures after the airway is secured with endotracheal intubation.

Enhanced elimination
- Not clinically useful.

Antidotes
- None available.

- Children may be observed at home following suspected unintentional ingestion of these agents. Referral for hospital assessment and management is required if they become symptomatic.
- Patients who remain asymptomatic 6 hours post ingestion are medically fit for discharge. Those who develop symptoms are admitted for further observation and supportive care until those symptoms resolve, usually within 24 hours.

Handy Tips

- Coma has been reported with large overdoses of some of these agents. However, other toxicological causes for coma should be sought in such cases, including other anticonvulsants such as carbamazepine, valproic acid or barbiturates.

Presentations

Gabapentin 100 mg, 300 mg, 400 mg, 600 mg, 800 mg capsules (100)
Levetiracetam 250 mg, 500 mg, 1000 mg tablets (60)
Levetiracetam 100 mg/1 mL oral solution (300 mL)
Levetiracetam 500 mg/5 mL vials
Oxcarbazepine 150 mg, 300 mg, 600 mg tablets (100)
Oxcarbazepine 60 mg/1 mL oral suspension (250 mL)
Tiagabine hydrochloride 5 mg, 10 mg, 15 mg tablets (50)
Topiramate 25 mg, 50 mg, 100 mg, 200 mg tablets (60)
Topiramate 15 mg, 25 mg, 50 mg sprinkle capsules (60)
Vigabatrin 500 mg (100)
Vigabatrin 500 mg sachets (60)

References

Fischer JH, Barr AN, Rogers SL et al. Lack of serious toxicity following gabapentin overdose. Neurology 1994; 44(5):982–983.

Klein-Schwartz W, Shepherd JG, Gorman S et al. Characterization of gabapentin overdose using a poison center case series. Journal of Toxicology–Clinical Toxicology 2003; 41(1):11–15.

Traub JS, Howland MA, Hoffman RS et al. Acute topiramate toxicity. Journal of Toxicology–Clinical Toxicology 2003; 41(7):987–990.

Wade JF, Dang CV, Nelson L et al. Emergent complications of the newer anticonvulsants. Journal of Emergency Medicine 2010; 38(2):231–237.

Wisniewski M, Lukasek-Glebocka M, Anand JS. Acute topiramate overdose – clinical manifestations. Clinical Toxicology 2009; 47:317–320.

3.11 ANTIHISTAMINES (NON-SEDATING)

Cetirizine, Desloratadine, Fexofenadine, Levocetirizine, Loratadine

See also Chapter 3.12: Antihistamines (sedating).

Overdose of non-sedating antihistamines is benign and has a good outcome with minimal supportive care. They cause only mild sedation and the risk of cardiac dysrhythmias is low unless there are pre-existing QT abnormalities.

RISK ASSESSMENT

- Mild sedation or anticholinergic effects may occur following overdose.

- QT prolongation following overdose is reported but rare.
- **Children:** accidental ingestion is unlikely to cause significant toxicity and the child may be observed at home unless symptoms develop. Referral for hospital assessment and management is required if they become symptomatic.

Toxic mechanism

Non-sedating antihistamines are mildly lipophilic and less able to cross the blood–brain barrier than sedating antihistamines. They are selective, competitive reversible inhibitors of peripheral H_1 receptors. Compared to sedating antihistamines, they have lower affinity for central H_1, muscarinic (M_1), α_1-adrenergic and serotonergic (5-HT) receptors. In overdose, selectivity may be lost and some sedation, anticholinergic effects and hypotension may be seen. QT interval prolongation is secondary to cardiac potassium channel blockade.

Toxicokinetics

Non-sedating antihistamines are well absorbed, reach peak effects in 1–3 hours and have volumes of distribution of less than 1.5 L/kg. Hepatic metabolism is minor and half-lives are variable, ranging from 8 to 24 hours.

CLINICAL FEATURES
- Minor sedation, nausea and ataxia
- Mild anticholinergic symptoms
- Symptoms develop within 2 hours of ingestion and resolve within 12 hours.

INVESTIGATIONS
Screening tests in deliberate self-poisoning
- 12-lead ECG, BGL and paracetamol level

MANAGEMENT
Resuscitation, supportive care and monitoring
- Resuscitation is rarely required.
- General supportive care measures are indicated, as outlined in **Chapter 1.4: Supportive care and monitoring**.
- Manage anticholinergic delirium as outlined in **Chapter 2.6: Anticholinergic toxicity**.
- Monitor for urinary retention with serial bladder scans and insert an indwelling urinary catheter if required.

Decontamination
- Activated charcoal is not indicated.

Enhanced elimination
- Not clinically useful.

Antidotes
- None indicated.

DISPOSITION AND FOLLOW-UP
- Patients who are clinically well 6 hours post ingestion are medically fit for discharge.

HANDY TIP
- Most ingestions are benign and have a good outcome with minimal supportive care.

PITFALL
- Failing to recognise the potential for QT prolongation in overdose.

Presentations
Cetirizine hydrochloride 10 mg tablets (7, 10, 30)
Cetirizine hydrochloride 1 mg/1 mL oral solution (75, 200 mL)
Cetirizine hydrochloride 10 mg/1 mL oral drops (20 mL)
Desloratadine 5 mg tablets (7, 28)
Fexofenadine hydrochloride 30 mg, 50 mg tablets (10, 20)
Fexofenadine hydrochloride 120 mg, 180 mg tablets (10, 20, 30, 50)
Fexofenadine hydrochloride 60 mg/pseudoephedrine 120 mg tablets (10)
Levocetirizine 5 mg tablets (10, 30)
Loratadine 10 mg tablets (10, 30, 50)
Loratadine 1 mg/1 mL syrup (100 mL, 150 mL, 200 mL)
Loratadine 5 mg/pseudoephedrine 120 mg modified-release tablets (6)

References
Ten Eick AP, Blumer JL, Reed MD. Safety of antihistamines in children. Drug Safety 2001; 24(2):119–147.
Thomas SHL. Antihistamine poisoning. Medicine 2012; 40(3):109–110.

3.12 ANTIHISTAMINES (SEDATING)

Brompheniramine, Chlorpheniramine, Cyproheptadine, Dexchlorpheniramine, Dimenhydrinate, Diphenhydramine, Doxylamine, Pheniramine, Promethazine

See also Chapter 3.11: Antihistamines (non-sedating).

Overdose is characterised by dose-dependent sedation and anticholinergic effects. The mainstay of treatment is supportive care.

RISK ASSESSMENT
- Sedation and anticholinergic delirium are dose-dependent, but the toxic dose is not clearly established for all agents.
- All agents lower seizure threshold, but seizures are infrequent.
- Cardiac conduction abnormalities (prolonged QRS or QT intervals) can occur but the risk of ventricular dysrhythmias is low.
- **Children:** children are more susceptible to the toxic effects of sedating antihistamines than adults. All accidental ingestions in children under the age of 2 require medical assessment.

Toxic mechanism
Antihistamines act by competitive inhibition of histamine (H_1) receptors. Side effects and toxicity are due to blockade at muscarinic (M_1), α_1-adrenergic and serotonergic (5-HT) receptors. Cardiac sodium and potassium channel blockade is reported in massive ingestions.

Toxicokinetics
Antihistamines are well absorbed orally, reaching peak levels in 2–3 hours. They are lipid soluble, have large volumes of distribution (>4 L/kg) and are metabolised in the liver. Half-lives are variable and range between 6 and 18 hours.

- CNS depression can result in coma requiring intubation. This is more likely if other sedative agents (including alcohol) are ingested.
- Anticholinergic effects including agitated delirium (see **Chapter 2.6: Anticholinergic toxicity**).
- Seizures, hyperthermia and rhabdomyolysis are rare.
- Tachycardia is common, but significant haemodynamic instability is unlikely.

Screening tests in deliberate self-poisoning
- 12-lead ECG, BGL and paracetamol level

Specific investigations
- An ECG should be performed on presentation and at 6 hours post ingestion to detect QRS or QT interval prolongation. Further ECGs are only necessary if an abnormality is noted.

Resuscitation, supportive care and monitoring
- Attention to airway, breathing and circulation are paramount. These priorities are managed along conventional lines, as outlined in **Chapter 1.2: Resuscitation**.
- General supportive care measures are indicated, as outlined in **Chapter 1.4: Supportive care and monitoring**.
- Manage anticholinergic delirium as outlined in **Chapter 2.6: Anticholinergic toxicity**.
- Monitor for urinary retention with serial bladder scans and insert an indwelling urinary catheter if required.
- Manage seizures as outlined in **Chapter 2.3: Seizures**.
- Hypotension usually responds to fluid administration.
- Ventricular dysrhythmias secondary to QRS or QT prolongation are very rare. In the unlikely event of this occurrence, management is as follows:
  - QRS prolongation complicated by ventricular dysrhythmias
    - IV bolus sodium bicarbonate, intubation and hyperventilation, as outlined in **Chapter 2.17: The 12-lead ECG in toxicology**.
  - QT prolongation complicated by ventricular dysrhythmias (torsades de pointes):
    - Electrical cardioversion may be required for persistent episodes that result in altered mental state or haemodynamic instability.
    - Magnesium 10 mmol IV bolus (0.05 mmol/kg in children) over 1–2 minutes, repeated once if torsades de pointes recurs.
    - Isoprenaline or overdrive electrical pacing are other treatment options to increase the resting heart rate to a target of >100 beats/min.
    - Ensure that all QT-dependent electrolytes (potassium, calcium, magnesium) are at the upper limit of normal (see **Chapter 2.17: The 12-lead ECG in toxicology**).
- Monitor for urinary retention with serial bladder scans and insert an indwelling urinary catheter if required.

Decontamination

- Activated charcoal can be considered in the asymptomatic patient presenting within 2 hours of ingestion of promethazine in order to decrease the incidence of anticholinergic delirium.
- Sedation can occur rapidly, and supportive care alone will ensure a good outcome. If the patient has a decreased level of consciousness, activated charcoal is only given once the airway is protected following intubation.

Enhanced elimination

- Not clinically useful.

Antidotes

- Physostigmine administration is considered in patients with severe anticholinergic delirium not controlled with benzodiazepines (see **Chapter 4.21: Physostigmine**).

DISPOSITION AND FOLLOW-UP

- Patients who remain asymptomatic and have a normal 12-lead ECG at 6 hours may be discharged. Discharge should not occur at night.
- Patients with mild sedation or anticholinergic features are managed supportively in a ward environment. They are fit for medical discharge when clinically well.
- Patients with significant agitation or delirium, and those requiring intubation, require management in a high-dependency or intensive care unit.
- Ongoing cardiac monitoring is required for patients with abnormal QRS or QT intervals until changes resolve.

HANDY TIP

- Antihistamines may be taken recreationally for their anticholinergic properties.

PITFALLS

- Failure to recognise anticholinergic delirium because of concomitant sedative effects.
- Failure to detect and relieve urinary retention. This exacerbates agitation and prevents control with benzodiazepine sedation.

Presentations

Alkylamines
Brompheniramine 2 mg/5 mL in decongestant elixirs
Chlorpheniramine 0.5–6 mg/tablet or 5 mL of elixir in cold and flu formulations
Dexchlorpheniramine maleate 2 mg, 6 mg modified-release tablets (20, 40)
Dexchlorpheniramine 2.5 mg/1 mL syrup (100 mL)
Ethanolamines
Dimenhydrinate 50 mg/hyoscine hydrobromide 0.2 mg/caffeine 20 mg tablets (10)
Diphenhydramine hydrochloride 50 mg capsules or tablets (10)
Diphenhydramine 2.5 mg/mL in cough syrup formulations
Doxylamine succinate 25 mg capsules (20)
Doxylamine succinate 6.25 mg per tablet in cold and flu preparations
Doxylamine 5–6.25 mg per tablet with paracetamol–codeine combination analgesics
Phenothiazines
Pheniramine maleate 43.5 mg tablets (10, 50)

Promethazine hydrochloride 10 mg, 25 mg tablets (50)
Promethazine hydrochloride 1 mg/1 mL elixir (100 mL)
Promethazine hydrochloride 25 mg/1 mL ampoules
Promethazine hydrochloride 50 mg/2 mL ampoules
Promethazine hydrochloride in cold and flu formulations and analgesics (e.g. Pain Stop)
Trimeprazine 7.5 mg/5 mL syrup (100 mL)
Trimeprazine 6 mg/1 mL syrup (100 mL)
Others
Cyproheptadine tablets 4 mg (50, 100)

References

Burns MJ, Linden CH, Graudins A et al. A comparison of physostigmine and
benzodiazepines for the treatment of anticholinergic poisoning. Annals of Emergency
Medicine 2000; 35(4):374–381.

Clark RF, Vance MV. Massive diphenhydramine poisoning resulting in a wide-complex
tachycardia: successful treatment with sodium bicarbonate. Annals of Emergency
Medicine 1992; 21:318–321.

Page CB, Duffull SB, Whyte IM et al. Promethazine overdose: clinical effects, predicting
delirium and the effect of charcoal. Quarterly Journal of Medicines 2009; 102(2):123–131.

Ten Eick AP, Blumer JL, Reed MD. Safety of antihistamines in children. Drug Safety 2001;
24(2):119–147.

Thomas SHL. Antihistamine poisoning. Medicine 2012; 40(3):109–110.

3.13 ARSENIC

Arsenic is a metalloid element found as a natural component of the
Earth's crust. It occurs as inorganic and organic compounds and can
exist in a trivalent (arsenite) or pentavalent (arsenate) state. Most
commercially available products are produced from arsenic trioxide, a
trivalent inorganic compound. Acute ingestion of inorganic arsenic
results in severe gastroenteritis and can be followed by progressive
life-threatening multiple organ failure. Subacute toxicity may occur from
industrial exposure, food contamination or ingestion of arsenic-
containing alternative medicines. The organic arsenoids found in seafood
are essentially non-toxic.

RISK ASSESSMENT

- Acute or subacute ingestion of inorganic arsenic can lead to a
  dose-dependent pattern of multiple organ toxicity. Ingestion of
  >1 mg/kg of inorganic arsenic compounds has resulted in death.
  - It may be difficult to quantify the amount of arsenic ingested
    for individual cases.
- The risk of systemic toxicity may be influenced by the
  physicochemical properties (e.g. particle size or solubility) of the
  inorganic arsenic compound.
- Chronic arsenic toxicity usually occurs secondary to long-term
  (>10 years) ingestion of contaminated artesian water.
- Organic arsenoids found in seafood (e.g. arsenobetaine) are
  non-toxic because the compounds are not significantly
  metabolised to release free arsenic.
- Arsine gas (AsH_3) can be generated when arsenic compounds
  react with an acid. Inhalation can result in the rapid onset of
  severe toxicity and death.

- **Children:** any ingestion of arsenic-containing insecticide is potentially lethal.

Toxic mechanism

Arsenic enters cells by active transport or passive diffusion, binds to sulfhydryl (–SH) groups and substitutes for phosphate in ATP. Toxicity results from disruption of multiple cellular enzymatic pathways, uncoupling of mitochondrial oxidative phosphorylation and impaired cellular respiration. Inhibition of DNA replication and repair, particularly in chronic exposure, results in an increased risk of bladder and lung malignancy. Arsine gas can cause rapid onset of severe haemolysis by generation of reactive oxygen species within erythrocytes.

Toxicokinetics

Absorption occurs predominantly via the gastrointestinal route, but inhalational absorption can occur, particularly with arsine gas. Dermal absorption is less likely to be significant unless the skin is broken or exposure is prolonged. Following acute ingestion, arsenic is rapidly cleared from the bloodstream and distributed to renal and hepatic tissue. Inorganic arsenic undergoes hepatic methylation and the metabolites are excreted in the urine, with an elimination half-life of 3–5 days. A small amount of inorganic arsenic is excreted in the urine unchanged.

In chronic ingestion, arsenic is distributed more widely to the lungs, nervous tissue and spleen. It will accumulate in highly keratinised tissue (nails, skin, hair) with prolonged exposure. The majority of organic arsenoids found in seafood are excreted unchanged.

CLINICAL FEATURES

Acute toxicity

- Following large ingestions there is rapid onset of severe watery diarrhoea, vomiting and abdominal pain.
- Gastrointestinal haemorrhage may occur.
- Encephalopathy, seizures and cardiovascular collapse may develop within hours.
- Hypersalivation and a characteristic garlic odour may be evident.
- Acute cardiomyopathy, ECG changes (prolonged QT) and cardiac ventricular dysrhythmias may occur.
- Acute adult respiratory distress syndrome, renal failure and hepatic injury follow.
- Bone marrow depression may develop within 24–72 hours, reaching a nadir in 2–3 weeks.
- Alopecia occurs in survivors of the initial phase.
- Peripheral neuropathy may develop with a delay of 1–3 weeks. It is an ascending sensorimotor neuropathy and may resemble Guillain–Barré syndrome if motor weakness predominates. Progression to respiratory failure has been reported.

Subacute toxicity

- Gastrointestinal symptoms related to the initial ingestion are usually reported.
- Hepatic and renal dysfunction may occur.
- Peripheral neuropathy may develop after several weeks.

Chronic toxicity

- Insidious onset over years of a multi-system disorder manifested by constitutional symptoms, cutaneous lesions (hyperkeratosis of palms and soles, hyperpigmentation), nail changes (Mees' lines), painful peripheral neuropathy (glove-stocking type distribution) and malignancies of the skin or bladder.

Screening tests in deliberate self-poisoning
- 12-lead ECG, BGL and paracetamol level

Specific investigations
- Spot urinary arsenic (normal <30 microgram/L or 400 nmol/L)
  - Helpful to confirm ingestion.
  - Levels after acute ingestion may be >1000 microgram/L (13 500 nmol/L).
- 24-hour urinary arsenic excretion (normal <50 microgram/24 hours or 675 nmol/24 hours)
  - Better reflection of body burden.
  - May be one or two orders of magnitude higher than normal following acute exposure.
  - 24-hour urine collection with speciation of non-toxic organic and toxic inorganic forms is useful in assessing chronic exposure.
- Blood levels
  - Limited utility due to rapid redistribution to tissue compartments (may be useful in the assessment of acute exposure in the anuric patient).
- FBC, EUC, Liver function tests, venous blood gas
- Chest and abdominal X-rays (inorganic arsenic compounds are radio-opaque)

Resuscitation, supportive care and monitoring
- Attention to airway, breathing and circulation are paramount. These priorities are managed along conventional lines, as outlined in **Chapter 1.2: Resuscitation**.
- The immediate life-threat in early acute arsenic poisoning is hypovolaemia and shock secondary to profound gastrointestinal fluid losses.
- General supportive care measures and meticulous fluid resuscitation are indicated, as outlined in **Chapter 1.4: Supportive care and monitoring.**
- The decision to administer chelation therapy may be based on the history of exposure and clinical features prior to confirmatory levels being obtained (see **Antidotes**).

Decontamination
- Activated charcoal does not bind arsenic and is not indicated.
- Cooperative patients who present following deliberate self-poisoning with inorganic arsenic confirmed on abdominal X-ray should undergo whole bowel irrigation with polyethylene glycol (see **Chapter 1.6: Gastrointestinal decontamination**). Therapy may be guided by monitoring arsenic transit on serial abdominal X-rays.

Enhanced elimination
- Not clinically useful.

Antidotes
- Chelation is indicated where there are objective clinical features of acute arsenic intoxication or where subacute intoxication is

diagnosed on the basis of history of exposure, clinical features and elevated urinary inorganic arsenic concentration (usually >200 microgram/L or 2700 nmol/L).

- DMSA, DMPS or dimercaprol (BAL) are the recommended agents for elemental and inorganic arsenic poisoning. Oral therapy with DMSA is the preferred option in most settings (see **Chapter 4.7: DMSA (succimer) and DMPS (unithiol)** and **Chapter 4.6: Dimercaprol)**.

DISPOSITION AND FOLLOW-UP
- Patients who remain clinically well without gastrointestinal symptoms at 12 hours following acute ingestion of arsenic are unlikely to develop clinical features of toxicity or require further medical management.
- Patients in whom clinical features develop following acute ingestion of inorganic arsenic require admission for observation, supportive care and chelation.
- Chronic intoxication can be managed on an outpatient basis.

HANDY TIPS
- Chelation therapy of acute arsenic intoxication is not delayed pending confirmatory levels. Animal data on acute arsenic poisoning indicate that the efficacy of chelation is greatest when administered within minutes to hours after arsenic exposure.
- Discovery of elevated arsenic levels in an asymptomatic patient undergoing a 'heavy metal screen' usually reflects increased excretion of non-toxic organic arsenic compounds contained in seafood. Speciation of urinary arsenic may differentiate between toxic and non-toxic forms.
  - Note: Patients should be instructed to avoid eating seafood or seaweed for several days prior to 24-hour urinary arsenic level.
- Brief exposure to burning or cutting wood products treated with copper chrome arsenate preservative is unlikely to cause significant acute toxicity. Elevated arsenic levels and chronic toxicity are associated with prolonged occupational or domestic exposure to this compound.

PITFALL
- Ordering 'heavy metal screens' on patients with non-specific symptoms without exposure assessment – these are rarely clinically useful.

CONTROVERSIES
- The relative efficacies of available chelating agents.
- Experimental data from animal models suggest a possible benefit of N-acetylcysteine as an antioxidant to minimise arsenic toxicity in addition to chelation agents.
- There is limited evidence to support benefit from treatment interventions for chronic arsenic poisoning. Prevention of exposure is the priority.
- Hair analysis for metal toxicity is unreliable as it is subject to environmental artefacts and may not reflect body burden. It should not be used for diagnostic or management purposes.

Presentations
Inorganic
Found naturally in ground water in some regions. Used in the production of semiconductors, glass, pesticides and wood preservatives. Used medically to induce remission in acute promyleocytic leukaemia. Found in many traditional and herbal remedies.
Organic
Found predominantly in fish and shellfish as non-toxic arsenobetaine and arsenocholine.

References
Graeme KA, Pollack CK. Heavy metal toxicity: arsenic and mercury. Journal of Emergency Medicine 1998; 16(1):45–46.

Kosnett MJ. The role of chelation in the treatment of arsenic and mercury poisoning. Journal of Medical Toxicology 2013; 9:347–354.

Ratnaike RN. Acute and chronic arsenic toxicity. Postgraduate Medical Journal 2003; 79:391–396.

Xu Y, Wang Y, Zheng Q. Clinical manifestations and arsenic methylation after a rare subacute arsenic poisoning accident. Toxicological Sciences 2008; 103(2): 278–284.

3.14 BACLOFEN

Baclofen use has increased significantly in recent years. It has a narrow therapeutic index and clinical presentations range from agitated delirium to profound coma. Supportive care should result in a favourable outcome.

RISK ASSESSMENT
- Ingestions >200 mg in adults are expected to cause significant CNS effects including delirium, respiratory depression or coma.
- Coma requiring intubation can occur with much lower doses, particularly in baclofen-naïve patients.
- Accumulation can occur with therapeutic dosing in the setting of renal dysfunction, resulting in significant toxicity.

Toxic mechanism
Baclofen is a synthetic analogue of GABA. It is an agonist at spinal $GABA_B$ receptors, inhibiting the release of excitatory neurotransmitters. It readily crosses the blood–brain barrier and increasing doses lead to sedation or coma. Paradoxical excitatory features such as delirium and seizures can occur and a withdrawal syndrome is recognised with abrupt cessation, particularly with intrathecal therapy.

Toxicokinetics
Baclofen is rapidly absorbed following oral administration, reaching peak serum concentrations within 2 hours. Volume of distribution is 0.7 L/kg and it is primarily excreted unchanged in the urine. The mean elimination half-life is 3.5 hours, but this can be significantly prolonged in renal failure.

CLINICAL FEATURES
- Clinical features of intoxication develop within 2 hours of overdose and include:
  - Central nervous system
    - Delirium
    - Respiratory depression
    - Profound and prolonged coma
    - Seizures

- — Cardiovascular
  - – Sinus bradycardia
  - – Hypotension.
- Delirium is often observed just prior to the onset of coma or on wakening.
- Following large ingestions, coma may be profound. The patient may appear brain dead with fixed dilated pupils, hypotonia and areflexia (including absent brainstem reflexes).
- The duration of coma is usually between 24 and 48 hours.

INVESTIGATIONS
Screening tests in deliberate self-poisoning
- 12-lead ECG, BGL and paracetamol level

MANAGEMENT
Resuscitation, supportive care and monitoring
- Baclofen poisoning is a potentially life-threatening emergency managed in an area equipped for cardiorespiratory monitoring and resuscitation.
- Respiratory depression and coma require prompt intubation and ventilation.
- Level of consciousness should be closely monitored during the first few hours.
- Seizures are managed with titrated doses of IV benzodiazepines.
- Hypotension usually responds to fluid boluses.
- Bradycardia is rarely severe enough to require specific treatment.

Decontamination
- Activated charcoal is only given to the comatose patient once the airway is protected by intubation.

Enhanced elimination
- Not clinically useful.

Antidotes
- None available.

DISPOSITION AND FOLLOW-UP
- Following baclofen overdose, all patients are observed for a minimum of 4 hours.
- Patients who are asymptomatic at 4 hours following ingestion are medically fit for discharge. Discharge should not occur at night.
- Patients with sedation or delirium require medical management until all clinical features resolve.

HANDY TIPS
- Baclofen overdose should be considered in any patient with access to this agent who presents with coma. It is not detected on routine drug screening.
- Baclofen is sometimes administered by continuous intrathecal infusion via a reservoir and pump system. Pump malfunctions resulting in even small intrathecal boluses can produce profound coma. Management recommendations in addition to standard resuscitation measures include:

- temporary cessation of baclofen infusion
- emptying reservoir
- lumbar puncture and removal of 30–50 mL of CSF.
- Baclofen withdrawal syndrome is recognised following abrupt cessation of intrathecal baclofen infusions. It manifests with altered mental state, rigidity and fevers.

PITFALL
- Failure to consider baclofen toxicity in the alcoholic patient presenting with an altered mental state.

CONTROVERSIES
- There is debate about the utility and safety of baclofen in alcohol abstinence programmes, particularly related to the narrow therapeutic index.
- The clinical significance of symptoms following abrupt cessation of oral baclofen therapy. They are likely to be not as severe as the withdrawal syndrome described with interruptions to intrathecal baclofen infusions.

Presentations
Baclofen 10 mg, 25 mg tablets (100)
Baclofen 0.05 mg/mL solution for intrathecal injection (1 mL, 20 mL)
Baclofen 2 mg/mL solution for intrathecal injection (5 mL)

References
Leung NY, Whyte IM, Isbister GK. Baclofen overdose: defining the spectrum of toxicity. Emergency Medicine Australasia 2006; 18:77–82.
Pelissier F, de Haro L, Cardona F. Self-poisoning with baclofen in alcohol-dependent patients: national reports to French Poison Control Centers, 2008–2013. Clinical Toxicology 2017; 55(4):275–284.

3.15 BARBITURATES

Pentobarbitone, Phenobarbitone, Primidone, Thiopentone

Barbiturate overdose can cause profound and prolonged coma. It is an uncommon presentation due to limited availability. Supportive care should result in a favourable outcome in the majority of patients, but haemodialysis is indicated in the setting of large ingestions of phenobarbitone.

RISK ASSESSMENT
- Ingestion of >8 mg/kg of phenobarbitone is expected to produce clinical features of toxicity in the non-tolerant individual.
- Self-administration of thiopentone or pentobarbitone by the intravenous route is likely to be lethal without immediate resuscitation.
- **Children:** accidental paediatric exposure is likely to cause toxicity.

Toxic mechanism
Barbiturates cause CNS depression by enhancing the inhibitory effects of gamma-aminobutyric acid (GABA)-mediated neurotransmission. They bind to the $GABA_A$ receptor complex and increase the duration of chloride channel opening (in contrast to benzodiazepines, which increase the frequency of opening). They also antagonise the

effect of the excitatory neurotransmitter glutamate in the CNS. Inhibition of medullary cardiorespiratory centres and hypothalamic autonomic nuclei results in hypothermia, peripheral vasodilatation, direct myocardial depression and respiratory arrest.

Toxicokinetics

All barbiturates are well absorbed from the gastrointestinal tract but only some agents are clinically effective after oral administration. The highly lipid-soluble barbiturates (thiopentone and pentobarbitone) are only useful if given intravenously. They have a short duration of action due to rapid redistribution from the CNS. In contrast, the less lipid-soluble 'long-acting' barbiturates (phenobarbitone and primidone) have a slower onset of action after oral ingestion and a prolonged effect due to slower redistribution. All barbiturates are metabolised by saturable hepatic microsomal pathways. Primidone has two active metabolites, phenobarbitone and phenylethylmalonamide (PEMA). Phenobarbitone undergoes both enterohepatic and enteroenteric recirculation, with 25–50% of an ingested dose excreted unchanged in the urine. The elimination half-life of phenobarbitone is long with considerable inter-individual variation. In overdose, the half-life is prolonged even further as a result of saturable kinetics.

CLINICAL FEATURES
- Barbiturate overdose can cause life-threatening coma, respiratory depression and hypotension.
- Clinical effects occur immediately following intravenous overdose of thiopentone or pentobarbitone, or within 1–2 hours of ingestion of phenobarbitone or primidone.
  - Central nervous system
    - Varying degrees of CNS depression can occur.
    - Profound coma may develop, with complete loss of neurological function. Clinical features can mimic brain death with absent pupillary responses, vestibulo-ocular and deep tendon reflexes.
    - Respiratory depression occurs, with Cheyne-Stokes respiration progressing to apnoea.
  - Cardiovascular system
    - Tachycardia
    - Hypotension
  - Other
    - Hypothermia
    - Ileus
    - Skin bullae over pressure areas can occur ('barbiturate blisters') but are not specific for barbiturate toxicity.
- The duration of coma from poisoning with the short-acting barbiturates (e.g. pentobarbitone) usually resolves within 24–48 hours. In contrast, poisoning from long-acting barbiturates (e.g. phenobarbitone, primidone) may last days or weeks, necessitating prolonged intensive care.

INVESTIGATIONS

Screening tests in deliberate self-poisoning
- 12-lead ECG, BGL and paracetamol level

Specific investigations
- Serum barbiturate levels
  - Phenobarbitone assays are readily available in most locations. Other barbiturate assays can be obtained at specialised centres.
  - CNS depression correlates well with serum phenobarbitone level (see **Table 3.15.1**).

TABLE 3.15.1 Correlation of serum phenobarbitone levels and clinical features

Level	Clinical features
15–25 mg/L (65–108 micromol/L)	Usual therapeutic range
30–80 mg/L (130–345 micromol/L)	Increasing sedation
>80 mg/L (>345 micromol/L)	Coma requiring intubation

- Serial levels are essential in the management of the comatose patient with barbiturate poisoning to guide the use of enhanced elimination techniques.
- A phenobarbitone level of >100 mg/L (>430 micromol/L) is an indication for haemodialysis.
- Other investigations may be required to exclude alternative causes of coma.
  - Note: The electroencephalogram (EEG) in barbiturate coma may demonstrate profound suppression of activity to the point of mimicking brain death.

MANAGEMENT

Resuscitation, supportive care and monitoring
- All patients are managed in an area equipped for cardiopulmonary monitoring and resuscitation.
- Attention to airway, breathing and circulation are paramount. These priorities are managed along conventional lines, as outlined in **Chapter 1.2: Resuscitation**.
- The need for intubation is anticipated and performed early in the patient with a declining level of consciousness.
- General supportive care measures are indicated, as outlined in **Chapter 1.4: Supportive care and monitoring**.

Decontamination
- Activated charcoal 50 g is administered via a nasogastric tube to the unconscious patient only after the airway is secured by endotracheal intubation.

Enhanced elimination
- Techniques of enhanced elimination are only considered for poisoning by long-acting barbiturates (phenobarbitone, primidone) where slow endogenous clearance can result in prolonged intensive care admission. The aim of instituting these interventions is to reduce the duration of coma and requirement for ventilation.
- Multiple-dose activated charcoal (MDAC) increases the rate of elimination of phenobarbitone by interrupting enterohepatic and enteroenteric circulation (see **Chapter 1.7: Enhanced elimination** for details on performing this intervention). It is indicated in the intubated comatose patient as long as bowel sounds are present.
- Haemodialysis, haemoperfusion and haemodiafiltration efficiently remove phenobarbitone. Indications include:
  - markedly elevated levels (>100 mg/L, >430 micromol/L)
  - levels that are rising or have plateaued despite MDAC
  - when MDAC is not feasible due to the presence of ileus.

Antidotes

- None available.

DISPOSITION AND FOLLOW-UP

- All children suspected of ingesting barbiturates must be referred to hospital for assessment and observation. They may be discharged home if they remain asymptomatic 6 hours post ingestion.
- Adult patients who deliberately self-poison with phenobarbitone or primidone should be observed in a closely monitored setting for a minimum of 6 hours. If they do not develop neurological signs or symptoms during that time, further medical management is not required.
- Patients who develop toxicity require admission for ongoing management.

HANDY TIPS

- Consider barbiturate poisoning in the patient with profound coma and hypotonia. Have a high index of suspicion if the patient has a medical or veterinary background or has a history of epilepsy.
- If intermittent haemodialysis is not available, continuous modalities are acceptable, although clearance will be lower.
- Haemoperfusion using a charcoal filter is not widely available and has a higher complication rate compared to intermittent haemodialysis or continuous modalities.

PITFALLS

- Failure to consider the diagnosis of barbiturate toxicity. Along with carbamazepine and valproate poisoning, it is an unusual but readily treatable cause of coma.
- Failure to institute appropriate enhanced elimination interventions at the earliest possible opportunity.

CONTROVERSIES

- Urinary alkalinisation has been shown to enhance elimination of phenobarbitone but it is inferior to MDAC and not recommended.
- Although MDAC enhances phenobarbitone elimination, it has not been shown to reduce duration of coma or length of stay in intensive care.
- There are no clinical trials that define an absolute threshold for haemodialysis or other enhanced elimination techniques for the treatment of barbiturate overdose. Recommendations are empiric and based on a risk–benefit analysis.

Presentations

Pentobarbitone sodium: available as a veterinary preparation (used to euthanase animals)
Phenobarbitone 15 mg/5 mL elixir (100 mL, 500 mL)
Phenobarbitone 30 mg tablets (200)
Phenobarbitone sodium 200 mg/1 mL ampoules
Primidone 250 mg tablets (100, 200)
Thiopentone sodium 500 mg ampoules for reconstitution

References

Ebid A-HIM, Abdel-Rahman HM. Pharmacokinetics of phenobarbital during certain enhanced elimination modalities to evaluate their clinical efficacy in management of drug overdose. Therapeutic Drug Monitoring 2001; 23(3):209–216.

Frenia ML, Schauben JL, Wears RL et al. Multiple-dose activated charcoal compared to urinary alkalinization for the enhancement of phenobarbital elimination. Clinical Toxicology 1996; 34(2):169–175.

Mactier R, Laliberté M, Mardini J et al. Extracorporeal treatment for barbiturate poisoning: recommendations from the EXTRIP workgroup. American Journal of Kidney Disease 2014; 64(3):347–358.

Pond SM, Olson KR, Osteroloh JD et al. Randomized study of the treatment of phenobarbital overdose with repeated doses of activated charcoal. Journal of the American Medical Association 1984; 251(23):3104–3108.

Roberts DM, Buckley NA. Enhanced elimination in acute barbiturate poisoning – a systematic review. Clinical Toxicology 2011; 49:2–12.

3.16 BENZODIAZEPINES

Alprazolam, Bromazepam, Clobazam, Clonazepam, Diazepam, Flunitrazepam, Midazolam, Nitrazepam, Oxazepam, Temazepam, Triazolam

Also covers the non-benzodiazepine sedative-hypnotics: Zolpidem, Zopiclone

Benzodiazepines are commonly involved in deliberate self-poisoning. Supportive care will result in a favourable outcome in the vast majority of cases.

RISK ASSESSMENT

- Isolated benzodiazepine overdose usually causes only mild sedation, irrespective of the dose ingested, and can be managed with basic supportive care.
- Alprazolam overdose is more likely to cause significant CNS depression that may require intubation and ventilation.
- Zolpidem and zopiclone rarely cause severe CNS or respiratory depression when taken alone.
- Co-ingestion of other CNS depressants (e.g. alcohol, opioids) increases the risk of secondary complications, including death.
- Patient factors such as extremes of age or pre-existing respiratory disease predispose to an increased risk of toxicity.
- **Children:** accidental ingestion of 1 or 2 benzodiazepine tablets usually causes ataxia and sedation within 2 hours.

Toxic mechanism

Benzodiazepines act by enhancing gamma-aminobutyric acid (GABA)-mediated neurotransmission. They bind to the $GABA_A$ receptor complex and increase the frequency of chloride channel opening. Zolpidem and zopiclone are non-benzodiazepine sedative-hypnotics that also act at the $GABA_A$ receptor complex.

Toxicokinetics

Benzodiazepines are rapidly absorbed following oral administration. They are highly lipophilic, with high protein binding. Benzodiazepines undergo hepatic metabolism and many have active metabolites. For example, diazepam is metabolised to N-desmethyldiazepam, oxazepam and temazepam, and alprazolam is metabolised to

1- and 4-hydroxyalprazolam. Although they can be classified as short-, medium- and long-acting agents, the duration of effect following overdose depends more on patient tolerance and redistribution than elimination. Clinical features of intoxication correlate poorly with serum benzodiazepine levels.

CLINICAL FEATURES

- Onset of symptoms occurs within 1–2 hours. Varying degrees of CNS depression can occur. Coma is rare, except with alprazolam or in mixed ingestions.
- Bradycardia and hypotension can occur but are not clinically significant.
- Resolution of CNS depression usually occurs within 12 hours. More prolonged coma is common in the elderly.

INVESTIGATIONS

Screening tests in deliberate self-poisoning

- 12-lead ECG, BGL and paracetamol level

MANAGEMENT

Resuscitation, supportive care and monitoring

- Attention to airway, breathing and circulation is paramount. These priorities are managed along conventional lines, as outlined in **Chapter 1.2: Resuscitation**.
- Monitor for urinary retention and place an indwelling catheter as required.

Decontamination

- Activated charcoal is not indicated because the onset of sedation occurs in the first few hours and basic supportive care ensures a good outcome.

Enhanced elimination

- Not clinically useful.

Antidotes

- Flumazenil is a competitive benzodiazepine antagonist with a specific role in benzodiazepine overdose. Its indications include:
  - management of coma with respiratory compromise when resources are not available to intubate and ventilate the patient safely
  - reversal of sedation in the benzodiazepine-naïve patient to prevent intubation, in particular for children and the elderly
  - reversal of excessive sedation from medically administered benzodiazepines.
- For further information on the indications, contraindications and administration see **Chapter 4.9: Flumazenil**.

DISPOSITION AND FOLLOW-UP

- Paediatric patients following accidental exposure may be observed at home. If significant ataxia or drowsiness occurs, referral to hospital for supportive care is required.
- Patients with mild sedation are managed supportively in a ward environment until clinically well. Ataxia may persist despite improvement in conscious state.

- Patients with CNS depression, or those who have received flumazenil, require ongoing assessment of their airway risk to prevent respiratory complications.

HANDY TIPS
- Profound coma, tachycardia or 12-lead ECG changes suggest a co-ingested agent and the need to reconsider the risk assessment.
- Flumazenil may be life-saving in selected patients when coma and respiratory depression cannot otherwise be managed.

PITFALL
- Administration of flumazenil when a history of benzodiazepine dependence or co-ingestants predicts a risk of seizure.

References
Buckley NA, Dawson AH, Whyte IM. Relative toxicity of benzodiazepines in overdose. British Medical Journal 1995; 310:219–221.

Garnier R, Guerault E, Muzard D et al. Acute zolpidem poisoning—analysis of 344 cases. Journal of Toxicology–Clinical Toxicology 1994; 32(4):391–394.

Isbister GK, O'Regan L, Sibbritt D et al. Alprazolam is relatively more toxic than other benzodiazepines in overdose. British Journal of Clinical Pharmacology 2004; 58(1):88–95.

3.17 BENZTROPINE

Benztropine is a potent anticholinergic agent and is frequently prescribed to patients on antipsychotic medications to manage symptoms of dystonia or dyskinesia. Like other anticholinergic agents, it is sometimes ingested for recreational purposes and can cause prolonged toxicity in overdose.

RISK ASSESSMENT
- Any overdose of this agent is likely to precipitate anticholinergic toxicity and require medical care.
- Anticholinergic toxicity can also occur with excessive therapeutic doses.

Toxic mechanism
Benztropine is a synthetic drug containing the active tropine component of atropine and the diphenylmethyl portion of diphenhydramine. It has anticholinergic and antihistamine activity and enhances dopaminergic effects by inhibiting dopamine re-uptake.

Toxicokinetics
There is limited information on the pharmacokinetics of benztropine and even less on its toxicokinetics. It is well absorbed following oral administration, with an onset of therapeutic action within 2 hours. A prolonged absorption phase can occur due to anticholinergic effects on gut transit. Metabolism is probably hepatic, with metabolites and unchanged drug excreted in the urine.

- The clinical features are those of the anticholinergic toxidrome (see **Chapter 2.6: Anticholinergic toxicity**) and include delirium, visual hallucinations, mydriasis, sinus tachycardia, warm flushed dry skin, urinary retention and ileus.
- Toxic effects are observed within 6 hours and may persist from 12 hours to several days.

INVESTIGATIONS
Screening tests in deliberate self-poisoning
- 12-lead ECG, BGL and paracetamol level

MANAGEMENT
Resuscitation, supportive care and monitoring
- Management is directed towards the specific features of anticholinergic toxicity.
- Control of delirium and agitation can be challenging. Initial sedation with titrated intravenous benzodiazepines or droperidol may be effective, but physical restraints or intubation and ventilation may be required in severe cases.
- Insert an indwelling urinary catheter as soon as possible. Urinary retention is almost universal in anticholinergic delirium and, if not relieved, will exacerbate the patient's agitation.
- Once adequate sedation is attained, one-to-one nursing in a calm, closely monitored environment is essential to ensure patient safety.
- General supportive care measures are indicated, as outlined in **Chapter 1.4: Supportive care and monitoring**.
- For a more detailed description of the management of anticholinergic toxicity, see **Chapter 2.6: Anticholinergic toxicity**.

Decontamination
- Activated charcoal may be useful to limit the duration of toxicity, if administered within 2 hours of ingestion.

Enhanced elimination
- Not clinically useful.

Antidotes
- Physostigmine is the specific antidote for central anticholinergic delirium. It can completely reverse the CNS features and is useful to confirm the diagnosis, but unfortunately is not widely available in most hospitals.
- Rapid administration of physostigmine can lead to bronchospasm, bradycardia or seizures (see **Chapter 4.21: Physostigmine** for details regarding administration).

DISPOSITION AND FOLLOW-UP
- The patient is admitted to a critical care area where one-to-one nursing care can be provided. Staff must be aware that the delirium can recur (even after dramatic improvement with physostigmine) and may persist for several days.

HANDY TIPS
- Complete resolution of anticholinergic delirium can occur with appropriate administration of physostigmine, confirming the

diagnosis and removing the requirement for further investigations such as CT head or lumbar puncture.
- The half-life of physostigmine is significantly shorter than that of benztropine, meaning that recurrence of anticholinergic toxicity (particularly delirium) can occur.

PITFALL
- Failure to exclude medical causes of the patient's presentation.

CONTROVERSY
- Other centrally acting cholinesterase inhibitors with a slower onset of action (e.g. rivastigmine) are suggested as antidotes for the management of anticholinergic delirium. There is limited evidence to support a clinically relevant benefit to these agents compared to the dramatic improvement in delirium that can be seen with titrated intravenous physostigmine.

3.18 BETA-BLOCKERS

Atenolol, Bisoprolol, Carvedilol, Esmolol, Metoprolol, Oxprenolol, Pindolol, Propranolol, Sotalol

Beta-blockers cause relatively mild toxicity in overdose and a good outcome is expected. The exceptions are propranolol and sotalol, which may cause life-threatening toxicity due to specific additional pharmacological effects.

RISK ASSESSMENT
- The following factors increase the risk of severe toxicity:
  - ingestion of propranolol or sotalol
  - pre-existing cardiac dysfunction
  - co-ingestion with other cardiac medications
  - advanced age.
- Significant toxicity from propranolol may occur with ingestions greater than 1 g.
- Propranolol has two properties responsible for toxicity in overdose:
  - sodium channel blockade (membrane stabilising activity)
  - high lipid solubility (enhanced CNS penetration).
- Sotalol has potassium channel blocking activity leading to QT prolongation and a risk of ventricular dysrhythmias and torsades de pointes.
- Toxicity usually occurs within the first few hours, with the exception of overdose with sotalol or controlled-release preparations of other beta-blockers.
- PR interval prolongation even in the absence of bradycardia is an early sign of toxicity.
- **Children:** there is risk of toxicity following ingestion of any dose of propranolol or sotalol. Accidental ingestion of 1 or 2 tablets of other agents does not cause significant toxicity.

Toxic mechanism

Competitive antagonists at beta-1 and beta-2 receptors. Excessive beta-adrenergic blockade leads to decreased intracellular cAMP concentration and resultant blunting of the chronotropic, inotropic and metabolic effects of catecholamines. Propranolol also has sodium-channel-blocking effects leading to cardiovascular toxicity (QRS widening and ventricular dysrhythmias) and CNS effects (seizures and coma). Sotalol also blocks cardiac potassium channels, leading to QT prolongation and the risk of torsades de pointes.

Toxicokinetics

Rapidly absorbed following ingestion with peak serum concentrations occurring within 4 hours of ingestion. Volumes of distribution, metabolism and elimination vary with the different agents. Propranolol is notable as it is highly lipophilic, readily crossing the blood–brain barrier, and has active metabolites.

CLINICAL FEATURES

Cardiovascular

- Bradycardia and hypotension
- Dysrhythmias include sinus bradycardia, 1st- to 3rd-degree heart block, junctional or ventricular escape rhythms
- QRS widening is observed following propranolol overdose and the magnitude is a predictor of ventricular dysrhythmias and seizures
- QT prolongation and torsades de pointes are observed following sotalol overdose

Central nervous system

- Delirium, seizures and coma (propranolol)

INVESTIGATIONS

Screening tests in deliberate self-poisoning

- 12-lead ECG, BGL and paracetamol level

Specific investigations

- EUC
- Calcium, magnesium (sotalol)

MANAGEMENT

Management of established beta-blocker toxicity is determined by the type of agent:

- Propranolol poisoning requires specific therapy for wide QRS, haemodynamic instability, seizures and coma.
- Sotalol poisoning requires specific therapy for QT prolongation.

Resuscitation, supportive care and monitoring

- Acute beta-blocker overdose is initially managed in an area equipped for cardiorespiratory monitoring and resuscitation.
- Bradycardia and hypotension
  - Usually responds to appropriate volume resuscitation and standard catecholamine therapy in the majority of cases. Treatment options include:
    - atropine (temporising measure)
    - adrenaline
    - isoprenaline
    - high-dose insulin has been used in severe poisonings with refractory cardiogenic shock (see **Chapter 4.14: Insulin (high-dose)**).
- **Propranolol**
  - The mainstays of treatment for both cardiovascular and CNS toxicity are:

- administration of IV sodium bicarbonate boluses
- intubation
- hyperventilation.
— Administer sodium bicarbonate 1–2 mmol/kg IV repeated every 1–2 minutes until:
  - restoration of perfusing rhythm
  - improvement in QRS widening.
— Intubation and hyperventilation to maintain a therapeutic endpoint of pH 7.5–7.55
— Hypotension may persist after initial resuscitation with sodium bicarbonate, hyperventilation and IV fluids, and titrated adrenaline infusion is indicated.

- **Sotalol**
  — QT prolongation
    - Correct QT-dependent electrolytes (potassium, calcium, magnesium) to the upper limit of normal
  — Torsades de pointes
    - Electrical cardioversion may be required for persistent episodes that result in altered mental state or haemodynamic instability
    - Magnesium 10 mmol IV bolus (0.05 mmol/kg in children) over 1-2 minutes, repeated once if torsades de pointes recurs
    - Isoprenaline or overdrive electrical pacing are other treatment options to increase the resting heart rate to a target of >100 beats/min.
    - Ensure that all QT-dependent electrolytes (potassium, calcium, magnesium) are at the upper limit of normal (see **Chapter 2.17: The 12-lead ECG in toxicology**).
- Close clinical observation and continuous ECG monitoring are mandatory for 6 hours post ingestion.

Decontamination
- Activated charcoal may be administered to patients who present within 2 hours but caution should be exercised following propranolol overdose because of the risk of imminent coma and seizures.

Enhanced elimination
- Not clinically indicated (see **Controversies**).

Antidotes
- High-dose insulin therapy may be considered for refractory cardiogenic shock (see **Chapter 4.14: Insulin (high-dose)**).

DISPOSITION AND FOLLOW-UP
- Patients who are clinically well with a normal ECG 6 hours following beta-blocker overdose do not require further medical management.
- Sotalol is an exception – the ECG must be normal 12 hours post ingestion.

HANDY TIPS
- Propranolol overdoses are managed effectively if approached in the same manner as tricyclic antidepressant overdoses.
- Beta-blockers are competitive antagonists at catecholamine receptors, and as such, standard catecholamines (adrenaline,

isoprenaline) can be expected to overcome bradycardia and
negative inotropic effects in most cases.

CONTROVERSIES

- Glucagon was historically regarded as a specific antidote for
  beta-blocker poisoning but it offers no advantage over standard
  inotropes and chronotropes. It is no longer recommended for
  beta-blocker poisoning.
- Precise indications for high-dose insulin therapy are undefined but
  it is warranted in the management of propranolol toxicity with
  refractory cardiogenic shock.
- Sotalol has a relatively small volume of distribution and dialysis
  may be justified to enhance clearance, particularly in the rare
  scenario of recurrent torsades de pointes in a patient with
  significant renal dysfunction.

Presentations

Atenolol 50 mg tablets (30)
Bisoprolol fumarate 2.5 mg, 5 mg, 10 mg tablets (28)
Carvedilol 3.125 mg tablets (30)
Carvedilol 6.25 mg, 12.5 mg, 25 mg tablets (60)
Esmolol hydrochloride 100 mg/10 mL ampoules
Metoprolol tartrate 50 mg tablets (100)
Metoprolol tartrate 100 mg tablets (60)
Metoprolol tartrate 5 mg/5 mL ampoules
Metoprolol succinate controlled-release 23.75 mg tablets (15)
Metoprolol succinate controlled-release 47.5 mg, 95 mg, 190 mg tablets (30)
Oxprenolol hydrochloride 20 mg, 40 mg tablets (100)
Pindolol 5 mg tablets (100)
Pindolol 15 mg tablets (50)
Propranolol hydrochloride 10 mg, 40 mg tablets (100)
Propranolol hydrochloride 160 mg tablets (50)
Sotalol hydrochloride 80 mg, 160 mg tablets (60)
Sotalol hydrochloride 40 mg/4 mL ampoules

References

DeWitt CR, Waksman JC. Pharmacology, pathophysiology and management of calcium
channel blocker and β-blocker toxicity. Toxicological Reviews 2004; 23(4):223–238.
Love J, Howell JM, Litovitz TL et al. Acute beta-blocker overdose: factors associated
with the development of cardiovascular morbidity. Journal of Toxicology–Clinical
Toxicology 2000; 38:275–281.
Reith DM, Dawson AH, Epid D et al. Relative toxicity of beta-blockers in overdose.
Journal of Toxicology–Clinical Toxicology 1996; 34:273–278.
Taboulet P, Cariou A, Berdeaux A et al. Pathophysiology and management of self-
poisoning with beta-blockers. Journal of Toxicology–Clinical Toxicology 1993;
31:531–551.

3.19 BUPROPION

This antidepressant agent is also used in smoking-cessation and
weight-management programmes and is only available as an extended-
release preparation. Bupropion has a narrow therapeutic index and
seizures can occur with any overdose. Life-threatening cardiotoxicity
may occur with massive ingestions.

RISK ASSESSMENT

- The significant risks following overdose are seizures, tachycardia and ventricular dysrhythmias.
- Seizures usually occur within 8 hours and are self-limiting, but may be recurrent. The onset of seizures may be delayed up to 24 hours.
- The risk of seizures is increased if there is a pre-existing lowered seizure threshold or co-ingestion of other centrally acting sympathomimetic or serotonergic agents.
- Severe cardiotoxicity can cause haemodynamic instability, and death has occurred at doses >9 g. See **Table 3.19.1**.
- **Children:** any child suspected of ingesting >10 mg/kg requires assessment and observation in hospital.

Toxic mechanism
Bupropion is a noradrenaline and dopamine reuptake inhibitor with a structure similar to amphetamines.

Toxicokinetics
It is well absorbed orally with peak plasma levels occurring within 6 hours. It has a large volume of distribution and active metabolites that are renally excreted.

CLINICAL FEATURES

- Clinical features develop progressively over 8 hours and include tachycardia, hypertension, tremors, agitation, hallucinations, altered mental state and seizures.
- Seizures can be heralded by agitation and tachycardia, but may occur without prodromal symptoms.
- Severe cardiotoxicity with hypotension and ECG manifestations (QRS widening) is reported after massive ingestions.

INVESTIGATIONS
Screening tests in deliberate self-poisoning
- 12-lead ECG, BGL and paracetamol level

Specific investigations
- ECGs
  - Perform a 12-lead ECG on all patients at presentation and at 6 and 12 hours post ingestion.
  - Symptomatic patients require serial ECGs until clinically well.

TABLE 3.19.1 Dose-related risk assessment: bupropion	
Dose	**Effect**
<4.5 g	Tachycardia, hypertension, agitation, hallucinations, GI symptoms Seizures can occur
>4.5 g	Seizure risk of 50% and first seizure usually within 8 hours of ingestion
>9 g	Risk of severe cardiovascular complications, including haemodynamic instability, prolonged QRS and QT intervals and ventricular dysrhythmias

MANAGEMENT
Resuscitation, supportive care and monitoring
- Bupropion overdose is managed in an area equipped for cardiorespiratory monitoring and resuscitation.
- Early intubation and ventilation is indicated when the history and clinical progression suggest ingestion of >9 g.
- Broad-complex tachycardias with haemodynamic compromise:
  - sodium bicarbonate 1–2 mEq/kg boluses titrated to clinical response (see **Chapter 4.24: Sodium bicarbonate**).
- Agitation and seizures are managed with titrated doses of IV benzodiazepines.
- General supportive care measures are indicated, as outlined in **Chapter 1.4: Supportive care and monitoring**.

Decontamination
- Activated charcoal or other attempts at decontamination are generally contraindicated because of the high risk of seizures, particularly if symptoms are already present.
- Asymptomatic patients presenting early after ingestion may be candidates for oral activated charcoal after consideration of the risk of secondary airway contamination in the event of seizures.

Enhanced elimination
- Not clinically useful.

Antidotes
- None available.

DISPOSITION AND FOLLOW-UP
- Because of the risk of seizures following bupropion overdose, all patients are observed with IV access in place for up to 24 hours and until symptom free. Discharge should not occur at night.
- Admission to ICU is indicated following massive ingestions (>9 g) and for patients manifesting signs of significant cardiotoxicity.

HANDY TIP
- Early administration of IV benzodiazepines may prevent seizures.

PITFALLS
- Failure to anticipate and prepare for delayed onset of symptoms and seizures.
- Failure to administer benzodiazepines early and in sufficient dose.

Presentations
Bupropion hydrochloride 90 mg/naloxone 8 mg modified-release tablets (112)
Bupropion hydrochloride 150 mg sustained-release tablets (10, 60, 100, 120)

References
Al-Abri SA, Orengo JP, Hayashi S et al. Delayed bupropion cardiotoxicity associated with elevated serum concentrations of bupropion but not hydroxybupropion. Clinical Toxicology 2013; 51(10):1230–1234.

Balit CR, Lynch CN, Isbister GK. Bupropion poisoning: a case series. Medical Journal of Australia 2003; 178:61–63.

Morazin F, Lumbroso A, Harry P. Cardiogenic shock and status epilepticus after massive bupropion overdose. Clinical Toxicology 2007; 45(7):794–797.

Shepherd G, Veliz LI, Keys DC. Intentional bupropion overdoses. Journal of Emergency Medicine 2004; 27(2):147–151.

Spiller HA, Bosic GM, Beuhler M et al. Unintentional ingestion of bupropion in children. Journal of Emergency Medicine 2010; 38(3):332–336.

Starr P, Klein-Schwartz W, Spiller H et al. Incidence and onset of delayed seizures after overdose of extended-release bupropion. American Journal of Emergency Medicine 2009; 27:911–915.

3.20 BUTTON BATTERIES

Ingestion of button batteries is almost exclusively a paediatric problem. The majority pass through the gastrointestinal tract without complication. Larger diameter batteries may lodge in the oesophagus, causing significant complications including death, particularly if diagnosis is delayed.

RISK ASSESSMENT

- Ingested batteries of 20 mm diameter or greater are more likely to lodge in the oesophagus and may cause severe local corrosive injury within 2 hours.
- Local corrosive injury may also occur after insertion of smaller batteries into the aural or nasal cavities.
- Most severe oesophageal injuries occur in children younger than 4 years old.
- Delayed diagnosis of oesophageal button battery ingestion is associated with worse outcome.
- Button batteries may contain manganese, silver, lithium or zinc but the quantities available for absorption are insufficient to cause systemic heavy metal toxicity.

Mechanism of injury

Electrical discharge from the button battery is the predominant mechanism of injury. Hydroxide ions are generated at the negative pole of the battery, causing localised alkaline corrosive injury with tissue liquefaction and necrosis within 2 hours of lodgement. Injury severity is directly related to the voltage of the battery and the duration of tissue contact. Potential complications include oesophageal perforation, trachea-oesophageal fistula, aorto-oesophageal fistula and stricture formation.

CLINICAL FEATURES

- Many children are asymptomatic initially and present to hospital because ingestion was witnessed or suspected by parents or carers, or only after signs and symptoms of oesophageal obstruction or injury develop.
- Where ingestion is unwitnessed, presentation may be delayed and symptoms relatively non-specific.
- Button battery ingestion should be considered in the presence of any of the following presenting complaints: airway obstruction, cough, fever, dysphagia, sore throat, chest discomfort, decreased oral intake, or coughing or choking with eating and drinking.

- Oesophageal perforations and fistulas may not be clinically evident for up to 28 days and strictures may present after weeks to months.

INVESTIGATIONS
- History or suspicion of possible button battery ingestion mandates plain anteroposterior (together with a lateral if an object is identified above the diaphragm) X-ray of the neck, chest and abdomen to localise the battery and guide further management.
- Mercury and other heavy metal levels are not required.

MANAGEMENT
Resuscitation and supportive care
- Resuscitation is rarely needed following acute ingestion unless airway obstruction occurs.
- Delayed presentation may require resuscitation following standard protocols for cardiovascular collapse secondary to haemorrhage or sepsis from oesophageal perforation, or for respiratory distress from tracheo-oesophageal fistula.

Decontamination
- A button battery lodged in the oesophagus requires endoscopic removal as soon as possible, and ideally within 2 hours of ingestion.
- Endoscopy allows both removal of the battery and examination for local complications to guide further management. The presence of a mucosal burn prompts consideration of further investigation to exclude perforation and associated injuries.
- A button battery located beyond the oesophagus in an asymptomatic child may be allowed to pass naturally following discussion with local gastroenterology services (see **Controversies**).
- Batteries lodged in the nose or ears should be removed urgently.

DISPOSITION AND FOLLOW-UP
- Children with a battery lodged in the oesophagus are referred for urgent upper GI endoscopy and removal.
- Children in whom the battery has passed beyond the pylorus are less likely to develop complications and can be discharged with advice to observe and return if symptoms develop. A follow-up X-ray to confirm passage is indicated if passage in the stool has not been observed.
- Decisions regarding the requirement for endoscopy to retrieve button batteries in the stomach benefit from involvement of the most experienced clinicians available, including consultation with the local gastroenterology service.

HANDY TIPS
- Batteries typically have a 'double ring' or 'halo' shape on anteroposterior view and a 'step-off' appearance on lateral view radiography.
- Magnet co-ingestion prompts urgent endoscopy and removal.

- Failure to consider the diagnosis in non-specific presentations where button battery ingestion was not witnessed.
- Mistaking a button battery on X-ray for a coin, ECG electrode or other external object. Batteries have a distinctive appearance and lateral X-ray may help to identify the object.
- Delayed referral for endoscopic removal.

CONTROVERSIES
- Management of established oesophageal burns. Currently there are no clearly established guidelines for management of established burns with regard to repeat endoscopy, use of steroids, antibiotic therapy and feeding.
- Management of button batteries located in the stomach.
- Recommendations for oral administration of honey or sucralfate to limit tissue injury prior to endoscopic removal have been extrapolated from animal studies. The outcome benefits for these interventions in human cases are unproven.
- Post-procedural irrigation of affected oesophageal mucosa with dilute acetic acid (pH neutralisation) after button battery removal is another intervention suggested to limit tissue damage, with limited high-quality evidence of outcome benefit.

Sources
Button batteries are found in numerous devices including watches, cameras, remote controls, electronic games and hearing aids. More recently, manufactured devices tend to have smaller button batteries.

References

Anfang RR, Jatana KR, Linn RL et al. pH-neutralizing esophageal irrigations as a novel mitigation strategy for button battery injury. Laryngoscope 2019; 129(1):49–57. doi:10.1002/lary.27312.

Birk M, Bauerfeind P, Deprez PH et al. Removal of foreign bodies in the upper gastrointestinal tract in adults: European Society of Gastrointestinal Endoscopy (ESGE) Clinical Guideline. Endoscopy 2016; 48:1–8.

Jatana KR, Barron CL, Jacobs IN. Initial clinical application of tissue pH neutralization after esophageal button battery removal in children. Laryngoscope 2019; 129:1772–1776.

Jatana KR, Litovitz T, Reilly JS et al. Pediatric button battery injuries: 2013 task force update. International Journal of Pediatric Otorhinolaryngology 2013; 77:1392–1399.

Litovitz T, Whitaker N, Clark L et al. Emerging battery-ingestion hazard: clinical implications. Pediatrics 2010; 125:1168–1177.

3.21 CALCIUM CHANNEL BLOCKERS (CCBs)

Non-dihydropyridines: **Diltiazem, Verapamil**

Dihydropyridines: **Amlodipine, Felodipine, Lercanidipine, Nifedipine, Nimodipine**

Diltiazem and verapamil are potent cardiotoxic agents with a significant risk of death in overdose. The dihydropyridine agents primarily cause vasodilatory shock and are less commonly associated with severe toxicity.

Diltiazem and verapamil

- All deliberate self-poisonings are regarded as potentially lethal.
- Toxicity can occur at twice the therapeutic daily dose in susceptible individuals.
- Onset of toxicity occurs early with standard-release preparations but can be delayed up to 16 hours following XR preparations.

Dihydropyridines

- Calcium channel blockers of this class are less likely to cause life-threatening toxicity.
- The risk of significant hypotension is increased by:
  - co-ingestion of other cardiotoxic drugs
  - pre-existing cardiac dysfunction
  - advanced age.
- **Children:** any ingestion of calcium channel blockers requires hospital assessment.

Toxic mechanism

Diltiazem and verapamil block L-type calcium channels in the myocardium, resulting in slowing of cardiac conduction and decreased contractility. In overdose, they also block pancreatic L-type calcium channels, resulting in drug-induced insulin resistance, which manifests as hyperglycaemia and elevated lactate.

Dihydropyridines preferentially block calcium channels in the peripheral vasculature, leading to smooth muscle relaxation and vasodilatation. They are less likely to cause severe bradycardia or decreased myocardial contractility.

Toxicokinetics

Calcium channel blockers are well absorbed orally; however, in overdose, peak levels may not occur until 6 hours for standard-release preparations and 22 hours for XR preparations. They have large volumes of distribution and are metabolised by the hepatic cytochrome system. Diltiazem and verapamil are particularly susceptible to accumulation in therapeutic dosing due to drug interactions, and both these agents have active metabolites.

- Cardiovascular
  - Bradycardia and 1st-degree heart block are early signs of toxicity.
  - Worsening bradycardia and high-grade heart blocks.
  - Hypotension with progression to refractory shock.
- Metabolic
  - Hyperglycaemia and lactic acidosis are hallmarks of toxicity.
- Central nervous system
  - Consciousness is usually preserved despite profound bradycardia and hypotension.

Screening tests in deliberate self-poisoning

- 12-lead ECG, BGL and paracetamol level

Specific investigations

- EUC, calcium, lactate and blood gas
- Serial ECGs based on clinical progression

- Echocardiography
- Cardiac output monitoring

MANAGEMENT

Management of established CCB toxicity is determined by the type of agent ingested:

- Diltiazem or verapamil poisoning requires early use of high-dose insulin therapy.
- Dihydropyridine toxicity requires volume resuscitation and titrated vasopressor therapy.

Resuscitation, supportive care and monitoring

- Acute CCB overdose is a time-critical emergency managed in an area equipped for cardiorespiratory monitoring and resuscitation.
- Potential early life-threats that require immediate intervention include:
  — hypotension
  — cardiac dysrhythmia
  — cardiac arrest.
- Airway protective reflexes and conscious state are usually preserved until cardiac arrest. Rapid-sequence endotracheal intubation and ventilation may be required in cases of severe established toxicity.
- Early invasive blood pressure monitoring is advised for evolving shock.
- Fluid resuscitation as required to optimise intravascular volume.
- High-dose insulin therapy is the mainstay of therapy in diltiazem and verapamil poisoning and should be started as soon as toxicity is evident (see **Chapter 4.14: Insulin (high-dose)**).
- Calcium therapy is unlikely to provide definitive benefit in severe poisoning. It can produce a transient increase in heart rate and blood pressure but there is limited evidence to support repeated doses (see **Chapter 4.2: Calcium**).
- Catecholamines have limited efficacy in severe diltiazem or verapamil poisoning, but are indicated as initial therapies in the haemodynamically unstable patient.
- Noradrenaline is the catecholamine vasopressor of choice in dihydropyridine toxicity.
- Ventricular pacing can be attempted, but mechanical capture is often difficult to achieve and may not be associated with improved perfusion.
- Consider interventions such as extracorporeal membrane oxygenation (ECMO), cardiopulmonary bypass or intra-aortic balloon pump.
  — Acute cardiovascular toxicity is frequently reversible once the poisoning has resolved. Supportive bridging therapy with mechanical assist devices is therefore warranted.

Decontamination

- Activated charcoal
  — Administer to all cooperative patients without established toxicity.
  — Administer to all intubated patients.

- Whole bowel irrigation (see **Chapter 1.6: Gastrointestinal decontamination**)
  - May be considered after a dose of activated charcoal in cooperative adult patients without evidence of established toxicity and who present within 4 hours of significant ingestion of diltiazem or verapamil XR tablets.

Enhanced elimination
- Not clinically useful.

Antidotes
- As discussed in **Resuscitation, supportive care and monitoring** above:
  - High-dose insulin therapy (see **Chapter 4.14: Insulin (high-dose)**) is the mainstay of therapy in diltiazem or verapamil poisoning and should be started as soon as toxicity is evident.
  - Calcium (see **Chapter 4.2: Calcium**).

DISPOSITION AND FOLLOW-UP
- Patients who are clinically well with normal vital signs and 12-lead ECG at 6 hours following standard preparations or 16 hours following XR preparations may be discharged. Discharge should not occur at night.
- Patients with manifestations of toxicity are managed in an intensive care unit. Haemodynamic instability may persist for greater than 48 hours.

HANDY TIPS
- Differentiation between vasodilatory and cardiogenic shock is best determined by echocardiography or cardiac output monitoring. In the absence of these modalities, it is possible to identify vasodilatory shock (the predominant feature in dihydropyridine poisoning) based on clinical grounds.
- Patients who ingest combination formulations of dihydropyridines with angiotensin-converting enzyme inhibitors or angiotensin II receptor blockers may have persistent hypotension poorly responsive to escalating vasopressor therapies.

PITFALLS
- Failure to anticipate potential for delayed onset of severe toxicity following ingestion of XR preparations.
- Failure to initiate prompt decontamination (activated charcoal followed by whole bowel irrigation) in patients who present early following life-threatening overdose of XR diltiazem or verapamil.
- Delay in institution of high-dose insulin therapy once evidence of toxicity develops.

CONTROVERSIES
- The clinical benefit of high-dose insulin therapy in dihydropyridine toxicity is not clearly established.

- There is limited evidence to support a role for intravenous lipid emulsion in CCB toxicity.
- Therapies such as methylene blue for persistent vasodilatory shock in dihydropyridine toxicity are of unproven benefit.

Presentations

Benzothiazepines
Diltiazem 60 mg tablets (90)
Diltiazem extended-release capsules 180 mg, 240 mg, 360 mg (30)

Phenylalkylamines
Verapamil hydrochloride immediate release tablets 40 mg, 80 mg, 120 mg, 160 mg (100)
Verapamil hydrochloride sustained-release 160 mg, 180 mg, 240 mg (30)
Verapamil hydrochloride 5 mg/2 mL ampoules
Verapamil hydrochloride 180 mg/trandolapril 2 mg sustained-release tablets (28)
Verapamil hydrochloride 240 mg/trandolapril 4 mg sustained-release tablets (28)

Dihydropyridines
Multiple dihydropyridine formulations exist, including combinations with ACE inhibitors, angiotensin receptor blockers (ARB) and thiazide diuretics.

References

Buckley N, Dawson A, Whyte I. Calcium channel blockers. Medicine 2007; 35(11):134–139.

DeWitt CR, Waksman JC. Pharmacology, pathophysiology and management of calcium channel blocker and β-blocker toxicity. Toxicological Reviews 2004; 23(4):223–238.

Huang J, Buckley NA, Isoardi KZ et al. Angiotensin axis antagonists increase the incidence of haemodynamic instability in dihydropyridine calcium channel blocker poisoning. Clinical Toxicology 2021; 59(6):464–471.

Mégarbane B, Karyo S, Baud FJ. The role of insulin and glucose (hyperinsulinaemia/euglycaemia) therapy in acute calcium channel antagonist and β-blocker toxicity. Toxicological Reviews 2004; 23(4):215–222.

Olsen KR, Erdman AR, Woolf AD et al. Calcium channel blocker ingestion: an evidence-based guideline for out-of-hospital management. Clinical Toxicology 2005; 43:797–822.

Pichon N, Dugard A, Clavel M et al. Extracorporeal albumin dialysis in three cases of acute calcium channel blocker poisoning with life-threatening refractory cardiogenic shock. Annals of Emergency Medicine 2012; 59:540–544.

Yuan TH, Kerns WP, Tomaszewski CA et al. Insulin-glucose as an adjunctive therapy for severe calcium channel antagonist poisoning. Clinical Toxicology 1999; 37(4):463–474.

3.22 CANNABINOIDS AND SYNTHETIC CANNABINOID RECEPTOR AGONISTS (SCRAs)

Delta-9-tetrahydrocannabinol (THC), delta-8-tetrahydrocannabinol, cannabinol, cannabidiol, numerous synthetic cannabinoids

Slang terms include cones, dope, grass, hash, pot and weed.

Cannabis is the most widely used recreational illicit drug in Australasia. It is a psychoactive drug that can cause unpleasant but generally benign symptoms in adults. Cannabis ingestion by children can lead to significant CNS depression.

RISK ASSESSMENT

- Cannabis poisoning rarely causes severe toxicity.
- Adults experience symptoms in a dose-dependent manner:
  - Low-dose effects: 50 microgram/kg (3–4 mg) are associated with mild sedation, disinhibition, mild disorientation and euphoria.
  - High-dose effects: 250 microgram/kg (15 mg) are associated with tachycardia, postural hypotension, CNS depression, anxiety, dysphoria, perceptual disturbances and psychotic symptoms.
- Co-ingestion of other CNS depressants has an additive effect.
- Chronic use leads to long-term neuropsychiatric sequelae and a withdrawal syndrome is described in habitually heavy users.
- Synthetic cannabinoids are formally categorised as synthetic cannabinoid receptor agonists (SCRAs). They are synthetic chemicals, typically dissolved in solvents and sprayed onto dried plant material, which is then smoked. The chemical properties of the SCRA itself, or adulterants added during the manufacturing process, are responsible for the more toxic clinical features.
  - In general, they have greater agonist activity at cannabinoid receptors than natural THC (delta-9-tetrahydrocannabinol). A number of these agents have structural similarities to serotonin and amphetamines, and as such have significant sympathomimetic and serotonergic effects in addition to psychoactive properties. The principles of management – most importantly benzodiazepines and supportive care – are detailed in **Chapter 3.7: Amphetamines and amphetamine-like substances** and **Chapter 2.5: Serotonin toxicity**.
- **Children:** ingestion may lead to life-threatening coma in a child.

Toxic mechanism

The cannabis plant (*Cannabis sativa*) contains numerous cannabinoids, of which delta-9-tetrahydrocannabinol (THC) is the principal psychoactive component. It acts on cannabinoid receptors in the central and peripheral nervous system (CB_1) and on immune cells (CB_2), and also augments dopamine release.

Synthetic cannabinoid receptor agonists in general have greater agonist activity at cannabinoid receptors than natural THC. A number of these agents have structural similarities to serotonin and amphetamines, and as such have significant sympathomimetic and serotonergic effects in addition to hallucinogenic properties.

Toxicokinetics

Cannabis is rapidly and completely absorbed by inhalation, but bioavailability is reduced if ingested. Cannabinoids are highly protein bound, lipid soluble and have large volumes of distribution (10 L/kg). They undergo hepatic metabolism to form active and inactive metabolites that are excreted in the urine. Elimination half-life of the metabolites is several days.

CLINICAL FEATURES

Patients may present with symptoms of acute intoxication, psychiatric sequelae or withdrawal. In adults, acute symptoms last up to 4 hours following inhalation and up to 8 hours following ingestion. Clinical features of intoxication include:

- Central nervous system
  - Ataxia, incoordination, impaired judgement
  - Sedation
  - CNS depression
  - Coma in children
- Cardiovascular
  - Tachycardia
  - Orthostatic hypotension
  - Syncope
- Psychiatric
  - Euphoria and relaxation
  - Agitation
  - Anxiety and panic attacks
  - Perceptual changes – time distortion or hallucinations
  - Acute psychosis
- Respiratory complications (rare)
  - Pneumothorax
  - Pneumomediastinum
- Cannabinoid hyperemesis syndrome
  - Chronic cannabis users may present repeatedly to emergency departments with cannabinoid hyperemesis syndrome. This syndrome is characterised by recurrent episodes of vomiting and symptoms can be difficult to control. Severe cases may be complicated by acid–base disturbances and acute renal failure. Patients often shower or bathe in hot water to achieve temporary relief from symptoms. The diagnosis should only be made after alternative aetiologies are excluded.
- Synthetic cannabinoid receptor agonists (SCRAs)
  - In addition to the clinical features noted above, SCRAs have an increased risk of dysphoria, agitation, tachycardia and seizures.
  - Renal failure has been described, either related to the SCRA itself or other chemical adulterants.

203

TOXICOLOGY HANDBOOK

INVESTIGATIONS
Screening tests in deliberate self-poisoning
- 12-lead ECG, BGL and paracetamol level

Specific investigations
- Urine cannabinoid levels are readily available but infrequently assist acute management. They are occasionally useful for psychiatric or forensic indications. Serum cannabinoid levels are not readily available.
- Urine screening tests may be positive for 1–3 days after acute use, or 10 days to 4 weeks after chronic use.
- Passive inhalation of cannabis may give positive results on some screening tests for several days after acute exposure.
- False positive urine tests can occur.

MANAGEMENT
Resuscitation, supportive care and monitoring
- Cannabis intoxication is usually benign and self-limiting.
- Tachycardia and hypotension are managed with fluids and sedation as appropriate.

- Treat severe agitation with IV benzodiazepines until adequate sedation is achieved. Additional or alternative agents include droperidol 5–10 mg IM or IV, or olanzapine 5–10 mg SL, IM or IV (see **Chapter 2.4: Approach to delirium**).
- Adult patients with mild dysphoria or agitation may be given PO benzodiazepines and reassured.
- Cannabinoid hyperemesis syndrome may require admission for intravenous fluids and symptomatic treatment. Standard anti-emetics are often ineffective and titrated agents such as IV droperidol or benzodiazepines are frequently required.

Decontamination
- Not clinically useful.

Enhanced elimination
- Not clinically useful.

Antidotes
- None available.

DISPOSITION AND FOLLOW-UP
- Children who may have ingested cannabis should be observed in hospital for 4 hours. If they do not develop symptoms during that period, they may then be safely discharged.
- Patients with intoxication adequately controlled with benzodiazepine sedation may be managed supportively in a ward environment. They may be discharged when asymptomatic. Patients with cannabinoid hyperemesis syndrome should be counselled and supported to achieve and maintain abstinence following discharge.

HANDY TIPS
- Cannabis poisoning is not life-threatening and severe toxicity is uncommon.
- Profound coma or 12-lead ECG changes suggest a co-ingested agent and the need to revise the risk assessment.
- The principles of management for serotonergic or amphetamine-like features of poisoning from SCRAs are detailed in **Chapter 3.7: Amphetamines and amphetamine-like substances** and **Chapter 2.5: Serotonin toxicity**.

PITFALL
- Failure to anticipate the potential in paediatric ingestions for rapid onset of hypotonia, abnormal movements, tachycardia or coma which may last more than 24 hours.

CONTROVERSY
- Capsaicin topical cream is suggested as an effective treatment for cannabinoid hyperemesis syndrome. There are limited data to support this claim.

Presentations
Any part or extract of the hemp plant (*Cannabis sativa*) can be dried or converted to a resin extract.

References

Allen JH, de Moore GM, Heddle R et al. Cannabinoid hyperemesis: cyclical hyperemesis in association with chronic cannabis abuse. Gut 2004; 53:1566–1570.

Hall W, Solowij N. Adverse effects of cannabis. Lancet 1998; 352:1611–1615.

Reece AS. Chronic toxicology of cannabis. Clinical Toxicology 2009; 47(6):517–524.

Richards JR, Lapoint JM, Burillo-Putze G. Cannabinoid hyperemesis syndrome: potential mechanisms for the benefit of capsaicin and hot water hydrotherapy in treatment. Clinical Toxicology 2018; 56(1):15–24.

Sydney S, Beck JE, Tekawa IE et al. Marijuana use and mortality. American Journal of Public Health 1997; 87:585–590.

Tait RJ, Caldicott D, Mountain D et al. A systematic review of adverse events arising from the use of synthetic cannabinoids and their associated treatment. Clinical Toxicology 2016; 54(1):1–13.

3.23 CARBAMAZEPINE

Deliberate self-poisoning with this anticonvulsant agent results in predictable dose-dependent coma and anticholinergic effects. Early recognition of the likelihood of prolonged coma guides the definitive management decision to intubate, ventilate and administer nasogastric activated charcoal with a protected airway.

RISK ASSESSMENT

- Clinical features are dose-dependent (see **Table 3.23.1**) and onset of toxicity may be delayed.
- Anticholinergic effects may be prominent prior to development of coma.
- Following massive ingestions, coma is anticipated to last several days, secondary to ongoing absorption, slow elimination and the presence of an active metabolite.
- **Pregnancy:** carbamazepine is teratogenic. Overdose in the first trimester warrants referral for further antenatal assessment.
- **Children:** ingestion of >20 mg/kg is likely to cause toxicity and warrants hospital assessment.

Toxic mechanism

Carbamazepine is structurally similar to the tricyclic antidepressant imipramine. It inhibits inactivated sodium channels, thus preventing the propagation of action potentials. It also blocks noradrenaline reuptake and is an antagonist at muscarinic, nicotinic and central N-methyl-D-aspartate and adenosine receptors.

TABLE 3.23.1	Dose-related risk assessment: carbamazepine
Dose	**Effect**
20–50 mg/kg	Mild-to-moderate CNS and anticholinergic effects
>50 mg/kg	Fluctuating mental status with intermittent agitation and risk of progression to coma Risk of hypotension and cardiotoxicity with massive doses

Toxicokinetics

Carbamazepine is slowly and erratically absorbed. Following large overdoses, ileus secondary to anticholinergic effects may result in ongoing absorption for several days. Carbamazepine has a small volume of distribution (0.8–1.2 L/kg) and is highly protein bound. It undergoes hepatic metabolism by cytochrome P450 3A4 to form an active metabolite (carbamazepine 10,11-epoxide).

CLINICAL FEATURES

Clinical features of intoxication are usually evident within 4 hours of ingestion, but peak effects including coma may be significantly delayed. Ongoing absorption and the presence of an active metabolite complicates large overdoses producing a prolonged, fluctuating clinical course (cyclical coma).

- CNS effects include nystagmus, dysarthria, ataxia, sedation, delirium, mydriasis, ophthalmoplegia and myoclonus.
- Anticholinergic effects such as urinary retention and tachycardia are common in the early stages.
- Large overdoses may be complicated by hypotension and recurrent seizures.
- Cardiac conduction abnormalities (QRS widening) can occur but ventricular dysrhythmias (VT, VF) are rarely seen, even with massive ingestions.

INVESTIGATIONS

Screening tests in deliberate self-poisoning

- 12-lead ECG, BGL and paracetamol level

Specific investigations

- Serum carbamazepine levels (see **Table 3.23.2**)
  - Confirm the diagnosis.
  - Patients without coma management can be guided by clinical features and serial levels are not essential.
  - In cases where coma develops, monitoring of carbamazepine levels every 6–8 hours is essential to guide management decisions.
- Serial 12-lead ECGs
  - Ingestions >50 mg/kg may be associated with evidence of sodium channel blockade.
  - An ECG should be evaluated at presentation and serial ECGs performed based on clinical progression.

TABLE 3.23.2 Correlation of serum levels and clinical features: carbamazepine

Carbamazepine level	Clinical features
8–12 mg/L (34–51 micromol/L)	Therapeutic range
>12 mg/L (51 micromol/L)	Nystagmus and ataxia
>20 mg/L (85 micromol/L)	CNS and anticholinergic effects
>40 mg/L (170 micromol/L)	Coma, seizures and cardiovascular effects

Resuscitation, supportive care and monitoring
- Attention to airway, breathing and circulation are paramount. These priorities are managed along conventional lines, as outlined in **Chapter 1.2: Resuscitation**.
- In the unlikely event of ventricular dysrhythmias, resuscitation should include the use of IV bolus sodium bicarbonate, as outlined in **Chapter 4.24: Sodium bicarbonate**.
- Monitor for urinary retention and insert an indwelling urinary catheter if required.
- General supportive care measures are indicated, as outlined in **Chapter 1.4: Supportive care and monitoring**.
- Seizures and agitated delirium are managed with intravenous benzodiazepines, as outlined in **Chapter 2.3: Seizures** and **Chapter 2.4: Approach to delirium**.

Decontamination
- Activated charcoal is recommended for all intentional ingestions of carbamazepine that present without established CNS toxicity.
- If there is evidence of CNS toxicity, activated charcoal is only administered after the patient is intubated.

Enhanced elimination
- Multiple-dose activated charcoal is indicated in intubated patients. It is not administered if bowel sounds are absent.
- Haemodialysis or continuous renal replacement therapies remove carbamazepine effectively and are warranted in severe intoxication. Indications include:
  - serum levels >80 mg/L (340 micromol/L)
  - prolonged coma, with serum levels >40 mg/L (170 micromol/L) after 48 hours
  - predicted prolonged coma based on ingested dose.

Antidotes
- None available.

DISPOSITION AND FOLLOW-UP
- Children suspected of ingesting >20 mg/kg of carbamazepine should be observed in hospital for 8 hours. Discharge should not occur at night.
- Patients who are clinically well without CNS or anticholinergic effects at 8 hours following ingestion do not require further medical management.
- Patients with clinical features of carbamazepine toxicity require ongoing management based on an accurate risk assessment.
- Patients with seizures or coma require management in an intensive care unit.

HANDY TIP
- In suspected paediatric ingestion, an undetectable serum carbamazepine level any time after the first hour excludes ingestion and allows immediate discharge.

PITFALLS
- Failure to appreciate the potential for delayed onset of toxicity.
- Failure to detect urinary retention and place an indwelling urinary catheter.

CONTROVERSY
- The indications for extracorporeal elimination. The decision remains one of clinical judgement involving a risk–benefit analysis.

Presentations
Carbamazepine tablets 100 mg, 200 mg (200)
Carbamazepine controlled-release tablets 200 mg, 400 mg (200)
Carbamazepine suspension 20 mg/mL (300 mL)

References
Ghannoum M, Yates C, Galvao TF et al. on behalf of the EXTRIP workgroup. Extracorporeal treatment for carbamazepine poisoning: systematic review and recommendations from the EXTRIP workgroup. Clinical Toxicology 2014; 52(10):993–1004.

Harder JL, Heung M, Vilay AM et al. Carbamazepine and the active epoxide metabolite are effectively cleared by hemodialysis followed by continuous venovenous hemodialysis in an acute overdose. Hemodialysis International 2011; 15:412–415.

Hojer J, Malmlund HO, Berg A. Clinical features in 28 consecutive cases of laboratory confirmed massive poisoning with carbamazepine alone. Journal of Toxicology–Clinical Toxicology 1993; 31:449–458.

Spiller HA. Management of carbamazepine overdose. Pediatric Emergency Care 2001; 17(6):452–456.

3.24 CARBON MONOXIDE

Carbon monoxide (CO) is a common cause of poisoning death. Acute effects are due to cellular hypoxia, particularly affecting the CNS and cardiovascular systems. Delayed neuropsychiatric sequelae frequently occur following significant toxicity.

RISK ASSESSMENT
- Death from CO poisoning almost always occurs pre-hospital.
- Patients who present to hospital after exposure to CO are particularly at risk of CNS or cardiovascular toxicity. Neurological features in particular may be vague and initially overlooked, especially in children.
- The risk assessment attempts to identify those at risk of significant myocardial injury and long-term neuropsychiatric sequelae.
- Evidence of myocardial ischaemia (chest pain, ECG changes, elevated troponin) is associated with increased mortality and worsened neurological outcomes.
- High-risk features include:
  - loss of consciousness or altered mental state
  - persistent neurological features

- severe metabolic acidosis
- evidence of myocardial ischaemia
- carboxyhaemoglobin (COHb) level >25%.
- Outcome, particularly neuropsychiatric sequelae, does not correlate directly with the documented carboxyhaemoglobin level.
- **Pregnancy:** fetal haemoglobin binds CO more avidly, rendering the fetus more susceptible to injury.
- **Children:** in the absence of definitive data guiding modification of the risk assessment, children should be assessed and managed as for adults.

Toxic mechanism

CO has greater than 200 times the affinity for haemoglobin than oxygen, resulting in impaired oxygen-carrying capacity and tissue oxygen delivery. Organs with high oxygen consumption such as the brain and heart are particularly susceptible to hypoxic injury. In addition, CO binds to intracellular molecules (myoglobin, mitochondrial cytochrome oxidase), leading to oxidative stress and mitochondrial dysfunction. CO also initiates endothelial oxidative injury, lipid peroxidation and an inflammatory cascade that is probably responsible for delayed neurological sequelae.

Methylene chloride (dichloromethane) is an industrial solvent metabolised to CO following inhalation, dermal exposure or ingestion. This process can occur over several hours.

Toxicokinetics

CO is rapidly absorbed from the pulmonary alveoli. The elimination half-life is determined by the partial pressure of oxygen as follows:
- room air: 240 min
- 100% oxygen: 90 min
- 100% oxygen at three atmospheres: 23 min.

CLINICAL FEATURES

Following acute exposure, most patients present with headache, nausea and altered mental state. A history of loss of consciousness is common. Clinical manifestations include:
- Central nervous system
  - Headache, nausea, dizziness
  - Confusion, poor concentration, mini mental status examination (MMSE) errors
  - Incoordination and ataxia
  - Seizures and coma
- Cardiovascular
  - Chest pain
  - Tachycardia
  - Hypotension
  - Dysrhythmias
  - Ischaemic ECG changes
  - Acute myocardial infarction
- Respiratory
  - Pulmonary oedema
- Metabolic
  - Lactic acidosis
  - Rhabdomyolysis
- Neurological sequelae can be characterised as persistent or delayed.
  - Persistent features are evident from the time of poisoning. Neuropsychiatric sequelae persist in 6–10% at 12 months.

- Delayed sequelae are the development of new clinical features attributable to CO poisoning which occur or become evident days to weeks after exposure. These either may not have been present on initial assessment or may not have been noted. A detailed neuropsychiatric examination is essential.
  - Symptoms may be subtle and include personality changes, mood disorders (anxiety, depression), poor concentration, cognitive deficits, psychosis, parkinsonism and ataxia. The majority of features improve or resolve within a year of onset.

INVESTIGATIONS

Screening tests in deliberate self-poisoning
- 12-lead ECG, BGL and paracetamol level

Specific investigations
- Carboxyhaemoglobin level (COHb)
  - Confirms exposure but does not correlate with symptoms or prognosis.
  - The COHb level in patients presenting to the emergency department does not reflect the peak blood level because of removal from the source, delay in attendance and administration of supplemental oxygen prior to arrival.
    - Note: Standard pulse oximetry does not reliably detect carboxyhaemoglobin and cannot be used to confirm or exclude CO poisoning.
- Serum lactate and blood gas
- Troponin
- FBC, EUC, liver function tests
- β-HCG
- Mini mental status examination (MMSE)
- Head CT or MRI
  - May demonstrate cerebral oedema, white matter subcortical demyelination, symmetrical hypoattenuation of the basal ganglia or thalamic nuclei, or delayed cerebral atrophy.
- Neuropsychiatric testing
  - Indicated to investigate persistent or delayed neurological symptoms.
- Biochemical neural markers have been investigated as predictors of an increased risk of delayed neurological sequelae but are not widely available or routinely used.

MANAGEMENT

Resuscitation, supportive care and monitoring
- Attention to airway, breathing and circulation are paramount. These priorities can usually be managed along conventional lines, as outlined in **Chapter 1.2: Resuscitation**.
- Patients with persistent coma require intubation and administration of 100% oxygen.
- All patients should receive 100% oxygen or high-flow oxygen via a non-rebreathing mask until all symptoms have resolved and for at least 6 hours.
- General supportive care measures are indicated, as outlined in **Chapter 1.4: Supportive care and monitoring**.

Decontamination
- Most patients will improve once removed from the exposure and receiving supplemental oxygen. Further decontamination is not required.

Enhanced elimination
- Elimination of CO is enhanced by:
  - Normobaric oxygen
    - All patients should receive 100% oxygen or high-flow oxygen via a non-rebreathing mask until all symptoms have resolved and for at least 6 hours.
  - Hyperbaric oxygen (HBO)
    - Patients with high-risk features following CO poisoning should be considered for HBO treatment (see **Controversies**).
    - All pregnant patients should be considered for HBO.

Antidotes
- None available.

DISPOSITION AND FOLLOW-UP
- All symptomatic patients immediately receive supplemental oxygen and are referred to hospital for assessment.
- Continue oxygen in hospital until all symptoms resolve and for at least 6 hours.
- Formal neuropsychiatric assessment is indicated 1–2 months after exposure.
- Patients exposed to methylene chloride require extended observation and documentation of a normal COHb level prior to discharge.

HANDY TIPS
- The patient who presents following accidental occupational or domestic poisoning represents an index case. Identification of the source and other potential victims is indicated.
- The decision regarding HBO therapy is best made in conjunction with the local hyperbaric unit. Logistical considerations including timely access, transport issues, patient suitability and staff safety are relevant to the decision-making process.

PITFALLS
- Failure to diagnose accidental occupational or domestic poisoning in patients who present with headache or other non-specific symptoms.
- Failure to perform and document a detailed neurological examination and MMSE.

CONTROVERSIES
- The duration of normobaric oxygen treatment is not clearly defined.
- The indications for and effectiveness of HBO. Randomised controlled trials give conflicting evidence. While HBO is not routinely recommended, there may be a subgroup of patients with poisoning for whom there is benefit. Clinical judgement and consideration of local logistics is required.

Sources

Incomplete combustion of hydrocarbon fuels

Methylene chloride (dichloromethane) is a solvent metabolised to CO in vivo.

References

Buckley NA, Juurlink DN, Isbister G et al. Hyperbaric oxygen for carbon monoxide poisoning. Cochrane Database of Systematic Reviews 2011; 4:CD002041.

Chiew AL, Buckley NA. Carbon monoxide poisoning in the 21st century. Critical Care 2014; 18:221.

Hampson NB, Piantodosi CA, Thom SR et al. Practice recommendations in the diagnosis, management, and prevention of carbon monoxide poisoning. American Journal of Respiratory and Critical Care Medicine 2012; 186:1095–1101.

Rose JJ, Wang L, Xu Q et al. Carbon monoxide poisoning: pathogenesis, management, and future directions of therapy. American Journal of Respiratory and Critical Care Medicine 2017; 195(5):596–606.

Scheinkestel CD, Bailey M, Myles PS et al. Hyperbaric or normobaric oxygen for acute carbon monoxide poisoning: a randomised controlled clinical trial. Medical Journal of Australia 1999; 170:203–210.

Weaver LK, Hopkins RO, Chan KJ et al. Hyperbaric oxygen for acute carbon monoxide poisoning. New England Journal of Medicine 2002; 347(14):1057–1067.

3.25 CHLORAL HYDRATE

Chloral hydrate is still available for use as a sedative in children undergoing procedures. It was withdrawn as a sedative-hypnotic for adults because of its narrow therapeutic index. In overdose, it causes rapid onset of CNS depression and cardiac dysrhythmias, and these are frequently lethal without intervention.

RISK ASSESSMENT

- Ingestion of >100 mg/kg, twice the upper limit of therapeutic dosing, is associated with high risk of coma and life-threatening cardiac dysrhythmias.

Toxic mechanism

Chloral hydrate has a direct irritant action on mucosal surfaces. The mechanism of action of the toxic metabolite trichloroethanol (TCE) on the CNS and cardiovascular system is unclear. Cardiac dysrhythmias are thought to be caused by sensitisation of the myocardium to circulating catecholamines. Chloral hydrate also decreases myocardial contractility and shortens the refractory period, which enhances cardiotoxicity.

Toxicokinetics

Chloral hydrate is rapidly absorbed following oral administration. It is then rapidly converted to the active metabolite TCE by hepatic alcohol dehydrogenase. TCE is conjugated with glucuronic acid and excreted in the urine and to a limited extent in the bile. Chloral hydrate has an elimination half-life of only 4–5 minutes whereas TCE has an elimination half-life of 8–12 hours after therapeutic doses and up to 35 hours after overdose.

CLINICAL FEATURES

Chloral hydrate overdose is characterised by rapid (<30 min) onset of life-threatening CNS and cardiovascular toxicity. Gastrointestinal effects and hypothermia complete the clinical profile.

- Central nervous system
  - Drowsiness, light-headedness and ataxia may rapidly progress to coma and respiratory depression.

- Cardiovascular
  - Cardiac dysrhythmias
    - Multifocal premature ventricular ectopics
    - Atrial fibrillation
    - Supraventricular tachycardia
    - Ventricular tachycardia
    - Ventricular fibrillation
    - Torsades de pointes
    - Asystole
  - Hypotension
- Hypothermia
- Gastrointestinal
  - Corrosive injury may be associated with gastro-oesophageal necrosis and even perforation.
  - Permanent stricture formation is a potential complication.

INVESTIGATIONS

Screening tests in deliberate self-poisoning
- 12-lead ECG, BGL and paracetamol level

Specific investigations
- Serial 12-lead ECGs are essential to monitor the effects on clinical conduction and response to therapy.
- TCE levels can be measured and correlate with toxicity, but are never available in a clinically useful time frame. They may be useful to retrospectively confirm the diagnosis in forensic cases.
- Gastroscopy may be indicated after a large ingestion to assess mucosal damage and potential for stricture formation.

MANAGEMENT

Resuscitation, supportive care and monitoring
- The patient is initially managed in an area equipped for cardiorespiratory monitoring and resuscitation.
- Attention to airway, breathing and circulation are paramount and managed along conventional lines, as outlined in **Chapter 1.2: Resuscitation**.
- Immediate endotracheal intubation and ventilation is indicated at the first signs of progressive CNS or cardiovascular toxicity.
- Beta-blockers are indicated for chloral-hydrate-induced cardiac tachydysrhythmias. Options include intravenous metoprolol or esmolol.
- Hypotension is managed with appropriate intravenous fluids.
- Catecholamines are avoided due to the risk of promoting ventricular dysrhythmias.
- General supportive care measures are indicated, as outlined in **Chapter 1.4: Supportive care and monitoring**.
- Corrosive effects of oral chloral hydrate, especially in large ingestions, may warrant evaluation with upper gastrointestinal endoscopy within 24 hours.

Decontamination
- Activated charcoal may be given once the airway is secured with endotracheal intubation, but never takes precedence over resuscitation and supportive care measures.

Enhanced elimination

- TCE elimination can be enhanced with haemodialysis, but patients are usually stabilised by the measures described above, rendering this intervention unnecessary.

Antidotes

- Not clinically useful.

DISPOSITION AND FOLLOW-UP

- All suspected paediatric ingestions and adult deliberate self-poisonings require immediate assessment and observation in hospital.
- All patients should be closely observed with cardiac monitoring in place for at least 2 hours and until recovery is complete.
- Development of CNS depression requiring intubation, cardiac dysrhythmias or hypotension is an indication for admission to an intensive care unit.

HANDY TIP

- Torsades de pointes is usually treated with IV magnesium and overdrive pacing, but beta blockade is the recommended treatment in the setting of chloral hydrate toxicity.

PITFALLS

- Exacerbation of ventricular dysrhythmias by the administration of catecholamines during resuscitation.
- Failure to administer beta-blockers to the patient with ventricular dysrhythmias.

CONTROVERSIES

- The administration of beta-blockers is based on the premise that ventricular dysrhythmias arise as a result of sensitisation of the myocardium to circulating catecholamines. Their efficacy is supported by clinical experience and multiple favourable case reports, but has not been evaluated in clinical trials.
- Flumazenil is reported to reverse the CNS depression of chloral hydrate, but its administration is not recommended. Given the life-threatening nature of the cardiovascular toxicity, early definitive control of airway and ventilation with endotracheal intubation is preferred.

Presentations

Chloral hydrate 1 g/10 mL syrup (200 mL)

References

Graham SR, Day RO, Lee R et al. Overdose with chloral hydrate: a pharmacological and therapeutic review. Medical Journal of Australia 1988; 149:686–688.

Pershad J, Palmisano P, Nichols M. Chloral hydrate: the good and the bad. Pediatric Emergency Care 1999; 15:432–435.

Sing K, Erickson T, Amitai Y et al. Chloral hydrate toxicity from oral and intravenous administration. Journal of Toxicology–Clinical Toxicology 1996; 34:101–106.

Zahedi A, Grant MH, Wong DT. Successful treatment of chloral hydrate cardiac toxicity with propranolol. American Journal of Emergency Medicine 1999; 17(5):490–491.

3.26 CHLOROQUINE AND HYDROXYCHLOROQUINE

Overdose with chloroquine or hydroxychloroquine produces initial gastrointestinal symptoms with rapid onset of hypotension, CNS depression, cardiac conduction defects and profound hypokalaemia. In severe cases, prompt intubation and immediate management of cardiotoxicity and hypokalaemia is imperative.

RISK ASSESSMENT
- Ingestion of >10 mg/kg of chloroquine is potentially toxic.
- Serious toxicity and increasing mortality is expected with ingested doses >30 mg/kg.
- Ingestion of >5 g of chloroquine in adults may be fatal without intervention.
- The dose-related risk assessment is less well defined for hydroxychloroquine, but appears to be similar to chloroquine.
- **Children:** ingestion of a single tablet of these agents requires hospital assessment.

Toxic mechanism

Chloroquine and hydroxychloroquine both have a narrow therapeutic index. They exert toxicity on the CNS via effects on voltage-dependent sodium channels. Hypotension and cardiogenic shock are due to a direct cardiodepressant effect. Cardiac conduction abnormalities are caused by blockade of inward sodium channels (QRS widening) and outward potassium channels (QT prolongation and torsades de pointes). Systemic hypokalaemia is a result of intracellular re-distribution of potassium due to blockade of tissue hERG potassium channels. Hypoglycaemia is reported, related to enhanced insulin release.

Toxicokinetics

Both agents have similar toxicokinetics. Absorption after ingestion is rapid and complete, with large volumes of distribution due to extensive tissue binding. They are partially metabolised by the liver and have prolonged half-lives.

CLINICAL FEATURES
Onset of symptoms occurs within 2 hours.
- Early symptoms:
  - Nausea, vomiting, dizziness
- Cardiovascular
  - Rapid onset of hypotension
  - Cardiac conduction defects (QRS widening, QT prolongation)
  - Cardiac arrest
- Central nervous system
  - Seizures
  - Coma
- Metabolic
  - Hypokalaemia
  - Hypoglycaemia

INVESTIGATIONS
Screening tests in deliberate self-poisoning
- 12-lead ECG, BGL and paracetamol level

Specific investigations
- EUC, calcium, magnesium
  - Detect abnormalities of QT-dependent electrolytes
- Serial ECGs
  - QRS and QT prolongation
  - Sinus arrest, varying degrees of heart block
- Specific levels are not routinely available and do not assist in management. They may be useful retrospectively to confirm the diagnosis.

MANAGEMENT
Resuscitation, supportive care and monitoring
- Chloroquine or hydroxychloroquine overdose is a life-threatening emergency and is managed in an area equipped for cardiorespiratory monitoring and resuscitation.
- Clinical features requiring immediate intervention include:
  - Coma:
    - Prompt intubation and ventilation is indicated at the first sign of a depressed conscious state.
  - Hypotension:
    - Manage initially with appropriate volume resuscitation, but inotropic and vasopressor support may be required. Options include adrenaline, noradrenaline and high-dose insulin therapy, guided by assessment of cardiovascular function.
    - Interventions such as ECMO, cardiopulmonary bypass or intra-aortic balloon pump may be required.
  - Torsades de pointes:
    - Electrical cardioversion may be required for persistent episodes that result in altered mental state or haemodynamic instability.
    - Magnesium 10 mmol IV bolus (0.05 mmol/kg in children) over 1–2 minutes, repeated once if torsades de pointes recurs.
    - Isoprenaline or overdrive electrical pacing are other treatment options to increase the resting heart rate to a target of >100 beats/min.
    - Ensure that all QT-dependent electrolytes (potassium, calcium, magnesium) are at the upper limit of normal (see **Chapter 2.17: The 12-lead ECG in toxicology**).
  - Broad complex tachycardias with haemodynamic compromise:
    - Manage initially with bolus IV sodium bicarbonate 1–2 mmol/kg IV, intubation and hyperventilation (see **Chapter 4.24: Sodium bicarbonate**). If there is no dynamic improvement in QRS widening following initial boluses of sodium bicarbonate, further IV doses are unlikely to be of benefit.
      - Note: Multiple doses of sodium bicarbonate can cause significant alkalaemia, exacerbating hypokalaemia and increasing the risk of torsades de pointes.

- Seizures are managed with IV benzodiazepines (see **Chapter 2.3: Seizures**).
- Hypokalaemia should be anticipated and the serum potassium monitored closely and maintained at the upper level of normal:
  - It may be difficult to achieve this with standard rates of IV potassium administration.
    - Note: In severe cases of hypokalaemia with recurrent torsades de pointes, haemodialysis may be required as part of intensive care management to correct serum potassium effectively.

Decontamination
- Administration of activated charcoal is withheld until the airway is protected.
- Following massive overdose of chloroquine or hydroxychloroquine, early intubation to facilitate safe administration of activated charcoal can be justified.

Enhanced elimination
- Due to their large volumes of distribution, haemodialysis will not effectively enhance drug clearance.

Antidotes
- None available.

DISPOSITION AND FOLLOW-UP
- All children suspected of ingesting even one chloroquine or hydroxychloroquine tablet must be assessed and observed in hospital.
- Patients who are asymptomatic at 6 hours following ingestion, with a normal ECG, are fit for medical discharge. Discharge should not occur at night.
- Admission to ICU is indicated following massive ingestions (>30 mg/kg) and for patients manifesting signs of significant toxicity.

HANDY TIPS
- Anticipate catastrophic deterioration in any patient presenting early following chloroquine overdose. Intubate and hyperventilate at the first sign of cardiotoxicity or clinical deterioration.
- Management of ventricular dysrhythmias can be challenging due to the presence of QRS widening and QT prolongation. Sodium channel blockade (QRS widening) may not respond to bolus sodium bicarbonate therapy, and excessive administration can lead to pulmonary and cerebral oedema, life-threatening hypokalaemia and catastrophic deterioration.

CONTROVERSIES
- Excessive IV administration of potassium may lead to rebound hyperkalaemia following resolution of toxicity. In practice, the risk of recurrent ventricular dysrhythmias due to hypokalaemia outweighs this potential and manageable risk.

- High-dose diazepam (0.5 mg/kg IV bolus then an infusion of 1 mg/kg IV over 24 hours) post intubation has historically been advocated to treat cardiovascular toxicity. However, the protective mechanism and efficacy of this intervention is unclear and it is not recommended as standard management.

Presentations
Chloroquine phosphate 250 mg tablets (no longer available in Australia)
Hydroxychloroquine sulfate 200 mg tablets (100)

References
Clemessy JL, Favier C, Borron SW et al. Hypokalaemia related to acute chloroquine ingestion. Lancet 1995; 346(8979):877–880.
Clemessy J-L, Taboulet P, Hoffman JR et al. Treatment of acute chloroquine poisoning: a 5-year experience. Critical Care Medicine 1996; 24:1189–1195.
Marquardt K, Albertson TE. The treatment of hydroxychloroquine overdose. Journal of Emergency Medicine 2005; 28(4):437–443.
Riou B, Barriot P, Rimailho A et al. Treatment of severe chloroquine poisoning. New England Journal of Medicine 1988; 318:1–6.
Smith ER, Klein-Schwartz W. Are 1–2 dangerous? Chloroquine and hydroxychloroquine exposure in toddlers. Journal of Emergency Medicine 2005; 28(4):437–443.

3.27 CLONIDINE AND OTHER CENTRAL α_2-ADRENERGIC AGONISTS

Clonidine overdose produces varying degrees of CNS depression and mild cardiovascular effects. The classical presentation is sedation, bradycardia, hypotension and miosis.

Other central α_2-adrenergic agonists include guanfacine, moxonidine and imidazoline derivatives. They are used for the management of ADHD and hypertension and as ophthalmological preparations, and have a similar toxicological profile to clonidine.

RISK ASSESSMENT
- Clinical effects correlate poorly with ingested dose. Significant CNS depression may occur with doses >20 microgram/kg, but large doses are sometimes tolerated with only minor effects.
- Onset of clinical features is rapid, usually within 2 hours of ingestion and always within 6 hours.
- **Children:** ingestion of 2 tablets is potentially lethal without supportive care:
  - >10 microgram/kg: bradycardia and hypotension
  - >20 microgram/kg: respiratory depression or apnoea.

Toxic mechanism
Clonidine stimulates central pre-synaptic α_2-adrenergic receptors, causing bradycardia and hypotension by a decrease in sympathetic outflow. It also increases endothelial-derived nitric oxide levels. Sedation is caused by augmentation of GABA in the CNS and endogenous β-endorphin release.

Toxicokinetics
Clonidine is rapidly absorbed with peak concentration occurring within 3 hours. Clonidine has a large volume of distribution, and the elimination half-life is up to 24 hours.

CLINICAL FEATURES
- Onset of toxicity is rapid. Transient early hypertension is reported but is not clinically significant.
- CNS depression ranging from sedation to coma is the most common clinical feature.
- Sinus bradycardia and hypotension are characteristic and can be profound. Transient heart block is reported.
- Respiratory depression and apnoea are prominent features of paediatric ingestion.

INVESTIGATIONS
Screening tests in deliberate self-poisoning
- 12-lead ECG, BGL and paracetamol level

Specific investigations
- Serial ECGs

MANAGEMENT
Resuscitation, supportive care and monitoring
- The patient is initially managed in an area equipped for cardiorespiratory monitoring and resuscitation.
- Basic resuscitative measures ensure the survival of the vast majority of patients.
- Coma and respiratory depression may respond to high-dose naloxone therapy (see **Antidotes**).
- Intubation and ventilation is required in severe intoxications not responding to antidotal therapy.
- Hypotension usually responds to appropriate IV fluid resuscitation. It seldom requires vasopressor support.
- Specific management for bradycardia (e.g. atropine, catecholamine infusion or pacing) is rarely required and only if there is hypotension unresponsive to fluid resuscitation or evidence of decreased end-organ perfusion.

Decontamination
- Activated charcoal is given only after the airway is protected with endotracheal intubation.

Enhanced elimination
- Not clinically useful.

Antidotes
- Naloxone in high doses has been shown to reverse CNS and respiratory depression caused by clonidine intoxication. Intubation and ventilation may still be required if naloxone is ineffective.
- Administration of naloxone is indicated in all children with established clonidine toxicity.
- The doses of naloxone required are significantly greater than for standard opioid reversal:
  - Paediatric: give an initial bolus dose of 2–5 mg IV, repeated every 1–2 minutes up to a maximum dose of 10 mg
  - Adult: consideration of IV naloxone boluses up to 10 mg see **Handy Tips**)

- If naloxone is effective, repeat boluses or an infusion of up to 5 mg/hr may be used.
- For further information on the indications, contraindications and administration see **Chapter 4.18: Naloxone**.

DISPOSITION AND FOLLOW-UP
- Paediatric patients should be observed in hospital following potential accidental exposure.
- Patients who are clinically well without symptoms at 6 hours following ingestion may be discharged. Discharge should not occur at night.
- Patients with mild symptoms may be managed supportively in a ward environment and can be discharged when clinically well.
- Bradycardia may persist for >24 hours, and the patient is at risk of postural hypotension when ambulating.

HANDY TIPS
- Consider the diagnosis of clonidine ingestion in any child who presents with lethargy, bradycardia and miosis.
- Adult patients have a lower incidence of respiratory depression or apnoea following clonidine ingestion and are more likely to have co-ingested opioids. Use of large doses of naloxone in this setting may precipitate acute opioid withdrawal.

PITFALLS
- Failure to recognise the potential lethality of accidental paediatric ingestion of clonidine.
- Failure to recognise respiratory depression in children, especially at night.
- Iatrogenic anticholinergic delirium from excessive doses of atropine administered in response to bradycardia.
- Patients may transiently respond to external stimuli, only to become re-sedated when undisturbed with an attendant risk of respiratory complications.

Presentations
Clonidine 100 microgram, 150 microgram tablets (100)
Clonidine 150 microgram/mL 1 mL ampoules

References

Erickson SJ, Duncan A. Clonidine poisoning – an emerging problem: epidemiology, clinical features, management and preventative strategies. Journal of Paediatrics and Child Health 1998; 34(3):280–282.

Fiser DH, Moss MM, Walker W. Critical care for clonidine poisoning in toddlers. Critical Care Medicine 1990; 18(10):1124–1128.

Isbister GK, Heppell SP, Page CB et al. Adult clonidine overdose: prolonged bradycardia and central nervous system depression, but not severe toxicity. Clinical Toxicology 2017; 55(3):187–192.

Seger DL. Clonidine toxicity revisited. Journal of Toxicology–Clinical Toxicology 2002; 40:145–155.

3.28 CLOZAPINE

Deliberate self-poisoning with this atypical antipsychotic agent is uncommon because its use is restricted and closely supervised. Sedation and coma are the predominant features in overdose.

RISK ASSESSMENT
- A clear dose–response is not defined but the threshold for severe poisoning including coma may be as low as 100 mg in adults.
- Small doses, particularly in naïve patients, may result in significant intoxication.
- Coma may persist >24 hours.
- **Children:** ingestion of a single tablet can cause profound coma. All ingestions require hospital assessment.

Toxic mechanism
Clozapine is an atypical dibenzodiazepine antipsychotic. It is an antagonist at mesolimbic dopamine (D_1 and D_2), serotonin (5-HT) and adrenergic receptors. Compared to other antipsychotic agents, it is a potent antagonist at muscarinic (M_1), histamine (H_1) and gamma-aminobutyric acid (GABA) receptors.

Toxicokinetics
Clozapine is rapidly absorbed following oral administration. It is highly protein bound and has a moderate volume of distribution. Clozapine is metabolised in the liver by cytochrome P450 enzymes, making it susceptible to drug interactions.

CLINICAL FEATURES
- CNS depression, including coma requiring intubation, can occur rapidly.
- Anticholinergic effects such as delirium and urinary retention are invariably present.
- Hypersalivation is a paradoxical but characteristic feature, and the precise mechanism in unknown.
- Seizures occur in 5–10% of patients.
- Extrapyramidal effects are more common in children and can persist for >24 hours.
- QT prolongation is uncommon and torsades de pointes has not been reported in overdose.

INVESTIGATIONS
Screening tests in deliberate self-poisoning
- 12-lead ECG, BGL and paracetamol level

Specific investigations
- Clozapine levels are used for therapeutic monitoring. They do not correlate well with the clinical features in acute overdose.
  - These are readily available and although not helpful in guiding management may be useful to confirm the diagnosis.

MANAGEMENT
Resuscitation, supportive care and monitoring
- Attention to airway, breathing and circulation are paramount. These priorities are managed along conventional lines, as outlined in **Chapter 1.2: Resuscitation.**

- Basic resuscitative measures ensure a good outcome in the vast majority of patients.
- Treat seizures with benzodiazepines, as outlined in **Chapter 2.3: Seizures**.
- General supportive care measures are indicated, as outlined in **Chapter 1.4: Supportive care and monitoring**.
- Monitor for urinary retention with serial bladder scans and insert an indwelling urinary catheter if required.

Decontamination
- Activated charcoal is only given after the airway is protected with endotracheal intubation.

Enhanced elimination
- Not clinically useful.

Antidotes
- None available.

DISPOSITION AND FOLLOW-UP
- Patients who are clinically well 6 hours following ingestion do not require further medical management.
- Paediatric patients are at risk of prolonged extrapyramidal effects.

HANDY TIP
- Therapeutic use of clozapine is associated with agranulocytosis and myocarditis. These are not clinical features of acute poisoning.

PITFALL
- Failure to recognise and correct urinary retention.

Presentations
Clozapine 25 mg tablets (28, 100)
Clozapine 50 mg tablets (100)
Clozapine 100 mg tablets (28, 100)
Clozapine 200 mg tablets (100)
Clozapine suspension 50 mg/mL 100 mL

References
Seger DL, Loden JK. Naloxone reversal of clonidine toxicity: dose, dose, dose. Clinical Toxicology 2018; 56(10):873–879.

Burns MJ. The pharmacology and toxicology of atypical antipsychotic agents. Clinical Toxicology 2001; 39(1):1–14.

Cobaugh DJ, Erdman AR, Booze LL et al. Atypical antipsychotic medication poisoning; an evidence based consensus guideline for out-of-hospital medication poisoning. Clinical Toxicology 2007; 45:918–942.

Isbister GK, Balit CR, Kilham HA. Antipsychotic poisoning in young children: a systematic review. Drug Safety 2005; 26(11):1029–1044.

Reith D, Monteleone JP, Whyte IM et al. Features and toxicokinetics of clozapine in overdose. Therapeutic Drug Monitoring 1998; 20(1):92–97.

Trenton A, Currier G, Zwemer F. Fatalities associated with therapeutic use and overdose of atypical antipsychotics. CNS Drugs 2003; 17(5):307–324.

Wong DC, Curtis LA. Are 1 or 2 dangerous? Clozapine and olanzapine exposure in toddlers. The Journal of Emergency Medicine 2004; 27:273–277.

3.29 COCAINE

Cocaine is a potent stimulant that also has local anaesthetic activity. Its use is associated with life-threatening complications: severe hypertension, myocardial ischaemia, tachydysrhythmias, stroke, seizures or coma.

RISK ASSESSMENT

- Ingestions of >1 g are potentially lethal. See **Table 3.29.1**.
- The toxic dose is highly variable and small doses, particularly in non-tolerant patients, may result in significant intoxication.
- The presence of hyperthermia, headache, cardiac conduction abnormalities, focal neurological signs or chest pain heralds potentially life-threatening complications.
- **Pregnancy:** cocaine is teratogenic and associated with an increased incidence of fetal and maternal morbidity and mortality.
- **Lactation:** cocaine is excreted in breast milk and can result in infant intoxication.
- **Children:** any ingestion is potentially lethal.

Toxic mechanism

Toxicity results from its sympathomimetic and sodium channel blocking (local anaesthetic) effects. Sympathomimetic effects are indirect, due to the blockade of pre-synaptic catecholamine reuptake, resulting in increased levels of noradrenaline, serotonin, dopamine and adrenaline at the adrenergic receptor site. Vasospasm and endothelial fissuring can result in acute coronary syndrome. Blockade of myocardial fast sodium channels may result in ventricular dysrhythmias. Central nervous system excitation is secondary to increased concentrations of the excitatory amino acids glutamate and aspartate in the brain.

Toxicokinetics

Cocaine is well absorbed through the mucous membranes of nasopharynx, pulmonary alveolar tree and gastrointestinal tract. Peak effects are achieved more rapidly by IV administration and smoking (3–5 minutes) compared to the intranasal route (20–30 minutes). It is a highly lipid soluble, with a volume of distribution of 2 L/kg. Cocaine is rapidly metabolised by liver and plasma cholinesterases to water-soluble metabolites. Only 1% of the drug appears unchanged in the urine. Metabolites may persist in the blood and urine for up to 36 hours. Clinical duration of effect is approximately 60 minutes, with serum half-lives between 0.5 and 1.5 hours.

CLINICAL FEATURES

Patients may present with symptoms of acute intoxication, medical complications of abuse or psychiatric sequelae. The onset of cocaine

TABLE 3.29.1 Dose-related risk assessment: cocaine	
Dose	**Effect**
1–3 mg/kg	Safe local anaesthetic dose
20–30 mg	Usual dose in a line of cocaine
1 g	Potentially lethal

intoxication is rapid, with major clinical manifestations occurring within the first hour and usually lasting 2–3 hours. They include:

- Central nervous system
  - Euphoria
  - Anxiety, dysphoria, agitation and aggression
  - Paranoid psychosis with visual and tactile hallucinations
  - Muscle rigidity and movement disorders
  - Seizures
- Cardiovascular
  - Tachycardia and hypertension
  - Dysrhythmias and cardiac conduction abnormalities
  - Chest pain
  - Acute coronary syndromes – vasospastic and/or thrombotic
  - Cardiomyopathy
  - Acute pulmonary oedema
- Other effects
  - Hyperthermia
  - Rhabdomyolysis
  - Renal failure
  - Aortic and carotid dissection
  - Subarachnoid and intracerebral haemorrhage
  - Ischaemic colitis
  - Pneumothorax or pneumomediastinum
  - Pulmonary infarction or pneumonitis

INVESTIGATIONS
Screening tests in deliberate self-poisoning
- 12-lead ECG, BGL and paracetamol level

Specific investigations
- EUC, creatine kinase
  - Detect electrolyte abnormalities, renal failure and rhabdomyolysis.
- ECG and troponin
  - Detect acute coronary syndromes and conduction abnormalities.
  - A Brugada-type pattern of ECG changes (RBBB with ST elevation in leads V1, V2 and V3) can occur in cocaine intoxication.
- Chest X-ray or CT angiogram
  - Detects cardiovascular or pulmonary complications.
- CT head
  - Detects intracranial haemorrhage.
- Echocardiogram
  - Assess cardiac function.
- Serum or urine cocaine levels are not readily available and do not assist acute management.

MANAGEMENT
Resuscitation, supportive care and monitoring
- Cocaine intoxication is a life-threatening emergency and is managed in an area equipped for cardiorespiratory monitoring and resuscitation.

- Clinical features requiring immediate intervention include:
  - tachydysrhythmias
  - chest pain
  - hypertension
  - hyperthermia
  - seizures
  - severe agitation.
- First-line treatment for all clinical features of cocaine intoxication is titrated parenteral benzodiazepines to reduce centrally mediated sympathetic stimulation.
- If hypertension is refractory to benzodiazepine administration, consider:
  - titrated vasodilator infusion (glyceryl trinitrate, sodium nitroprusside) or phentolamine IV titrated to effect (if available).
- Broad complex tachycardias may be caused by sodium channel blockade. In addition to benzodiazepines, an initial dose of IV sodium bicarbonate 8.4% 50–100 mL (1–2 mL/kg) aiming for a dynamic improvement in QRS prolongation is indicated (see **Chapter 2.17: The 12-lead ECG in toxicology**).
- Acute coronary syndrome is largely managed according to standard protocols with the following caveats:
  - Beta-blockers are contraindicated (see **Controversy**).
  - Verapamil or diltiazem are alternative agents but should be administered cautiously as they may cause haemodynamic deterioration due to negative inotropic effects.
  - Thrombolysis may not be appropriate as the pathophysiology is frequently vasospasm.
- Urgent coronary angiography is indicated in the setting of ST elevation that persists after nitroglycerine and calcium channel blockers.
- Seizures and agitation are managed with IV benzodiazepines titrated to effect (see **Chapter 2.3: Seizures** and **Chapter 2.4: Approach to delirium**).
- Hyperthermia
  - Temperature >38.5°C is an indication for continuous core-temperature monitoring, benzodiazepine administration and cooling measures.
  - Temperature >39.5°C requires rapid external cooling to prevent multiple organ failure and neurological injury. Paralysis, intubation and ventilation may be required.

Decontamination
- Gastrointestinal decontamination with activated charcoal is not indicated except in the specific instance of cocaine body packers as discussed in **Chapter 2.14: Body packers and stuffers**.

Enhanced elimination
- Not clinically indicated.

Antidotes
- None available.

DISPOSITION AND FOLLOW-UP
- Children with potential ingestions should be observed in hospital for 4 hours. If they remain asymptomatic, they can be safely discharged.

- Patients whose intoxication is adequately controlled with benzodiazepine administration and have a normal blood pressure and 12-lead ECG may be managed supportively in a ward environment. They are discharged when clinically well.
- Patients with significant clinical features require management in a high-dependency or intensive care unit.

HANDY TIPS
- Benzodiazepines are the mainstay of treatment for cocaine toxicity and early use is recommended for all clinical features.
- Ongoing chest pain or headache requires further investigation.
- CT scanning should be performed prior to anticoagulation if vascular dissection or haemorrhage is a clinical concern.

PITFALL
- Failure to administer adequate benzodiazepines to a patient with significant cocaine intoxication.

CONTROVERSY
- Administration of beta-blockers in the management of cocaine intoxication is contraindicated in most guidelines as unopposed alpha-adrenergic stimulation may cause severe vasoconstriction. This includes agents with combined alpha- and beta-blocking effects (labetalol).

Presentations
Prescription medications
Cocaine eye drops 15 mL bottles
Illicit cocaine derivatives
Cocaine hydrochloride powder or paste: processed from the alkaloid extracted from coca leaves, it cannot be smoked as it decomposes at high temperatures.
Cocaine base (crack cocaine) or free-base: created by combining cocaine hydrochloride with an alkaline substance to render it heat stable.

References
Afonso L, Mohammad T, Thatai D. Crack whips the heart: a review of the cardiovascular toxicity of cocaine. American Journal of Cardiology 2007; 100(6):1040–1043.
Lange RA, Hillis LD. Cardiovascular complications of cocaine use. New England Journal of Medicine 2001; 345(5):351–358.
Zimmerman JL. Cocaine intoxication. Critical Care Clinics 2012; 28:517–526.

3.30 COLCHICINE

Colchicine overdose is uncommon but potentially lethal. Toxicity is characterised by severe gastroenteritis followed by multi-system organ failure. Immediate decontamination and supportive care are the cornerstones of management.

RISK ASSESSMENT
- Any intentional ingestion of colchicine is considered potentially lethal. The doses outlined in **Table 3.30.1** are useful in predicting

TABLE 3.30.1	Dose-related risk assessment: colchicine
Dose	**Effect**
<0.2 mg/kg	Gastrointestinal symptoms
0.2–0.5 mg/kg	Potential for systemic toxicity and death
0.5–0.8 mg/kg	Systemic toxicity with multi-system organ effects and increasing risk of death
>0.8 mg/kg	Severe poisoning with cardiovascular collapse and multi-system organ failure Approaching 100% mortality

outcome, although fatalities are reported with acute ingestion of as little as 0.2 mg/kg.

- **Children:** any paediatric ingestion of colchicine requires prompt hospital assessment.

Toxic mechanism
Colchicine is a naturally occurring alkaloid found in the autumn crocus (*Colchicum autumnale*) and glory lily (*Gloriosa superba*). It is used in the treatment of acute gout, pericarditis and rare conditions such as familial Mediterranean fever. It binds tubulin and prevents microtubule formation, thus inhibiting mitosis and leucocyte migration into inflamed tissue (diapedesis). Following overdose, tissues with high cellular turnover (gastrointestinal, bone marrow) are preferentially affected.

Toxicokinetics
Colchicine is rapidly absorbed, with peak levels occurring within 2 hours post ingestion. Bioavailability is 45% as a result of extensive first-pass metabolism. Colchicine is extensively tissue bound with a volume of distribution of 2 L/kg. Elimination is by hepatic metabolism, with an elimination half-life up to 30 hours. Colchicine exhibits biliary excretion with the potential for entero-hepatic recirculation.

CLINICAL FEATURES
Colchicine overdose usually presents with severe gastroenteritis followed by onset of multi-organ toxicity in the subsequent 24 hours (see **Table 3.30.2**).

TABLE 3.30.2	Clinical progression of severe colchicine toxicity
Time	**Effect**
2–24 hours	Nausea, vomiting, diarrhoea, abdominal pain. Severe GI fluid losses can result in haemodynamic instability. Peripheral leucocytosis commonly seen on blood film
2–7 days	Bone marrow suppression and pancytopenia, rhabdomyolysis, renal failure, progressive metabolic acidosis, respiratory insufficiency, ARDS, cardiac dysrhythmias and risk of sudden cardiac death
>7 days	Rebound leucocytosis and transient alopecia. Complete recovery may occur in patients who survive to this stage

INVESTIGATIONS
Screening tests in deliberate self-poisoning
- 12-lead ECG, BGL and paracetamol level

Specific investigations
- Specific colchicine levels are not routinely available.
- Appropriate investigations to assess and monitor multi-organ toxicity:
  - FBC, EUC, liver function tests, coagulation studies, troponin, creatine kinase and venous blood gas.

MANAGEMENT
Resuscitation, supportive care and monitoring
- Immediate gastrointestinal decontamination is a priority following deliberate self-poisoning with colchicine and should be instituted as soon as possible after ingestion (see **Decontamination**).
- Patients may present in hypovolaemic shock due to significant GI fluid losses. They require appropriate resuscitation with intravenous crystalloid solutions.
- Management in an intensive care environment offers the best chance of survival in severe colchicine poisoning. Meticulous clinical, physiological and laboratory monitoring is required.
- Ventilatory and haemodynamic support are implemented as indicated.
- Granulocyte colony-stimulating factor (GCSF) is indicated for bone marrow depression with established neutropenia.

Decontamination
- Administer activated charcoal 50 g (1 g/kg in children) as soon as possible to **ANY** patient presenting with an acute overdose or supratherapeutic ingestion of colchicine because prevention of absorption of even a small amount may be life-saving.

Enhanced elimination
- Multiple-dose oral activated charcoal may enhance elimination by preventing enterohepatic recirculation and should be offered to all patients with the potential for significant toxicity.

Antidotes
- Colchicine-specific antibodies were used in a single case of colchicine overdose but are not commercially available.

DISPOSITION AND FOLLOW-UP
- All cases of deliberate self-poisoning are admitted for observation.
- Patients who are clinically well without gastrointestinal symptoms within 24 hours of ingestion and have stable biochemical and haematological parameters do not require ongoing medical management.
- Patients with significant toxicity require admission to an intensive care unit.

HANDY TIPS
- Admit **ALL** colchicine overdoses. Arrange early transfer to intensive care if more than 0.5 mg/kg is ingested or any symptoms develop.

- Interactions with CYP3A4 and P-glycoprotein inhibitors such as macrolide antibiotics, azole antifungals, cyclosporin, calcium channel blockers (diltiazem, verapamil) or grapefruit juice can increase colchicine concentrations and the risk of toxicity.

PITFALLS
- Failure to identify ingestion of colchicine at presentation.
- Failure to anticipate the severity of colchicine poisoning.

CONTROVERSY
- Due to the potential lethality of colchicine following acute overdose, it may be justified to intubate a non-compliant patient to facilitate administration of activated charcoal in a timely fashion.

Presentations
Colchicine 500 microgram tablets (30)

References
Finkelstein Y, Aks SE, Hutson JR et al. Colchicine poisoning: the dark side of an ancient drug. Clinical Toxicology 2010; 48(5):407–414.

Jayaprakash V, Ansell G, Galler D. Colchicine overdose: the devil is in the detail. New Zealand Medical Journal 2007; 120(1248):81–88.

Wijerathna TM, Gawarammana IB, Fahim Mohamed F et al. Epidemiology, toxicokinetics and biomarkers after self-poisoning with Gloriosa superba. Clinical Toxicology 2017; 57(11):1080–1086.

Zawahir S, Gawarammana I, Dargan PI et al. Activated charcoal significantly reduces the amount of colchicine released from Gloriosa superba in simulated gastric and intestinal media. Clinical Toxicology 2017; 55(8):914–918.

3.31 CORROSIVES

Alkalis: **Ammonia, Potassium hydroxide, Sodium hydroxide, Sodium hypochlorite**

Acids: **Hydrochloric acid, Sulfuric acid**

See also Chapter 3.20: Button Batteries, Chapter 3.38: Glyphosate and Chapter 3.63: Paraquat.

Ingestion of corrosive agents causes injury to the upper airway and gastrointestinal tract. Upper airway injury is a life-threatening emergency. Endoscopy and CT scanning stratify the immediate and long-term risks in symptomatic patients.

RISK ASSESSMENT
- The risk of severe injury following ingestion of a corrosive agent is determined by five major factors:
  - chemical properties of the agent
  - concentration
  - volume
  - pH
  - intent (deliberate versus accidental).

- Ingestions of strong alkalis such as sodium hydroxide (NaOH) or potassium hydroxide (KOH) result in severe corrosive injury to the pharynx, upper airway, oesophagus and stomach.
- Strong acids such as sulfuric acid (H_2SO_4) or hydrochloric acid (HCl) also cause severe injury, particularly to the stomach and duodenum. In addition, an early severe metabolic acidosis can occur with these agents, with rapid onset of multi-organ failure and death.
- Sodium hypochlorite is the most common component of household bleach and is less likely to cause significant corrosive injury.
- The absence of lip or oral burns does not exclude significant gastro-oesophageal injury.
- Corrosive agents such as glyphosate or paraquat are more likely to cause severe systemic toxicity as their predominant clinical feature.
- **Children:** accidental ingestion of household drain and oven cleaners or automatic dishwashing powders can cause severe corrosive injury. Accidental ingestion of household bleach containing sodium hypochlorite is usually less toxic, but all corrosive ingestions in children mandate medical assessment and observation.

Toxic mechanism
Corrosive agents cause direct chemical injury to tissues. The extent of injury is determined by the pH, concentration and volume of the agent ingested. Alkaline agents cause liquefactive necrosis, resulting in deep and progressive mucosal damage. Acids cause protein denaturation and coagulative necrosis.

CLINICAL FEATURES
- Stridor, dysphonia, throat pain or dyspnoea indicate airway injury or aspiration and an immediate threat to life.
- Gastrointestinal features include oropharyngeal lesions, vomiting, dysphagia, drooling, haematemesis and abdominal pain. The likelihood of significant gastro-oesophageal injury increases proportional to the number of clinical features.
- Oesophageal perforation and mediastinitis are associated with chest pain, dyspnoea, fever, subcutaneous emphysema and a pleural rub.
- Perforation of the stomach or small intestine may result in clinical features of peritonitis.
- Oesophageal or gastric strictures develop most commonly 6–12 weeks after ingestion.
- Higher-grade injuries are associated with development of oesophageal carcinoma many decades later.

INVESTIGATIONS
Screening tests in deliberate self-poisoning
- 12-lead ECG, BGL and paracetamol level

Specific investigations
All patients with ongoing symptoms require further investigation to assess the extent of injury and the risk for immediate (perforation) and delayed (stricture) complications.

- Endoscopy should ideally be performed within 24 hours of ingestion to minimise the risk of perforation.
- CT scanning is advocated as an alternative to endoscopy (see **Tables 3.31.1** and **3.31.2** and **Controversies**).
- The main sign of transmural digestive necrosis on CT imaging is the absence of post-contrast wall enhancement, and its presence at any level (oesophagus, stomach, duodenum, bowel, colon) is an indication for emergency surgery.

TABLE 3.31.1 Endoscopic grading of corrosive injury

Endoscopic grading	Appearance
Grade 0	Normal
Grade I	Mucosal oedema and hyperaemia
Grade IIA	Superficial ulcers, bleeding and exudates
Grade IIB	Deep focal or circumferential ulcers
Grade IIIA	Focal necrosis
Grade IIIB	Extensive necrosis

Adapted from Zargar SA, Kochhar R, Mehta S et al. The role of fiberoptic endoscopy in the management of corrosive ingestion and modified endoscopic classification of burns. Gastrointestinal Endoscopy 1991; 37(2):165–169.

TABLE 3.31.2 CT grading of oesophageal and gastric caustic injury – adults

CT grading	Appearance
Grade I	Homogeneous post-contrast wall enhancement No wall oedema or mediastinal fat stranding
Grade IIa	Enhancement of oesophageal mucosa Wall oedema Increased post-contrast wall enhancement Mediastinal fat stranding is present Note: 'Target' appearance of oesophagus may be present due to concentric contrast enhancement of mucosa and wall
Grade IIb	No enhancement of necrotic mucosa Wall oedema Fine rim of external wall enhancement Mediastinal fat stranding is present
Grade III	Transmural necrosis as shown by the absence of post-contrast wall enhancement

Adapted from Chirica M, Kelly MD, Siboni S et al. Esophageal emergencies: WSES guidelines. World Journal of Emergency Surgery 2019; 14(26). https://doi.org/10.1186/s13017-019-0245-2

Resuscitation, supportive care and monitoring

- Symptomatic corrosive ingestion is a time-critical emergency managed in an area equipped for resuscitation.
- The immediate life-threat is rapid loss of airway. Early endotracheal intubation or surgical airway may be required.
- General supportive care measures are indicated, as outlined in **Chapter 1.4: Supportive care and monitoring**.
- The symptomatic patient remains nil by mouth and no nasogastric tube is inserted until the extent of injury is defined by either endoscopy or CT scan.
- Urgent surgical intervention is indicated if there is evidence of full-thickness necrosis or perforation.
- Broad-spectrum antibiotics are not indicated unless there is evidence of perforation.
- It is reasonable to treat with intravenous proton pump inhibitors, but there are limited data to show definite outcome benefit.

Decontamination

- The mouth may be rinsed with water as an immediate first aid measure, but other interventions are not indicated:
  - Do not induce vomiting.
  - Do not administer oral fluids.
  - Do not administer activated charcoal.
  - Do not attempt pH neutralisation.

Enhanced elimination

- Not clinically useful.

Antidotes

- None available.

DISPOSITION AND FOLLOW-UP

- Patients who are asymptomatic and tolerating oral fluids at 4 hours post ingestion are medically fit for discharge.
- Symptomatic patients remain nil by mouth and are admitted for observation and further investigation within 24 hours. Further management and disposition is directed by endoscopic or CT findings.
- Patients with airway compromise require intensive care admission once the airway is controlled.

HANDY TIPS

- Signs and symptoms may correlate poorly with the extent of gastro-oesophageal injury.
- Decisions regarding the requirement for endoscopy or CT scanning in the presence of ongoing symptoms, particularly in children, benefit from involvement of the most experienced clinicians available, as well as consultation with the local gastroenterology service.

PITFALL

- Underestimating the possibility of gastrointestinal injury, particularly in the absence of oropharyngeal burns.

CONTROVERSIES

- Relative benefits of CT scanning versus endoscopy to determine the extent of gastro-oesophageal injury and requirement for surgery and whether the two investigations are complementary.
  - CT scanning with a standard protocol including intravenous contrast (see Chirica et al. in **References**) is advocated as a more reliable alternative than endoscopy regarding decisions for surgical intervention – decreasing the rate of unnecessary oesophagectomy and preserving the native gastrointestinal tract. The benefits of CT scanning include widespread availability, but successful interpretation of the results may be dependent on the degree of radiological and surgical expertise. CT scanning is certainly indicated where endoscopy cannot be performed safely.
  - Endoscopy is a safe procedure if performed within 24 hours and by experienced practitioners and provides the opportunity for placement of an enteral feeding tube under direct visual control. Currently, endoscopy is recommended for initial assessment of symptomatic paediatric patients due to concerns regarding excessive radiation exposure. However, even in the paediatric population, CT scanning may be appropriate to further refine the decision for gastro-oesophageal surgery in the presence of severe endoscopically confirmed injury.
- The role of steroids in the prevention of delayed gastrointestinal complications following corrosive ingestion.
  - In paediatric patients with visualised Grade IIB endoscopic injury (excluding minor or higher-grade injuries injuries), high-dose methylprednisolone (1000 mg/1.73 m^2 for 3 days) reduced the rate of stricture formation without increasing the risk of sepsis or perforation (see **References**). However, there is limited evidence to support a similar benefit in adult patients.
- The role of steroids in cases of upper airway corrosive injury to limit oedema and inflammation or decrease the duration of intubation.
  - In the absence of definitive data showing benefit, standard institutional approaches for dosing of agents such as dexamethasone are reasonable and can be determined on a case-by-case basis.

Sources

Ammonia – anti-rust products, jewellery and metal cleaners
Hydrochloric acid – metal cleaners
Sodium hydroxide – button batteries, detergents, drain and oven cleaners
Sodium hypochlorite – bleaches and household cleaners
Sulfuric acid – automotive batteries, drain cleaners

References

Betalli P, Falchetti D, Stefano Giuliani S et al. Caustic ingestion in children: is endoscopy always indicated? Gastrointestinal Endoscopy 2008; 68(4):34–39.

Chirica M, Kelly MD, Siboni S et al. Esophageal emergencies: WSES guidelines. World Journal of Emergency Surgery 2019; 14(26). https://doi.org/10.1186/s13017-019-0245–2.

Cowan T, Foster R, Isbister GK. Acute esophageal injury and strictures following corrosive ingestions in a 27 year cohort. American Journal of Emergency Medicine 2017; 35(3):488–492. doi:10.1016/j.ajem.2016.12.002.

Isbister GK, Page CB. Early endoscopy or CT in caustic injuries. Clinical Toxicology 2011; 49(7):641–642.

Lurie Y, Slotky M, Fischer D et al. The role of chest and abdominal computed tomography in assessing the severity of acute corrosive ingestion. Clinical Toxicology 2013; 51:834–837.

Munoz EM, Garcia-Domingo MI, Santiago JR et al. Massive necrosis of the gastrointestinal tract after ingestion of hydrochloric acid. European Journal of Surgery 2001; 67:195–198.

Pelclová D, Navrátil T. Do corticosteroids prevent oesophageal stricture after corrosive ingestion? Toxicological Reviews 2005; 24(2):125–129.

Ryu HH, Jeung KW, Lee BK et al. Caustic injury: can CT grading system enable prediction of esophageal stricture? Clinical Toxicology 2010; 48:137–142.

Usta M, Erkan T, Cokugras FC et al. High doses of methylprednisolone in the management of caustic esophageal burns. Pediatrics 2014; 33(6):1518–1524.

Wightman RS, Read KB, Hoffman RS. Evidence-based management of caustic exposures in the emergency department. Emergency Medicine Practice 2016; 18(5):1–17.

Zargar SA, Kochhar R, Mehta S et al. The role of fiberoptic endoscopy in the management of corrosive ingestion and modified endoscopic classification of burns. Gastrointestinal Endoscopy 1991; 37(2):165–169.

3.32 CYANIDE

Acute cyanide poisoning is a rare, dramatic and lethal presentation. Rapid removal from the source, attention to the principles of critical care and timely administration of an antidote in selected cases provides the best opportunity for survival.

RISK ASSESSMENT

- Acute cyanide exposure, whether by ingestion of cyanide salts or inhalation of hydrogen cyanide gas, can be rapidly lethal. Death may occur before arrival at hospital.
- The lethal oral dose in adults is 50 mg of hydrogen cyanide or 200 mg of potassium cyanide.
- Patients who arrive alive at hospital following inhalational exposure will likely survive with supportive care alone, even if antidotal therapy is not available.
- Ingestion of acetonitrile can lead to delayed onset (up to 2 hours) of life-threatening cyanide toxicity.
- Ingestion of amygdalin (cyanogenic-containing plant material, usually seeds) can result in toxicity but rarely causes serious poisoning because of lower bioavailability.
- Chronic occupational intoxication leads to non-specific symptoms such as headache and fatigue.
- **Children:** any exposure to cyanide is potentially lethal.

Toxic mechanism

Cyanide acts at several sites. It binds to the ferric ion (Fe^{3+}) of cytochrome oxidase and inhibits oxidative metabolism, leading to lactic acidosis. It stimulates release of biogenic amines, resulting in pulmonary and coronary vasoconstriction. In the CNS, cyanide triggers neurotransmitter release, particularly N-methyl-D-aspartate (NMDA), which leads to seizures.

Toxicokinetics

Cyanide is rapidly absorbed and taken up into cells. It has a volume of distribution of 1.5 L/kg and is protein bound. The metabolism of cyanide is not fully understood. The main mechanism is thought to involve hepatic transfer of sulfane sulfur to cyanide, forming thiocyanate, which is non-toxic and excreted in the urine. This reaction is catalysed by the enzyme rhodanese. Cyanide elimination half-life is 2–3 hours.

Acetonitrile (methyl cyanide), an industrial solvent, undergoes hepatic metabolism in vivo to yield cyanide. The process takes place slowly, with the conversion half-life estimated to be greater than 30 hours.

CLINICAL FEATURES

- Acute inhalation of hydrogen cyanide gas leads to loss of consciousness within seconds to minutes.
- Symptoms develop within minutes of ingestion of cyanide salts.
- Early features include nausea, vomiting, headache, dyspnoea, hypertension, tachycardia, agitation, collapse and seizures.
- Progressive features include hypotension, bradycardia, confusion, respiratory depression and coma.
- Delayed neurological toxicity may be observed weeks to months after severe poisoning.

INVESTIGATIONS

Screening tests in deliberate self-poisoning

- 12-lead ECG, BGL and paracetamol level

Specific investigations

- Arterial blood gases and serum lactate
  - Serum lactate strongly correlates with severity of intoxication.
  - In smoke inhalation victims without severe burns, the sensitivity, specificity and positive predictive values of a serum lactate >10 mmol/L for cyanide levels >40 micromol/L (0.1 mg/dL) are: 87%, 94% and 95%, respectively.
- EUC, LFT and FBC
- ECG and troponin
  - Detect myocardial ischaemia.
- Cyanide levels (see **Table 3.32.1**).
  - Do not aid acute management but confirm diagnosis in retrospect.
  - Do not correlate directly with survival.
  - Take blood before antidotes are commenced (heparinised tube).

TABLE 3.32.1 Correlation of blood levels and clinical effects: cyanide

Level	Effect
<12 micromol/L (0.5 mg/L)	Asymptomatic
23–58 microml/L (1–2.5 mg/L)	Systemic multi-organ effects
>58 micromol/L (2.5 mg/L)	Coma and potentially lethal

Resuscitation, supportive care and monitoring

- Cyanide poisoning is a life-threatening emergency and patients should be managed in an area capable of cardiorespiratory monitoring and resuscitation.
- Immediate threats to life include seizures, coma, shock and profound lactic acidosis.
- Immediate intubation and ventilation with 100% oxygen is indicated in severe poisoning.
- Immediate administration of a cyanide antidote is indicated in a patient with suspected cyanide poisoning and severe toxicity as detailed above.
- Resuscitation otherwise proceeds along conventional lines, as outlined in **Chapter 1.2: Resuscitation**.
- General supportive care measures are indicated, as outlined in **Chapter 1.4: Supportive care and monitoring**.
- Administration of 100% oxygen or high-flow oxygen via a non-rebreathing mask is essential during initial management of all cases of cyanide poisoning.

Decontamination

- Removal from the source of hydrogen cyanide gas exposure is vital.
- Remove clothes and wash skin with soap and water. Clothing should be bagged.
- Cyanide is rapidly absorbed and the onset of symptoms occurs within minutes. Resuscitation takes priority over decontamination.

Enhanced elimination

- Not clinically useful.

Antidotes

- Hydroxocobalamin is the preferred antidote for severe cyanide poisoning.
- Sodium thiosulfate acts to enhance cyanide elimination, usually in combination with hydroxocobalamin (see **Chapter 4.13: Hydroxocobalamin** and **Chapter 4.26: Sodium thiosulfate**).
- Other antidotes (amyl nitrite, sodium nitrite, dicobalt edetate) are rarely used because of significant side effects and limited availability.

DISPOSITION AND FOLLOW-UP

- Patients who are clinically well at 4 hours may be discharged.
- Patients with a history of acetonitrile ingestion must be observed for at least 24 hours.
- Patients who have received oxygen and supportive care (without antidote administration) and show rapid clinical improvement with normal mental status and vital signs may be managed in a ward environment.
- Patients with severe cyanide intoxication and cardiovascular instability require management in an intensive care setting.

HANDY TIPS

- Consider the diagnosis of cyanide poisoning in the patient presenting with seizure, coma and haemodynamic instability with persistent severe lactic acidosis.
- Early administration of 100% oxygen and good supportive care may be sufficient to achieve a good outcome in most cases without the requirement for specific antidotes.
- The decision to give an antidote can be made empirically based on clinical judgement.

PITFALL

- Failure to recognise cyanide intoxication.

CONTROVERSY

- The requirement for specific antidote administration is not clearly defined for patients with mild symptoms and no significant cardiorespiratory instability.

Sources
Industrial
Cyanide salts are used in metallurgy and ore extraction
Hydrogen cyanide is a fumigant (aeroplanes, buildings, ships)
Nitriles that yield cyanide are used in manufacture of plastics and synthetic fibres
Non-industrial
Cyanide is the product of combustion of natural substances and synthetic material and therefore commonly produced in fires
Solvent in artificial nail remover
Natural
Amygdalin (apple, apricot and peach pips)
Foodstuffs (almonds, cabbage, spinach, tapioca, white lima beans)
Iatrogenic
Chemical warfare agent
Sodium nitroprusside therapy

References
Baud FJ, Borron SW, Mégarbane B et al. Value of lactic acidosis in the assessment of the severity of acute cyanide poisoning. Critical Care Medicine 2002; 30(9):2044–2050.

Braitberg G, Vanderpyl MMJ. Treatment of cyanide poisoning in Australasia. Emergency Medicine 2000; 12(3):232–240.

Hall A, Saiers J, Baud F. Which cyanide antidote? Critical Reviews in Toxicology 2009; 39(7):541–552.

Reade MC, Davies SR, Morley PT et al. Review article: management of cyanide poisoning. Emergency Medicine Australasia 2012; 24:225–238.

3.33 DIGOXIN: ACUTE OVERDOSE

See also 3.34: Digoxin: Chronic poisoning.

Acute digoxin poisoning presents with early onset of vomiting and hyperkalaemia and can progress to life-threatening cardiac dysrhythmias. Cardiovascular toxicity may be refractory to conventional resuscitation measures. Digoxin immune Fab is the definitive antidote.

- Acute digoxin intoxication is likely if more than 10 times the daily defined dose is ingested.
- **Automaticity** is a hallmark of cardiac toxicity. It refers to an increased frequency of spontaneous cardiac ectopic beats caused by changes in resting membrane potentials due to intracellular calcium excess. Any cardiac tissue can be affected – the significant mortality risk is the development of malignant ventricular dysrhythmias (VT or VF).
- Bradycardia or atrioventricular blocks can result in significant haemodynamic instability, but mortality is more often related to ventricular dysrhythmias.
- Hyperkalaemia occurs due to inhibition of the membrane Na^+–K^+-ATPase pump and, in the setting of acute overdose, is a marker of significant toxicity.
- Potentially lethal acute digoxin intoxication is predicted by:
  — dose ingested >10 mg (adult) or >4 mg (child)
  — serum digoxin level >15 nmol/L (12 ng/mL) at any time
  — serum potassium >5.5 mmol/L.
- Potentially lethal cardiac glycoside intoxication can occur following ingestion of certain plants or infusions brewed using glycoside-containing plants or toad skins.
- **Children:** ingestion of up to 75 microgram/kg is safe and does not require hospital observation or treatment unless symptoms develop.

Toxic mechanism

Digoxin inhibits the membrane Na^+–K^+-ATPase pump, resulting in increased intracellular sodium and leading to a secondary increase in intracellular calcium via the Na^+–Ca^{2+} exchange pump. The elevated intracellular calcium results in the therapeutic positive inotropic effect but is also responsible for the enhanced automaticity causing cardiac ectopic beats and the risk of dysrhythmias. Digoxin also can increase serum potassium levels (particularly with acute toxicity) and enhances vagal tone, leading to a decrease in sinoatrial and atrioventricular node conduction velocities.

Toxicokinetics

Digoxin is well absorbed after oral administration, with bioavailability of 60–80% and a large volume of distribution (5–10 L/kg). Equilibration with tissue compartments occurs around 6 hours after an ingested dose. Hepatic metabolism is minimal and it is eliminated unchanged by the kidneys. The elimination half-life is 30–40 hours and will be prolonged in the setting of renal impairment. Drug interactions with inhibitors of the P-glycoprotein efflux membrane transporter (e.g. amiodarone, verapamil, macrolide antibiotics) will cause an increase in serum digoxin concentration.

Nausea and vomiting are early clinical features of acute digoxin poisoning and develop within 2–4 hours. Peak clinical effects occur 6–8 hours following ingestion and death secondary to cardiovascular collapse may follow at 8–12 hours. Specific clinical features include:

- Gastrointestinal
  — Nausea, vomiting and abdominal pain
- Cardiovascular
  — Bradycardias
    – 1st-, 2nd- or 3rd-degree AV block
    – AF with ventricular response <60

- Automaticity
    - Atrial or ventricular ectopic beats
    - Accelerated supraventricular or junctional tachycardias with or without AV block
    - Ventricular tachycardia
- Syncope
- Central nervous system
    - Lethargy
    - Confusion and delirium.
- Note: Acute natural cardiac glycoside intoxication (e.g. oleander) has similar clinical features. However, onset may be more rapid if liquid preparations are ingested.

INVESTIGATIONS
Screening tests in deliberate self-poisoning
- 12-lead ECG, BGL and paracetamol level

Specific investigations
- Serum digoxin levels
    - Confirm poisoning.
    - Provide indication for antibody treatment.
    - Perform level 4–6 hours post ingestion and then serial measurements 2–4 hourly until definitive antidotal therapy is given or toxicity resolves.
        - Note: For other cardiac glycoside poisoning (e.g. oleander), the serum digoxin level in these scenarios may not be reliable due to variability in laboratory assays.
- EUC
    - Hyperkalaemia of any magnitude is an important early sign of severe digoxin toxicity.
    - Assess renal function.
- Serial 12-lead ECGs
    - Essential to monitor progression or resolution of cardiotoxicity (see **Figure 3.33.1**).

MANAGEMENT
Resuscitation, supportive care and monitoring
- Acute digoxin poisoning is a potentially life-threatening emergency managed in an area equipped for cardiorespiratory monitoring and resuscitation. Cardiac monitoring must be continued until resolution of toxicity.
- Early life-threats that require immediate intervention include:
    - cardiac arrest
    - cardiac dysrhythmias
    - hypotension.
- In cardiac arrest, standard resuscitation measures are likely futile. Advanced cardiac life support measures are initiated while 5 ampoules (or as many as are available) of digoxin immune Fab are sourced and administered. Resuscitation should continue for at least 30 minutes after the administration of digoxin immune Fab.

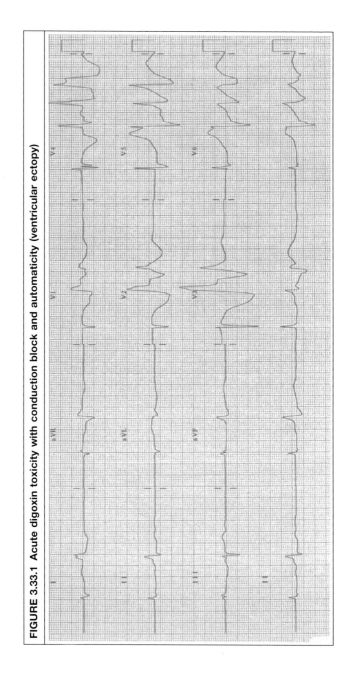

FIGURE 3.33.1 Acute digoxin toxicity with conduction block and automaticity (ventricular ectopy)

- If digoxin immune Fab is not immediately available, temporising measures are instituted to manage imminent life-threats:
  - Hyperkalaemia
    - Administer sodium bicarbonate 100 mEq IV bolus (1 mEq/kg in children).
    - Give insulin 10 units and 50 mL 50% dextrose simultaneously as an IV bolus (0.1 units/kg insulin and 5 mL/kg 10% glucose in children).
      - Notes:
        - Calcium is relatively contraindicated in the acute management of hyperkalaemia with digoxin toxicity due to a theoretical risk of exacerbating intracellular calcium overload and cardiac dysrhythmias. However, available data suggest use of calcium salts does not exacerbate toxicity.
        - Magnesium sulphate may exert similar beneficial effects to that of calcium on the transmembrane potential in the setting of hyperkalaemia.
  - Bradycardia or atrioventricular block
    - Give atropine 0.6 mg IV bolus. Repeat until desired clinical effect is achieved to a maximum of 1.8 mg (20 microgram/ kg/dose in children).
    - Isoprenaline or adrenaline infusions may be required to manage bradycardia if digoxin immune Fab is not available, although there is an attendant risk of provoking ventricular tachydysrhythmias.
    - Electrical pacing is an additional temporising option.
  - Ventricular tachydysrhythmias
    - Administer lidocaine 1 mg/kg (max 100 mg) IV over 2 minutes.
- Correct hypokalaemia and hypomagnesaemia if present.
- Correct hypovolaemia if present.
  - Note: For other cardiac glycoside poisoning (e.g. oleander), the spectrum of toxicity may not exhibit the same risk of ventricular dysrhythmias as digoxin toxicity – treatment of bradycardia or atrioventricular block may respond well to atropine or isoprenaline.

Decontamination
- Oral activated charcoal should be offered to cooperative adults who present within the first 2 hours following overdose. Administration may be problematic due to persistent vomiting.
- Multiple-dose activated charcoal may be associated with improved outcomes in plant glycoside poisoning, particularly where digoxin immune Fab is not immediately available.

Enhanced elimination
- Not clinically useful.

Antidotes
- Digoxin immune Fab is the definitive treatment for acute digoxin poisoning. It is indicated whenever potentially life-threatening toxicity is present or predicted:
  - cardiac arrest
  - life-threatening cardiac dysrhythmias

- automaticity (significant ventricular ectopy)
- ingested dose >10 mg (adult) or >4 mg (child)
- serum digoxin level >15 nmol/mL (12 ng/mL)
- serum potassium >5.5 mmol/L.
- Digoxin immune Fab dosing is empirical or based on the dose of digoxin known to be ingested (see **Chapter 4.5: Digoxin immune Fab**).

DISPOSITION AND FOLLOW-UP
- Patients with serial serum digoxin levels falling into the non-toxic range, normal serum potassium and renal function, no gastrointestinal symptoms and no evidence of cardiotoxicity at 12 hours after ingestion do not require ongoing medical care or management.
- Patients who have received digoxin immune Fab and remain clinically well over the next 24 hours with normal serum potassium and renal function and manifest no significant cardiac dysrhythmia do not require ongoing medical management. If available, free serum digoxin levels provide additional objective evidence of resolving intoxication.

HANDY TIPS
- Early accurate risk assessment allows administration of digoxin immune Fab before life-threatening toxicity develops.
- Serum K >5.5 mmol/L in acute digoxin poisoning predicts high mortality without digoxin immune Fab.
- Digoxin may be co-ingested with other cardiotropic medications, such as calcium channel or beta-blockers. The aetiology of bradycardia or AV block may not be solely attributable to one agent. Therapeutic trial of digoxin immune Fab may assist diagnosis and management.
- Serum digoxin levels following treatment may paradoxically increase because most assays measure both free and Fab-bound digoxin. Some laboratories are able to assay free digoxin levels – these provide better guidance for the subsequent administration of Fab, particularly in the setting of poor renal clearance.
- Standard digoxin assays can confirm ingestion of plant or animal glycosides but may not accurately reflect the total serum level of all glycosides or the risk of severe toxicity.

PITFALLS
- Failure to appreciate the potential life-threatening nature of acute digoxin poisoning.
- Failure to treat with digoxin immune Fab because of underestimation of potential mortality risk and concerns about cost.

CONTROVERSY
- Precise indications and dosing for digoxin immune Fab. The threshold for antidotal therapy requires a consideration of the risk of cardiovascular deterioration in an individual patient and the clinician's ability or willingness to manage that risk with or without antidotal therapy (see **Chapter 4.5: Digoxin immune Fab**).

Presentations
Digoxin 62.5 microgram tablets (200)
Digoxin 250 microgram tablets (100)
Digoxin 50 microgram/mL elixir (60 mL)
Digoxin 50 microgram/2 mL ampoules
Digoxin 500 microgram/2 mL ampoules
Note: Natural sources of cardiac glycosides with similar toxicity:
- Plants: foxglove, lily of the valley, oleander, rhododendron
- Animals: toad (*Bufo* spp.) venom and body parts – used in some traditional Chinese medicines.

References
Antman EM, Wenger TL, Butler VP et al. Treatment of 150 cases of life-threatening digitalis intoxication with digoxin-specific Fab antibody fragments: final report of a multicenter study. Circulation 1990; 81(6):1744–1752.
Bateman DN. Digoxin-specific antibody fragments: how much and when? Toxicological Reviews 2004; 23(3):135–143.
Chan B, Buckley N. Digoxin-specific antibody fragments in the treatment of digoxin toxicity. Clinical Toxicology 2014; 52(8):824–836.
De Silva HA, Fonseka MM, Pathmeswaran A et al. Multiple-dose activated charcoal for treatment of yellow oleander poisoning: a single-blind, randomised, placebo-controlled trial. Lancet 2003; 361:1935–1938.
Eddleston M, Rajapakse S, Rajakanthan JS et al. Anti-digoxin Fab fragments in cardiotoxicity induced by ingestion of yellow oleander: a randomised controlled trial. Lancet 2000; 355(9208):967–972.
Woolf AD, Wenger T, Smith TW et al. The use of digoxin-specific Fab fragments for severe digitalis intoxication in children. New England Journal of Medicine 1992; 326:1739–1744.

3.34 DIGOXIN: CHRONIC POISONING

See also 3.33: Digoxin: Acute overdose.

Chronic digoxin poisoning is an underdiagnosed condition that carries significant morbidity and mortality. Digoxin has a narrow therapeutic index and intoxication commonly develops in elderly patients with multiple co-morbidities. Appropriate use of digoxin immune Fab reduces mortality and may reduce hospital length of stay and cost of care.

RISK ASSESSMENT
- Chronic digoxin poisoning, although variable in severity, is a life-threatening condition.
- The mortality risk is difficult to predict accurately for individual patients.
- The duration of the increased mortality risk is prolonged in the presence of renal impairment.
- **Automaticity** is the hallmark of cardiac toxicity. It refers to an increased frequency of spontaneous cardiac ectopic beats caused by changes in resting membrane potentials due to intracellular calcium excess. Any cardiac tissue can be affected – the significant mortality risk is the development of malignant ventricular dysrhythmias (VT or VF).
- Bradycardia or atrioventricular blocks can result in significant haemodynamic instability, but mortality is most often related to ventricular dysrhythmias.

TABLE 3.34.1 Probability of digoxin toxicity		
Clinical features	Serum digoxin level 1.5 ng/mL (1.9 nmol/L)	Serum digoxin level 2.5 ng/mL (3.2 nmol/L)
Bradycardia only	10%	50%
GI symptoms only	25%	60%
GI symptoms and bradycardia	60%	90%
Automaticity alone	70%	90%
Automaticity plus any other feature	>80%	100%

Adapted from Abad-Santos F, Carca AJ, Ibanez C et al. Digoxin level and clinical manifestations as determinants in the diagnosis of digoxin toxicity. Therapeutic Drug Monitoring 2000; 22(2):163–168.

- The probability of digoxin toxicity can be estimated by considering the serum digoxin level and three major clinical features: gastrointestinal symptoms, bradycardia and automaticity (particularly ventricular ectopic beats) – see **Table 3.34.1**.

Toxic mechanism

Digoxin inhibits the membrane Na^+–K^+-ATPase pump, resulting in increased intracellular sodium and leading to a secondary increase in intracellular calcium via the Na^+–Ca^{2+} exchange pump. The elevated intracellular calcium results in the therapeutic positive inotropic effect but is also responsible for the enhanced automaticity causing cardiac ectopic beats and the risk of dysrhythmias. Digoxin also can increase serum potassium levels (particularly with acute toxicity) and enhances vagal tone, leading to a decrease in sinoatrial and atrioventricular node conduction velocities.

Toxicokinetics

Digoxin is well absorbed after oral administration, with bioavailability of 60–80% and a large volume of distribution (5–10 L/kg). Steady-state levels are most reliable 6 hours following a therapeutic dose. Hepatic metabolism is minimal and it is eliminated unchanged by the kidneys. The elimination half-life is 30–40 hours and will be prolonged in the setting of renal impairment.

CLINICAL FEATURES

The clinical manifestations of chronic digoxin toxicity may be non-specific. Digoxin intoxication commonly develops in elderly patients in the context of an intercurrent illness, particularly where this leads to impaired renal function and decreased digoxin elimination. Patients with potential chronic digoxin toxicity are often on other cardiotropic medications, such as calcium channel or beta-blockers. The aetiology of bradycardia or AV block may not solely be attributable to one agent (see **Controversies**).

Therapeutic trial of digoxin immune Fab may assist diagnosis and management.

Onset is insidious over days or weeks. Clinical features include:

- Cardiovascular
  - Bradycardias
    - 1st-, 2nd- or 3rd-degree AV block
    - AF with slow ventricular response (<60/minute)
  - Automaticity
    - Atrial or ventricular ectopic beats
    - Accelerated supraventricular or junctional tachycardias with or without AV block
    - Ventricular tachycardia
  - Syncope
- Gastrointestinal
  - Nausea, vomiting, abdominal pain
- Central nervous system
  - Lethargy
  - Confusion and delirium
- Visual
  - Decreased visual acuity
  - Aberration of colour vision (chromatopsia)
  - Yellow haloes (xanthopsia).

INVESTIGATIONS

Screening tests in deliberate self-poisoning
- 12-lead ECG, BGL and paracetamol level

Specific investigations
- Serum digoxin level
  - The diagnosis of chronic digoxin intoxication is based on a steady-state level 6 or more hours after the last dose.
  - Serum digoxin levels near the therapeutic range of 0.5–1.0 ng/mL (0.6–1.3 nmol/L) correlate poorly as isolated markers of toxicity (see **Table 3.34.1**).
- Other investigations
  - EUC, magnesium.
  - Investigations as indicated to assess intercurrent illnesses.
- Serial 12-lead ECGs
  - Essential to monitor progression or resolution of cardiotoxicity (see **Figure 3.34.1**).

MANAGEMENT

Resuscitation, supportive care and monitoring
- Chronic digoxin poisoning is a potentially life-threatening emergency managed in an area equipped for cardiorespiratory monitoring and resuscitation. Cardiac monitoring continues until resolution of toxicity.
- Early life-threats that require immediate intervention include:
  - cardiac arrest
  - cardiac dysrhythmias
  - hypotension.
- In cardiac arrest, standard resuscitation measures are likely futile. Advanced cardiac life support measures are initiated while 5 ampoules (or as many as are available) of digoxin immune Fab are

FIGURE 3.34.1 Chronic digoxin toxicity with automaticity (ventricular ectopy)

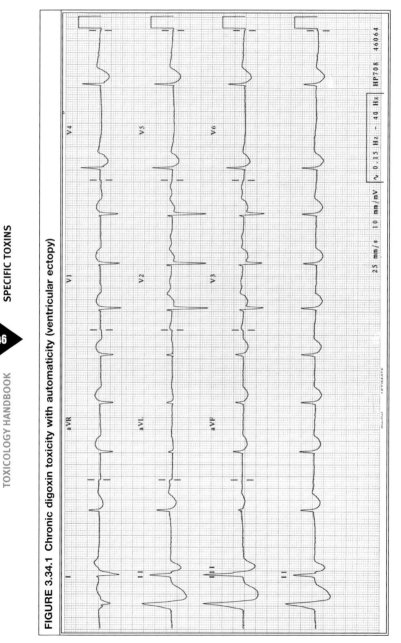

sourced and administered. Resuscitation should continue for at
least 30 minutes after the administration of digoxin immune Fab.
- If digoxin immune Fab is not immediately available, temporising
  measures are instituted to deal with imminent life-threats.
  — Hyperkalaemia
    – Administer sodium bicarbonate 100 mEq IV bolus (1 mEq/kg
      in children).
    – Give insulin 10 units and 50 mL 50% dextrose
      simultaneously as an IV bolus (0.1 units/kg insulin and
      5 mL/kg 10% dextrose in children).
    – Note: Calcium is relatively contraindicated in the acute
      management of hyperkalaemia with digoxin toxicity due to
      a theoretical risk of exacerbating intracellular calcium
      overload and cardiac dysrhythmias. However, available
      data suggest use of calcium salts does not exacerbate
      toxicity.
    – Magnesium sulphate may exert similar beneficial effects to
      that of calcium on the transmembrane potential in the
      setting of hyperkalaemia.
  — Bradycardia or atrioventricular block
    – Give atropine 0.6 mg IV bolus. Repeat until desired clinical
      effect is achieved to a maximum of 1.8 mg (20 microgram/
      kg/dose in children).
    – Isoprenaline or adrenaline infusions may be required to
      manage bradycardia if digoxin immune Fab is not
      available, although there is an attendant risk of provoking
      ventricular tachydysrhythmias.
    – Electrical pacing is an additional temporising option.
  — Ventricular tachydysrhythmias
    – Administer lidocaine 1 mg/kg (max 100 mg) IV over
      2 minutes.
- Correct hypovolaemia if present.
- Correct hypokalaemia and hypomagnesaemia if present.
- Assess and manage contributing intercurrent illnesses.

Decontamination
- Not indicated.

Enhanced elimination
- Not clinically useful.

Antidotes
- Digoxin immune Fab is indicated whenever clinical features of
  digoxin intoxication are associated with an elevated steady-state
  serum digoxin level. A dose of 1–2 ampoules is usually sufficient
  to reverse features of toxicity within 4–6 hours (see **Chapter 4.5:
  Digoxin immune Fab**).

DISPOSITION AND FOLLOW-UP
- If significant cardiac dysrhythmias do not occur over a 12-hour
  observation period following treatment with digoxin immune Fab,
  ongoing cardiac monitoring may not be required.
- There is the possibility of a rebound increase in free serum
  digoxin levels due to movement from the tissue compartment

down a concentration gradient. Patients with abnormal renal function are at risk of a delay in the recurrence of digoxin toxicity due to decreased clearance of digoxin antibody complexes, and prolonged observation and monitoring is warranted (see **Duration of treatment** in **Chapter 4.5: Digoxin immune Fab**).

- The vast majority of patients with chronic digoxin poisoning require admission to hospital for management of intercurrent illnesses, even after treatment with digoxin immune Fab.

HANDY TIPS

- Consider the diagnosis of chronic digoxin intoxication in any patient on digoxin who presents with collapse, hypotension, bradycardia, dysrhythmia, gastrointestinal symptoms, altered mental status or general deterioration.
- Appropriate early treatment with digoxin immune Fab should be considered cost effective because it may decrease the requirement for prolonged cardiac monitoring, decrease hospital length of stay and improve mortality.
- If a serum digoxin level is not readily available, patients with suspected chronic digoxin intoxication are safely treated with an initial empirical dose of 1–2 ampoules of digoxin immune Fab.
- If cardiac dysrhythmias continue 12 hours after a definitive dose of digoxin immune Fab, an alternative cause is likely.
- Serum digoxin levels following treatment may paradoxically increase because most assays measure both free and Fab-bound digoxin.
  - Some laboratories are able to assay free digoxin levels
  - These provide better guidance for the subsequent administration of Fab, particularly in the setting of poor renal function, when recurrence of digoxin toxicity can occur.
- Drug interactions with inhibitors of P-glycoprotein (macrolide antibiotics, verapamil, amiodarone) may lead to increased risk of digoxin toxicity.

PITFALLS

- Failure to appreciate the potential life-threatening nature of chronic digoxin poisoning.
- Failure to treat with digoxin immune Fab because of underestimation of potential mortality risk and concerns about cost.

CONTROVERSIES

- Precise indications and dosing for digoxin immune Fab. The threshold for antidotal therapy requires a consideration of the risk of cardiovascular deterioration in an individual patient and the clinician's ability or willingness to manage that risk with or without antidotal therapy (see **Chapter 4.5: Digoxin immune Fab**).
- Recent medical literature has proposed recognition of BRASH syndrome (bradycardia, renal failure, AV blockade, shock and hyperkalaemia). It is useful to consider the multiple pathophysiological processes affecting a patient with likely chronic digoxin toxicity (see **References**).

Presentations

Digoxin 62.5 microgram tablets (200)
Digoxin 250 microgram tablets (100)
Digoxin 50 microgram/mL elixir (60 mL)
Digoxin 50 microgram/2 mL ampoules
Digoxin 500 microgram/2 mL ampoules

References

Abad-Santos F, Carca AJ, Ibanez C et al. Digoxin level and clinical manifestations as determinants in the diagnosis of digoxin toxicity. Therapeutic Drug Monitoring 2000; 22(2):163–168.

Antman EM, Wenger TL, Butler VP et al. Treatment of 150 cases of life-threatening digitalis intoxication with digoxin-specific Fab antibody fragments: final report of a multicenter study. Circulation 1990; 81(6):1744–1752.

Chan B, Buckley N. Digoxin-specific antibody fragments in the treatment of digoxin toxicity. Clinical Toxicology 2014; 52(8):824–836.

Chan BS, Isbister GK, Page CB et al. Clinical outcomes from early use of digoxin-specific antibodies versus observation in chronic digoxin poisoning (ATOM-4). Clinical Toxicology 2019; 57(7):638–643. doi:10.1080/15563650.2018.1546010.

DiDomenico RJ, Walton SM, Sanoski CA et al. Analysis of the use of digoxin immune Fab for the treatment of non-life-threatening digoxin toxicity. Journal of Cardiovascular Pharmacology and Therapeutics 2000; 5(2):77–85.

Farkas JD, Long B, Koyfman A et al. BRASH syndrome: bradycardia, renal failure, AV blockade, shock, and hyperkalemia. The Journal of Emergency Medicine 2020; 59(2):216–223. https://doi.org/10.1016/j.jemermed.2020.05.001.

Lapostolle F, Borron SW, Verdier C et al. Digoxin-specific Fab fragments as single first-line therapy in digitalis poisoning. Critical Care Medicine 2008; 36:3014–3018.

3.35 DIPHENOXYLATE–ATROPINE

This combination antidiarrhoeal drug causes delayed onset of opioid and anticholinergic effects when ingested, even in small amounts. Fatalities have been reported, particularly in children.

RISK ASSESSMENT

- Ingestions have the potential to cause significant opioid or anticholinergic poisoning.
- Adults are less susceptible than children to toxic effects.
- **Children:**
  - Any child under the age of 2 years who may have ingested diphenoxylate-atropine should be assessed in hospital.
  - Acute ingestion of more than 1 tablet in any child over the age of 2 years may cause opioid and/or anticholinergic poisoning and should be assessed and observed in hospital.

Toxic mechanism

Combination synthetic opioid (diphenoxylate) and anticholinergic (atropine) preparation used as treatment for diarrhoea. Atropine is added to discourage illicit misuse of the opioid component. Diphenoxylate is an opioid agonist and atropine is a competitive antagonist of acetylcholine at muscarinic receptors.

Toxicokinetics

Diphenoxylate is well absorbed following oral administration. It is rapidly metabolised to difenoxin, a compound five times more active than diphenoxylate and which undergoes enterohepatic circulation, with a prolonged elimination half-life of 12 hours. Atropine is rapidly absorbed following oral administration, with peak plasma levels occurring at 2 hours and an elimination half-life of up to 12 hours. The co-administration of atropine in this compound preparation may significantly slow the absorption of diphenoxylate, with a resultant delay in onset of toxic effects.

CLINICAL FEATURES

The clinical features are those of opioid intoxication and anticholinergic poisoning.

- Opioid intoxication
  - Decreased level of consciousness
  - Respiratory depression
  - Miosis
  - Note: Opioid effects usually manifest within the first few hours but may develop over 12–24 hours.
- Anticholinergic poisoning
  - Delirium, agitation
  - Tachycardia, dry skin
  - Urinary retention
  - Note: Not all patients develop anticholinergic effects. If these do occur, they may precede or be obscured by the opioid effects. Occasionally, the anticholinergic effects may predominate.

INVESTIGATIONS

Screening tests in deliberate self-poisoning

- 12-lead ECG, BGL and paracetamol level

MANAGEMENT

Resuscitation, supportive care and monitoring

- Attention to airway, breathing and circulation is paramount. These priorities are managed along conventional lines, as outlined in **Chapter 1.2: Resuscitation**.
- Basic resuscitative measures ensure the survival of the vast majority of patients.
- General supportive care measures are indicated, as outlined in **Chapter 1.4: Supportive care and monitoring**.
- Monitor for urinary retention with serial bladder scans and insert an indwelling urinary catheter if required.

Decontamination

- Consider administration of oral activated charcoal to the cooperative alert patient who presents within 2 hours. Decontamination is not necessary to ensure a favourable outcome but may reduce naloxone requirement and length of stay.

Enhanced elimination

- Not clinically useful.

Antidotes

- Naloxone is indicated to reverse clinical manifestations of opioid intoxication. Repeated doses or an infusion may be necessary (see **Chapter 4.18: Naloxone**).

DISPOSITION AND FOLLOW-UP

- Children who may have ingested diphenoxylate-atropine should be observed in hospital for a minimum of 12 hours. Discharge should not occur at night.
- Adults are observed for at least 8 hours following deliberate self-poisoning.
- Symptomatic patients require admission until clinical manifestations resolve. This may take up to 48 hours.

PITFALLS

- Failure to recognise the potential lethality of diphenoxylate-atropine, particularly in children.
- Failure to observe in hospital for delayed onset of toxicity.
- Failure to detect urinary retention and place a urinary catheter when indicated.

Presentations

Diphenoxylate hydrochloride 2.5 mg/atropine sulfate 25 microgram tablets (8, 20, 100)

References

McCarron MM, Chalhower KR, Thompson GA. Diphenoxylate–atropine (Lomotil) overdose in children: an update (report of 8 cases and review of the literature). Pediatrics 1991; 87(5):694–700.

Thomas TJ, Pauze D, Love JN. Are one or two dangerous? Diphenoxylate–atropine exposure in toddlers. Journal of Emergency Medicine 2008; 34(1):71–75.

3.36 DIRECT ORAL ANTICOAGULANTS

Apixaban, Dabigatran, Rivaroxaban

The direct oral anticoagulants (DOACs) are widely used for the prevention and treatment of thromboembolic disease. They differ from other anticoagulants by directly inhibiting thrombin or factor Xa. Most DOAC-related bleeding occurs in the context of therapeutic administration, and published data on deliberate self-poisoning is limited. Risk assessment is complicated by the poor correlation between anticoagulant activity and classic coagulation tests. Patients with active bleeding require urgent reversal therapy.

RISK ASSESSMENT

- The risk of bleeding is difficult to quantify reliably for individual patients. Limited evidence suggests that the risk of significant bleeding following acute overdose of these agents is relatively low.
- Standard coagulation studies correlate poorly with the anticoagulant effect of these agents and have a limited role in defining the bleeding risk.
- The role for coagulation factor replacement and antidotal therapy is less clearly established than it is for toxicity from warfarin or other vitamin K antagonists.

- Based on available literature, the most important determinants in the risk assessment to guide therapeutic interventions are:
  - presence or absence of active bleeding
  - time since last ingestion
  - increased risk of bleeding (including older age and presence of co-morbidities)
  - renal and hepatic dysfunction.
- Following acute overdose in patients with normal renal and hepatic function, the anticoagulant effect can be expected to resolve in a time frame determined by the clearance of the specific agent:
  - apixaban: 1.5–3 days
  - dabigatran: 2.5–3.5 days
  - rivaroxaban: 1–2 days.
- Decisions to administer coagulation factors or antidotes require a consideration of the risk of haemorrhage for an individual patient and the likelihood of clinically relevant anticoagulant activity (based on the time of overdose or last therapeutic dose), weighed against the risk of prothrombotic complications following reversal therapies.
- **Children:** accidental paediatric ingestion of DOACs is unlikely to cause significant bleeding.

Toxic mechanism

Dabigatran is a direct inhibitor of free and fibrin-bound thrombin, preventing the conversion of fibrinogen to fibrin.

Apixaban and rivaroxaban directly inhibit free and clot-bound factor Xa, resulting in an anticoagulant effect by preventing the conversion of prothrombin to thrombin.

Toxicokinetics

Dabigatran has a bioavailability of only 6% following oral administration but this is increased to 75% if the granules are removed from the capsules prior to ingestion. Peak concentrations occur 2–4 hours after ingestion. The volume of distribution is small and protein binding is 35%. Dabigatran is metabolised by the liver to active metabolites but elimination is predominantly renal, with a terminal half-life of 12–24 hours. This is significantly prolonged in the presence of renal impairment.

Apixaban and rivaroxaban have similar kinetics. Bioavailability is >50% following oral ingestion and peak concentrations are reached 3–4 hours later. Volumes of distribution are small and both agents are highly protein bound. Elimination is renal and hepatic with terminal elimination half-lives of 5–14 hours.

Notes: Patients with severe renal or hepatic disease will have prolonged anticoagulant effects for any given ingestion. This is particularly relevant for dabigatran in the setting of renal dysfunction.

DOACs are susceptible to accumulation in therapeutic dosing due to drug interactions, particularly related to P-glycoprotein and CYP3A4 inhibition.

CLINICAL FEATURES

- Most patients with an acute overdose are asymptomatic at presentation, and bleeding is more likely to occur in patients who have become over-anticoagulated on therapeutic dosing.
- Coagulopathy may result in manifestations ranging in severity from purpura, gingival bleeding and epistaxis to haematuria, gastrointestinal bleeding or intracerebral haemorrhage.

INVESTIGATIONS

Screening tests in deliberate self-poisoning
- 12-lead ECG, BGL and paracetamol level

Specific investigations
- FBC, EUC, liver function tests, blood cross-match
  - The effects of DOACs on commonly available coagulation tests (INR, aPTT) are variable (see **Table 3.36.1**) and do not correlate well with drug levels or risk of bleeding.
  - More sensitive assays are useful (see **Table 3.36.1**) but less readily available.

TABLE 3.36.1   Effects of DOACs on coagulation studies

Parameter	Dabigatran effect	Factor Xa inhibitor effect (apixaban, rivaroxaban)
INR	Mild and unpredictable elevation Does not correlate with anticoagulant effect	Variable elevation A normal INR is reassuring but does not guarantee absent Xa inhibitor activity
aPTT	Prolonged but poor correlation with drug concentration aPTT >90 seconds suggests high drug level Normal aPTT suggests minimal drug present	Variable
Thrombin clotting time (TT, TCT)	Very sensitive to even trace amount of drug Normal value excludes presence of dabigatran	Not useful
Dilute thrombin time (Haemoclot assay)	Useful to derive levels but does not predict bleeding risk	Not useful
Factor Xa assay	Not useful	Provides estimate of drug level but does not predict bleeding risk

Notes:
1 Combination of INR >2 and aPTT >90 seconds suggests high plasma levels of dabigatran.
2 Combination of normal INR and normal aPTT suggests low plasma levels of dabigatran.
3 Combination of normal INR and normal aPTT suggests low plasma levels of apixaban and rivaroxaban.
4 Factor Xa and thrombin time assays are not available in all hospitals.
5 Thromboelastography can detect anticoagulant activity of DOACs but specific, validated assays have not been developed.

Resuscitation, supportive care and monitoring
- In patients with evidence of haemorrhage, attention to airway, breathing and circulation are paramount. These priorities can usually be managed along conventional lines, as outlined in **Chapter 1.2: Resuscitation**.
- If active bleeding is evident, measures include:
  - Local haemostatic control – compression, suturing.
  - Volume resuscitation, blood transfusion and haemodynamic support are determined by clinical and laboratory assessment.
- Administration of coagulation factors is indicated for significant active bleeding. Early consultation with haematology is recommended.
  - Prothrombin complex concentrate (PCC) and fresh frozen plasma (FFP) are the replacement therapies of choice in most institutional protocols but the efficacy of these agents is not well established.
  - Other coagulation factor therapies such as factor VIII inhibitor bypass activity (FEIBA) have also been recommended, but there are limited data and clinical experience to support its use.
  - Recombinant factor VIIa is not recommended as a therapeutic option due to lack of evidence for clinical benefit and an unacceptable risk of thrombotic complications.
- Tranexamic acid may have a role as antifibrinolytic therapy and is considered to have low thrombotic potential in this setting.
- Antidotal therapy with idarucizumab or andexanet alfa may be indicated for active bleeding (see **Antidotes** below).
- General supportive care measures are indicated, as outlined in **Chapter 1.4: Supportive care and monitoring**.

Decontamination
- Following deliberate self-poisoning in cooperative patients presenting within 4 hours of ingestion, administer 50 g oral activated charcoal.

Enhanced elimination
- Dabigatran is effectively removed by haemodialysis and this can be considered in patients with significantly impaired renal function to optimise drug clearance. The potential complications of placing a dialysis catheter in a coagulopathic patient limit the usefulness of this intervention (see **Antidotes** below).
- Haemodialysis is not useful in apixaban or rivaroxaban overdose or toxicity.

Antidotes
- Idarucizumab is the specific reversal agent for dabigatran. It is a monoclonal antibody fragment that binds to and neutralises dabigatran.
- Andexanet alfa is a recombinant modified form of factor Xa that acts as a decoy molecule, able to bind and neutralise both apixaban and rivaroxaban.
- Routine administration of these antidotal reversal agents for acute overdose without active bleeding is not supported by available literature.

- Indications for administration include life-threatening or uncontrolled bleeding, or requirement for emergency surgery, in a patient likely to have clinically relevant plasma DOAC levels. Optimal dosing schedules are not clearly defined for *either agent* in all scenarios, but standard recommendations are available for each agent:
  - idarucizumab: 5 g as an IV bolus or infusion
  - andexanet alfa:
    - low dose – a bolus of 400 mg given at 30 mg/minute, followed by an infusion of 480 mg given at 4 mg/minute for up to 120 minutes.
    - high dose – a bolus of 800 mg given at 30 mg/minute, followed by an infusion at 960 mg given at 8 mg/minute for up to 120 minutes.

DISPOSITION AND FOLLOW-UP
- All patients who overdose on DOACs are admitted to hospital for observation and until serial coagulation studies have normalised.
- All patients with DOAC-related bleeding are admitted to hospital for active treatment as above.
- Dagibatran overdose should be managed in a hospital with capacity for haemodialysis.
- Following dabigatran overdose, patients are medically fit for discharge if the INR and aPTT remain normal at 12 hours post ingestion.
- Following factor Xa inhibitor overdose, patients are medically fit for discharge if the INR and aPTT remain normal at 12 hours post ingestion.

HANDY TIP
- Do not rely on point-of-care (POC) coagulation testing because correlation with DOAC levels or bleeding risk is not validated.

PITFALLS
- Failure to prevent falls in patients with significant anticoagulation.
- Administration of coagulation factors in the absence of significant bleeding. This is associated with a risk of thromboembolic complications.

CONTROVERSY
- Thresholds for administration of coagulation factors or antidotes. There is no evidence that these interventions are associated with clinical benefit in the absence of active bleeding.

Presentations
Dabigatran etexilate 75 mg, 110 mg, 150 mg capsules (10, 60)
Apixaban 2.5 mg tablets (20, 30, 60)
Apixaban 5 mg tablets (60)
Rivaroxaban 10 mg tablets (10, 15, 30, 100)
Rivaroxaban 15 mg (28, 42)
Rivaroxaban 20 mg (28)

References

Chiew AL, Khamoudes D, Chan BS. Use of continuous veno-venous haemodiafiltration therapy in dabigatran overdose. Clinical Toxicology 2014; 52:283–287.

Cuker A, Burnett A, Triller D et al. Reversal of direct oral anticoagulants: guidance from the Anticoagulation Forum. American Journal of Hematology 2019; 94:697–709.

Koscielny J, Rutkauskaite E. Rivaroxaban and hemostasis in emergency care. Emergency Medicine International 2014. doi:10.1155/2014/935474.

Kumar R, Smith RE, Henry BL. A review of and recommendations for the management of patients with life-threatening dabigatran-associated hemorrhage: a single-center university hospital experience. Journal of Intensive Care Medicine 2014; 30(8):462–472.

Majeed A, Schulman S. Bleeding and antidotes in new oral anticoagulants. Best Practice and Research. Clinical Haematology 2013; 26:191–202.

Pernod G, Albaladejo P, Godier A. Management of major bleeding complications and emergency surgery in patients on long-term treatment with direct oral anticoagulants, thrombin or factor-Xa inhibitors: proposals of the Working Group on Perioperative Haemostasis (GIHP) – March 2013. Archives of Cardiovascular Disease 2013; 106:382–393.

Piran S, Khatib R, Schulman S et al. Management of direct factor Xa inhibitor-related major bleeding with prothrombin complex concentrate: a meta-analysis. Blood Advances 2019; 3(2):158–167. doi:10.1182/bloodadvances.2018024133.

Tran H, Joseph J, Young L et al. New oral anticoagulants: a practical guide on prescription, laboratory testing and peri-procedural/bleeding management. Australasian Society of Thrombosis and Haemostasis. Internal Medicine Journal 2014; 44(6):525–536. doi:10.1111/lmj.12448.

3.37 GAMMA-HYDROXYBUTYRATE (GHB)

Includes GHB precursors: Gamma-butyrolactone, 1,4-butanediol.

Slang terms: Fantasy, G, Georgia homeboy, GHB, Liquid ecstasy, Liquid G.

When taken in excessive doses, this illicit drug causes rapid onset of CNS and respiratory depression, myoclonic jerking and bradycardia. Management of intoxication is supportive. The duration of toxic effects is short, with complete recovery occurring within 4–8 hours. Gamma-butyrolactone and 1,4-butanediol are precursor drugs that are rapidly metabolised to GHB and cause similar toxicity.

RISK ASSESSMENT

- GHB is frequently distributed at a strength of 1 g/mL, but concentrations can vary widely.
- Overdose usually occurs because the concentration supplied was higher than anticipated by the recreational user or the user is naïve to the drug.
- Standard recreational doses are up to 30 mg/kg.
- Ingestion of >50 mg/kg can cause coma and respiratory depression.
- Overdose is life-threatening without timely support of airway and ventilation.
- Maximal toxicity is usually evident by the time of arrival at the emergency department.
- Co-ingestion of ethanol or other CNS depressants increases the risk of respiratory depression, apnoea and death.
- **Children:** any ingestion may be associated with rapid onset of coma and is regarded as potentially fatal.

Toxic mechanism

GHB is a short-chain carboxylic acid that occurs naturally in the brain. It is both a precursor and metabolite of gamma-aminobutyric acid (GABA) and is a neurotransmitter itself. The mechanisms of action include agonism activity at GABA$_B$ receptors, activity at specific GHB receptors and dopaminergic modulation promoting addiction and withdrawal syndromes.

Toxicokinetics

GHB is rapidly absorbed following oral administration with peak plasma concentrations occurring 25–60 minutes post ingestion. Gamma-butyrolactone (GBL) is rapidly transformed to GHB in the liver and 1,4-butanediol (BD) is metabolised rapidly to GHB by alcohol dehydrogenase. Alcohol competitively inhibits metabolism and can delay the onset of clinical effect. GHB is rapidly oxidised to carbon dioxide and water, with saturable kinetics. The elimination half-life is usually less than 1 hour and elimination is complete within 4–8 hours.

CLINICAL FEATURES

Clinical effects of GHB occur within 20 minutes of ingestion and peak at 30–60 minutes. Standard recreational doses produce rapid onset of euphoria, and in overdose this can be followed by rapid onset of coma. The patient may rouse to an external stimulus, only to become deeply somnolent again when not disturbed. Sudden recovery of consciousness occurs, usually within 2–3 hours. Recovery is characterised by a short period of agitation or delirium. Complete recovery is expected within 8 hours.

Deaths are reported and occur from airway obstruction, pulmonary aspiration or respiratory arrest.

Typical clinical features observed following overdose include:
- Central nervous system
  - CNS depression
  - Agitation and delirium
  - Miosis
  - Myoclonic movements may occur, but epileptiform seizures are uncommon.
- Respiratory
  - Airway obstruction
  - Respiratory depression
  - Periodic breathing (Cheyne-Stokes respiration)
- Cardiovascular
  - Bradycardia
  - Mild hypotension responsive to intravenous fluids
  - Non-specific ECG changes
- General
  - Mild hypothermia
  - Vomiting
  - Sweating.
- Withdrawal syndrome
  - Tolerance to GHB develops with regular use and a withdrawal syndrome is described. Clinical features of GHB withdrawal include hallucinations, paranoia, insomnia, anxiety, sweating, palpitations and agitation. Clinical features of withdrawal may develop within hours of the last dose of GHB and persist for several days.

INVESTIGATIONS
Screening tests in deliberate self-poisoning
- 12-lead ECG, BGL and paracetamol level

Specific investigations
- Other investigations as indicated to exclude alternative diagnoses for coma.
- Standard urine drug screens do not detect GHB. Specific blood and urine levels may be indicated in forensic cases; however, GHB is rapidly cleared from the blood and may not be detected in biological samples taken later in the clinical course.

MANAGEMENT
Resuscitation, supportive care and monitoring
- Acute GHB intoxication is a potentially life-threatening emergency managed in an area equipped for cardiorespiratory monitoring and resuscitation. Basic resuscitative measures ensure the survival of the vast majority of patients.
- Potential early life-threats that require immediate intervention include:
  — coma
  — respiratory depression
  — loss of airway protective reflexes.
- Attention to airway, breathing and circulation are paramount. These priorities can usually be managed along conventional lines, as outlined in **Chapter 1.2: Resuscitation**.
- General supportive care measures are indicated, as outlined in **Chapter 1.4: Supportive care and monitoring**.
- Bradycardia is common. Specific management (e.g. atropine, catecholamine infusion or pacing) is not usually required.
- Myoclonic movements do not require specific management. If seizures are suspected, they should be managed as outlined in **Chapter 2.3: Seizures**.
- Close clinical and physiological monitoring is indicated.

Decontamination
- Activated charcoal is not indicated because absorption and onset of CNS depression occurs rapidly.

Enhanced elimination
- Not clinically useful.

Antidotes
- None available.

DISPOSITION AND FOLLOW-UP
- Patients who are clinically well 2 hours following ingestion may be discharged.
- Patients with mild symptoms are managed supportively in a ward environment. They are fit for medical discharge when clinically well.
- Patients with significant CNS depression requiring intubation are admitted to an intensive care unit. Short-term ventilation in the emergency department is an alternative when the diagnosis is certain.

HANDY TIPS

- The resolution of coma may be abrupt. Care is required as patients may be agitated and forcefully extubate themselves.
- The diagnosis of GHB intoxication is frequently made in retrospect. It should be suspected in any young person found collapsed at a music festival or dance party, although alternative diagnoses should be sought.
- Symptoms of significant withdrawal from GHB may be treated with titrated doses of benzodiazepine or baclofen as required.

PITFALL

- Coma lasting longer than 8 hours suggests an alternative diagnosis (e.g. co-ingested agent or complication) and should prompt further investigation.

Presentations and sources

GHB is a white crystalline powder. It is usually distributed dissolved in water to form a clear colourless liquid.

Precursors are found in several household solvents:
- Gamma-butyrolactone (GBL) is an oily liquid.
- 1,4-butanediol (BD) is a water-soluble liquid.

References

Chin RL, Sporer KA, Cullison B et al. Clinical course of gamma-hydroxybutyrate overdose. Annals of Emergency Medicine 1998; 31:716–722.

Schep LJ, Knudsen K, Slaughter RJ et al. The clinical toxicology of gamma-hydroxybutyrate, gamma-butyrolactone and 1,4-butanediol. Clinical Toxicology 2012; 50:458–470.

Snead 3rd OC, KM Gibson. Gamma-hydroxybutyric acid. New England Journal of Medicine 2005; 352(26):2721–2732.

3.38 GLYPHOSATE

Glyphosate is a widely used herbicide. Severe toxicity occurs as result of deliberate ingestion of a concentrated formulation. It manifests with gastrointestinal corrosive symptoms and, in large ingestions, severe metabolic acidosis, hyperkalaemia and cardiovascular collapse can occur.

RISK ASSESSMENT

- Ingestion of concentrated formulations (30–50% glyphosate) poses the greatest risk.
- Ready-to-use pre-diluted formulations (1–5% concentration) generally cause only mild gastrointestinal symptoms.
- Dose is frequently difficult to quantify but correlates to severity (see **Table 3.38.1**).
- Corrosive injury to the upper airways poses a potential threat to life.
- Tachycardia, abnormal chest X-ray, metabolic acidosis, hyperkalaemia, acute renal impairment and older age are associated with poorer prognosis.
- Cutaneous exposures cause skin irritation but do not cause systemic toxicity.

TABLE 3.38.1   Dose-related risk assessment: glyphosate

Dose	Effect
<50 mL	Asymptomatic or minor gastrointestinal symptoms
50–100 mL	Severe gastrointestinal symptoms. Risk of early upper airways swelling. May develop multi-system toxicity, especially metabolic acidosis, hyperkalaemia and hypotension
>100 mL	Potentially fatal. Death occurs due to metabolic acidosis and refractory shock

- **Children:** accidental exposures to dilute formulations can be observed at home unless symptoms develop. Ingestion of concentrated formulations requires medical assessment. Do not need hospital assessment unless symptoms develop.

Toxic mechanism
The mechanism of toxicity is poorly understood. It is likely an intracellular toxin uncoupling mitochondrial oxidative phosphorylation. Toxicity may also be due to the surfactant co-formulant (typically polyoxyethyleneamine) rather than glyphosate itself. Concentrated glyphosate solutions also cause direct corrosive injury to mucosal surfaces when ingested. Glyphosate (glycine phosphonate) is not an organophosphate insecticide and does not inhibit cholinesterase enzymes.

Toxicokinetics
Glyphosate is poorly but rapidly absorbed following ingestion with peak concentrations occurring within 4 to 6 hours. It is not metabolised but eliminated unchanged by the kidneys, with an elimination half-life of 4 to 6 hours. The elimination half-life is prolonged in renal impairment.

CLINICAL FEATURES
- Gastrointestinal
  - Corrosive injury to the oropharynx, oesophagus, stomach and duodenum manifests with nausea, vomiting, diarrhoea and abdominal pain.
  - Corrosive injury is rarely severe and Grade III injuries (see **Chapter 3.31: Corrosives**) are not reported after glyphosate ingestion.
- Cardiovascular
  - Myocardial depression
  - Hypotension
  - Cardiovascular collapse
- Respiratory
  - Aspiration pneumonitis and non-cardiogenic pulmonary oedema have been reported.
- Metabolic
  - Hyperkalaemia
  - Metabolic acidosis
- Patients may develop hepatic and renal dysfunction.
- Multi-organ dysfunction secondary to myocardial depression and systemic acidosis can also occur.

INVESTIGATIONS
Screening tests in deliberate self-poisoning
- 12-lead ECG, BGL and paracetamol level

Specific investigations
- Glyphosate levels are not readily available and not clinically useful.
- EUC, LFTs
  - Detect and monitor hyperkalaemia.
  - Detect and monitor hepatic and renal dysfunction.
- Venous blood gas and lactate
  - Detect and monitor metabolic acidosis.
- Chest X-ray
  - Detects aspiration pneumonitis, pulmonary oedema.
- Endoscopy/CT chest
  - This is not routinely required as severe corrosive injury of the gastrointestinal tract is unusual.

MANAGEMENT
Resuscitation, supportive care and monitoring
- Manage the patient in an area equipped for cardiorespiratory monitoring and resuscitation.
- Intubate and ventilate if any evidence of airway compromise from oropharyngeal corrosive injury.
- Treat hypotension initially with 20 mL/kg of crystalloid solution IV. Those patients unresponsive to fluid challenge are likely to require invasive monitoring and vasopressor therapy.
- General supportive care measures are indicated, as outlined in **Chapter 1.4: Supportive care and monitoring**.

Decontamination
- Offer activated charcoal to cooperative patients who have ingested large volumes of concentrated formulations.
- Activated charcoal should be administered by nasogastric tube after initial aspiration of stomach contents if the patient is intubated.

Enhanced elimination
- Haemodialysis enhances the elimination of glyphosate and is considered early in patients with rapid clinical deterioration or multi-organ toxicity, or at high risk of developing these complications (older age, ingestions >100 mL of concentrated formulations).

Antidotes
- None available.

DISPOSITION AND FOLLOW-UP
- Patients who have ingested <100 mL of concentrated glyphosate and remain asymptomatic 6 hours after ingestion may be discharged. Discharge should not occur at night.
- Patient known to have ingested >100 mL of concentrated glyphosate are admitted to a high-dependency or intensive unit in anticipation of multiple organ effects within 24 hours.
- Adult patients with dermal occupational exposure do not require referral to hospital unless they are symptomatic.

PITFALLS
- Failure to appreciate potential for cardiovascular compromise following large ingestions.
- Confusion between glyphosate and organophosphate poisoning. These are two distinct clinical entities.

CONTROVERSY
- Threshold for initiation of haemodialysis in glyphosate poisoning.

Presentations and sources
Numerous glyphosate formulations are available.
Concentrated preparations are usually 36–50% glyphosate while ready-to-use diluted preparations are approximately 10%.
All preparations also contain polyoxyethyleneamine surfactant.

References
Bradberry SM, Proudfoot AT, Vale JA. Glyphosate poisoning. Toxicological Reviews 2004; 23(3):159–167.

Chen H-H, Lin J-L, Huang W-H et al. Spectrum of corrosive esophageal injury after intentional paraquat or glyphosate-surfactant herbicide ingestion. International Journal of General Medicine 2013; 6:677–683.

Garlich FM, Goldman M, Pepe J et al. Hemodialysis clearance of glyphosate following a life-threatening ingestion of glyphosate-surfactant herbicide. Clinical Toxicology 2014; 52(1):66–71.

Lee CH, Shih CP, Hsu KH et al. The early prognostic features of glyphosate-surfactant intoxication. American Journal of Emergency Medicine 2008; 26:275–281.

Lee HL, Chen KW, Chi CH et al. Clinical presentations and prognostic factors of glyphosate-surfactant herbicide intoxication: a review of 131 cases. Academic Emergency Medicine 2000; 7(8):906–910.

Roberts DM, Buckley NA, Mohamed F et al. A prospective observational study of the clinical toxicology of glyphosate-containing herbicides in adults with acute self-poisoning. Clinical Toxicology 2010; 48:129–136.

3.39 HYDROCARBONS

Aliphatic: **Essential oils (includes eucalyptus, clove and pennyroyal oils), Kerosene, Petroleum Distillates, Turpentine**

Aromatic: **Benzene, Toluene, Xylene**

Halogenated: **Carbon tetrachloride, Chloroform, Methylene chloride, Tetrachloroethylene, Trichloroethylene**

See also Chapter 2.13: Solvent abuse.

Hydrocarbons, whether ingested or inhaled, can cause rapid onset of CNS depression, seizures and (rarely) cardiac dysrhythmias. Aspiration can lead to chemical pneumonitis. Other end-organ effects are uncommon and usually associated with long-term occupational exposure.

RISK ASSESSMENT
- The major risks following acute ingestion are early CNS depression and seizures.
- Ingestion may be complicated by aspiration, resulting in a pneumonitis that can evolve over hours; however, mortality is rare.

- Prolonged inhalational exposure to hydrocarbon gases (e.g. butane, propane) can produce asphyxia due to physical displacement of oxygen.
- Significant toxicity can occur following dermal absorption of hydrocarbons – particularly aromatic or halogenated compounds. The risk is proportional to the duration and extent of exposure.
- Compounds that are highly viscous and have low volatility (e.g. motor oil, petroleum jelly) have a low risk of systemic toxicity or chemical pneumonitis after ingestion.
- **Children:** there is a risk of pulmonary aspiration and chemical pneumonitis following ingestion of any hydrocarbon. Ingestion of 5 mL of eucalyptus oil or other essential oils can cause rapid onset of coma.

Toxic mechanism

The vast majority of hydrocarbons act as CNS depressants. However, the exact mechanisms through which they exert their effects on the CNS are unknown. Inhaled hydrocarbon causes disruption of lung surfactant and direct pulmonary injury, leading to a chemical pneumonitis. Ventricular dysrhythmias can occur secondary to myocardial sensitisation to endogenous catecholamines. Halogenated hydrocarbons (e.g. carbon tetrachloride, chloroform) can cause hepatotoxicity either directly or via a cytotoxic metabolite.

Toxicokinetics

Inhalation is the primary route of exposure for compounds with high volatility (e.g. petrol, kerosene). Absorption following inhalational exposure is by passive diffusion, determined by the concentration, duration of exposure and partition coefficient of the agent. Distribution to the CNS is determined primarily by lipid solubility. Absorption following ingestion is inversely related to the molecular weight of the hydrocarbon. Minimal absorption occurs following dermal exposure for most agents, but prolonged exposure (e.g. immersion) can result in significant local dermal or systemic toxicity. Most hydrocarbons are eliminated unchanged through expired air. Some compounds produce metabolites that are excreted in the bile or urine.

CLINICAL FEATURES

- Respiratory
    - Immediate coughing and choking after ingestion indicates aspiration.
    - The development of chemical pneumonitis is heralded by wheeze, tachypnoea, hypoxia, haemoptysis and pulmonary oedema. In some cases, pulmonary signs may be delayed several hours. Features may resolve promptly or worsen over 24–72 hours and resolve over 5–7 days.
- Cardiovascular
    - Ventricular dysrhythmias typically occur early in poisoning (pre-hospital).
- Neurological
    - Altered mental state, CNS depression, seizures and coma may occur early after ingestion.
    - Chronic toluene abuse results in ataxia, cerebral atrophy, dementia and peripheral neuropathy (see **Chapter 2.13: Solvent abuse**).
- Gastrointestinal
    - Nausea, vomiting and diarrhoea can be severe following ingestion of hydrocarbons.

- Other
  - Chemical phlebitis and local tissue injury occur following IV or SC injection.
  - High-pressure injection injuries can produce extensive tissue injury involving tendons and deep structures.
  - Hepatic and renal injury can occur from various hydrocarbons
    - Halogenated (carbon tetrachloride, chloroform), essential oils (clove, pennyroyal).
  - Toluene causes renal tubular acidosis.
  - Benzene is associated with haemolysis and leukaemia.

INVESTIGATIONS
Screening tests in deliberate self-poisoning
- 12-lead ECG, BGL and paracetamol level

Specific investigations
- Serial ECGs and continuous cardiac monitoring if ectopy or bigeminy are noted at initial assessment.
- FBC, EUC, LFTs, venous blood gases.
- Chest X-ray: radiographic changes may lag behind clinical features of pneumonitis.
- Chronic toluene abuse leads to a renal tubular acidosis characterised by hypokalaemic hyperchloraemic non-anion gap metabolic acidosis.

MANAGEMENT
Resuscitation, supportive care and monitoring
- Attention to airway, breathing and circulation are paramount. These priorities are managed along conventional lines, as outlined in **Chapter 1.2: Resuscitation**.
- Resuscitation proceeds along conventional lines, as outlined in **Chapter 1.2: Resuscitation**.
- In the event of ventricular dysrhythmias (VT, VF):
  - Beta-blockers are the agent of choice to reduce catecholamine-induced myocardial toxicity:
    - Options include metoprolol 1–5 mg IV (0.1 mg/kg in children) titrated to response.
  - Correct hypokalaemia and hypomagnesaemia.
  - Withhold catecholamine inotropes if possible.
- Manage seizures along conventional lines, as outlined in **Chapter 2.3: Seizures**.
- General supportive care measures are indicated, as outlined in **Chapter 1.4: Supportive care and monitoring**.
- Chemical pneumonitis is managed supportively with supplemental oxygen, and bronchodilators if bronchospasm is present. Non-invasive ventilation or intubation and ventilation may be required in severe cases. There is no proven benefit from corticosteroids or prophylactic antibiotics.
- Fever is common following significant aspiration pneumonitis. Antibiotics are indicated if there is objective evidence of infection.

Decontamination
- Remove patient from the exposure, remove clothing and wash skin.
- Activated charcoal does not bind hydrocarbons and is not indicated.

- Gastrointestinal decontamination of any kind is not indicated following ingestion because induction of vomiting increases the risk of hydrocarbon aspiration.

Enhanced elimination
- Not clinically useful.

Antidotes
- N-acetylcysteine is recommended as a non-specific antioxidant for patients who develop hepatotoxicity, typically from halogenated hydrocarbons or certain essential oils (clove or pennyroyal oil). The treatment regimen is the same as for paracetamol toxicity (see **Chapter 4.17: N-acetylcysteine**).

DISPOSITION AND FOLLOW-UP
- Children suspected of ingesting small amounts of hydrocarbons may be observed at home providing they remain asymptomatic. Essential oils are an exception and hospital assessment and observation is warranted for all cases.
- Patients who are clinically well without cough, dyspnoea, wheeze or any alteration in vital signs (including pulse oximetry) at 6 hours are fit for medical discharge.
- Symptomatic patients are admitted for observation and supportive care.
- Patients with high-pressure injection injuries require surgical referral for urgent debridement.

HANDY TIP
- Coughing or choking following ingestion suggests aspiration.

PITFALL
- Failure to recognise dry cough as a symptom of evolving pneumonitis.

CONTROVERSY
- The requirement for treatment with N-acetylcysteine as prophylaxis for all exposures to potentially hepatotoxic hydrocarbons (e.g. clove or pennyroyal oil, halogenated hydrocarbons) in adults and children.

Sources
Most commercial hydrocarbon products are mixtures. Hydrocarbons are organic compounds derived from many sources, including petroleum, plant oils and animal fats. They are widely used in both commercial and household settings as fuel, lubricants, paint thinners and solvents.

References
Flanagan RJ, Ruprah M, Meredith TJ et al. An introduction to the toxicology of volatile substances. Drug Safety 1990; 5(5):359–383.

Kopec KT, Brent J, Banner W et al. Management of cardiac dysrhythmias following hydrocarbon abuse: clinical toxicology teaching case from NAACT acute and intensive care symposium. Clinical Toxicology 2014; 52:141–145.

Tibballs J. Clinical effects and management of eucalyptus oil ingestion in infants and young children. Medical Journal of Australia 1995; 163(4):177–180.

Tormoehlen LM, Tekulve KJ, Nañagas KA. Hydrocarbon toxicity: a review. Clinical Toxicology 2014; 52(5):479–489.

Hydrofluoric acid (HF) is a highly corrosive agent with numerous industrial applications. Accidental dermal exposure is the most common presentation. Toxicity ranges from minor dermal injury to life-threatening systemic fluorosis, which can be rapidly fatal.

RISK ASSESSMENT

- Any dermal exposure can cause chemical burns, characteristically with delayed presentation. Concentrated solutions are likely to cause immediate symptoms.
- Inhalational exposure can lead to pulmonary injury.
- Systemic life-threatening fluorosis is associated with oral ingestion or extensive dermal exposures proportional to the concentration of HF acid and body surface area (BSA) affected:
  - dermal exposure with 100% HF solution to 2.5% BSA
  - dermal exposure with 70% HF to 8% BSA
  - dermal exposure with 23% HF to 11% BSA
  - ingestion of $\geq$ 100 mL of low-concentration HF (6%) by an adult
  - ingestion of any volume of higher concentrations of HF.
- **Children:** any exposure to an HF-containing product is potentially lethal.

Toxic mechanism

HF molecules penetrate readily through skin, soft tissues and lipid membranes and dissociate to form hydrogen cations and fluoride anions. Corrosive hydrogen ions cause local tissue injury and immediate pain. Cytotoxic fluoride anions are responsible for delayed local effects – they react with cellular calcium and magnesium to form insoluble chelates (CaF_2 and MgF_2), inhibiting the Na^+–K^+-ATPase pump and resulting in local hyperkalaemia. Systemic fluorosis occurs when fluoride absorbed into the bloodstream is carried to all body organs in proportion to their vascularity, inducing liquefactive necrosis and cellular death by the same mechanism. Systemic toxicity causes hypocalcaemia, hypomagnesaemia, hyperkalaemia and metabolic acidosis, leading to ventricular dysrhythmias and cardiac arrest.

Toxicokinetics

HC is well absorbed through skin and mucous membranes.

CLINICAL FEATURES

- Dermal exposure
  - Skin contact with HF in concentrations <15% is not immediately painful and may go unnoticed for several hours.
  - Gradual onset of severe deep unremitting pain develops at the contact site over hours without obvious erythema or blistering.
  - Pallor and blanching appear after several hours.
  - Blistering or tissue loss is delayed many hours or days.
  - More concentrated solutions will cause immediate pain.
  - Large exposures will result in systemic fluorosis.
- Inhalational exposure
  - Immediate onset of mucosal irritation followed by delayed onset of dyspnoea, cough and wheeze.
  - Non-cardiogenic pulmonary oedema can occur in severe cases.

- Ingestion
  - Any concentration of ingested HF can cause corrosive injury.
  - Cardiac arrest from systemic fluorosis may occur within 6 hours of exposure.
- Systemic toxicity (fluorosis)
  - Hypocalcaemia, hypomagnesaemia and hyperkalaemia can manifest as tetany and weakness.
  - QT prolongation may be evident.
  - Ventricular dysrhythmias and cardiac arrest.

INVESTIGATIONS

Screening tests in deliberate self-poisoning
- 12-lead ECG, BGL and paracetamol level

Specific investigations
- Serial ECGs
  - Indicated in all patients with potential systemic HF poisoning every 2 hours while monitored.
  - Degree of QT prolongation is a useful marker of hypocalcaemia.
- EUC, calcium and magnesium
  - Measure at presentation and 2 hourly in all patients with potential systemic HF poisoning.
- Endoscopy or CT scan
  - May be indicated to assess the extent of corrosive injury.

MANAGEMENT

Resuscitation, supportive care and monitoring
- Systemic HF poisoning is a time-critical emergency and is managed in an area equipped for cardiopulmonary monitoring and resuscitation.
- Attention to airway, breathing and circulation are paramount. These priorities are managed along conventional lines, as outlined in **Chapter 1.2: Resuscitation**.
- The presence of QT prolongation, ventricular dysrhythmias or clinical features of hypocalcaemia prompt immediate administration of calcium intravenously:
  - Calcium gluconate 10% 20 mL (0.6 mL/kg in children) or calcium chloride 10% 10 mL (0.2 mL/kg) IV and repeat every 5 minutes based on response. Multiple doses may be required to maintain serum calcium concentrations.
  - In cardiac arrest, larger doses are indicated.
  - Administer magnesium sulfate 10 mmol IV (0.05 mmol/kg in children).
  - Hyperkalaemia and acidosis are managed along conventional lines.
- General supportive care measures are indicated, as outlined in **Chapter 1.4: Supportive care and monitoring**.
- Hydrofluoric acid burns are treated with topical, intralesional, intravenous or intra-arterial formulations of calcium. See **Antidotes** for details.
- Administer oral and parenteral analgesia as required.
- Continuous cardiac monitoring is indicated if there is potential for systemic fluorosis.

Decontamination
- Dermal exposure
  - Remove clothing.
  - Irrigate thoroughly with copious amounts of water prior to antidotal therapy with calcium.
- Ingestion
  - Do not induce vomiting.
- Ocular exposure
  - Irrigate thoroughly with water or saline.

Enhanced elimination
- Not clinically useful.

Antidotes
- Calcium (see **Chapter 4.2: Calcium**).
  - Calcium gluconate or calcium chloride is given by IV infusion as described above to correct systemic hypocalcaemia. Large doses may be required.
  - Calcium gluconate gel is indicated for all symptomatic patients following dermal exposure. Administer repeatedly to all affected areas until pain resolves.
  - If local tissue pain is refractory to topical application, calcium gluconate is administered by subcutaneous infiltration, regional IV infusion or intra-arterial infusion as described in **Chapter 4.2: Calcium**.
  - **WARNING:** Do not give calcium chloride by SC injection, regional IV infusion or arterial infusion as it will cause tissue damage.

DISPOSITION AND FOLLOW-UP
- Minor skin exposure to low-concentration preparations may be managed in the outpatient setting with calcium gluconate gel.
- Patients are instructed to return if pain is not controlled with repeated applications of gel.
- Outpatient follow-up in a burns clinic may be required.
- Formal ophthalmological review is recommended for ocular injuries.
- Patients who require calcium administration by regional intravenous or intra-arterial infusion are not discharged until pain has resolved.
- All patients at risk of systemic HF poisoning require cardiac monitoring for at least 8 hours post ingestion or 12 hours after extensive dermal exposure and until serum calcium and 12-lead ECG are normal without calcium administration.

HANDY TIPS
- Onset of pain is delayed after dermal HF exposure; the less concentrated the product, the greater is the delay.
- Patients often present with pain in the evening or night after using an HF product during the previous day.
- Use of a surgical glove filled with calcium gluconate gel is an effective means of providing topical treatment for burns to the fingers or hand.
- Pain is out of proportion to local signs and frequently requires parenteral opioids until calcium can be effectively delivered.

- Local anaesthetic techniques are not recommended as relief of pain is used as an end point to determine adequacy of calcium delivery.
- If not available, 2.5% calcium gluconate gel may be made by mixing:
  - 30 g of amorphous hydrogel wound dressing with 10 mL of calcium gluconate 10% solution. The resultant product will make approximately 40 g of calcium gluconate gel 2.5%.
- Do not use calcium gluconate to irrigate after ocular exposures – use normal saline or water.

PITFALLS
- Failure to appreciate the severity of dermal injury due to lack of local signs.
- Administration of calcium chloride by subcutaneous injection, IV regional or intra-arterial routes.

CONTROVERSIES
- The role of prophylactic calcium and magnesium administration in patients at risk of systemic HF poisoning.
- There are limited data to support the use of topical calcium gluconate for ocular injuries or nebulised solution for inhalational injuries.

Presentations
Exists in two forms, aqueous and anhydrous:
- Aqueous HF is available in a wide range of concentrations up to 40%.
- Anhydrous form is more concentrated (>50%) and used in industry.

Products for domestic use typically contain 5–12% aqueous HF.

References
Bajraktarova-Valjakova E, Korunoska-Stevkovska V, Georgieva S et al. Hydrofluoric acid: burns and systemic toxicity, protective measures, immediate and hospital medical treatment. Macedonian Journal of Medical Sciences 2018; 6(11):2257–2269.

Kao W, Dart RC, Kuffner E et al. Ingestion of concentrated hydrofluoric acid: an insidious and potentially fatal poisoning. Annals of Emergency Medicine 1999; 34(1):35–41.

Kirkpatrick JR, Enion DS, Burd DAR. Hydrofluoric acid burns: a review. Burns 1995; 21:483–493.

Vohra R, Velez LI, Rivera W et al. Recurrent life-threatening ventricular dysrhythmias associated with acute hydrofluoric acid ingestion: observations in one case and implications for mechanism of toxicity. Clinical Toxicology 2008; 46(1):79–84.

Wightman RS, Read KB, Hoffman RS. Evidence-based management of caustic exposures in the emergency department. Emergency Medicine Practice 2016; 18(5):1–17.

3.41 HYDROGEN PEROXIDE

Hydrogen peroxide (H_2O_2) is an oxidising agent with a wide range of domestic and industrial applications. Ingestion of concentrated solution can cause serious toxicity and death due to corrosive effects or gas embolism resulting from the generation of oxygen gas in the arterial or venous circulation.

RISK ASSESSMENT

- Ingestion of 3% H_2O_2 causes a spectrum of toxicity ranging from mild gastrointestinal effects to more severe systemic effects depending on the volume ingested.
- Life-threatening toxicities (severe corrosive injury to airway and gastrointestinal tract, gas embolism) are more likely with ingestion of concentrated (>10%) H_2O_2 solutions.
- Topical exposure to concentrated H_2O_2 solutions will result in local tissue injury.
- Gas embolism can arise where H_2O_2 solutions are used medically to irrigate closed body cavities.
- **Children:** minor exposures to domestic products containing 3% H_2O_2 are unlikely to cause significant injury. Any exposure to concentrated H_2O_2 solutions (>10%) or where symptoms develop requires hospital assessment.

Toxic mechanism

Hydrogen peroxide causes toxicity by three mechanisms: direct corrosive injury, oxygen gas formation and lipid peroxidation. Hydrogen peroxide is corrosive and exposure can cause local tissue damage to the skin, mucosal membranes or cornea. Metabolism of ingested H_2O_2 liberates large quantities of oxygen. Once the amount of oxygen produced exceeds its solubility in the blood, oxygen gas emboli form in the venous or arterial circulation. Rapid accumulation of oxygen in closed body cavities can cause mechanical distension and complications such as rupture of a hollow viscus. Intravascular foaming may occur and can seriously impede left ventricular output.

Toxicokinetics

Following ingestion, H_2O_2 is readily absorbed through the gastrointestinal mucosa into the portal venous system. Metabolism by serum or tissue catalase generates oxygen and water; 30 mL of 35% H_2O_2 solution liberates almost 3.5 L of oxygen at standard temperature and pressure. Arterial emboli can occur due to the presence of intra-cardiac or intra-pulmonary shunts.

CLINICAL FEATURES

- Ingestion
  - Stridor, dysphonia, throat pain or dyspnoea indicate airway injury or aspiration and an immediate threat to life.
  - Severe pulmonary injury may progress to pulmonary oedema and respiratory failure.
  - The likelihood of significant gastro-oesophageal injury is increased by the presence of two or more of the following: vomiting, drooling or abdominal tenderness.
  - Foaming at the mouth and abdominal distension may occur secondary to liberation of large volumes of gas in the gastrointestinal tract.
  - Portal venous gas embolism may result in progressive or persistent abdominal pain.
  - Cerebral gas embolism causes progressive neurological disturbance. The symptoms or signs may initially be subtle and a high index of suspicion must be maintained.
  - Tachycardia, hypotension, confusion, seizures, coma and cardiac arrest may occur within minutes following large ingestions of highly concentrated H_2O_2 solutions.

- Dermal
  - Inflammation, blistering and skin necrosis can occur following exposure to concentrated solutions.
- Ocular
  - Exposure of the cornea to 3% H_2O_2 solution produces immediate pain and irritation.
  - Transient corneal injury is reported after insertion of soft contact lenses stored in 3% H_2O_2 solution without neutralisation.
  - Concentrated solutions may cause corneal ulceration and perforation.

INVESTIGATIONS

Screening tests in deliberate self-poisoning
- 12-lead ECG, BGL and paracetamol level

Specific investigations
- Chest and abdominal X-ray or CT
  - Evidence of gastrointestinal perforation, oxygen gas embolism, pneumonitis or pulmonary oedema.
- Cerebral CT or MRI
  - May demonstrate cerebral gas embolism or infarction.
- Upper gastrointestinal endoscopy or CT
  - If there are clinical features of corrosive injury to the airway or gastrointestinal tract (see **Chapter 3.31: Corrosives**).

MANAGEMENT

Resuscitation, supportive care and monitoring
- Early definitive airway management is critical for patients with corrosive airway injury. Endotracheal intubation or a surgical airway may be required.
- The patient is initially managed in an area equipped for cardiorespiratory monitoring and resuscitation.
- High-flow oxygen via a tight-fitting mask is administered to all patients.
- Hyperbaric oxygen therapy is indicated for treatment of cerebral or venous gas embolism.
- If systemic gas embolism is suspected, the patient should be placed supine, avoiding the head-up position.
- General supportive care measures are indicated, as outlined in **Chapter 1.4: Supportive care and monitoring**.

Decontamination
- Gastrointestinal decontamination is not indicated due to the rapid decomposition of H_2O_2.
- Immediate eye irrigation with copious amounts of water or saline for at least 15 minutes is indicated after ophthalmic exposure.
- Clothing should be removed and the exposed skin washed with copious amounts of water following dermal exposure.

Enhanced elimination
- Not useful.

Antidotes
- None available.

DISPOSITION AND FOLLOW-UP

- Minor unintentional exposures to 3% solutions in either children or adults do not require hospital evaluation unless symptoms develop.
- Any symptomatic patient following ingestion of H_2O_2 is admitted for observation.
- Patients in whom arterial or venous gas embolism is suspected or confirmed require hyperbaric oxygen therapy.
- Patients with eye exposures and any signs or symptoms of corneal injury should be referred for formal ophthalmological evaluation.

HANDY TIP

- A normal CT head in the presence of neurological symptoms does not exclude cerebral gas embolism. MRI is a more sensitive modality in this setting.

PITFALL

- Discharge of a patient with vague neurological symptoms or signs without recognition of the possibility of cerebral gas embolism.

Presentations

Solutions ranging in concentration from 3% to 90% are used in various applications:

- household products (mostly 3% H_2O_2): disinfectants, bleaches, fabric stain removers, contact lens disinfectants, hair dyes, tooth-whitening products
- industrial products: bleaching agent in paper industry
- medical products: wound irrigation solutions, sterilising solutions for ophthalmic and endoscopic instruments.

References

Byrne B, Sherwin R, Courage C et al. Hyperbaric oxygen therapy for systemic gas embolism after hydrogen peroxide ingestion. Journal of Emergency Medicine 2014; 46:171–175.

French LK, Horowitz BZ, McKeown NJ. Hydrogen peroxide ingestion associated with portal venous gas and treatment with hyperbaric oxygen: a case series and review of the literature. Clinical Toxicology 2010; 48:533–538.

Smedley BL, Gault A, Gawthrope IC. Cerebral arterial gas embolism after pre-flight ingestion of hydrogen peroxide. Diving and Hyperbaric Medicine 2016; 46(2):117–119.

Watt BE, Proudfoot AT, Vale JA. Hydrogen peroxide poisoning. Toxicological Reviews 2004; 23:51–57.

3.42 INSULIN

Deliberate self-administered insulin overdose causes profound and prolonged hypoglycaemia that may result in life-threatening seizures, coma and permanent neurological injury.

RISK ASSESSMENT

- The severity and duration of hypoglycaemia following intentional overdose of insulin is unpredictable and correlates poorly with the dose and formulation injected.
- Hypoglycaemia may last for days; patients require prolonged monitoring and treatment until toxicity has resolved.
- Poor outcome is associated with delayed presentation or established hypoglycaemic coma. The prognosis is excellent with early effective glucose resuscitation.

Toxic mechanism

Insulin is released from the beta pancreatic islet cells at a low basal rate, which increases in response to various stimuli. Exogenous insulin is used for the treatment of type 1 and type 2 diabetes mellitus, severe hyperkalaemia and calcium-channel-blocker overdose. Insulin stimulates the transfer of glucose, potassium, phosphate and magnesium into cells. It promotes synthesis and storage of glycogen, protein and triglycerides.

Toxicokinetics

In overdose, the pharmacokinetic properties of insulin change. The duration of action is prolonged and does not depend on the type of insulin preparation administered. Instead, it is determined by the slow and erratic release from subcutaneous adipose tissue at the injection site, in addition to the prolonged clearance of the absorbed insulin. Insulin undergoes hepatic metabolism (60%) and renal clearance (40%).

CLINICAL FEATURES

The clinical features are those of hypoglycaemia. They usually manifest within 2 hours of administration.

- Autonomic symptoms
  - Nausea and vomiting
  - Diaphoresis
  - Tachycardia and palpitations
- Central nervous system
  - Agitation and tremor
  - Confusion and visual disturbances
  - Seizures
  - Neurological deficits
  - Coma
- The hyperinsulinaemic state commonly persists for >2 days.
- Prolonged untreated hypoglycaemia may cause permanent neurological injury and death.

INVESTIGATIONS

Screening tests in deliberate self-poisoning

- 12-lead ECG, BGL and paracetamol level

Specific investigations

- Serial blood glucose levels (BGLs)
  - Perform every 15 minutes during the resuscitation phase and until the glucose infusion requirement has stabilised. Frequency may then be reduced to 1–2 hourly.
- EUC, serum phosphate and magnesium
- Insulin levels
  - Insulin levels will be elevated but do not guide the duration of glucose administration and are not clinically useful.

— Insulin and C-peptide levels are helpful in the rare circumstance where it is necessary to exclude alternative diagnoses (e.g. insulinoma, factitious hypoglycaemia).

MANAGEMENT
Resuscitation, supportive care and monitoring
- Insulin overdose is a life-threatening emergency and the patient should be managed in an area capable of detecting and managing hypoglycaemia with close clinical and physiological monitoring.
- If symptoms of hypoglycaemia occur or BGL is <4.0 mmol/L (bedside or laboratory value) administer concentrated IV glucose:
  - **Adult**
    - 50-mL bolus of 50% glucose IV
    - Repeat if no immediate clinical improvement.
  - **Child**
    - 2-mL/kg bolus of 10% glucose IV
    - Repeat if no immediate clinical improvement.
- Hyperinsulinaemia resulting in hypoglycaemia requires ongoing exogenous glucose administration. The infusion concentration and rate are titrated to maintain serum glucose at or just above the normal range.
- Commence a 10% glucose infusion at 100 mL/hour and monitor bedside BGL frequently.
- Any further episodes of symptomatic hypoglycaemia are treated with an IV bolus of concentrated glucose (25–50 mL of 50% glucose).
- If the above infusion fails to maintain normoglycaemia, obtain central venous access and commence a titrated infusion of 50% glucose to maintain normoglycaemia (or mild hyperglycaemia).
- Infusion rates of >100 mL/hour of 50% glucose may be required for several days.
- Manage asymptomatic hypoglycaemia by increasing the rate of infusion without bolus therapy.
- Monitor serum potassium and supplement as required to keep in the low-to-normal range (e.g. 20 mmol/hour).
- Enteral supplementation with complex carbohydrates should be encouraged as early as feasible based on the patient's clinical status.

Decontamination
- Not clinically useful.

Enhanced elimination
- Not clinically useful.

Antidotes
- Glucose as outlined in **Chapter 4.12: Glucose**.
- Glucagon is not indicated in the hospital management of hypoglycaemia.

DISPOSITION AND FOLLOW-UP
- Patients who are clinically well with normal BGL at 6 hours following exposure have not administered a significant insulin dose and do not require further medical care.

- Confirmed significant deliberate self-poisoning with insulin requires admission to an intensive care or high-dependency unit for several days of ongoing exogenous IV glucose administration via a central line and careful monitoring of BGL and serum potassium levels.

HANDY TIPS
- Anticipate the need for large ongoing glucose requirement and insert a central line early so that 50% glucose infusion may commence.
- Withdrawal of glucose infusion should be gradual and should not take place at night.
- Monitor patients for 6 hours after glucose cessation.
- Non-diabetic patients are at particular risk of hypoglycaemia during weaning of glucose infusions because exogenous glucose administration stimulates endogenous pancreatic insulin release, prolonging the hyperinsulinaemic state. Attempts should be made to limit bolus IV glucose therapy in response to borderline hypoglycaemia unless significant clinical features are evident.
- Consider the diagnosis of deliberate insulin overdose in any patient who presents with profound and recurrent hypoglycaemia.

PITFALLS
- Failure to anticipate ongoing glucose requirement after initial hypoglycaemia in a patient with deliberate self-poisoning.
- Attempts to manage with an infusion of 5% glucose solution.
- Premature, rapid weaning of glucose infusion with subsequent occurrence of hypoglycaemia.

CONTROVERSY
- Excision of the insulin injection site has been attempted, but benefit is unproven and such an invasive procedure is not justified.

Presentations
Numerous insulin formulations are available.

References
Haskell RJ, Stapczynski JS. Duration of hypoglycaemia and need for intravenous glucose following intentional overdoses of insulin. Annals of Emergency Medicine 1984; 13:505–511.

Klein-Schwartz W, Stassinos GL, Isbister GK. Treatment of sulfonylurea and insulin overdose. British Journal of Clinical Pharmacology 2016; 81(3):496–504.

Megarbane B, Deye N, Bloch V et al. Intentional overdose with insulin: prognostic factors and toxicokinetic/toxicodynamic profiles. Critical Care 2007; 11(5):R115.

3.43 IRON

Oral: **Ferrous chloride, Ferrous fumarate, Ferrous gluconate, Ferrous phosphate, Ferrous sulfate, Iron amino acid chelates**

Parenteral: **Ferric carboxymaltose, Ferric derisomaltose, Iron polymaltose, Iron sucrose**

Iron poisoning occurs primarily by ingestion of oral formulations. The toxicity is dose-related, based on the elemental iron content. Most acute overdoses result in only minor gastrointestinal effects. Large overdoses are potentially lethal, and early gastrointestinal decontamination and consideration of chelation with desferrioxamine are warranted.

RISK ASSESSMENT

Oral ingestion

- It is essential to determine the dose of elemental iron ingested (see **Table 3.43.1**).
- The amount of elemental iron in a ferrous or ferric salt is detailed in the product information or can be calculated as follows:
  - ferric chloride dose divided by 3.5
  - ferrous chloride dose divided by 4
  - ferrous fumarate dose divided by 3
  - ferrous gluconate dose divided by 9
  - ferrous sulfate (dried) dose divided by 3.3
  - ferrous sulfate (heptahydrate) dose divided by 5.
- The threshold for therapeutic interventions is determined by two key investigations:
  - abdominal X-ray
  - serum iron level (or venous blood gas as a surrogate marker if iron level is unavailable).
- Patients presenting with established systemic iron toxicity have a poor prognosis and chelation therapy may not improve outcome.

Supratherapeutic parenteral administration

- Supratherapeutic dosing of parenteral formulations (e.g. from dose miscalculations) are unlikely to cause significant toxicity. The iron is formulated as stable complexes and released into the systemic circulation slowly.
- In this setting, the serum iron level is expected to be markedly elevated and does not correlate directly with the development of toxicity.
- **Children:** most paediatric ingestions are below the threshold expected to result in systemic toxicity. Patients ingesting a dose confirmed <40 mg/kg may be observed at home if they remain asymptomatic.

Toxic mechanism

Iron toxicity is mediated by the oxidised ferric ion (Fe^{3+}) which liberates oxygen free radicals causing lipid peroxidation of cell membranes and cell death. Iron also causes intracellular toxicity due to mitochondrial damage and impaired oxidative phosphorylation.

TABLE 3.43.1 Elemental iron: dose-related risk assessment	
Elemental iron dose	**Effect**
<20 mg/kg	Asymptomatic
20–60 mg/kg	Gastrointestinal symptoms
>60–120 mg/kg	Systemic toxicity anticipated
>120 mg/kg	Potentially lethal

Initial cytotoxic damage affects gastrointestinal mucosa. Progressive systemic cellular toxicity results in multi-system organ effects. Metabolic acidosis is caused by lactic acid production due to mitochondrial dysfunction and the liberation of free hydrogen ions in the plasma from hydration of ferric ions. Coagulopathy results from hepatic dysfunction and direct impairment of the coagulation cascade.

Toxicokinetics

Iron homeostasis is normally finely regulated. Iron is absorbed from the upper GI tract in the ferrous (2+) state and oxidised to the ferric (3+) state in enterocytes. In overdose, the physiological transport and storage proteins (transferrin and ferritin) are overwhelmed, with a marked increase in free serum iron levels. Iron is transported by active processes to intracellular compartments and the liver is particularly susceptible due to passive accumulation into hepatocytes. Elimination is by gastrointestinal losses via sloughed intestinal cells and, in women, by menstrual losses.

Parenteral iron preparations are formulated as stable carbohydrate complexes, which are taken up by the reticuloendothelial system and release iron slowly into the systemic circulation. This limits the potential for iron toxicity following inadvertent supratherapeutic dosing.

CLINICAL FEATURES

Iron toxicity following oral ingestion was historically described as having five stages, but this is an artificial classification. Not all patients experience all stages and the duration of each stage is imprecise and they usually overlap. Iron toxicity is more accurately conceptualised as two overlapping stages with a pathophysiological basis: gastrointestinal and systemic toxicity (see **Table 3.43.2**).

Systemic features are unlikely in the absence of GI symptoms.

INVESTIGATIONS
Screening tests in deliberate self-poisoning
- 12-lead ECG, BGL and paracetamol level

TABLE 3.43.2 Stages of iron toxicity: oral ingestion

Time post ingestion	Clinical features
0–6 hours	Direct corrosive effect on GI tract characterised by vomiting, diarrhoea and abdominal pain. Large GI fluid losses may cause significant hypovolaemia
6–12 hours	Ongoing absorption and redistribution. Gastrointestinal symptoms may improve, with apparent resolution of toxicity
12–48 hours	Progressive mitochondrial toxicity resulting in metabolic acidosis, vasodilatory shock and multi-organ failure
2–5 days	Hepatic failure with jaundice, coma, hypoglycaemia and coagulopathy. This phase has a high mortality
2–6 weeks	GI tract fibrosis and strictures can occur during the recovery phase

Specific investigations
- Abdominal X-ray
  - Iron preparations are radio-opaque and may be visible on abdominal X-ray to confirm or quantify ingestion.
  - The presence of a significant amount of ingested iron may justify decontamination with whole bowel irrigation.
- Serum iron concentration
  - Iron levels peak 4–6 hours following ingestion, with subsequent redistribution to the intracellular compartment.
  - Peak levels may be delayed further with slow-release formulations or in large ingestions, and serial iron levels can be considered.
  - A clear correlation between iron levels and clinical toxicity is not established, but peak levels >90 micromol/L (500 microgram/dL) are thought to be predictive of systemic toxicity.
- Venous blood gas
  - If a serum iron level is not available, a venous blood gas can be used as a surrogate marker.
    - A decrease in serum bicarbonate, elevated serum lactate or metabolic acidosis are markers of systemic toxicity.
- FBC, EUC, LFT, coagulation studies
  - To monitor and treat multi-system organ toxicity.
- Note: Hyperglycaemia and elevated white cell counts are frequently observed in iron poisoning but do not correlate directly with toxicity.

MANAGEMENT
Resuscitation, supportive care and monitoring
- An early priority is the restoration of adequate circulating volume. Give boluses of 10–20 mL/kg of crystalloid and assess response.
- Ongoing fluid replacement is essential in the face of continuing gastrointestinal and third-space losses.

Decontamination
- Iron is not adsorbed to activated charcoal.
- Whole bowel irrigation (WBI) is the decontamination method of choice and recommended for ingestions >60 mg/kg with evidence of tablet residue on abdominal X-ray (see **Chapter 1.6: Gastrointestinal decontamination**).

Enhanced elimination
- Not clinically useful.

Antidotes
- Desferrioxamine chelation therapy is indicated if systemic toxicity (shock, metabolic acidosis, altered mental status) is present or predicted by a serum iron level >90 micromol/L (500 microgram/dL) at 4–6 hours post ingestion. For further details, see **Chapter 4.4: Desferrioxamine**.

DISPOSITION AND FOLLOW-UP
- Children accidentally ingesting <40 mg/kg may be managed at home provided they remain asymptomatic.

- Larger accidental ingestions, intentional overdoses or symptomatic patients are assessed in hospital with appropriate investigations.
- If the assessment and investigations exclude significant risk of toxicity and the patient remains clinically well, ongoing medical management is not required.
- Patients presenting with established systemic iron toxicity or requiring intravenous chelation therapy are managed in an intensive care environment.

HANDY TIPS

- Where serum iron levels are not readily available, progressively decreasing serum bicarbonate concentration or increasing lactate are good surrogate markers of systemic iron poisoning and, in conjunction with worsening clinical features, would justify desferrioxamine administration.
- Iron supplements are readily accessible to pregnant women and thus are frequently taken in overdose. The fetus is relatively protected unless maternal cardiovascular instability develops. Therapy is directed towards care of the mother and does not differ from the care of the non-pregnant patient.

PITFALLS

- Over-treatment of trivial ingestions.
- Failure to perform an initial risk assessment leading to delays in initiation of appropriate therapy following overdose.
- Failure to consider systemic iron toxicity in the patient who presents late with minimal elevation in serum iron level.

CONTROVERSIES

- Threshold serum iron level that mandates chelation with desferrioxamine.
- Duration and endpoints for desferrioxamine therapy.

Presentations

There are numerous over-the-counter vitamin preparations containing relatively small amounts of elemental iron – usually iron amino acid chelates, ferrous phosphate or ferrous fumarate. The important preparations containing large amounts of elemental iron are:

- ferrous sulfate 325 mg (105 mg elemental iron) slow-release tablets (30)
- ferrous sulfate 250 mg (80 mg elemental iron)/folic acid 300 mg combination controlled-release tablets (30)
- ferrous sulfate 6 mg/mL oral liquid (250 mL).

References

Chang TP, Rangan C. Iron poisoning: a literature-based review of epidemiology, diagnosis, and management. Pediatric Emergency Care 2011; 27(10):978–985. http://dx.doi:10.1097/pec.0b013e3182302604.

Chyka PA, Butler AY. Assessment of acute iron poisoning by laboratory and clinical observations. American Journal of Emergency Medicine 1993; 11(2):99–103.

Pearn J, Nixon J, Ansford A et al. Accidental poisoning in childhood: five year urban population study with 15 year analysis of fatality. British Medical Journal 1984; 288:44–46.

Singhi SC, Baranwal AK, Jayashree M. Acute iron poisoning: clinical picture, intensive care needs and outcome. Indian Pediatrics 2003; 40(12):1177–1182.

Tenenbein M. Benefits of parenteral deferoxamine for acute iron poisoning. Journal of Toxicology–Clinical Toxicology 1996; 34(5):485–489.

Isoniazid overdose is rare but potentially fatal. Severe poisoning presents with rapid onset of seizures, coma and severe metabolic acidosis. Pyridoxine is the specific antidote.

RISK ASSESSMENT
- Toxicity is of rapid onset, occurring within 30 min to 2 hours of ingestion and follows a predictable dose–response (see **Table 3.44.1**).

TABLE 3.44.1 Dose-related risk assessment: isoniazid

Dose	Effect
>1.5 g (20 mg/kg)	May develop symptoms
>3 g (40 mg/kg)	Seizures, metabolic acidosis and coma
>10 g (130 mg/kg)	May be fatal without intervention

Toxic mechanism
Isoniazid is structurally related to pyridoxine, nicotinic acid and NAD, and induces a state of functional pyridoxine deficiency by multiple mechanisms - it inhibits the enzyme responsible for the conversion of pyridoxine to its active form, pyridoxine-5-phosphate (P5P); binds to and inactivates P5P; and enhances urinary excretion of P5P. Because P5P is an essential co-factor for the conversion of glutamic acid to gamma-aminobutyric acid (GABA) in the CNS, an acute deficiency of GABA develops resulting in generalised tonic-clonic seizures. Severe lactic acidosis is due to recurrent seizures and also caused by direct isoniazid inhibition of the conversion of lactate to pyruvate.

Toxicokinetics
Absorption following oral administration is rapid and complete. Peak serum levels occur within 1–2 hours. Volume of distribution is 0.6 L/kg. Isoniazid undergoes hepatic metabolism by either acetylation to form acetyl-isoniazid or hydrolysis by cytochrome P450 to form hydrazine derivatives. Some drug is excreted unchanged in the urine. There are 'fast' and 'slow' acetylators such that the elimination half-life varies from 1 to 4 hours.

CLINICAL FEATURES
- Initial symptoms include light-headedness, blurred vision, photophobia, nausea and vomiting.
- Progressive toxicity results in confusion, coma, recurrent seizures, severe lactic acidosis and death.
- Seizures are typically generalised tonic–clonic and may be recurrent. Complications of status epilepticus include hyperpyrexia, pulmonary aspiration and rhabdomyolysis.

INVESTIGATIONS
Screening tests in deliberate self-poisoning
- 12-lead ECG, BGL and paracetamol level

Specific investigations

- Blood gas
  - Severe anion gap metabolic acidosis with a high serum lactate is a major feature of isoniazid overdose.
- Isoniazid levels
  - Not routinely available and do not aid in acute management. They may be useful to confirm the diagnosis retrospectively.

MANAGEMENT

Resuscitation, supportive care and monitoring

- Isoniazid overdose is a life-threatening emergency and managed in an area equipped for cardiorespiratory monitoring and resuscitation.
- Attention to airway, breathing and circulation is paramount. These priorities are managed along conventional lines, as outlined in **Chapter 1.2: Resuscitation**.
- The patient presenting with coma or recurrent seizures requires prompt rapid-sequence intubation and ventilation.
- Seizures are managed with escalating doses of intravenous benzodiazepines and intravenous pyridoxine.
- Barbiturates are alternative agents for refractory seizures.
- Intravenous pyridoxine is the specific antidote (see below).

Decontamination

- Activated charcoal is only given once the airway is secured with endotracheal intubation and never takes precedence over resuscitation and supportive care.

Enhanced elimination

- Haemodialysis can enhance elimination of isoniazid and may be considered in the setting of recurrent seizures, particularly if sufficient doses of pyridoxine are not available.

Antidotes

- Urgent administration of IV pyridoxine is indicated if coma or seizures develop (see **Chapter 4.23: Pyridoxine**).
- Give 1 g for each gram of isoniazid ingested, to a maximum dose of 5 g.
- If the ingested dose is unknown, give 5 g of pyridoxine and review response.

DISPOSITION AND FOLLOW-UP

- Patients are observed for 6 hours and are fit for medical discharge if they remain asymptomatic.
- All patients who develop neurological toxicity should be managed in an intensive care or high-dependency unit.

HANDY TIPS

- Always consider isoniazid overdose in the differential diagnosis of status epilepticus, particularly if the patient or a household member has a history of tuberculosis.
- Appropriate resuscitation and intravenous benzodiazepines may be sufficient to achieve a good outcome even in the absence of pyridoxine.

- There is no evidence to support a beneficial role for other anticonvulsants such as levetiracetam or phenytoin.
- EEG monitoring may be required in an intubated patient.

CONTROVERSY
- The beneficial effect of oral or nasogastric pyridoxine in the absence of intravenous formulations.

Presentations
Isoniazid 25 mg, 100 mg tablets (100)

Reference
Bateman DN, Page CB. Antidotes to coumarins, isoniazid, methotrexate and thyroxine, toxins that work via metabolic processes. British Journal of Clinical Pharmacology 2016; 81(3):437-445. doi:10.1111/bcp.12736.
Maw G, Aitken P. Isoniazid overdose: a case series, literature review and survey of antidote availability. Clinical Drug Investigation 2003; 23:479–485.

3.45 LAMOTRIGINE

Lamotrigine is an anticonvulsant that is also prescribed for mood disorders, neuropathic pain and migraine. In overdose, the principal toxic effects are sedation, but more significant effects such as seizures, respiratory depression, serotonin toxicity and cardiovascular collapse can occur. Management is principally supportive.

RISK ASSESSMENT
- A dose-related risk assessment has not been clearly defined, but doses exceeding 10 mg/kg are likely to cause toxic effects.
- Most overdoses cause only mild sedation but seizures and coma can occur at relatively low doses.
- CNS effects develop within 4 hours of ingestion and may be prolonged.
- Cardiovascular toxicity is a feature of lamotrigine toxicity, particularly in doses greater than 4 g. Broad complex tachydysrhythmias and profound hypotension can result in cardiovascular collapse.
- Serotonin toxicity can occur, particularly in combination with other serotonergic agents.
- **Children:** accidental ingestion can result in sedation, altered mental status and myoclonus, which may persist for 24–48 hours. Seizures occur in a significant percentage of patients and any accidental ingestion requires medical assessment.

Toxic mechanism
Lamotrigine blocks voltage-gated sodium channels in neural and cardiac tissue. In the CNS, it inhibits the release of excitatory neurotransmitters (principally glutamate). In cardiac tissue, it is associated with QRS widening and intraventricular conduction delays. It also inhibits serotonin, noradrenaline and dopamine reuptake. Reversible blockade of monoamine oxidase enzymes can contribute to serotonergic toxicity.

Toxicokinetics

Lamotrigine is rapidly and completely absorbed, with a moderate volume of distribution of 1.1 L/kg and approximately 50% protein binding. Hepatic metabolism is by glucuronidation with renal excretion of inactive metabolites and a half-life in therapeutic use of approximately 24 hours. Metabolism is affected by numerous drug interactions – plasma levels and half-life are increased by valproic acid and decreased by phenytoin, carbamazepine and oral contraceptives.

CLINICAL FEATURES

- Central nervous system
  - Sedation, ataxia and dysarthria are typical
  - Seizures and status epilepticus
  - Coma
  - Serotonin toxicity
- Cardiac
  - Sinus tachycardia
  - Hypotension
  - Broad-complex tachydysrhythmias

INVESTIGATIONS
Screening tests in deliberate self-poisoning

- BGL and paracetamol level

Specific investigations

- Serial ECGs
  - Evidence of sodium channel blockade (prolongation of QRS interval, R wave in aVR)
- Lamotrigine levels are not readily available and are not useful to guide management.

MANAGEMENT
Resuscitation, supportive care and monitoring

- All patients are managed in an area equipped for cardiopulmonary monitoring and resuscitation.
- Attention to airway, breathing and circulation are paramount. These priorities are managed along conventional lines, as outlined in **Chapter 1.2: Resuscitation**.
- Seizures are treated with intravenous benzodiazepines. Recurrent seizures will require intubation and propofol or barbiturate infusions.
- Broad complex tachyarrhythmias with haemodynamic compromise:
  - Manage initially with bolus IV sodium bicarbonate 1–2 mmol/kg IV, intubation and hyperventilation. If there is no dynamic improvement in QRS widening following initial boluses of sodium bicarbonate, and the pH is maintained at >7.5 by appropriate ventilation, further IV doses are unlikely to be of benefit.
  - Note: Multiple doses of sodium bicarbonate can cause significant alkalaemia, with resultant hypokalaemia and increasing the risk of ventricular dysrhythmias (torsades de pointes).

- Hypotension: manage initially with appropriate volume resuscitation, but inotropic and vasopressor support may be required. Options include adrenaline or noradrenaline, guided by assessment of cardiovascular function.
- Serotonin toxicity is treated as outlined in **Chapter 2.5: Serotonin toxicity**.

Decontamination
- Activated charcoal should be given to all comatose patients following lamotrigine overdose once the airway is protected by endotracheal intubation.

Enhanced elimination
- Haemodialysis effectively removes lamotrigine but is not routinely indicated even in the presence of coma. It has been considered in cases of severe poisoning to shorten the duration of toxicity, but there is no clear evidence of clinical benefit.

Antidotes
- None available.

DISPOSITION AND FOLLOW-UP
- Paediatric patients following accidental ingestion who are clinically well at 4 hours do not require ongoing medical management. Discharge should not occur at night.
- Adult patients with deliberate self-poisoning are observed for 6 hours. If they remain clinically well with a normal ECG, further medical management is not required.
- Patients with clinical features of toxicity can usually be managed in a ward environment for 12–24 hours. They are fit for medical discharge when clinical features resolve.
- Patients with significant sedation or cardiotoxicity require management in an intensive care unit.

HANDY TIPS
- Intraventricular conduction delay can occur, which may not reflect direct sodium channel blockade. Treatment with IV sodium bicarbonate boluses does not lead to dynamic improvement in QRS duration as it does in tricyclic antidepressant poisoning, and repeated administration once the pH has reached 7.5 may lead to complications such as pulmonary or cerebral oedema.
- Recurrent seizures are associated with an increased risk of haemodynamic deterioration and must be controlled immediately.

CONTROVERSY
- A beneficial role for haemodialysis in the management of lamotrigine toxicity is not clearly established.

Presentations
Lamotrigine 5 mg, 25 mg, 50 mg, 100 mg, 200 mg tablets (56)

References
Alyahya B, Friesen M, Nauche B et al. Acute lamotrigine overdose: a systematic review of published adult and pediatric cases. Clinical Toxicology 2018; 56(2):81–89.

Becker T, Chiew AL, Chan BSH. Intermittent haemodialysis in lamotrigine poisoning. Journal of Clinical Toxicology 2019; 9(4):1–4.

Lofton AL, Klein-Schwartz W. Evaluation of lamotrigine toxicity reported to poison centers. Annals of Pharmacotherapy 2004; 38(11):1811–1815. doi:10.1345/aph.1E192.

Moore PW, Donovan JW, Burkhart KK et al. A case series of patients with lamotrigine toxicity at one center from 2003 to 2012. Clinical Toxicology 2013; 51(7):545–549. doi:10.3109/15563650.2013.818685.

Nogar JN, Minns AB, Savaser DJ et al. Severe sodium channel blockade and cardiovascular collapse due to a massive lamotrigine overdose. Clinical Toxicology 2011; 49(9):854–857. doi:10.3109/15563650.2011.617307.

Roberts D, Premachandra K, Priyadarshini S. Dialyzability of lamotrigine by continuous venovenous haemodiafiltration. Clinical Toxicology 2021. doi:10.1080/15563650.2021.1916517.

3.46 LEAD

Acute lead intoxication is rare, but potentially life-threatening. Chronic environmental lead exposure remains a major issue in some regions and occupations, and prevention of lead exposure is the most important public health intervention. Evaluation of patients with possible lead poisoning requires a detailed exposure history and whole blood levels to guide the risk assessment and subsequent management decisions.

RISK ASSESSMENT

- Acute or subacute lead poisoning occurs in the context of inhalation or oral ingestion of lead. Severe toxicity is rare but can cause seizures, encephalopathy, cerebral oedema and death.
- Chronic occupational or environmental exposure usually leads to a non-specific multi-system disorder with the potential for permanent neurological and neuropsychiatric sequelae.
- Clinical effects and risk of long-term neurological sequelae correlate with whole blood lead levels; however, there is wide inter-individual variability. Patients may remain asymptomatic with significantly elevated blood levels.
- **Pregnancy:** lead is readily transferred across the placenta. Major malformations are reported in children born to mothers with elevated lead levels.
- **Children:** children are more susceptible to neurological toxicity than adults and any elevated blood level is associated with impaired neurological development.

Toxic mechanism

Lead has no physiological function and any exposure is detrimental. It causes toxicity through two major mechanisms – oxidative stress (formation of reactive oxygen species and impairment of antioxidant pathways) and ionic binding to sulfhydryl groups and substitution for other bivalent cations (particularly $Ca2^+$). These processes result in impairment of cell wall integrity, haem synthesis and neurotransmitter systems. The major toxic effects are on the neurological, renal, haematopoietic and reproductive systems.

Toxicokinetics

Absorption is via inhalational, oral and topical routes. Fumes from lead smelting or inhaled lead dust are rapidly absorbed by the lungs. Oral absorption is greater in children than adults (bioavailability 50% and 20% respectively) and is enhanced in the presence of iron or calcium deficiencies. Absorption of organic lead compounds can occur through intact skin or from lead foreign bodies such as shotgun pellets. Lead is absorbed and bound by red cells, then distributed widely throughout the body. The bony skeleton acts as the major lead reservoir but other sites of deposition are the liver, kidneys, central and peripheral nervous systems and bone marrow. Bone stores can remobilise long after exposure has ceased, resulting in persistently high levels for months to years. Lead easily crosses the placenta and significant fetal transfer can occur. Urinary and biliary excretion are the principal elimination pathways (65% and 35% respectively).

CLINICAL FEATURES
- Acute
  - Acute ingestion of lead leads to abdominal pain, nausea, vomiting, haemolytic anaemia and hepatitis.
  - Seizures, encephalopathy, cerebral oedema and coma are features of severe toxicity.
- Chronic
  - Non-specific multi-system effects include anorexia, abdominal pain, headache, impaired concentration, emotional lability, weight loss, arthralgia and impaired coordination.
  - Neurocognitive impairment and psychiatric manifestations (anxiety, depression).
  - Peripheral, predominantly motor neuropathies.
  - Anaemia.

INVESTIGATIONS
Screening tests in deliberate self-poisoning
- 12-lead ECG, BGL and paracetamol level

Specific investigations
- Whole blood lead level
  - Most useful indicator of lead exposure and guides management decisions
- FBC
  - Normochromic, normocytic anaemia with basophilic stippling of erythrocytes
- EUC, liver function tests
  - Nephritis, Fanconi syndrome, liver injury, LFTs
- Free erythrocyte protoporphyrin (FEP) or zinc protoporphyrin (ZPP)
  - Reflects abnormal haemoglobin synthesis; however, this is not specific for lead toxicity and can occur with anaemia from other causes
  - Can remain elevated for longer than whole blood levels and may be indicated if the whole blood lead level is low but the clinical suspicion for lead poisoning remains
- X-ray (e.g. abdominal or soft tissue)
  - identifies ingested lead foreign bodies or retained bullets
- Nerve conduction and psychomotor testing
  - May be useful in chronic exposures to demonstrate objective evidence of lead neurotoxicity

MANAGEMENT
Resuscitation, supportive care and monitoring
- Acute resuscitation is rarely required.

- In cases of acute lead-induced encephalopathy, management of airway, breathing and circulation are managed along conventional lines, as outlined in **Chapter 1.2: Resuscitation**.
- Seizures are treated with benzodiazepines, as outlined in **Chapter 2.3: Seizures**.
- Decisions regarding management interventions are based on clinical features and the whole blood level (see **Antidotes**).

Decontamination
- Lead foreign body ingestion
  - Endoscopic retrieval if located in the oesophagus or stomach.
  - If beyond the pylorus and the patient is asymptomatic, commence a high-residue diet plus oral polyethylene glycol to drink at home. Repeat abdominal X-rays to confirm passage of the foreign body within 72 hours.
  - Suppression of stomach acid with a proton pump inhibitor may decrease lead absorption.
  - If the foreign body is still present at 72 hours, admit the patient for formal whole bowel irrigation with polyethylene glycol (see **Chapter 1.6: Gastrointestinal decontamination**).
- Bullet fragments
  - Surgical excision to prevent ongoing absorption is considered in the symptomatic patient or those with elevated lead levels.

Enhanced elimination
- Not clinically useful.

Antidotes
- Chelation therapy is indicated in symptomatic lead poisoning, in the presence of elevated whole blood levels or if long-term neurological injury is anticipated.
- DMSA (2,3-dimercaptosuccinic acid; succimer) is an oral analogue of dimercaprol used as a chelating agent in patients without encephalopathy.
- DMPS (2,3-dimercapto-1-propanesulfonic acid; unithiol) is the intravenous formulation of dimercaprol indicated if oral therapy is not feasible. For administration see **Chapter 4.7: DMSA (succimer) and DMPS (unithiol))**.
- Dimercaprol (British anti-Lewisite; BAL) is the original intramuscular formulation of this chelating agent.
- Sodium calcium edetate is an alternative intravenous chelating agent. These latter two agents are indicated as combination therapy in the rare setting of severe lead encephalopathy. See **Chapter 4.25: Sodium calcium edetate** and **Chapter 4.6: Dimercaprol** for more detailed information regarding indications for use.

HANDY TIPS
- Diagnosis of chronic lead intoxication identifies an index case. Family members and work colleagues should be screened and all potential exposures considered.
- Lead levels <25 microgram/dL are usually asymptomatic. However, any level >5 microgram/dL mandates strenuous efforts to identify the source and prevent further exposure, especially in children.
- Lead intoxication is a notifiable disease in most jurisdictions.

PITFALL

- Failure to identify and remove the source of lead exposure in chronic poisoning to prevent further toxicity.

CONTROVERSIES

- Value of chelation therapy for children with lead levels <45 microgram/dL. Despite theoretical benefit, there is limited evidence to support a measurable improvement in neuropsychiatric outcomes.
- The optimal duration of chelation therapy is best determined by consideration of the individual patient's response based on clinical features, improvement in blood lead levels and (ideally) assessment of urinary lead excretion. The minimum effective duration appears to be 5 days, but repeated courses may be indicated.
- Based on historical evidence, the recommendation for treatment of severe lead encephalopathy is combination therapy with BAL and sodium calcium edetate (due to concerns that EDTA preferentially mobilises lead bone stores which could re-distribute to the CNS and transiently worsen encephalopathy). The relative efficacies and clinical benefits of the newer agents (DMSA or DMPS) as monotherapy in this setting have not been definitively studied but case series suggest that the outcomes are similar and may be appropriate alternative regimens (see **References**).

Sources

Smelting and metal recycling
Atmospheric lead due to leaded petrol
Occupations and hobbies (e.g. soldering metal, lead galvanising and painting, jewellery, stained glass, radiator repairs, battery recycling, plumbing, injection moulding of plastics, sports shooting)
Lead paint used in housing prior to 1960s (tastes sweet and attractive to children)
Soil contamination – often idiopathic
Fishing sinkers
Antique toys painted with lead paint
Pottery glazes
Lead-containing alternative medications (e.g. Ayurvedic) available in many developing countries
Cosmetics (especially from the Indian subcontinent)
Retained bullet fragments

References

Agency for Toxic Substances and Disease Registry. Toxicological profile for Lead. ATSDR; 2020. Available at http://www.atsdr.cdc.gov/toxprofiles/tp13.pdf.

Arnold J, Morgan B. Management of lead encephalopathy with DMSA after exposure to lead-contaminated moonshine. Journal of Medical Toxicology 2015; 11:464–467.

Bradberry S, Vale A. Dimercaptosuccinic acid (succimer; DMSA) in inorganic lead poisoning. Clinical Toxicology 2009; 47:617–631.

Canfield RL, Henderson CR, Cory-Slechta DA et al. Intellectual impairment in children with blood lead concentrations below 10 microg per deciliter. New England Journal of Medicine 2003; 348(16):1517–1526.

Centers for Disease Control and Prevention (Atlanta) 2010. Centers for Disease Control and Prevention (Atlanta). Guidelines for the identification and management of lead exposure in pregnant and lactating women: CDC; 2010. Available at. https://www.cdc.gov/nceh/lead/publications/leadandpregnancy2010.pdf.

Dietrick KN, Ware JH, Salganik M et al. Effect of chelation therapy on neuropsychological and behavioural development of lead-exposed children after school entry. Pediatrics 2004; 114:19–26.

National Health and Medical Research Council (Canberra) 2016. National Health and Medical Research Council (Canberra). Managing individual exposure to lead in Australia – a guide for health professionals: NHMRC; 2016. Available at. www.nhmrc. gov.au/guidelines/publications/eh58.

Rogan WJ, Dietrich KN, Ware JH et al. The effect of chelation therapy with succimer on neuropsychological development in children exposed to lead. New England Journal of Medicine 2003; 44(19):1421–1426.

Thurtle N, Greig J, Cooney L et al. Description of 3,180 courses of chelation with dimercaptosuccinic acid in children ≤5 y with severe lead poisoning in Zamfara, Northern Nigeria: a retrospective analysis of programme data. PLoS Med 2014; 11(10). doi:10.1371/journal.pmed.1001739 pmed.1001739.

3.47 LITHIUM: ACUTE OVERDOSE

See also Chapter 3.48: Lithium: Chronic poisoning.

Acute lithium overdose commonly causes early gastrointestinal effects – nausea, vomiting, abdominal pain and diarrhoea. The majority of acute overdoses will have a good outcome without significant neurotoxicity provided that adequate renal elimination of lithium is maintained.

RISK ASSESSMENT

- Acute ingestions up to 25 g of lithium, in the setting of normal renal function, are expected to cause predominantly gastrointestinal symptoms.
- Once lithium is absorbed from the gut, the blood–brain barrier slows entry into the CNS.
- Doses exceeding 25 g carry an increasing risk of neurotoxicity. In order to reduce this risk, it is imperative to optimise renal excretion of lithium.
- The presence of volume depletion or renal impairment will reduce urinary clearance of lithium, promoting distribution into the CNS from the vascular compartment.
- Patients with established neurotoxicity have a risk assessment similar to that of chronic lithium toxicity (see **Chapter 3.48: Lithium: Chronic poisoning**).
- **Children:** minor paediatric ingestions do not cause toxicity and do not require hospital assessment unless symptoms develop.

Toxic mechanism

Lithium is a monovalent cation primarily used in the management of bipolar disorder. Like other metal salts, lithium carbonate acts as a direct irritant to the GI tract. Once absorbed, lithium ions substitute for sodium and potassium ions and are thought to modulate intracellular second messengers. They may also affect neurotransmitter (including serotonin) production and release.

Toxicokinetics

Lithium carbonate is well absorbed orally, with peak serum levels occurring within 6 hours for immediate-release and up to 12 hours for slow-release preparations. Lithium is slowly distributed from the intravascular compartment to tissue compartments, most importantly the CNS, with a steady-state volume of distribution of 0.7–0.9 L/kg. Elimination is almost entirely by the kidney. Clearance is dependent on glomerular filtration and will be reduced if renal function is impaired. Elimination half-life is approximately 24 hours in a normal adult.

CLINICAL FEATURES
- Small acute overdoses are often asymptomatic.
- Following larger ingestions, symptoms of acute gastroenteritis occur early and significant fluid losses may occur.
- The most common neurological sign is tremor. Neurotoxicity rarely progresses beyond this provided adequate lithium excretion is maintained.
- Patients occasionally develop more significant neurotoxicity (see **Chapter 3.48: Lithium: Chronic poisoning** for description).

INVESTIGATIONS
Screening tests in deliberate self-poisoning
- 12-lead ECG, BGL and paracetamol level

Specific investigations
- EUC
  - Monitor electrolyte status and renal function.
- Serum lithium levels
  - Useful to confirm ingestion and, following larger overdoses, monitor progress and determine appropriateness for medical discharge.
  - Peak levels >5 mmol/L occurring 4–8 hours post ingestion are not unusual following acute overdose.

MANAGEMENT
Resuscitation, supportive care and monitoring
- Patients may present with hypovolaemia due to significant GI fluid losses. They require appropriate resuscitation with intravenous crystalloid solutions.
- It is imperative to optimise clearance of lithium by the administration of normal saline to maintain effective renal perfusion. Large volumes may be required to ensure volume repletion and adequate urinary output.
- Assess the patient's intravascular volume status frequently and correlate with the cadence of clinical features.
- Serum lithium levels must decrease rapidly (within 24–48 hours) to prevent progression of neurotoxicity.

Decontamination
- Activated charcoal does not adsorb lithium and is not indicated.

Enhanced elimination
- Haemodialysis will effectively remove lithium from the intravascular compartment; however, in the patient with normal renal function managed appropriately with intravenous fluids, this invasive intervention is seldom indicated for acute overdoses.
- Haemodialysis is warranted in patients with established renal failure or those with persistently elevated serum lithium levels and progressive neurotoxicity.

Antidotes
- None available.

DISPOSITION AND FOLLOW-UP
- Patients with no clinical evidence of neurotoxicity and a serum lithium level <1 mmol/L do not require further medical care or monitoring.

HANDY TIPS
- Patients on long-term lithium therapy are likely to develop nephrogenic diabetes insipidus. They may continue to produce large volumes of dilute urine even if intravascularly volume deplete, predisposing to the development of hypernatraemia.
- Patients on long-term lithium therapy do not have a significantly increased risk of developing severe neurotoxicity following an acute lithium overdose. The approach to management does not require modification.

PITFALL
- Underestimating the importance of appropriate intravenous fluid administration to promote renal excretion of lithium.

CONTROVERSIES
- Whole bowel irrigation has been advocated following overdose of sustained-release preparations. The additional outcome benefit of this intervention is unproven.
- The threshold serum lithium level for initiating haemodialysis is undefined. Recent references suggest an acute level >5 mmol/L. However, a good clinical outcome can be expected without haemodialysis if the level decreases to <1 mmol/L within 24–48 hours.
- A nomogram derived from a retrospective case series predicts the likelihood of the serum lithium level falling below 1 mmol/L within 36 hours. The combination of serum lithium concentration and eGFR is suggested as an indication for haemodialysis (see Buckley et al. in **References**). However, the nomogram calculation is one component of the multi-factorial clinical decision to institute invasive therapeutic modalities.

Presentations
Lithium carbonate 250 mg standard-release tablets (200)
Lithium carbonate 450 mg slow-release tablets (100)

References
Baird-Gunning J, Lea-Henry T, Hoegberg LCG et al. Lithium poisoning. Journal of Intensive Care Medicine 2017; 32(4):249–263.

Buckley NA, Cheng S, Isoardi K et al. Haemodialysis for lithium poisoning: translating EXTRIP recommendations into practical guidelines. British Journal of Clinical Pharmacology 2020; 86:999–1006.

Decker BS, Goldfarb DS, Dargan PI et al. Extracorporeal treatment for lithium poisoning: systematic review and recommendations from the EXTRIP workgroup. Clinical Journal of the American Society of Nephrology 2015; 10(5):875–887.

Waring WS. Management of lithium toxicity. Toxicology Reviews 2006; 25(4):221–230.

See also Chapter 3.46: Lithium: Acute overdose.

Chronic lithium toxicity differs from acute overdose in that neurological features are more prominent as equilibration between serum and CNS levels of lithium has occurred. Neurotoxicity develops in patients on lithium therapy when renal lithium excretion is impaired for any reason.

RISK ASSESSMENT

- Consider lithium toxicity in any patient on lithium therapy who presents with neurological signs or symptoms.
- Significant coma or seizure activity is an indication of severe toxicity that carries a risk of permanent neurological sequelae.
- Serum lithium levels may not be markedly elevated even in the presence of significant neurotoxicity because there has been sufficient time for lithium to cross the blood–brain barrier and accumulate in the CNS.
- The severity of toxicity is determined by the degree and duration of elevated lithium levels in the CNS.

Toxic mechanism

Lithium ions substitute for sodium and potassium ions and are thought to modulate intracellular second messengers. They may also affect neurotransmitter (including serotonin) production and release. Prolonged therapeutic use is associated with other toxic effects – nephrogenic diabetes insipidus and the development of hypernatraemia, hypothyroidism, and hyperparathyroidism.

Toxicokinetics

Following therapeutic administration, lithium absorbed from the GI tract is slowly distributed from the intravascular compartment to tissue compartments, most importantly the CNS. The steady-state volume of distribution is 0.7–0.9 L/kg and elimination is almost entirely by the kidney. Clearance is dependent on glomerular filtration and will be reduced if renal function is impaired. Elimination half-life is approximately 24 hours in a normal adult.

CLINICAL FEATURES

- The clinical features are principally neurological. There is a spectrum of clinical manifestations ranging from tremor, myoclonus, hyperreflexia and ataxia to altered mental state with confusion, sedation, seizures and coma.
- Gastrointestinal symptoms are not a prominent feature of chronic lithium toxicity.
- The clinical presentation may be complicated by features of the underlying precipitating illness.
- Nephrogenic diabetes insipidus is associated with long-term lithium therapy. Patients may continue to produce large volumes of dilute urine even when intravascularly volume depleted, worsening renal function and leading to hypernatraemia.

INVESTIGATIONS
Specific investigations
- Serum lithium levels
  - Confirm toxicity and monitor progress in response to management.

- EUC
  - Monitor electrolyte status and renal function.
- Thyroid function tests, serum calcium
  - Exclude associated toxicity.

Resuscitation, supportive care and monitoring
- Acute resuscitation is unlikely to be necessary except in cases of severe neurotoxicity with coma and seizures.
- Volume resuscitation may be required to adequately restore and maintain effective renal perfusion.
- It is imperative to optimise clearance of lithium by the administration of normal saline to maintain effective renal perfusion. This may not be achievable in the setting of established renal failure or pre-existing cardiovascular disease.
- Cease lithium and any drugs that impair lithium excretion (e.g. non-steroidal anti-inflammatories, angiotensin-converting enzyme inhibitors and diuretics).
- Ongoing management is guided by frequent re-assessment of clinical status, renal function and monitoring of lithium levels and electrolytes.

Decontamination
- No role in chronic toxicity.

Enhanced elimination
- Haemodialysis will effectively remove lithium from the intravascular compartment. The threshold serum level mandating haemodialysis is not fixed.
  - It is warranted in patients presenting with severe neurotoxicity, established renal failure or those who do not respond adequately to initial intravenous fluid management.

Antidotes
- None available.

DISPOSITION AND FOLLOW-UP
- Patients with significant lithium toxicity require prolonged admission to ensure effective management and treatment of any intercurrent precipitating illness.
- Resolution of neurological symptoms may be very slow (weeks) and persistent neurological deficits (particularly cerebellar or cognitive) may occur.

HANDY TIPS
- Nephrogenic diabetes insipidus is a result of lithium-induced unresponsiveness of the renal tubules to antidiuretic hormone. This decreases the patient's ability to concentrate urine and promotes free water loss.
- Patients may depend on the daily ingestion of large volumes of fluids to maintain electrolyte and volume homeostasis, and if their habitual oral intake is reduced, they may become significantly dehydrated.

- Delay in recovery from lithium neurotoxicity is due to slow redistribution and clearance of lithium from the CNS.

PITFALL
- Disregarding a normal or minimally elevated serum lithium level in the presence of neurological features consistent with lithium toxicity.

CONTROVERSIES
- A nomogram derived from a retrospective case series predicts the likelihood of the serum lithium level falling below 1 mmol/L within 36 hours. The combination of serum lithium concentration and eGFR is suggested as an indication for haemodialysis (see Buckley et al. in **References**). However, the nomogram calculation is one component of the multi-factorial clinical decision to institute invasive therapeutic modalities.
- The effect of haemodialysis on outcome has not been evaluated in controlled trials. Intermittent haemodialysis will provide most rapid clearance from the intravascular compartment but continuous modalities are more readily available and may minimise osmotic and electrolyte shifts.

Presentations
Lithium carbonate 250 mg standard-release tablets (200)
Lithium carbonate 450 mg slow-release tablets (100)

References
Baird-Gunning J, Lea-Henry T, Hoegberg LCG et al. Lithium poisoning. Journal of Intensive Care Medicine 2017; 32(4):249–263.

Buckley NA, Cheng S, Isoardi K et al. Haemodialysis for lithium poisoning: translating EXTRIP recommendations into practical guidelines. British Journal of Clinical Pharmacology 2020; 86(5):999–1006.

Decker BS, Goldfarb DS, Dargan PI et al. Extracorporeal treatment for lithium poisoning: systematic review and recommendations from the EXTRIP workgroup. Clinical Journal of the American Society of Nephrology 2015; 10(5):875–887.

Hansen HE, Amdisen A. Lithium intoxication. Quarterly Journal of Medicine 1978; 47:123–144.

Oakley P, Whyte IM, Carter GL. Lithium toxicity: an iatrogenic problem in susceptible individuals. Australian and New Zealand Journal of Psychiatry 2001; 35:833–840.

Waring WS. Management of lithium toxicity. Toxicology Reviews 2006; 25(4):221–230.

3.49 LOCAL ANAESTHETIC AGENTS

Amethocaine, Articaine, Benzocaine, Bupivacaine, Levobupivacaine, Lidocaine, Mepivacaine, Prilocaine, Ropivacaine

Local anaesthetic systemic toxicity (LAST) usually occurs due to inadvertent intravascular administration or excessive dosing. Significant CNS and cardiovascular toxicity (seizures, hypotension and ventricular dysrhythmias) can occur and require immediate resuscitation. Intravenous lipid emulsion is indicated for the management of severe cases.

- The clinical manifestations of LAST correspond to the peak concentration in the systemic circulation.
- Toxicity typically occurs rapidly after injection of local anaesthetic (LA), but the onset can be delayed greater than 60 minutes or occur even later in the setting of anaesthetic infusions.
- Patients at the extremes of age (infants, elderly) are most susceptible to the development of LAST.
- Maximum recommended doses for selected agents are listed in **Table 3.49.1** but toxicity can occur when lower doses are delivered by intravascular injection or by enhanced absorption through mucous membrane surfaces. Larger doses can safely be given when co-administered with adrenaline.
- Methaemoglobinaemia is not dose-related and is more likely to occur following administration of benzocaine, lidocaine or prilocaine.
- **Children:** accidental ingestion of lidocaine-containing teething gels or other topical preparations is unlikely to cause toxicity due to poor oral bioavailability. Hospital assessment is not required unless >6 mg/kg may have been ingested or symptoms develop. Children are more likely than adults to develop methaemoglobinaemia after LA administration, including topical administration.

Toxic mechanism

LAs bind reversibly to the intracellular domain of open voltage-gated sodium channels in neural and cardiac tissue. Once bound, they maintain the sodium channel in the inactivated state, inhibiting sodium influx and the propagation of action potentials. Additional toxic effects may include blockade of potassium and calcium channels, inhibition of intracellular metabolic pathways and methaemoglobinaemia.

Toxicokinetics

Amide LAs are the agents most commonly used in clinical practice. Systemic toxic effects correspond to peak concentrations achieved in the systemic circulation. Toxicity is rare following ingestion because of extensive first-pass metabolism. Some preparations contain adrenaline to cause local vasoconstriction, delaying absorption of the LA and prolonging the duration of anaesthesia. The amide LAs have small volumes of distribution and most are eliminated by hepatic metabolism. Accumulation can occur in the presence of hepatic dysfunction or reduced hepatic blood flow. Bupivacaine and ropivacaine have the longest elimination half-lives. Ester LAs such as benzocaine, procaine and tetracaine have short half-lives due to rapid hydrolysis by plasma cholinesterases.

TABLE 3.49.1 Maximum dose of selected local anaesthetic agents (without adrenaline)	
Local anaesthetic	**Maximum dose (mg/kg)**
Bupivacaine	2.5
Lignocaine	5
Mepivacaine	5
Prilocaine	7
Ropivacaine	3

CLINICAL FEATURES

- Earliest symptoms of LA toxicity are neurological and include anxiety, confusion, perioral paraesthesias, tinnitus or dizziness.
- More severe toxicity is characterised by:
  - CNS effects – seizures, coma
  - cardiovascular effects – bradycardia, hypotension, ventricular dysrhythmias and asystole.
- CNS toxicity normally occurs before cardiovascular toxicity, except following massive intravenous overdose where cardiac arrest may be the first clinical manifestation.
- Bupivacaine is particularly cardiotoxic due to prolonged binding to myocardial tissue.
- Methaemoglobinaemia presents with blue discolouration of the mucous membranes, progressing to CNS and cardiovascular manifestations of cellular hypoxia, resulting in death as methaemoglobin concentrations rise above 70%.

INVESTIGATIONS

Specific investigations

- EUC, venous blood gas, methaemoglobin concentration
- Serial ECGs
  - Sodium channel blockade (prolongation of PR and QRS intervals, large terminal R wave in aVR).

MANAGEMENT

Resuscitation, supportive care and monitoring

- Attention to airway, breathing and circulation are paramount. These priorities are managed along conventional lines, as outlined in **Chapter 1.2: Resuscitation**. Immediate intubation and hyperventilation to correct respiratory and metabolic acidosis is indicated in the presence of seizures, coma or haemodynamic instability.
- Intravenous lipid emulsion (Intralipid) is indicated for significant CNS or cardiovascular toxicity. The initial dose is 1–1.5 mL/kg IV of 20% intralipid (see **Chapter 4.15: Intravenous lipid emulsion**).
- Ventricular dysrhythmias can be treated with sodium bicarbonate 100 mEq (1 mEq/kg in children) IV repeated every 1–2 minutes until restoration of perfusing rhythm (see **Chapter 4.24: Sodium bicarbonate**).
- Seizures are treated with benzodiazepines, as described in **Chapter 2.3: Seizures**.
- Hypotension is treated with administration of intravenous crystalloid 10–20 mL/kg followed by inotropic support as necessary.

Decontamination

- Not indicated.

Enhanced elimination

- Not clinically useful.

Antidotes
- Intravenous lipid emulsion is indicated in severe CNS or cardiovascular toxicity. For full details on mechanism of action, dosing and administration, see **Chapter 4.15: Intravenous lipid emulsion**.
- Sodium bicarbonate for ventricular dysrhythmias secondary to sodium channel blockade as described above.
- Methylene blue is the specific antidote for methaemoglobinaemia and is administered to all symptomatic patients. For details on administration, see **Chapter 4.16: Methylene blue**.

DISPOSITION AND FOLLOW-UP
- Children who ingest >6 mg/kg of lidocaine-containing anaesthetic preparations would be expected to develop symptoms within 2 hours. If they are clinically well after this, further medical observation is not required.
- LA toxicity usually occurs in a hospital or clinic setting. Once resuscitated, the patient should be managed in an intensive care setting until toxicity resolves.

HANDY TIP
- The development of any neurological symptoms during or shortly after administration of a LA prompts close observation in an area equipped for cardiorespiratory monitoring and resuscitation.

CONTROVERSIES
- The threshold indications for administration of intravenous lipid emulsion in the management of CNS or cardiovascular manifestations of LA toxicity. Supporting data is derived from case reports and animal studies, but it is considered the recommended antidotal therapy in this clinical scenario.
- Cardiovascular and CNS toxicity is mediated by sodium channel blockade and will likely respond to prompt intubation, hyperventilation to correct respiratory or metabolic acidosis and titrated administration of sodium bicarbonate.

References
Balit CR, Lynch AM, Gilmore SP et al. Lignocaine and chlorhexidine toxicity in children resulting from mouthpaint ingestion: a bottling problem. Journal of Paediatrics and Child Health 2006; 42(6):350–353.

Curtis LA, Dolan TS, Seibert HE. Are one or two dangerous? Lidocaine and topical anesthetics exposure in children. Journal of Emergency Medicine 2009; 37:32–39.

Felice KL, Schumann HM. Intravenous lipid emulsion for local anesthetic toxicity: a review of the literature. Journal of Medical Toxicology 2008; 4(3):184–191.

Weinberg G. Lipid rescue resuscitation from local anaesthetic cardiac toxicity. Toxicological Reviews 2006; 25(3):139–145.

3.50 MERCURY

Elemental mercury, Inorganic mercury, Organic mercury, Merbromin

Mercury poisoning is rare, but occupational and environmental exposures or deliberate self-poisoning may cause serious clinical features. Patterns

of toxicity differ according to the dosage, degree of exposure and the physical or chemical state – elemental, inorganic or organic.

RISK ASSESSMENT

- Liquid elemental mercury is insoluble in water or organic solvents and is not significantly absorbed by the oral or cutaneous routes. Accidental ingestion of a small volume (e.g. from a broken thermometer bulb) does not cause toxicity.
- Inhalation of mercury vapour (heating of elemental mercury) or aerosol (after vacuuming) can result in severe pneumonitis and neurological injury.
- Inorganic mercury salts exist in either mercury(I) or mercury(II) oxidation states:
  - Mercury(I) chloride is insoluble in water and lipid and has low toxicity following oral ingestion.
  - Mercury(II) chloride is soluble in water and organic solvents and is toxic following ingestion, resulting in haemorrhagic gastroenteritis, acute renal failure and shock. The potential lethal dose of mercury(II) chloride is 30–50 mg/kg.
- Organic mercury compounds always exist in the mercury(II) state and have variable toxicity:
  - The laboratory reagent 'methylmercury' refers to dimethylmercury (CH_3HgCH_3), a compound with high lipid solubility that is rapidly absorbed through intact skin or latex gloves and is highly toxic.
  - Methylmercury found in fish or seafood refers to the methylmercury ion (CH_3Hg^+) which is ingested primarily as sulfhydryl compounds and has relatively low toxicity. Clinical effects can occur from bioaccumulation due to localised industrial water pollution or frequent ingestion of mercury-containing species (e.g. shark, swordfish).
- Injection of liquid mercury results in subcutaneous or pulmonary vascular deposition which can persist as insoluble, relatively inert droplets for many years.
- Dental amalgams containing mercury release vapour during chewing that can be inhaled and enter the bloodstream. The inhaled dose is generally negligible and not associated with clinical effects.
- The mercury component of some vaccines (the preservative thimerosal) is not considered a significant health risk.
- Merbromin (mercurochrome, a topical antiseptic) is poorly absorbed through intact skin, but mucosal absorption or intentional ingestion can result in elevated mercury levels. However, significant toxicity is unlikely as the compound is relatively stable and renal excretion is rapid.
- **Pregnancy:** mercury readily crosses the placenta and enters the fetal brain, potentially causing significant neurological injury.
- **Children:** minor unintentional ingestion or skin exposure to elemental mercury or mercurochrome antiseptic solution does not warrant medical assessment, observation or investigation.

Toxic mechanism

Mercury is a metal with no natural cellular function. It binds to sulfhydryl (–SH) groups at multiple sites, inhibiting protein synthesis and enzyme function and causing injury to cellular membranes, transport mechanisms and intracellular organelles.

Toxicokinetics

There is minimal absorption of **elemental** mercury from an intact gastrointestinal tract. In contrast, elemental mercury is well absorbed from the respiratory tract when inhaled as either an aerosol (produced when it is vacuumed) or vapour (when heated). Elemental mercury readily crosses the blood–brain barrier, where it is oxidised by the enzyme catalase to the mercury(II) state, resulting in toxicity to the cerebral and cerebellar cortices.

Ingested **inorganic** mercury salts mostly remain bound to mucosal surfaces and intestinal contents, and only 10% of the dose is absorbed, more readily in the mercury(II) state.

Organic mercury compounds are better absorbed orally (up to 90% for methylmercury) and freely enter the CNS. Slow dissociation of the covalent bond releases mercury(II) ions, which are responsible for the delayed and progressive toxic effects on neural tissue.

Dermal absorption of inorganic and organic mercury species is highly variable and difficult to quantify. Once absorbed, mercury in any form is initially bound to sulfhydryl groups (cysteine) in erythrocytes or carried in the plasma and rapidly distributed throughout the body to all tissues. The higher lipid solubility of elemental and organic mercury favours distribution to the CNS, whereas inorganic mercury does not readily cross the blood–brain barrier and is sequestered in the kidneys bound to cysteine-containing proteins such as metallothionein. Elemental and inorganic mercury are excreted primarily by the kidney and across the GI tract into the faeces, with a half-life around 40 days. Organic mercury has little renal excretion and is eliminated primarily in the faeces (including enterohepatic circulation), with a half-life of up to 70 days.

CLINICAL FEATURES

- **Acute exposure to elemental mercury** – acute intoxication develops following inhalational exposure to vapour or aerosolised mercury. Within a few hours, there is the abrupt onset of dyspnoea, cough, fever, metallic taste, headache and visual disturbances. Respiratory failure secondary to interstitial pneumonitis may occur over the following days.
- **Acute exposure to inorganic mercury** – acute ingestion may cause severe haemorrhagic gastroenteritis within hours, with oropharyngeal or abdominal pain, metallic taste, nausea, vomiting and diarrhoea. Grey discolouration of the mucous membranes may be noted. Hypotension, shock and renal failure can occur.
- **Exposure to organic mercury** – acute manifestations include gastrointestinal symptoms and dermatitis, but neurotoxicity is the most significant feature. This may develop weeks or months after initial exposure and is usually permanent. Severe neurodevelopmental and cognitive deficits can occur following prenatal exposure. Organic mercury is excreted in breast milk and can produce toxicity in infants. Neurological sequelae include:
  — Neuropsychiatric: poor concentration, memory loss, constriction of visual fields, emotional lability, depression, seizures, coma
  — Cerebellar: ataxia, incoordination and dysdiadochokinesis
  — Sensorimotor: tremor, spasticity, weakness, paralysis, peripheral paraesthesias, scanning speech and dysarthria.
- **Chronic mercury toxicity** – chronic low-level exposure to elemental mercury vapour or inorganic mercury leads to the insidious onset of a multi-system disorder. CNS accumulation related to prolonged exposure and slow elimination results in prominent neuropsychiatric symptoms:
  — Neurological: tremor, fatigue, headaches, decreased concentration, erethism (blushing and intense shyness), emotional lability, insomnia, delirium, mixed sensorimotor neuropathy, ataxia, tunnel vision, anosmia

- Gastrointestinal: metallic taste, burning pain in the mouth, gingivostomatitis, loose teeth, nausea, hypersalivation
- Renal dysfunction: proximal tubular atrophy, membranous nephropathy
- Acrodynia (usually children) – erythematous, oedematous, hyperkeratotic indurated rash of the palms, soles and face. It often progresses to desquamation and ulceration.

INVESTIGATIONS

Screening tests in deliberate self-poisoning
- 12-lead ECG, BGL and paracetamol level

Specific investigations
- Mercury concentrations in blood or urine may not correlate well with clinical features, depending on the time between exposure and sample collection. Whole blood levels become less reliable following tissue redistribution and 24-hour urine collections may provide more useful information.
- **Whole blood mercury level** (normal <20 microgram/L (100 nmol/L))
  - Reflects recent exposure and is expected to be elevated in a patient with acute toxicity.
  - Level >200 microgram/L (1000 nmol/L) is associated with symptoms.
- **24-hour urine mercury level** (normal <10 microgram/L (50 nmol/L))
  - More reliable indicator of chronic or low-level exposure to elemental or inorganic mercury.
  - Limited use following organic mercury exposure as most is faecally excreted.
  - Level >100 microgram/L (500 nmol/L) is associated with neuropsychiatric features.
  - Useful in assessing response to chelation therapy.
- Note: Hair analysis is unreliable as it does not reflect body burden and should not be used for diagnostic or management purposes.
- X-rays
  - Elemental mercury is radio-opaque and X-rays confirm ingestion, subcutaneous or intravenous injection.
  - Intravenous injection produces multiple mercuric pulmonary emboli and a characteristic 'milky way' appearance on chest X-ray.
- Endoscopy
  - May be indicated to assess corrosive GI injury.

MANAGEMENT

Resuscitation, supportive care and monitoring
- Accidental oral or skin exposure to elemental mercury does not require medical assessment or management.
- Following other acute exposure, attention to airway, breathing and circulation are paramount. These priorities are managed along conventional lines, as outlined in **Chapter 1.2: Resuscitation**.
- Inhalational exposure to mercury vapour requires close clinical and physiological monitoring and general supportive care

measures, as outlined in **Chapter 1.4: Supportive care and monitoring**.

- Ingestion of inorganic mercury requires appropriate fluid resuscitation and general supportive care measures.
- Exposure to organic mercury requires general supportive care measures, as outlined in **Chapter 1.4: Supportive care and monitoring**.
- The decision to administer chelation therapy may be based on the history of exposure and clinical features prior to confirmatory levels being obtained (see **Antidotes**).

Decontamination

The primary aim of decontamination is to prevent further exposure to mercury.

- Environmental
  - Seek advice from local authorities regarding clean-up and disposal of mercury spills.
  - Cardboard, adhesive tape or eye droppers can be used to clean-up liquid mercury spills.
  - Avoid vacuuming.
  - Discard contaminated carpets or coverings in double wrapped bags in hazardous waste facility.
  - Mercury decontamination kits contain calcium polysulfide which forms insoluble mercuric sulfide.
  - Specific scenarios
    - Elemental mercury
      - Remove contaminated clothing.
      - Remove mercury from skin (soap, water).
      - Surgical excision of subcutaneous mercury deposits following SC injection where feasible.
    - Inorganic
      - Administer activated charcoal if feasible (inorganic mercuric salts are substantially adsorbed to charcoal).
    - Organic
      - Although the benefit is unknown, administer activated charcoal to cooperative patients with 2 hours of ingestion.

Enhanced elimination

- N-acetylcysteine enhances the renal clearance of mercury, particularly if started early after exposure. Although there are limited published outcome data, the theoretical benefit and low adverse effects of this agent justify its use at the same dosing regimen as for paracetamol toxicity.
- Administration of oral polythiol resin (if available) may interrupt enterohepatic circulation of organic mercury compounds.

Antidotes

- Chelation therapy is indicated when there is a history of exposure to mercury and objective clinical features of intoxication or where markedly elevated blood or urine mercury levels indicate potential for significant morbidity.
- Case studies suggest clinical benefit from increased renal clearance of mercury in symptomatic patients. However,

established neurotoxicity may not improve, particularly that caused by organic mercury.

- Chelation is only useful once ongoing exposure to mercury is removed.
- DMSA, DMPS or dimercaprol (BAL) are the recommended agents for elemental and inorganic mercury poisoning. Oral therapy with DMSA is the preferred option in most settings (see **Chapter 4.7: DMSA (succimer) and DMPS (unithiol)** and **Chapter 4.6: Dimercaprol**).
- Note: Dimercaprol is supposedly contraindicated following organic mercury exposure due to concern that it increases distribution of mercury to the brain. There is limited evidence to support this, but DMSA or DMPS are preferred agents in this setting.

DISPOSITION AND FOLLOW-UP

- Patients exposed to mercury vapour or aerosol are counselled regarding appropriate measures to cease exposure and clean up remaining environmental contamination.
- Symptomatic patients require admission for further management.
- Patients with potential ingestion of inorganic or organic mercury require admission for observation and appropriate management should clinical features develop.

HANDY TIPS

- Intentional ingestion of a large volume of elemental mercury poses significant logistical issues. Prolonged exposure and transit through the gut may result in oxidation to the absorbable divalent form or vaporisation of elemental mercury. Attempts at gastrointestinal decontamination with laxatives or whole-bowel irrigation are warranted, with radiological confirmation of improvement in gastrointestinal load. Mercurial waste must be disposed of safely.
- DMPS is formulated as an intravenous preparation but has also been given orally (at a higher dose due to decreased oral bioavailability).

PITFALL

- Ordering 'heavy metal screens' on patients with non-specific symptoms without exposure assessment – these are rarely clinically useful.

CONTROVERSIES

- The benefits of chelation in patients following inhalational exposure to mercury. A small case series documents increased urinary mercury excretion following the use of DMPS in this setting, but there are no data showing improvement in neurological outcomes.
- The benefits of chelation therapy in established neurotoxicity, particularly from organic mercury poisoning. DMSA or DMPS can increase urinary excretion of mercury, but this may in part reflect mobilisation of existing renal mercury deposits and not removal of charged mercury(II) ions retained in the CNS. Chelation may not alter prognosis or outcome, particularly when initiation is delayed.

- The value of chelation therapy following IV or subcutaneous injection of mercury where excision of mercurial deposits is not feasible. Liberation of toxic mercury(II) ions from these depots is slow and clinical toxicity may not occur.
- The literature does not support the routine replacement of mercury dental amalgams.

Sources

Elemental mercury (Hg^0): dental amalgam, thermometers, barometers, manufacture of chlorine and caustic soda, paints, pigments and gold mining

Inorganic mercury (mercuric acetate, mercuric arsenate, mercuric bromide, mercuric chloride, mercuric potassium cyanide, mercuric sulfide): disinfectants, fireworks and explosives, processing of fur and leather, waterproofing and antifouling paints, photographic plates, batteries, alternative medications (e.g. Ayurvedic) or cosmetics available in many developing countries

Organic mercury (alkoxyalkyl mercury, alkyl mercury, methyl mercury): embalming fluid, fungicides, pesticides, wood preservatives, seafood

Merbromin

References

Bernhoft RA. Mercury toxicity and treatment: a review of the literature. Journal of Environmental and Public Health 2012; 2012:460508. doi:10.1155/2012/460508.

Brownawall AM, Berent S, Brent RL et al. The potential adverse effects of dental amalgam. Toxicological Reviews 2005; 24(1):1–10.

Clarkson TW, Magos L. The toxicology of mercury and its chemical compounds. Critical Reviews in Toxicology 2006; 36(8):609–662.

Clarkson TW, Magos L, Myers GJ. The toxicology of mercury: current exposures and clinical manifestations. New England Journal of Medicine 2003; 349:1731–1737.

Kales SN, Goldman RH. Mercury exposure: current concepts, controversies, and a clinic's experience. Journal of Occupational and Environmental Medicine 2002; 44:143–154.

Kosnett MJ. The role of chelation in the treatment of arsenic and mercury poisoning. Journal of Medical Toxicology 2013; 9:347–354.

Nierenberg DW, Nordgren RE, Chang MB et al. Delayed cerebellar disease and death after accidental exposure to dimethylmercury. New England Journal of Medicine 1998; 338(23):1672–1676.

Nuttall KL. Interpreting mercury in blood and urine of individual patients. Annals of Clinical and Laboratory Science 2004; 34(3):235–250.

3.51 METFORMIN

Metformin can cause life-threatening lactic acidosis. This may occur in patients on therapeutic doses who develop renal failure or intercurrent illness, or following large acute ingestions. Early recognition and haemodialysis are life-saving.

RISK ASSESSMENT

- Metformin-associated lactic acidosis (MALA) in a patient on therapeutic metformin usually occurs in the context of acute renal failure or intercurrent illness and carries a significant mortality risk.
- Acute metformin overdose is usually benign, but severe lactic acidosis can occur and is more likely in the presence of renal dysfunction from any cause. The threshold dose of concern is not clearly defined but is thought to be >10 g.

- The prognosis for severe lactic acidosis from metformin toxicity is improved is there is early recognition and appropriate institution of haemodialysis.
- Metformin overdose is not expected to cause significant hypoglycaemia as a direct effect.
- **Children:** accidental paediatric ingestion of up to 2 tablets does not cause significant toxicity and hospital assessment is not required.

Toxic mechanism

Metformin inhibits hepatic gluconeogenesis and stimulates peripheral glucose uptake by potentiating insulin effect. In overdose or toxic accumulation, metformin has inhibitory effects on mitochondrial pathways leading to both increased production and decreased metabolism of lactate.

Toxicokinetics

Metformin is rapidly absorbed following oral administration, with peak levels occurring at 2 hours for immediate-release and 6–8 hours for extended-release preparations. It is not metabolised to any significant extent and elimination is entirely dependent on renal excretion.

CLINICAL FEATURES

- Acute metformin overdose is usually asymptomatic.
- The development of significant lactic acidosis will result in clinical features such as nausea, vomiting, dyspnoea, tachycardia, hypotension and confusion.
- Lactic acidosis may progress to coma, shock and death.

INVESTIGATIONS

Screening tests in deliberate self-poisoning
- 12-lead ECG, BGL and paracetamol level

Specific investigations
- EUC, venous blood gas and serum lactate
  - Confirm diagnosis of lactic acidosis and monitor progress.

MANAGEMENT

Resuscitation, supportive care and monitoring
- Attention to airway, breathing and circulation are paramount. These priorities are managed along conventional lines, as outlined in **Chapter 1.2: Resuscitation**.
- General supportive care measures, as outlined in **Chapter 1.4: Supportive care and monitoring** ensure a good outcome in the majority of patients.
- It is essential to optimise volume status and renal perfusion by appropriate administration of intravenous fluids.
- Administration of sodium bicarbonate may have beneficial effects as a temporising measure in patients with severe metabolic acidosis awaiting haemodialysis (see **Chapter 4.24: Sodium bicarbonate**).

Decontamination
- Administer oral activated charcoal to the cooperative patient who presents within 2 hours of deliberately self-poisoning with >10 g of metformin.

Enhanced elimination
- Haemodialysis rapidly corrects acidosis and also removes metformin, thereby preventing further lactate accumulation. It is urgently indicated in:
  - any patient with significant lactic acidosis from therapeutic administration
  - acute overdose with progressive lactic acidosis and worsening clinical features.
- Haemodialysis may need to be prolonged to maintain resolution of the acid–base disturbance and clear metformin effectively.

Antidotes
- None available.

DISPOSITION AND FOLLOW-UP
- Deliberate self-poisoning with >10 g of metformin mandates observation for at least 8 hours. Patients who remain clinically well with a normal serum lactate (or stable serum bicarbonate as a surrogate marker) are fit for medical discharge.
- Patients at risk of developing lactic acidosis should have ready access to haemodialysis in the event of clinical or biochemical deterioration.

HANDY TIP
- Consider the diagnosis of metformin-associated lactic acidosis in any unwell patient with access to metformin.

PITFALLS
- Treating metformin overdose as a sulfonylurea overdose – they are both antidiabetic medications but belong to different classes and have different toxicities and risk assessments.
- Failure to consider the diagnosis of metformin-associated lactic acidosis.

CONTROVERSIES
- Precise indications for initiating haemodialysis in metformin-associated lactic acidosis following overdose. It may be reasonable to tolerate serum lactate levels up to 10 mmol/L provided the patient remains clinically well with normal renal function and no significant acidosis.
- Relative efficacies of various haemodialysis methods. If intermittent haemodialysis is not available, continuous modalities are acceptable, although clearance will be lower.

Presentations
Metformin hydrochloride 500 mg tablets (100)
Metformin hydrochloride 850 mg tablets (60)
Metformin hydrochloride 1000 mg tablets (90)
Metformin hydrochloride 500 mg controlled-release tablets (120)
Metformin hydrochloride 1000 mg controlled-release tablets (60)
Metformin hydrochloride 250 mg/glibenclamide 1.25 mg tablets (90)
Metformin hydrochloride 500 mg/glibenclamide 2.5 mg tablets (90)
Metformin hydrochloride 250 mg/glibenclamide 5 mg tablets (90)

References

Calello DP, Liu KD, Wiegand TJ et al. Extracorporeal treatment for metformin poisoning: systematic review and recommendations from the Extracorporeal Treatments in Poisoning Workgroup. Critical Care Medicine 2015; 43(8):1716–1730.

Seidowsky A, Nseir S, Houdret N et al. Metformin-associated lactic acidosis: a prognostic and therapeutic study. Critical Care Medicine 2009; 37(7):2191–2196.

Spiller HA, Weber JA, Winter ML et al. Multicenter case series of pediatric metformin ingestion. Annals of Pharmacotherapy 2000; 34:1385–1388.

3.52 METHOTREXATE

Methotrexate toxicity occurs most commonly in the setting of inadvertent supratherapeutic dosing. Intentional acute overdoses are less likely to cause significant toxicity. Folinic acid is used as an antidote in selected cases.

RISK ASSESSMENT

- Acute overdose
  - Toxicity is unlikely following most intentional acute ingestions, particularly for doses <500 mg (<5 mg/kg in children).
  - Doses >500 mg (>5 mg/kg in children) require further risk stratification. Timed methotrexate levels and assessment of renal function are useful to guide the requirement for antidotal therapy (see **Table 3.52.1**).
- Supratherapeutic ingestion
  - May cause potentially lethal bone marrow suppression.
  - Toxicity may develop if the weekly therapeutic oral dose is taken on as few as 3 consecutive days.
  - Patients with renal impairment are more susceptible to methotrexate-induced bone marrow suppression.
  - The serum methotrexate level is not useful in determining the risk of toxicity or requirement for antidotal therapy in this scenario because it does not reflect the active intracellular form of methotrexate.
- Intrathecal overdose
  - Potentially lethal.
- **Children:** toxicity is not reported after accidental ingestion but single ingestion >5 mg/kg warrants referral to hospital for assessment including a methotrexate level.

TABLE 3.52.1 Threshold methotrexate levels for antidotal therapy following acute ingestion

Time since ingestion (h)	Methotrexate level (micromol/L)
6	5
12	1
24	0.1

Toxic mechanism

Methotrexate is a structural analogue of folate. It acts by competitive inhibition of dihydrofolate reductase and thymidylate synthetase, resulting in decreased DNA and RNA synthesis, and hence decreased cell replication. Methotrexate toxicity primarily affects rapidly dividing cells (e.g. gastrointestinal tract, bone marrow). Renal and hepatic injuries are also noted.

Toxicokinetics

Methotrexate has variable absorption after oral ingestion and bioavailability decreases at higher ingested doses as active transporter proteins become saturated. Peak levels occur 1–2 hours post ingestion and the volume of distribution is small. Methotrexate is a weak acid and it is primarily excreted by the kidney unchanged or as a hepatic metabolite (7-hydroxymethotrexate). Elimination half-life increases with dose, accounting for the accumulation and severe toxicity seen with inadvertent daily dosing. In supratherapeutic toxicity, intracellular polyglutamated forms of methotrexate mediate prolonged anti-metabolite effects even after serum levels have declined.

CLINICAL FEATURES

- Most patients remain asymptomatic after acute ingestion.
- Following supratherapeutic ingestion, patients can present with clinical features and complications of multi-organ toxicity.
- Stomatitis is an early sign.
- Nausea, vomiting and diarrhoea are common.
- Haematological toxicity can affect any cell line with clinical features secondary to anaemia, neutropenia or thrombocytopenia.

INVESTIGATIONS

Screening tests in deliberate self-poisoning

- 12-lead ECG, BGL and paracetamol level

Specific investigations

- Methotrexate level and renal function
  - Following acute single overdose, a timed methotrexate level and renal function tests help determine the need for folinic acid therapy.
  - In supratherapeutic toxicity, the serum methotrexate level may be below the limit for detection and should not be relied upon to determine the requirement for folinic acid therapy.
- FBC, EUC, liver function tests

MANAGEMENT

Resuscitation, supportive care and monitoring

- Resuscitation is required only in the rare instances of patients with established methotrexate toxicity who present with volume depletion or sepsis.
- Attention to airway, breathing and circulation are paramount and managed along conventional lines, as outlined in **Chapter 1.2: Resuscitation**.
- Supportive care includes appropriate intravenous fluids to optimise renal excretion of methotrexate.

Acute overdose
- Ingestion <500 mg (<5 mg/kg in children)
  - Ensure adequate hydration.
  - Check renal function and assess methotrexate level 6 or more hours post ingestion.
- Ingestion >500 mg (>5 mg/kg in children)
  - Commence folinic acid.
  - Check renal function and assess methotrexate level 6 or more hours post ingestion.
- If renal function is normal and the serum methotrexate level is below thresholds for likely toxicity (see **Table 3.52.1**), further folinic acid is not indicated and the patient is fit for medical discharge if otherwise well. A follow-up FBC is recommended at 7 days.

Supratherapeutic ingestion or established methotrexate toxicity
- Commence folinic acid.
- Monitor clinical status and laboratory parameters.
- Granulocyte-colony-stimulating factor (GCSF) is indicated for bone marrow suppression with established neutropenia.

Decontamination
- Oral activated charcoal 50 g (1 g/kg in children) is indicated in cooperative patients who present within 2 hours of acute overdose of >500 mg (>5 mg/kg in children).
- Some authorities recommend decontamination with oral folinic acid 15 mg as a competitive antagonist for intestinal transporter absorption, rather than activated charcoal. This preparation may not be readily available in an acute overdose presentation.

Enhanced elimination
- Not clinically useful.
- Methotrexate and its metabolites may precipitate within the acidic environment of the renal tubule. Urinary alkalinisation may provide added benefit to standard intravenous fluids to limit crystal deposition within the nephron and optimise renal clearance (see **Chapter 4.24: Sodium bicarbonate** for further detail on administration).

Antidotes
- Folinic acid is indicated for patients if toxicity is present or predicted:
  - clinical features of methotrexate toxicity
  - renal impairment
  - ingested dose >500 mg (>5 mg/kg in children)
  - a methotrexate level cannot be obtained within 24 hours following acute overdose
  - the methotrexate level is above the threshold for likely toxicity following acute overdose.
- With toxicity from supratherapeutic dosing, therapy is continued until clear resolution of toxicity (especially bone marrow recovery) is documented. This may take several days.
- Refer to **Chapter 4.10: Folinic acid** for further detail on administration and therapeutic end points.

DISPOSITION AND FOLLOW-UP

- Most patients with acute oral overdose will not require ongoing antidotal therapy with folinic acid following biochemical assessment of renal function and methotrexate level. A follow-up FBC is recommended 7 days following discharge.
- Patients who require folinic acid but are clinically well with normal haematological and biochemical parameters may be treated as an outpatient. They require close supervision to complete antidotal therapy and monitor clinical and laboratory parameters.
- Patients with established methotrexate toxicity are admitted for supportive care, laboratory monitoring and folinic acid therapy. It may take several days for clinical and laboratory features to resolve.

HANDY TIPS

- Methotrexate levels are not available in all hospitals. A result can usually be obtained within 24 hours by sending blood (rather than the patient) elsewhere.
- If a methotrexate level is not readily available following acute overdose, empirical treatment with folinic acid is justified as a low-risk and potentially beneficial therapy.

PITFALLS

- Failure to recognise the potential lethality of supratherapeutic dosing.
- Administration of folic acid instead of folinic acid as an antidote.

CONTROVERSIES

- Risk assessment and management plans for acute methotrexate overdose have been extrapolated from experience with high-dose intravenous dosing and clinical outcomes from case series involving small numbers of acute ingestions.
- The threshold methotrexate levels for antidotal therapy in acute overdose detailed in **Table 3.52.1** are based on limited published evidence but remain useful to guide management decisions. Poor outcomes associated with acute overdose remain uncommon.
- Glucarpidase is a recombinant bacterial enzyme that cleaves methotrexate into inactive metabolites. It has a role as rescue therapy following high-dose intravenous methotrexate used to treat malignancies in patients with impaired renal function or following inadvertent intrathecal overdose. It has not been used in other settings to treat methotrexate toxicity.

Presentations

Methotrexate 2.5 mg tablets (30)
Methotrexate 10 mg tablets (15, 50)
Methotrexate 2.5 mg/mL injectable (2 mL)
Methotrexate 25 mg/mL injectable (2 mL, 20 mL)
Methotrexate 100 mg/mL injectable (10 mL, 50 mL)

References

Bebarta VS, Hensley MD, Borys DJ. Acute methotrexate ingestions in adults: a report of serious clinical effects and treatments. Journal of Toxicology 2014; 2014:214574.

Chan BS, Dawson AH, Buckley NA. What can clinicians learn from therapeutic studies about the treatment of acute oral methotrexate poisoning? Clinical Toxicology 2017; 55(2):88–96.

Isoardi KZ, Harris K, Carmichael KE et al. Acute bone marrow suppression and gastrointestinal toxicity following acute oral methotrexate overdose. Clinical Toxicology 2018; 56(12):1204–1206.

Lovecchio F, Katz K, Watts D et al. Four-year experience with methotrexate exposures. Journal of Medical Toxicology 2008; 4(3):149–150.

Ramsey LB, Balis FM, O'Brien MM et al. Consensus guideline for use of glucarpidase in patients with high-dose methotrexate induced acute kidney injury and delayed methotrexate clearance. The Oncologist 2018; 23(1):52-61. doi:10.1634/theoncologist.2017-0243.

3.53 MIRTAZAPINE

Deliberate self-poisoning with this tetracyclic antidepressant usually follows a benign course. Mild CNS depression and tachycardia are the most frequently reported clinical features. Care is supportive.

RISK ASSESSMENT

- Mirtazapine overdose causes relatively minor clinical effects, even after large ingestions.
- **Children:** accidental ingestion of mirtazapine is unlikely to cause significant effects. Referral to hospital is not required unless symptoms occur.

Toxic mechanism

Mirtazapine enhances release of noradrenaline and serotonin by antagonism at pre-synaptic α_2-adrenergic receptors. It is also an antagonist at serotonin (5-HT$_2$, 5-HT$_3$) and histamine (H$_1$) receptors.

Toxicokinetics

Mirtazapine is rapidly absorbed following oral ingestion, and peak plasma concentrations occur at 2 hours. It undergoes hepatic metabolism by cytochrome P450 and the elimination half-life is 20–40 hours.

CLINICAL FEATURES

- Most patients remain asymptomatic. If symptoms occur, onset is within the first 4 hours.
- Mild tachycardia, hypertension and sedation may occur particularly with larger ingestions.
- Cardiovascular and CNS effects are rarely significant enough to require specific interventions.

INVESTIGATIONS

Screening tests in deliberate self-poisoning

- 12-lead ECG, BGL and paracetamol level

MANAGEMENT

Resuscitation, supportive care and monitoring

- General supportive care measures are indicated, as outlined in **Chapter 1.4: Supportive care and monitoring**.

- Intubation for airway control is unlikely to be required.

Decontamination
- Activated charcoal is not indicated.

Enhanced elimination
- Not clinically useful.

Antidotes
- None available.

DISPOSITION AND FOLLOW-UP
- Patients who are clinically well 4 hours post ingestion are fit for medical discharge.
- Patients with sedation require observation until clinical features have resolved.

HANDY TIP
- Development of coma or seizures prompts consideration of alternative diagnoses and revision of the risk assessment.

Presentations
Mirtazapine 15 mg, 30 mg, 45 mg tablets (30)

References
Berling I, Isbister GK. Mirtazapine overdose is unlikely to cause major toxicity. Clinical Toxicology 2014; 52:20–24.
Waring WS, Good AM, Bateman DN. Lack of significant toxicity after mirtazapine overdose: a five-year review of cases admitted to a regional toxicology unit. Clinical Toxicology 2007; 45:45–50.

3.54 MONOAMINE OXIDASE INHIBITORS (MAOIs)

Irreversible non-selective: Phenelzine, Tranylcypromine
Irreversible selective: Selegiline
Reversible selective: Moclobemide

Irreversible non-selective MAOIs can cause severe serotonin toxicity in overdose. They are also associated with significant adverse reactions at therapeutic dosing, and a withdrawal syndrome is described. Reversible or selective agents are less toxic in overdose but can cause significant clinical effects, particularly in combination with other serotonergic agents or following large ingestions.

RISK ASSESSMENT
- Phenelzine and tranylcypromine are associated with dose-dependent, potentially lethal serotonin and sympathomimetic toxicity. Symptoms may be delayed in onset and are prolonged in duration.
- Overdose of moclobemide as a single agent usually causes only mild symptoms, even in large ingestions.
  - Mild serotonin toxicity occurs in <5%.
  - QT prolongation may occur with ingestions >3 g but torsades de pointes is not reported.

- Co-ingestion of moclobemide with other serotonergic agents is associated with a high risk of severe serotonin toxicity, irrespective of dose (see **Chapter 2.5: Serotonin toxicity**).
- Phenelzine and tranylcypromine are associated with dose-dependent, potentially lethal serotonin and sympathomimetic toxicity. Symptoms may be delayed in onset and are prolonged in duration.
  - Dose-related risk assessment for severe phenelzine and tranylcypromine:
    - >2 mg/kg associated with severe toxicity and fatalities.
- **Children:** any ingestion of phenelzine or tranylcypromine tablets requires assessment in hospital. Accidental ingestion of moclobemide alone is less likely to cause toxicity and referral to hospital is only required if symptoms develop.

Toxic mechanism
This class of drugs can selectively or non-selectively inhibit monoamine oxidase (MAO) A and B, in either a reversible or irreversible manner. MAO-A metabolises serotonin and noradrenaline, and MAO-B metabolises dopamine and phenylethylamine. Irreversible blockade requires the synthesis of new enzymes to re-establish MAO activity, meaning that serotonergic and sympathomimetic toxicity can persist for several days.

Toxicokinetics
All MAOIs are well absorbed after oral administration and reach peak levels within 2–3 hours. They undergo hepatic metabolism and are renally excreted.

CLINICAL FEATURES
- Phenelzine or tranylcypromine overdose
  - The onset of toxicity may be delayed several hours.
  - Serotonin toxicity is likely to be severe and prolonged (see **Chapter 2.5: Serotonin toxicity**).
  - Multi-organ dysfunction occurs in patients with severe toxicity.
- Moclobemide overdose (as single agent)
  - Minimal symptoms are expected.
  - Serotonin toxicity is rare.
  - QT prolongation may occur.
- Moclobemide overdose in combination with another serotonergic or sympathomimetic agent
  - Serotonin toxicity frequently develops within 6–12 hours (see **Chapter 2.5: Serotonin toxicity**).
- MAOI adverse reactions at therapeutic dosing
  - Drug–drug interactions (serotonergic or sympathomimetic agents).
  - Tyramine reaction: following ingestion of a tyramine-containing food (e.g. cheese, cured meats, wine), patients can develop an acute hypertensive crisis with end-organ damage.

INVESTIGATIONS
Screening tests in deliberate self-poisoning
- 12-lead ECG, BGL and paracetamol level

Specific investigations
- Serial ECGs (moclobemide)
  - A 12-lead ECG should be repeated 6 hours after ingestion to exclude significant QT prolongation.

Resuscitation, supportive care and monitoring
- Attention to airway, breathing and circulation is paramount (see **Chapter 1.2: Resuscitation**).
- Severe serotonergic or sympathomimetic toxicity require specific management as outlined in **Chapter 2.5: Serotonin toxicity** and **Chapter 3.7: Amphetamines and amphetamine-like substances**.
- Immediate life-threats are severe rigidity compromising ventilation, hyperthermia and altered mental status. Rapid sequence intubation, ventilation and neuromuscular paralysis are indicated for patients with established severe toxicity or if there is no immediate response to intravenous benzodiazepines and fluids.
- Intravenous benzodiazepines are the initial treatment of choice with paralysis.
- Hypertension and tachycardia are initially managed with titrated intravenous benzodiazepines. Severe or refractory hypertension (including tyramine reactions) may require parenteral vasodilator therapy. Caution is required as autonomic instability may rapidly produce hypotension. Options include:
  - titrated vasodilator infusion (glyceryl trinitrate, sodium nitroprusside)
  - labetalol 10–20 mg IV repeated every 10 minutes to a maximum of 300 mg (or as an infusion).
  - Note: Beta-blockers are theoretically contraindicated as unopposed α-adrenergic stimulation may cause severe vasoconstriction; however, there is limited evidence for adverse outcomes due to this effect.
- Seizures and agitated delirium are managed with benzodiazepines, as outlined in **Chapter 2.3: Seizures** and **Chapter 2.4: Approach to delirium**.
- Hyperthermia resulting from MAOI toxicity requires immediate therapy.
  - Temperature >38.5°C is an indication for continuous core-temperature monitoring, benzodiazepine sedation and fluid resuscitation.
  - Temperature >39.5°C requires rapid treatment to prevent multiple-organ failure and neurological injury. Paralysis, intubation, ventilation and active cooling are indicated.
- General supportive care measures are indicated, as outlined in **Chapter 1.4: Supportive care and monitoring**.
- A basic level of supportive care and monitoring is sufficient for pure moclobemide overdose.

Decontamination
- Moclobemide overdose has a good prognosis and decontamination is not indicated.
- Patients who are alert and cooperative and who have ingested >2 mg/kg of phenelzine or tranylcypromine are given 50 g oral activated charcoal if they present within 2 hours. Activated charcoal is contraindicated in the unintubated symptomatic patient due to the potential for rapid onset of seizures and coma.

Enhanced elimination
● Not clinically useful.

Antidotes
● Antidotal therapies for serotonin toxicity can be considered, as outlined in **Chapter 2.5: Serotonin toxicity**.

DISPOSITION AND FOLLOW-UP
● Patients who are clinically well without features of serotonin toxicity at 12 hours do not require further medical management. Discharge should not occur at night.
● Patients with moclobemide overdose are observed for 6 hours. If they remain clinically well at that stage, with a normal ECG, they do not require further medical management.

HANDY TIPS
● The toxic effects following overdose of an irreversible MAOI can persist for several days.
● Phentolamine 1–5 mg IV (repeated as necessary up to 15 mg) is an effective treatment for hypertension but it is not readily available.

PITFALLS
● Failure to appreciate the potential severity of phenelzine or tranylcypromine ingestions.
● Failure to observe a patient for a sufficient period of time following deliberate self-poisoning with phenelzine or tranylcypromine.

CONTROVERSY
● The role of specific serotonin antagonists (cyproheptadine, olanzapine) in the management of MAOI toxicity.

Presentations
Moclobemide 150 mg, 300 mg tablets (60)
Phenelzine sulfate 15 mg tablets (100)
Selegiline hydrochloride 5 mg tablets (100)
Tranylcypromine sulfate 10 mg tablets (50)

References
Downes MA, Whyte IM, Isbister GK. QTc abnormalities in deliberate self-poisoning with moclobemide. Internal Medicine Journal 2005; 35:388–391.
Isbister GK, Hackett LP, Dawson AH et al. Moclobemide poisoning: toxicokinetics and occurrence of serotonin toxicity. British Journal of Clinical Pharmacology 2003; 56(4):441–450.
Kaplan RF, Feinglass NG, Webster W. Phenelzine overdose treated with dantrolene sodium. Journal of the American Medical Association 1986; 255:642–644.
Mills KC. Monoamine oxidase inhibitor toxicity. Emergency Medicine 1993; 15:58–71.

3.55 NON-STEROIDAL ANTI-INFLAMMATORY DRUGS (NSAIDS)

Celecoxib, Diclofenac, Etoricoxib, Ibuprofen, Indomethacin, Ketoprofen, Ketorolac, Mefenamic Acid, Meloxicam, Naproxen, Parecoxib, Piroxicam, Sulindac, Tiaprofenic acid

Acute overdose of NSAIDs is generally benign. The exceptions are mefenamic acid or massive ingestions of the other agents. Medical interventions are not usually required.

RISK ASSESSMENT

- Dose-related risk assessment is best defined for ibuprofen but can be extrapolated to other agents (see **Table 3.55.1**).
- Massive overdose is associated with seizures and coma.
- Renal dysfunction and metabolic acidosis, if they occur, are transient and reversible.
- Overdose with any amount of mefenamic acid is associated with seizures.
- **Children:** significant symptoms usually are not observed until the dose ingested approaches 300 mg/kg of ibuprofen (or equivalent of other NSAID). Accidental ingestion of <100 mg/kg of ibuprofen does not require referral to hospital for assessment or observation. All mefenamic acid ingestions are referred to hospital because of the increased seizure risk.

Toxic mechanism

NSAIDs exert their pharmacological effects through the competitive inhibition of cyclooxygenase-1 and -2 and consequent blockade of prostaglandin synthesis. The NSAIDs are directly irritant to the gastrointestinal tract. Prostaglandin inhibition leads to renal glomerular vasoconstriction and mild reversible renal dysfunction. The mechanism by which NSAIDs cause seizures and coma is unclear.

Toxicokinetics

NSAIDs are rapidly absorbed following oral administration, although sustained-release formulations will have a delayed peak plasma level. Most are highly protein bound and have small volumes of distribution. They undergo hepatic metabolism and are excreted in the urine. Most agents have elimination half-lives of less than 4 hours (exceptions are naproxen and piroxicam, which have half-lives of 12 and 45 hours, respectively).

CLINICAL FEATURES

- Following acute overdose, most patients are asymptomatic or experience minor self-limiting gastrointestinal symptoms such as nausea, vomiting and epigastric discomfort.
- Minor CNS symptoms such as lethargy and drowsiness are sometimes observed.
- Massive ibuprofen overdose can result in rapid onset of seizures, coma, acute renal dysfunction and metabolic acidosis.
- Self-limiting seizures commonly occur within hours of mefenamic acid overdose.

TABLE 3.55.1	Dose-related risk assessment: ibuprofen
Dose	**Effect**
<100 mg/kg	Asymptomatic
100–300 mg/kg	Mild GI and CNS symptoms
>300 mg/kg	Risk of seizures, coma and metabolic acidosis

- Chronic use of ibuprofen is associated with renal tubular acidosis and the potential for life-threatening hypokalaemia.

INVESTIGATIONS
Screening tests in deliberate self-poisoning
- 12-lead ECG, BGL and paracetamol level

Specific investigations
- EUC, LFTs and FBC in symptomatic patients.
- A mild anion gap metabolic acidosis is commonly observed and of no clinical significance. It usually resolves within 24–48 hours.

MANAGEMENT
Resuscitation, supportive care and monitoring
- Attention to airway, breathing and circulation are paramount. These priorities are managed along conventional lines, as outlined in **Chapter 1.2: Resuscitation**.
- Seizures are managed with benzodiazepines, as outlined in **Chapter 2.3: Seizures**.
- General supportive care measures are indicated, as outlined in **Chapter 1.4: Supportive care and monitoring**.

Decontamination
- Not indicated.
- Oral activated charcoal is contraindicated following mefenamic overdose because of the risk of seizures.

Enhanced elimination
- Not clinically useful.

Antidotes
- None available.

DISPOSITION AND FOLLOW-UP
- Children may be observed at home following possible unintentional ingestion, unless symptoms occur.
- Adult patients following deliberate self-poisoning who are asymptomatic with normal vital signs at 4 hours post ingestion are fit for medical discharge.
- Symptomatic patients with mild-to-moderate gastrointestinal or CNS symptoms are managed supportively in a ward environment. They are fit for medical discharge when clinically well.

HANDY TIP
- Anticipate seizures following mefenamic acid overdose.

Preparations
Numerous non-steroidal anti-inflammatory products are commercially available, including combination formulations with other analgesics and decongestants.

References
Balali-Mood M, Critchley JA, Proudfoot AT et al. Mefenamic acid overdose. Lancet 1981; 1:1354–1356.
Hall AH, Smolinske SC, Stover B et al. Ibuprofen overdose in adults. Journal of Toxicology–Clinical Toxicology 1992; 30(1):23–27.

Hunter LJ, Wood DM, Dargan PI. The patterns of toxicity and management of acute nonsteroidal anti-inflammatory drug (NSAID) overdose. Open Access Emergency Medicine 2011; 6(3)39–48. https://doi.org/10.2147/OAEM.S22795.

McElwee NE, Veltri JC, Bradford DC et al. A prospective, population-based study of acute ibuprofen overdose: complications are rare and routine serum levels not warranted. Annals of Emergency Medicine 1990; 19(6):657–662.

Ng JL, Morgan DJR, Loh NKM et al. Life-threatening hypokalaemia associated with ibuprofen-induced renal tubular acidosis. Medical Journal of Australia 2011; 194:313–316.

3.56 OLANZAPINE

Deliberate self-poisoning with this commonly prescribed second-generation (atypical) antipsychotic agent is characterised by agitated delirium fluctuating with sedation and coma. Thorough supportive care ensures a good outcome.

RISK ASSESSMENT

- Olanzapine overdose is associated with predictable dose-dependent clinical features (see **Table 3.56.1**).
- Co-ingestion of ethanol or other sedative-hypnotic agents increases the risk of coma and loss of airway protective reflexes.
- **Children:** accidental ingestion of olanzapine requires hospital assessment and observation. Delayed extrapyramidal effects may occur over the following days.

Toxic mechanism

Olanzapine is an antagonist at dopamine (D_2), serotonin (particularly 5-HT_2), histamine (H_1), muscarinic (M_1) and peripheral alpha (α) receptors.

Toxicokinetics

Olanzapine is well absorbed after oral or sublingual administration. It is highly lipophilic and metabolised by cytochrome P450 enzymes to inactive metabolites. There is a large first-pass effect after oral dosing.

CLINICAL FEATURES

- Onset of toxicity occurs within 2 hours.
- Sedation, miosis and tachycardia are common.
- Fluctuating mental status with episodic agitated delirium is characteristic.
- Urinary retention frequently complicates this presentation.
- Duration of toxic effects lasts from 12 to 48 hours.

TABLE 3.56.1 Dose-related risk assessment: olanzapine

Dose (adult)	Effect
40–100 mg	Mild-to-moderate sedation with possible anticholinergic effects
100–300 mg	Sedation with episodic agitated delirium
>300 mg	Increasing likelihood of coma requiring intubation Hypotension secondary to peripheral alpha blockade

- QT prolongation can occur but torsades de pointes has not been reported.
- Extrapyramidal effects are uncommon in adults.
- Seizures are rare.

INVESTIGATIONS
Screening tests in deliberate self-poisoning
- 12-lead ECG, BGL and paracetamol level

MANAGEMENT
Resuscitation, supportive care and monitoring
- Attention to airway, breathing and circulation are paramount. These priorities are managed along conventional lines, as outlined in **Chapter 1.2: Resuscitation**.
- General supportive care measures are indicated, as outlined in **Chapter 1.4: Supportive care and monitoring**.
- Severe agitated delirium is managed with titrated doses of intravenous benzodiazepines, as outlined in **Chapter 2.4: Approach to delirium**. This may be challenging due to co-existing CNS depression, and intubation and ventilation may be required to protect the airway.
- Monitor for urinary retention and insert an indwelling urinary catheter if required.

Decontamination
- Activated charcoal should be given to all comatose patients following olanzapine overdose once the airway is protected by endotracheal intubation.

Enhanced elimination
- Not clinically useful.

Antidotes
- None available.

DISPOSITION AND FOLLOW-UP
- All paediatric patients are observed in hospital following accidental ingestion. If they remain clinically well 4–6 hours later, they can be discharged. Discharge should not occur at night. Parents are advised that abnormal (extrapyramidal) movements may occur up to 3 days after ingestion.
- Patients who are clinically well 4–6 hours after ingestion do not require further medical management.

HANDY TIP
- The combination of sedation, episodic agitated delirium and miosis is highly suggestive of olanzapine intoxication.

PITFALL
- Undetected urinary retention can exacerbate agitation and requires placement of an indwelling catheter.

Presentations
Olanzapine 2.5 mg, 5 mg, 7.5 mg, 10 mg, 15 mg, 20 mg tablets (28)

Olanzapine 5 mg, 10 mg, 15 mg, 20 mg wafers (28)
Olanzapine 10 mg powder, injectable
Olanzapine pamoate monohydrate 210 mg, 300 mg, 405 mg depot.

References

Burns MJ. The pharmacology and toxicology of atypical antipsychotic agents. Journal of Toxicology–Clinical Toxicology 2001; 39(1):1–14.

Isbister GK, Balit CR, Kilham HA. Antipsychotic poisoning in young children: a systematic review. Drug Safety 2005; 26(11):1029–1044.

Palenzona S, Meier PJ, Kupferschmidt H et al. Clinical picture of olanzapine poisoning with special reference to fluctuating mental status. Journal of Toxicology–Clinical Toxicology 2004; 42(1):27–32.

Wong DC, Curtis LA. Are 1 or 2 dangerous? Clozapine and olanzapine exposure in toddlers. The Journal of Emergency Medicine 2004; 27(3):273–277.

3.57 OPIOIDS

Buprenorphine, Codeine, Dextropropoxyphene, Fentanyl, Heroin, Hydromorphone, Methadone, Morphine, Oxycodone, Pethidine

Opioid toxicity is the leading cause of death from poisoning. CNS and respiratory depression are the primary toxic effects and death is secondary to hypoxic end-organ injury.

RISK ASSESSMENT

- There is considerable inter-individual variability in the response to opioids. This variability is multi-factorial, including the agent itself, genetic polymorphism, age, tolerance and co-ingestants.
- Life-threatening CNS and respiratory depression may occur just above the analgesic dose.
- Opioid-naïve patients (no tolerance) or co-ingestion of other CNS depressants (antidepressants, benzodiazepines, ethanol) increases the severity of CNS depression and the likelihood of a fatal outcome without supportive care.
- Certain agents have additional toxic effects (see **Table 3.57.1**).
- Administration of a partial opioid agonist (e.g. buprenorphine) or antagonist (naloxone or naltrexone) to a patient with opioid dependence can result in symptoms of acute severe opioid withdrawal (see **Chapter 2.11: Opioid use disorder**).

TABLE 3.57.1 Opioid risk assessment: special cases	
Drug	**Effect**
Dextropropoxyphene	Sodium channel blockade leading to seizures and ventricular dysrhythmias
Methadone and oxycodone	QT prolongation
Pethidine	Seizures due to norpethidine metabolite

- **Children:** opioid toxicity is the leading cause of death by poisoning in children. Ingestion of a single opioid tablet or a mouthful of liquid preparations can cause death. All opioid ingestions require assessment and observation in hospital.

Toxic mechanism

Opioid effects are mediated by central and peripheral opioid receptors (mu, kappa, delta). Agonist activity at mu receptors is responsible for the major toxic effects – sedation and respiratory depression. Opioids can be full or partial agonists and have differing potencies which influence their clinical effects.

Toxicokinetics

Most opioids are absorbed rapidly, with the exception of controlled-release preparations. The half-life can vary significantly both therapeutically and in overdose. Most opioids undergo hepatic metabolism, and many have active metabolites. They have large volumes of distribution and are primarily renally excreted. Codeine is an example of genetic polymorphism affecting toxicity – ultra-rapid metabolisers are at increased risk of toxicity.

Administration also occurs via intravenous, inhalational or transdermal routes.

CLINICAL FEATURES

- The opioid toxidrome consists of:
  - CNS depression
  - respiratory depression (respiratory rate and tidal volume)
  - miosis.
- The duration of effects depends on the pharmacokinetics of the individual agent. Heroin intoxication is typically short (e.g. less than 6 hours), while methadone and oxycodone intoxication may last more than 24 hours.
- Apnoea and loss of airway protective reflexes result in hypoxia.
- Nausea and vomiting may occur, promoting pulmonary aspiration.
- Bradycardia is common. Tachycardia may occur as a response to hypoxia and hypercarbia.
- Hypothermia, skin necrosis, compartment syndrome, rhabdomyolysis and hypoxic brain injury may complicate prolonged intoxication.
- Methadone and oxycodone are associated with QT prolongation, although torsades de pointes is rare.
- Dextropropoxyphene toxicity can cause seizures and ventricular dysrhythmias.

INVESTIGATIONS

Screening tests in deliberate self-poisoning

- 12-lead ECG, BGL and paracetamol level

Specific investigations

- Blood or urine opioid levels rarely assist acute management. They may be useful to confirm use, particularly for forensic evaluation.
- Investigations as indicated to diagnose and assess secondary complications.

MANAGEMENT

Resuscitation, supportive care and monitoring

- Attention to airway, breathing and circulation are paramount and ensure the survival of the vast majority of patients.

- These priorities are managed along conventional lines, as outlined in **Chapter 1.2: Resuscitation**.
- General supportive care measures are indicated, as outlined in **Chapter 1.4: Supportive care and monitoring**.
- Close clinical and physiological monitoring is indicated.
- In the rare event of ventricular dysrhythmias in dextropropoxyphene intoxication, resuscitation includes serum alkalinisation by the administration of IV bolus sodium bicarbonate, as outlined in **Chapter 4.24: Sodium bicarbonate**.

Decontamination
- Oral activated charcoal may reduce length of stay if administered to a patient presenting early after overdose with controlled-release opioids.

Enhanced elimination
- Not clinically useful.

Antidotes
- Respiratory and CNS depression can be reversed with titrated doses of naloxone (see **Chapter 4.18: Naloxone**). Continuous naloxone infusion may be required following overdose of long-acting opioids or slow-release preparations.

DISPOSITION AND FOLLOW-UP
- The period of observation required to detect CNS depression varies with the opioid. For most standard-release oral preparations, 4 hours is sufficient.
- A patient who ingests controlled-release opioid preparations must be observed for at least 12 hours before medical discharge. Patients who have received naloxone should be observed for at least 2 hours to ensure that opioid toxicity does not recur.
- Symptomatic patients require close physiological monitoring in an area able to manage respiratory depression until they are clinically well.
- Any child who has potentially ingested an opioid is admitted for 12 hours of close observation in an area equipped and staffed to detect and manage respiratory depression. Discharge must not occur at night.
- Patients with significant CNS depression requiring intubation or naloxone infusion require management in an intensive care unit.

HANDY TIPS
- Patients must be admitted to an area with staff and resources capable of detecting CNS and respiratory depression.
- It is vital that the adequacy of ventilation is measured by assessing both respiratory rate and tidal volume.
- Respiratory depression can be delayed up to 12 hours following ingestion of controlled-release preparations.
- Respiratory effort should be assessed while the patient is sleeping or otherwise unroused.
- Routine administration of supplemental oxygen will mask desaturation from hypoventilation, with the risk that significant respiratory acidosis can occur.

PITFALLS

- Failure to recognise the potential lethality of unintentional paediatric ingestion of opioids.
- Failure to detect opioid-induced respiratory depression due to inadequate observation (in-hospital deaths have occurred).

Presentations
Multiple pharmaceutical and illicit preparations

Reference
Sachdeva DK, Stadnyk JM. Are one or two dangerous? Opioid exposure in toddlers. Journal of Emergency Medicine 2005; 29(1):77–84.

3.58 ORGANOCHLORINES

Aldrin, Chlordane, Dichlorodiphenyltrichloroethane (DDT), Dieldrin, Endosulfan, Endrin, Ethylan, Heptachlor, Hexachlorobenzene, Isobenzan, Lindane, Methoxychlor

Chlorinated pesticides are widely used in agriculture. Lindane is used medically as a treatment for lice infestations. Acute ingestion or repeated large dermal exposure causes neurological toxicity, including seizures and coma. Rarely, ventricular dysrhythmias occur due to sensitisation of the myocardium to catecholamines. Management is supportive.

RISK ASSESSMENT

- The risk assessment for lindane is relatively well documented (see **Table 3.58.1**). There is a paucity of data regarding acute and chronic exposures to other organochlorines. As a general guide endrin, aldrin, dieldrin and chlordane have the lowest LD50s in animal models.
- Toxicity occurs in three main settings:
  - acute deliberate self-poisoning by ingestion – rapid onset of neurological symptoms, seizures and coma
  - excessive dermal application or accidental ingestion of lindane – agitation and seizures
  - occupational exposures via dermal or inhalational routes – usually no acute symptoms.
- **Children:** ingestion is potentially life-threatening. Topical lindane used as a lice treatment can cause agitation and seizures, particularly with repeat use or prolonged application.

TABLE 3.58.1	Dose-related risk assessment: lindane
	Effect
Child	Ingestion of >50 mg (5 mL of 1% solution) causes symptoms
Adult	Estimated mean lethal ingested dose is 125 mg/kg Dose required to induce toxicity from dermal absorption not defined

Toxic mechanism

Lindane and the cyclodienes (aldrin, dieldrin, heptachlor, endrin, chlordane, endosulfan) are non-competitive antagonists acting at the chlorine ion channel of GABA$_A$ receptors. DDT acts by inhibiting sodium channel closure following depolarisation. Both mechanisms are neuroexcitatory.

Toxicokinetics

These agents are rapidly absorbed following ingestion. The degree of dermal absorption depends on the agent, concentration, solvent (usually hydrocarbon) and skin integrity. Lindane and the cyclodienes are well absorbed across skin. Organochlorines are highly lipid soluble and widely distributed to fat stores. Accumulation may occur with repeated occupational exposure. Organochlorines undergo hepatic microsomal metabolism prior to elimination in the urine. They have non-linear kinetics due to slow redistribution from fat stores. Elimination of some organochlorines may take weeks to months.

CLINICAL FEATURES

- Principal clinical features of toxicity are:
  - nausea and vomiting
  - anxiety, agitation and confusion
  - perioral paraesthesia, fasciculation and myoclonic movements
  - seizures – these are usually of short duration but may be recurrent
  - sedation and coma.
- Clinical features develop within 1–2 hours of acute ingestion and over hours to days following excessive dermal application.
- Hypotension, cardiac dysrhythmias and ventricular ectopy are rare complications of severe intoxication.
- Hypoxaemia and acidosis contribute to myocardial sensitisation to catecholamines.
- Hepatitis and renal dysfunction are reported following acute intoxication.
- Vomiting and aspiration may be complicated by a severe chemical pneumonitis from the hydrocarbon vehicle in which many of these agents are formulated.

INVESTIGATIONS

Screening tests in deliberate self-poisoning
- 12-lead ECG, BGL and paracetamol level

Specific investigations
- Arterial blood gases
  - Hypoxaemia and acidosis.
- Serial 12-lead ECGs
  - Increased ventricular ectopy may herald the onset of ventricular tachydysrhythmias.
- EUC, liver function tests
  - Hepatic and renal injury.
- Serum and fat organochlorine levels
  - Not readily available and do not assist management.

MANAGEMENT

Resuscitation, supportive care and monitoring
- Organochlorine poisoning is a potentially life-threatening emergency managed in an area equipped for cardiorespiratory monitoring and resuscitation.

- Potential life-threats that require immediate intervention include:
  - coma (see **Chapter 2.1: Coma**)
  - seizures (see **Chapter 2.3: Seizures**)
  - ventricular dysrhythmias.
- Control agitation with titrated intravenous doses of benzodiazepines.
- In the event of ventricular dysrhythmias (VT, VF):
  - Beta-blockers are the agent of choice to reduce catecholamine-induced myocardial toxicity.
  - Options include metoprolol 1–5 mg IV (0.1 mg/kg in children) titrated to response.
- Institute general supportive care, as outlined in **Chapter 1.4: Supportive care and monitoring**.

Decontamination
- Resuscitation takes priority over decontamination and activated charcoal is not indicated until the airway is secured by endotracheal intubation.
- Following excessive dermal exposure, wash the skin with soap and water.

Enhanced elimination
- Not clinically useful.

Antidotes
- None available.

DISPOSITION AND FOLLOW-UP
- Children with potential ingestions should be observed in hospital for 4 hours. If they do not develop symptoms during that period, they may then be discharged.
- Excessive dermal exposure only warrants referral to hospital if symptoms occur.
- Patients with objective evidence of organochlorine intoxication as evidenced by gastrointestinal or neurological symptoms are managed in a hospital location capable of managing seizures. Those that develop features of major intoxication (recurrent seizures or coma) require admission to the intensive care unit for ongoing supportive care.
- Patients may be safely discharged once all symptoms resolve. Follow-up is not necessary if asymptomatic.

HANDY TIPS
- The seizures associated with acute intoxication are usually rapid in onset, short duration and controlled with benzodiazepines.
- Ventricular dysrhythmias associated with organochlorines are rare and may respond to IV beta-blockers (e.g. metoprolol or propranolol).

PITFALL
- Failure to recognise the onset of acute toxicity, manifested by vomiting, agitation or perioral paraesthesia.

- The chronic subclinical effect of the organochlorines, including their carcinogenic potential.

Presentations
Most organochlorines are solid at room temperature and dissolved in hydrocarbon for ease of application.

Industrial formulations
Aldrin, chlordane, dichlorodiphenyltrichloroethane (DDT), dieldrin, endosulfan, endrin, ethylan, heptachlor, hexachlorobenzene, isobenzan, lindane, methoxychlor

Medical formulations
Lindane 1% shampoo or lotion

References
Aks SE, Krantz A, Hryhorczuk DO et al. Acute accidental lindane ingestion in toddlers. Annals of Emergency Medicine 1995; 26(5):647–651.

Baselt R. Disposition of toxic chemicals and drugs in man. 5th edn Foster City, California: Chemical Toxicology Institute; 2000.

CDC 2005. CDC. Unintentional topical lindane ingestions – United States, 1998–2003. MMWR Morbidity Mortality Weekly Report 2005; 54(21):533–535.

3.59 ORGANOPHOSPHORUS AGENTS (ORGANOPHOSPHATES AND CARBAMATES)

Organophosphates: Chlorpyrifos, Coumaphos, Diazinon, Dichlorvos, Dimethoate, Fenthion, Malathion, Parathion, Trichlorfon

Carbamates: Aldicarb, Carbendazim, Carbendazole, Carbazine, Propoxur

Chemical nerve agents: Sarin (GB), Soman (GD), Tabun (GA), VX

Deliberate self-poisoning with organophosphate and carbamate insecticides is responsible for more than 200 000 deaths worldwide each year, but presentations in Australasia are infrequent. Inhibition of acetylcholinesterase enzymes leads to profound cholinergic toxicity, and death results primarily from respiratory failure. Prompt resuscitation, intensive care management and early antidotal therapy may be life-saving.

RISK ASSESSMENT
- Deliberate self-poisoning by ingestion of organophosphates invariably produces life-threatening toxicity.
- Mortality rates range from 10 to 30% for those who survive to hospital admission.
- Carbamate poisoning causes similar cholinergic toxicity, but the clinical effects are usually of shorter duration.
- The onset of clinical features may be delayed several hours, depending on the agent ingested.
- Accidental dermal or inhalational exposure to these agents may cause cholinergic effects but is unlikely to be life-threatening.
- Secondary organophosphorus poisoning of staff (nosocomial poisoning) does not occur provided standard precautions for exposure to bodily fluids are followed.

- **Children:** any ingestion of organophosphates or carbamates is potentially lethal.

Toxic mechanism

Organophosphates bind to and inhibit acetylcholinesterase (AChE) enzymes, thereby increasing acetylcholine (ACh) concentration at both muscarinic and nicotinic cholinergic receptors. Clinical features are secondary to the widespread effects of increased ACh at CNS, autonomic (parasympathetic and sympathetic) and skeletal muscle neuromuscular synapses.

Formation of a permanent covalent bond between the organophosphate and AChE ('ageing') causes irreversible inhibition of the enzyme and prevents reactivation by the antidote pralidoxime. The time taken for ageing to occur depends on the individual agent. Carbamates cause reversible inhibition of the cholinesterase enzyme, and ageing does not occur. Organophosphates and carbamates are frequently formulated with hydrocarbon solvents (e.g. xylene). Inhalation of solvent fumes can produce symptoms such as headache and dizziness but this does not represent organophosphate poisoning. The insecticides themselves have very low vapour pressures and are only inhaled when aerosolised.

Toxicokinetics

All agents are well absorbed after ingestion. Dermal and inhalational absorption do occur but are less likely to be clinically significant unless exposure is prolonged. Organophosphates generally have large volumes of distribution and redistribution from lipid stores may result in delayed or recurrent toxicity ('intermediate syndrome'). A number of organophosphates are indirect agents requiring metabolism to their active forms. Metabolism is by serum HDL-bound esterase enzymes (paraoxonases) or hepatic microsomal (cytochrome P450) systems, with excretion of inactive metabolites in the urine. Carbamates have lower lipid solubility and are distributed less to the CNS. Most carbamates are hepatically metabolised and excreted renally.

CLINICAL FEATURES

- The onset of symptoms depends on the agent, dose and route of exposure. Symptoms may occur within minutes following ingestion of some agents (e.g. dimethoate, parathion) or be delayed by many hours.
- The clinical features are variable and either muscarinic or nicotinic features can predominate.
- Dimethoate has low lipid solubility and poisoning is characterised by the early onset of coma, cardiovascular collapse and death within 24 hours.
- Chlorpyrifos may present with early muscarinic features.
- Fenthion is associated with few early symptoms but delayed onset of paralysis and respiratory failure.
- Typical clinical syndromes include:

Acute intoxication
- Muscarinic effects
  - Diarrhoea, urination, miosis, bronchorrhoea, bronchospasm, emesis, lacrimation, salivation ('DUMBBELS' mnemonic)
  - Bradycardia and hypotension
- Nicotinic effects
  - Tremor, fasciculations, weakness, respiratory muscle paralysis
  - Tachycardia and hypertension
    - Note: Tachycardia rather than bradycardia may predominate related to hypoxia, hypotension or nicotinic stimulation of adrenal tissue, leading to catecholamine release.

- Central nervous system
  - Agitation, coma, seizures
- Respiratory
  - Chemical pneumonitis caused by aspiration of hydrocarbon solvent
    - Note: For further detail on the cholinergic features, see **Chapter 2.7: Cholinergic toxicity**.

Intermediate syndrome
- Delayed onset of paralysis occurring 2–4 days after apparent recovery from initial symptoms. This syndrome is associated with particular agents (e.g. fenthion, diazinon, malathion) but the pathophysiology is not well understood. The likely causes are delayed redistribution from tissue lipid stores; prolonged motor end-plate stimulation leading to muscle dysfunction; or inadequate pralidoxime dosing.

Delayed neurotoxicity
- Organophosphate-induced delayed neuropathy (OPIDN) is rare and occurs 1–5 weeks following acute exposure to particular agents (e.g. fenthion, chlorpyrifos, parathion). It is an ascending sensorimotor polyneuropathy thought to be secondary to inhibition of axonal neuropathy target esterase (NTE).

Chronic organophosphate-induced neuropsychiatric disorder
- Long-term neuropsychiatric disorder, which may occur following acute intoxication or chronic low-level exposure.

INVESTIGATIONS
Screening tests in deliberate self-poisoning
- 12-lead ECG, BGL and paracetamol level

Specific investigations
- Red cell and plasma cholinesterase levels
  - The diagnosis and management of acute anticholinesterase poisoning is primarily clinical but measures of cholinesterase activity can be useful in making a definitive diagnosis and to monitor therapy.
  - Access to these assays can be difficult and samples must be processed promptly due to ongoing in vitro reactions.
  - Significant clinical features generally occur at levels <25% of normal activity.
  - Plasma cholinesterase activity is a sensitive biomarker of anticholinesterase exposure. It falls more rapidly and recovers more quickly (4–6 weeks) than red cell cholinesterase activity. It may be undetectable on plasma assay but does not correlate directly with clinical severity. Once it starts to increase, it suggests that the plasma concentration of the anticholinesterase compound is negligible.
  - Red cell cholinesterase activity correlates better with severity of anticholinesterase poisoning and may take longer to recover. It returns to normal following successful oxime therapy and can be used to monitor progress when oximes are withdrawn.

— The mixed cholinesterase test has been advocated as a method to assess adequacy of therapy but has not been validated. Patient and control serum are mixed in a 50:50 ratio. A plasma cholinesterase activity of the mixed sample that is less than the mean of the two unmixed samples suggests the patient's plasma contains unbound organophosphate and increased oxime administration is considered.

MANAGEMENT
Resuscitation, supportive care and monitoring
- Acute organophosphate poisoning is a life-threatening emergency managed in an area equipped for cardiorespiratory monitoring and resuscitation.
- Early life-threats that require immediate intervention include:
  - respiratory failure
  - coma
  - seizures
  - hypotension.
- Resuscitation must not be delayed by external decontamination procedures, which should proceed simultaneously. Staff should use standard precautions, ensuring that the room is well ventilated to minimise symptoms of hydrocarbon vapour inhalation. More sophisticated personal protective equipment is not required.
- Atropine is the resuscitation antidote required for muscarinic features causing respiratory failure or haemodynamic compromise – bronchorrhoea, cough, wheeze, respiratory crackles, bradycardia or hypotension. Start escalating doses as detailed below in **Antidotes** and **Chapter 4.1: Atropine**.
- Control agitation or seizures with titrated doses of benzodiazepines.
- Institute general supportive care, as outlined in **Chapter 1.4: Supportive care and monitoring**.

Decontamination
- Remove clothes and wash skin with soap and water. Clothing should be bagged.
- Insertion of a nasogastric tube is warranted to attempt aspiration of ingested liquid preparations, particularly if the patient is intubated.
- Activated charcoal adsorbs organophosphorus compounds, but a clear outcome benefit has not been proven. However, it is reasonable to administer by nasogastric tube after initial aspiration of stomach contents.

Enhanced elimination
- Not clinically useful.

Antidotes
- Atropine
  - Atropine in escalating doses is indicated to control the muscarinic features of cholinergic excess: diaphoresis, bronchorrhoea, wheeze, cough, reduced breath sounds, bradycardia or hypotension.

— Administer 1.2 mg (50 microgram/kg in children) IV and double the dose every 5 minutes until there is improvement in airway secretions, breath sounds and bradycardia. Large doses may be required. Continuing administration of repeat bolus doses or an infusion is frequently required.
  – Note: Atropine has no effect on the nicotinic receptors of the neuromuscular junction to improve muscle weakness.
— For more information on indications, administration and therapeutic end points, see **Chapter 4.1: Atropine**.
- Pralidoxime
  — Pralidoxime may reverse neuromuscular blockade by reactivating inhibited AChE before ageing occurs. However, the clinical utility of pralidoxime is debated (see **Controversies** below).
  — Give 2 g IV then continue an infusion of 0.5 g/hour for at least 24 hours.
  — Pralidoxime is not indicated for carbamate poisoning as irreversible binding to the acetylcholinesterase enzyme does not occur.
  — For more information on indications, administration and therapeutic end points, see **Chapter 4.22: Pralidoxime**.

DISPOSITION AND FOLLOW-UP
- Any patient who has ingested an organophosphate or carbamate insecticide is admitted for intensive monitoring for a minimum of 12 hours. Discharge does not occur at night.
- Patients with objective evidence of organophosphate or carbamate intoxication requiring antidote administration are admitted to an intensive care unit to detect and manage respiratory and neuromuscular complications and monitor response to therapy.
- Patients are observed for at least 24 hours after the cessation of oxime therapy to detect and manage intermediate syndrome.
- Adult patients with potential occupational exposure do not require referral to hospital unless they develop cholinergic symptoms.

PITFALLS
- Failure to appreciate the risk of life-threatening poisoning in the patient who presents asymptomatic.
- Failure to recognise the features of cholinergic toxicity.
- Excessive concern about risks of nosocomial poisoning. This is not documented following exposure to the organophosphate poisoned patient and unwarranted concerns should not compromise patient care. Standard precautions and management in a well-ventilated room to minimise the strong odours of the hydrocarbon solvent are appropriate.

CONTROVERSIES
- The value of pralidoxime in improving clinical outcomes from organophosphate poisoning is debated.
  — Pralidoxime reactivates red cell acetylcholinesterase, particularly following poisoning from diethyl compounds such as

chlorpyrifos, but there is limited published evidence of clinical benefit such as decreased intubation rates or improved survival.
— However, published studies are difficult to interpret as they include diethyl and dimethyl organophosphate compounds with variable speeds of ageing and responses to pralidoxime. Further research may lead to the development of more effective cholinesterase reactivators or identify specific management recommendations for individual organophosphates.

• Research continues for additional therapies, but as yet there are no strong recommendations. Non-depolarising muscle relaxants may reduce prolonged muscle weakness by protecting the neuromuscular junction from repetitive stimulation; and calcium channel blockers and magnesium sulfate are currently under investigation as adjunctive treatments.

• Association between long-term occupational exposure and the development of malignancies is unclear.

Presentations

These agents may be in both solid and liquid forms. They are frequently formulated with organic solvents such as xylene, toluene or toxic alcohols, in varying concentrations.

References

Eddleston M, Buckley NA, Eyer P et al. Management of acute organophosphorus pesticide poisoning. Lancet 2008; 3(9612):597–607.

Eddleston M, Eyer P, Worek F et al. Differences between organophosphorus insecticides in human self-poisoning: a prospective cohort study. Lancet 2005; 366:1452–1459.

Eddleston M, Eyer P, Worek F et al. Pralidoxime in acute organophosphorus insecticide poisoning: a randomised controlled trial. PLoS Medicine 2009; 6(6):e1000104.

Eyer P. The role of oximes in the management of organophosphorus pesticide poisoning. Toxicological Reviews 2003; 22(3):165–190.

Pawar KS, Bholte RR, Pillay CP et al. Continuous pralidoxime infusion versus repeated bolus injection to treat organophosphorus pesticide poisoning: a randomized controlled trial. Lancet 2006; 368:2136–2141.

Worek F, Thiermann H, Wille T. Organophosphorus compounds and oximes: a critical review. Archives of Toxicology 2020; 94:2275–2292.

3.60 PARACETAMOL: IMMEDIATE-RELEASE PREPARATIONS (ACUTE OVERDOSE)

Paracetamol, N-acetyl-p-aminophenol (APAP)

See also Chapter 3.61: Paracetamol: Modified-release preparations, Chapter 3.62: Paracetamol: Repeated supratherapeutic ingestion.

This chapter refers to a single or staggered ingestion of immediate-release paracetamol. The decision to treat with N-acetylcysteine is determined by a timed serum paracetamol level plotted on the modified Rumack–Matthew nomogram. If the nomogram cannot be applied, a biochemical risk assessment (serum paracetamol and hepatic transaminase levels) guides the decision to treat with N-acetylcysteine. Treatment within 8 hours ensures survival in the vast majority of cases.

RISK ASSESSMENT

- The threshold dose for paracetamol-induced hepatic injury in adults is variable but considered to be ≥200 mg/kg or ≥10 g, whichever is less.
- Life-threatening hepatotoxicity is uncommon but fatalities do occur.
- The risk of hepatotoxicity following a single or staggered ingestion of immediate-release preparations is predicted by plotting a serum paracetamol level on the modified Rumack–Matthew nomogram (see **Figure 3.60.1**).
- The risk of hepatotoxicity is determined primarily by time from overdose to commencement of N-acetylcysteine.
  — Survival is essentially guaranteed when N-acetylcysteine is commenced within 8 hours of ingestion (a percentage of patients develop elevation of hepatic transaminases).
  — Hepatotoxicity is more likely if treatment with N-acetylcysteine is delayed >8 hours post ingestion.
  — There is still a role for N-acetylcysteine with established hepatic injury as it decreases morbidity (cerebral oedema and inotropic requirements) and mortality.
- Patients presenting within 8 hours of ingestion have a paracetamol level taken at 4 hours or later plotted on the nomogram. Treatment with N-acetylcysteine can be deferred until the paracetamol result is available, provided it can be initiated within 8 hours.

FIGURE 3.60.1 Paracetamol treatment nomogram recommended for use in Australia and New Zealand

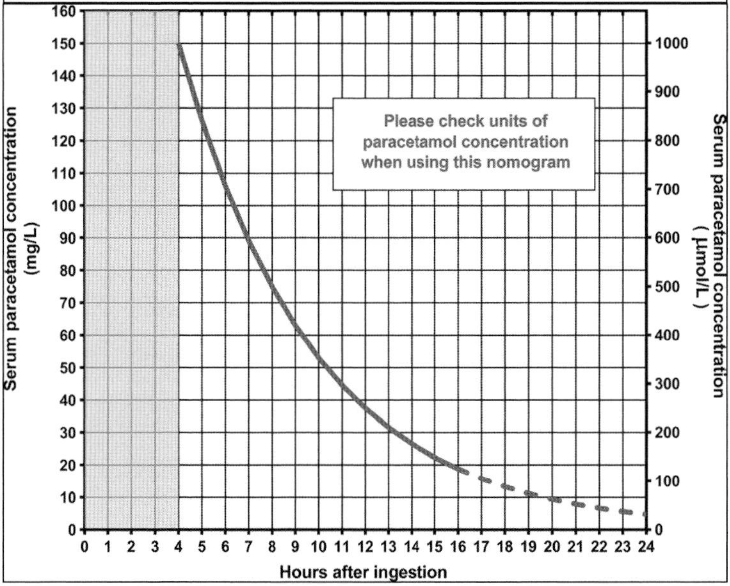

- Patients presenting >8 hours after ingestion; who have an unknown time of ingestion; or whose paracetamol level will not be available within 8 hours are commenced on N-acetylcysteine immediately until the biochemical risk assessment (serum paracetamol and hepatic transaminase (ALT) levels) is available.
- For staggered ingestions, the risk assessment can safely be performed by time-anchoring strategies using the earliest possible time of ingestion as the point of reference for the entire ingested dose (see **Handy Tips** below).
- Patients with a massive ingestion (e.g. ≥30 g or ≥500 mg/kg) and a paracetamol level > double the nomogram line should receive an increased dose of N-acetylcysteine.
- N-acetylcysteine is a safe and effective antidote. If there is any confusion regarding interpretation of paracetamol levels and a perceived risk of hepatotoxicity, it is always justified to initiate therapy with N-acetylcysteine and monitor the patient's progress.
- **Children:** there are no reports of death following acute ingestion in children under 6 years of age. Ingestion of <200 mg/kg as a single dose or over a period of <8 hours does not warrant intervention or referral to hospital. Paediatric liquid preparations are absorbed rapidly and a 2 (to 4) hour level below the 4-hour nomogram treatment line allows safe early discharge. If the 2-hour paracetamol level is above 150 mg/L (1000 micromol/L) it should be repeated at 4 hours post-ingestion and N-acetylcysteine commenced if it remains above this threshold.

Toxic mechanism
Elevated production of N-acetylparabenzoquinone imine (NAPQI) following paracetamol overdose leads to depletion of hepatic glutathione stores. Once glutathione levels reach a critical threshold (30% of normal), NAPQI binds to cellular proteins, causing hepatocyte injury. The hallmark of paracetamol-induced hepatotoxicity is centrilobular necrosis.

Toxicokinetics
Paracetamol is well absorbed from the small intestine following oral administration; peak levels occur within 1–2 hours for standard tablets or capsules and within 30 minutes for liquid preparations. The volume of distribution is 0.9 L/kg. Ninety per cent of paracetamol undergoes hepatic glucuronidation or sulfation to conjugates that are excreted in the urine. Most of the remainder is oxidised by the cytochrome P450 system to form NAPQI, a potentially toxic intermediate. Under normal circumstances, NAPQI is immediately bound by intracellular glutathione and eliminated in the urine as mercapturic adducts.

CLINICAL FEATURES
- Early gastrointestinal symptoms are common.
- Clinical features of progressive hepatic injury develop in a minority of patients.
- Sedation, coma and early metabolic acidosis are rare but are reported following massive paracetamol ingestion.
- The four classically described clinical stages of paracetamol hepatotoxicity are described in **Table 3.60.1**.

INVESTIGATIONS
Screening tests in deliberate self-poisoning
- 12-lead ECG, BGL and paracetamol level.
- Following deliberate self-poisoning with paracetamol, the serum paracetamol level is a specific investigation (see below).

TABLE 3.60.1 Clinical stages of acute paracetamol overdose

Stage 1 (<24 hours)	Patients are frequently asymptomatic but may have nausea and vomiting
Stage 2 (24–72 hours)	Right upper quadrant tenderness is common. Hepatotoxicity is formally defined as an ALT or AST >1000 U/L. Transaminases rise rapidly and may exceed 10 000 U/L. The INR elevation usually reaches its highest level within hours of the peak increase in transaminases. Hypoglycaemia and hyperbilirubinaemia also occur and renal function may be impaired.
Stage 3 (72–96 hours)	In severe cases, fulminant hepatic failure is clinically evident with jaundice and encephalopathy. Death can occur and is associated with worsening lactic acidosis, progressive renal failure, severe coagulopathy and cerebral oedema.
Stage 4 (4 days–2 weeks)	Recovery phase during which hepatic structure and function return to normal

Specific investigations
- Serum paracetamol
  - Used to determine the need for treatment.
- Hepatic transaminases
  - In paracetamol poisoning, an ALT ≤50 U/L is considered normal.
  - An ALT can be taken for baseline assessment for patients presenting <**8 hours** after paracetamol ingestion but is not essential for the decision to initiate N-acetylcysteine treatment.
  - An ALT is performed for all patients presenting >**8 hours** after ingestion.
- In all cases treated with N-acetylcysteine, the ALT is repeated shortly before completion of the infusion to determine the requirement for ongoing therapy.
- In addition, for patients with a massive ingestion (e.g. ≥30 g or ≥500 mg/kg) and a paracetamol level > double the nomogram line, a repeat paracetamol level is required in combination with the ALT to determine the need for continuation of the N-acetylcysteine infusion.
- Hepatic transaminases, coagulation studies, blood glucose, platelet count, renal function and acid–base status are useful to monitor clinical status and prognosis in the setting of established hepatotoxicity.
- A recommended approach to initial investigations is outlined in **Figure 3.60.2**.

MANAGEMENT
Resuscitation, supportive care and monitoring
- Resuscitation is required only in the rare instances of coma due to massive acute ingestion or delayed presentation with

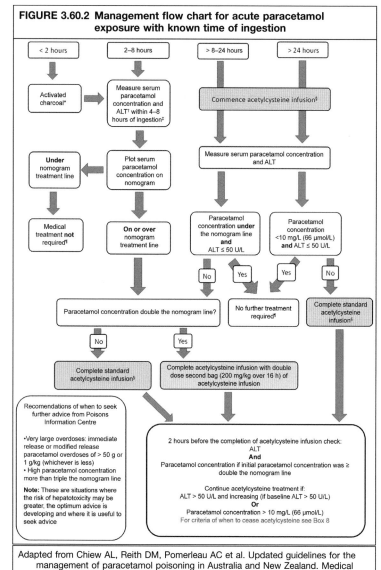

FIGURE 3.60.2 Management flow chart for acute paracetamol exposure with known time of ingestion

Adapted from Chiew AL, Reith DM, Pomerleau AC et al. Updated guidelines for the management of paracetamol poisoning in Australia and New Zealand. Medical Journal of Australia 2019; 212(4):175–183.

established hepatic failure. In such cases, urgent attention to airway, breathing and circulation, plus correction of hypoglycaemia, is required.
- General supportive care and monitoring measures are indicated, as outlined in **Chapter 1.4: Supportive care and monitoring**.
- A management flow chart for acute paracetamol exposure with known time of ingestion is shown in **Figure 3.60.2**.

Decontamination
- Activated charcoal is recommended for all patients with a toxic ingestion of paracetamol who present within 2 hours as it may sufficiently reduce the 4-hour paracetamol level to such an extent that N-acetylcysteine is not required.
- Activated charcoal is recommended for massive ingestions ($\geq$30 g or $\geq$500 mg/kg) within 4 hours.
- Activated charcoal is not indicated for children under the age of 6 because the incidence of toxic serum levels is very low even following ingestion of $\geq$200 mg/kg.

Enhanced elimination
- Not routinely indicated.

Antidotes
- Intravenous N-acetylcysteine is required for all patients in whom the risk assessment indicates the potential for hepatotoxicity and in patients who present late with clinical or biochemical evidence of hepatic injury (see **Chapter 4.17: N-acetylcysteine** for full details on dosing and administration).
- Presentation <8 hours following a defined time of ingestion:
  — The decision to initiate N-acetylcysteine can be deferred until the result of a paracetamol level taken at 4 hours or later is plotted on the nomogram.
- Presentation 8–24 hours following a defined time of ingestion:
  — N-acetylcysteine is initiated immediately and continued if a paracetamol level is above the nomogram treatment line or the ALT is >50 U/L.
- Presentation >24 hours post ingestion:
  — N-acetylcysteine is indicated if paracetamol is detectable or hepatic transaminases are elevated (ALT >50 U/L). It is continued until hepatic transaminases are stable or falling and the patient is clinically well.
- Unknown time of ingestion:
  — This scenario commonly occurs if a reliable history is not available due to coma or delirium. A biochemical risk assessment is required to exclude potential or established toxicity. N-acetylcysteine is commenced if paracetamol is >10 mg/L (66 micromol/L) or hepatic transaminases are >50 U/L. It may be ceased if:
    – a reliable history can be obtained to allow appropriate use of the nomogram
    – the paracetamol level is negative and hepatic transaminases are $\leq$50 U/L (or unchanged from baseline) at the end of the N-acetylcysteine infusion.
- A management flow chart for acute paracetamol exposure with known time of ingestion is shown in **Figure 3.60.2**.

DISPOSITION AND FOLLOW-UP

- Most patients treated with N-acetylcysteine will remain well and antidotal therapy can be stopped when the ALT is ≤50 U/L (or stable) at the end of the infusion.
- Patients in whom the ALT is increasing or who have clinical symptoms suggestive of hepatotoxicity (abdominal pain, tenderness or vomiting) require continuation of the N-acetylcysteine infusion at 100 mg/kg over 16 hours, with serial assessment of ALT and clinical status until improving.
- Patients with clear evidence of resolving hepatotoxicity (undetectable paracetamol, falling ALT, INR <2 and who are clinically well) do not require further N-acetylcysteine treatment and are fit for medical discharge.
- Patients with fulminant hepatic failure require management in an intensive care unit and referral to a liver transplant service. Appropriate referral criteria include:
  - INR >3.0 at 48 hours or >4.5 at any time
  - oliguria or creatinine >200 micromol/L
  - acidosis with pH <7.3 after resuscitation
  - systolic hypotension with BP <80 mmHg, or lactate >3 mmol/L
  - hypoglycaemia
  - severe thrombocytopenia
  - encephalopathy of any degree.

HANDY TIPS

- A minor rise in INR (<2) early in the course of overdose, without evidence of elevated transaminases, is a direct effect of paracetamol on Factor VII and not due to hepatic injury. The INR in this setting typically recovers promptly to the normal range.
- Time-anchoring strategies may be used to determine risk of hepatotoxicity and need for N-acetylcysteine where the ingestion is staggered. If multiple ingestions have occurred over several hours (e.g. at 1 pm, 3 pm and 4 pm), a worst-case scenario may be constructed. A serum paracetamol level is plotted on the nomogram, assuming that the entire dose was taken at the earliest time. If it is above the line, N-acetylcysteine is commenced.
- Between 16 and 24 hours post ingestion the paracetamol assay approaches the limits of detection. Most laboratories will not report a level less than 10 mg/L (66 micromol/L), which equates to just above 20 hours on the nomogram line.
  - A biochemical risk assessment (paracetamol level and hepatic transaminase (ALT) level) increases the reliability of using laboratory markers to exclude the risk of significant hepatotoxicity due to possible errors in the estimated time of ingestion.

PITFALLS

- Failure to commence N-acetylcysteine immediately in the patient who presents more than 8 hours following a paracetamol overdose.
- N-acetylcysteine dosing errors (see **Chapter 4.17: N-acetylcysteine** for advice on safe charting of infusions).

- Failure to check paracetamol units. Different units are used to report paracetamol levels (mg/L and micromol/L). Incorrect plotting of the level may lead to a potentially lethal error.

CONTROVERSIES
- The threshold for treatment with N-acetylcysteine. The modified Rumack–Matthew nomogram uses a line extending from 150 mg/L at 4 hours using a semi-logarithmic scale. The United Kingdom's Medicines and Healthcare products Regulatory Agency (MHRA) lowered the treatment threshold to a line extending from 100 mg/L (662 micromol/L) at 4 hours, but improvement in outcomes has not been established.
- The duration of treatment with N-acetylcysteine. Research is ongoing regarding modified or shortened treatment regimens in selected cases.

Presentations
Numerous paracetamol products are commercially available, including combination formulations with other analgesics, decongestants, antihistamines and antitussives.

References
Chiew AL, Isbister GK, Kirby KA et al. Massive paracetamol overdose: an observational study of the effect of activated charcoal and increased acetylcysteine dose (ATOM-2). Clinical Toxicology 2017; 55(10):1055–1065.

Chiew AL, Reith DM, Pomerleau AC et al. Updated guidelines for the management of paracetamol poisoning in Australia and New Zealand. Medical Journal of Australia 2019; 212(4):175–183.

O'Grady JG. Acute liver failure. Postgraduate Medical Journal 2005; 81:148–154.

Prescott LF, Illingworth RN, Critchley JA. Intravenous N-acetylcysteine: the treatment of choice for paracetamol poisoning. British Medical Journal 1979; 2:1097.

Rumack BH, Bateman DH. Acetaminophen and acetylcysteine dose and duration: past, present and future. Clinical Toxicology 2012; 50:91–98.

Rumack BH, Matthew H. Acetaminophen poisoning and toxicity. Pediatrics 1975; 55:871–876.

3.61 PARACETAMOL: MODIFIED-RELEASE FORMULATIONS

Paracetamol, N-acetyl-p-aminophenol (APAP)

See also Chapter 3.60: Paracetamol: Immediate-release preparations (acute overdose), Chapter 3.62: Paracetamol: Repeated supratherapeutic ingestion.

Modified-release tablets contain immediate- and delayed-release paracetamol formulations, with a higher total dose per tablet than standard immediate-release preparations. Due to the different pharmacokinetic profile, standard risk-assessment is not applicable and modification of the treatment algorithm for immediate-release preparations is required.

RISK ASSESSMENT
- Risk assessment for the development of hepatotoxicity is not clearly defined and a conservative approach is recommended.

- The threshold dose for the development of toxicity is considered to be the same as for acute ingestions of immediate-release paracetamol preparations (≥200 mg/kg or ≥10 g).
- Initial management differs compared to the approach for immediate-release preparations:
  — **Above the threshold dose**
    – N-acetylcysteine is started immediately and a full course is completed.
    – Serial paracetamol levels 4 and 8 hours post ingestion determine the requirement for an increased dose of N-acetylcysteine or further decontamination with activated charcoal.
  — **Below the threshold dose**
    – Serial paracetamol levels 4 and 8 hours post ingestion determine the requirement for antidotal therapy.
- Prolonged and erratic absorption of modified-release paracetamol formulations may require extended duration of antidotal therapy well beyond the standard 20-hour protocol.
- Patients with a massive ingestion (e.g. ≥30 g or ≥500 mg/kg) and a paracetamol level > double the nomogram line should receive an increased dose of N-acetylcysteine.
- N-acetylcysteine is a safe and effective antidote. If there is any confusion regarding interpretation of paracetamol levels and a perceived risk of hepatotoxicity, it is always justified to initiate therapy with N-acetylcysteine and monitor the patient's progress.
- **Children:** in the absence of definitive data to guide the risk assessment, ingestions of modified-release paracetamol in children should be assessed and managed as for adults.

Toxic mechanism
See Chapter 3.60: Paracetamol: Immediate-release preparations (acute overdose).

Toxicokinetics
Australian modified-release preparations consist of 665 mg of paracetamol, of which 69% is slow-release and 31% immediate-release, arranged in a bilayer tablet. This formulation results in a prolonged absorption phase compared to standard preparations. Peak levels usually occur within 2–3 hours of ingestion but may be delayed up to 20 hours following overdose. Metabolism and elimination are as described in **Chapter 3.60: Paracetamol: Immediate-release preparations (acute overdose).**

CLINICAL FEATURES
Patients who develop toxicity following overdose manifest the clinical features of paracetamol toxicity as described in **Table 3.60.1.** Timely treatment with N-acetylcysteine prevents or minimises subsequent hepatotoxicity.

INVESTIGATIONS
Screening tests in deliberate self-poisoning
- 12-lead ECG and BGL. An untimed 'screening' paracetamol level is not useful following deliberate self-poisoning with modified-release paracetamol and should be replaced by specific timed levels (see below).

Specific investigations (see Figure 3.60.2)

- A single timed paracetamol level is insufficient to determine the risk of hepatoxicity following overdose of modified-release preparations.
  - If the time of ingestion is known, a timed paracetamol level is taken at least 4 hours after ingestion and repeated 4 hours later.
  - If the time of ingestion is unknown, a biochemical risk assessment (negative paracetamol level and ALT ≤50 U/L) is required to exclude the risk of hepatotoxicity.
- In all cases treated with N-acetylcysteine, paracetamol and ALT levels are repeated shortly before completion of the infusion to determine the requirement for ongoing therapy.
- Hepatic transaminases, coagulation studies, blood glucose, platelet count, renal function and acid–base status are useful to monitor clinical status and prognosis of established hepatotoxicity.

MANAGEMENT

Resuscitation, supportive care and monitoring

- Resuscitation is required only for rare instances of coma due to massive acute ingestion and for delayed presentation with established hepatic failure. In such cases, urgent attention to airway, breathing and circulation, plus correction of hypoglycaemia, are required.
- General supportive care and monitoring measures are indicated, as outlined in **Chapter 1.4: Supportive care and monitoring**.
- A management flow chart for acute modified-release paracetamol ingestion exposure with known time of ingestion is shown in **Figure 3.61.1**.

Decontamination

- Activated charcoal should be given to all patients presenting with potentially toxic overdose of modified-release paracetamol who present within 4 hours.
- Patients with a massive ingestion (e.g. ≥30 g or ≥500 mg/kg) may benefit from activated charcoal beyond 4 hours, or from multiple doses.

Enhanced elimination

- Not routinely indicated.

Antidotes

- Start N-acetylcysteine immediately if the history suggests ingestion of ≥200 mg/kg or ≥10 g, or the dose is unknown.
- The full course of N-acetylcysteine is completed regardless of the paracetamol levels.
- Paracetamol and ALT levels are performed shortly before completion of the 20-hour infusion. N-acetylcysteine is continued if:
  - paracetamol ≥10 mg/L (≥66 micromol/L)
  - ALT >50 U/L (or increasing if baseline >50 U/L).
- N-acetylcysteine is ceased when the following criteria are met:
  - paracetamol <10 mg/L
  - ALT is decreasing
  - INR <2
  - patient is clinically well.

FIGURE: 3.61.1 Management flow chart for ingestion of modified-release paracetamol preparations

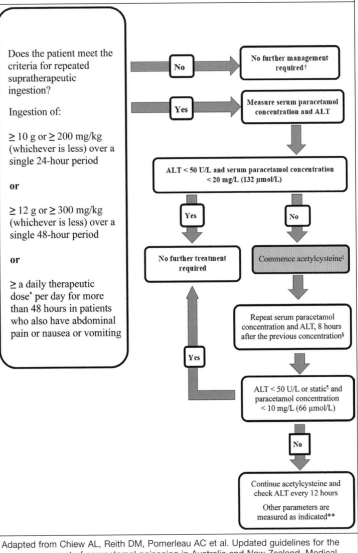

Does the patient meet the criteria for repeated supratherapeutic ingestion?

Ingestion of:

≥ 10 g or ≥ 200 mg/kg (whichever is less) over a single 24-hour period

or

≥ 12 g or ≥ 300 mg/kg (whichever is less) over a single 48-hour period

or

≥ a daily therapeutic dose* per day for more than 48 hours in patients who also have abdominal pain or nausea or vomiting

No → No further management required†

Yes → Measure serum paracetamol concentration and ALT

↓

ALT < 50 U/L and serum paracetamol concentration < 20 mg/L (132 µmol/L)

Yes → No further treatment required

No → Commence acetylcysteine‡

↓

Repeat serum paracetamol concentration and ALT, 8 hours after the previous concentration§

↓

ALT < 50 U/L or static¶ and paracetamol concentration < 10 mg/L (66 µmol/L)

Yes → (No further treatment required)

No ↓

Continue acetylcysteine and check ALT every 12 hours

Other parameters are measured as indicated**

Adapted from Chiew AL, Reith DM, Pomerleau AC et al. Updated guidelines for the management of paracetamol poisoning in Australia and New Zealand. Medical Journal of Australia 2019; 212(4):175–183.

- See **Chapter 4.17: N-acetylcysteine** for full details on dosing and administration of N-acetylcysteine.

DISPOSITION AND FOLLOW-UP
- Patients with clear evidence of resolving hepatotoxicity (undetectable paracetamol, falling ALT, INR <2 and who are clinically well) do not require further N-acetylcysteine treatment and are fit for medical discharge.
- Patients with fulminant hepatic failure require management in an intensive care unit and consideration for referral to a liver transplant service (see **Chapter 3.60: Paracetamol: Immediate-release preparations (acute overdose)** for referral criteria).

HANDY TIP
- Consider the possibility of ingestion of modified-release preparations of paracetamol where history suggests the ingestion of multiples of 12 tablets or large packets containing 96 or 192 tablets.

PITFALLS
- Failure to recognise ingestion of a modified-release formulation.
- Failure to commence and complete a full course of N-acetylcysteine based on history of ingested dose.
- Failure to check paracetamol units. Different units are used to report paracetamol levels (mg/L and micromol/L). Incorrect plotting of the level may lead to a potentially lethal error.

CONTROVERSY
- Requirement for completion of the 20-hour infusion for all patients who present within 8 hours, have ingested more than 200 mg/kg or 10 g but have serial paracetamol levels below the nomogram treatment line.

Presentations
Paracetamol controlled-release tablets 665 mg (96, 192)

References

Chiew A, Day P, Salonikas C et al. The comparative pharmacokinetics of modified-release and immediate-release paracetamol in a simulated overdose model. Emergency Medicine Australasia 2010; 22:548–555.

Chiew AL, Reith DM, Pomerleau AC et al. Updated guidelines for the management of paracetamol poisoning in Australia and New Zealand. Medical Journal of Australia 2019; 212(4):175–183.

Roberts DM, Buckley NA. Prolonged absorption and delayed peak paracetamol concentration following poisoning with extended-release formulation. Medical Journal of Australia 2008; 188:310–311.

3.62 PARACETAMOL: REPEATED SUPRATHERAPEUTIC INGESTION

Paracetamol, N-acetyl-p-aminophenol (APAP)

See also Chapter 3.60: Paracetamol: Immediate-release preparations (acute overdose), Chapter 3.61: Paracetamol: Modified-release formulations.

Repeated supratherapeutic ingestion refers to the administration of paracetamol in excess of recommended daily dosing (>4 g/day in adults or >60 mg/kg/day in children). In adults, it usually occurs in the context of self-medication for pain conditions. In children, it is usually a therapeutic error. Repeated supratherapeutic ingestion is responsible for all deaths related to paracetamol in children less than 6 years of age and up to 15% of those in adults. Standard nomograms do not apply – the decision to treat is based on a biochemical risk assessment (serum paracetamol and hepatic aminotransferase levels).

RISK ASSESSMENT

- The modified Rumack–Matthew nomogram is not applicable in this setting.
- Risk assessment is based on dose history and biochemical testing.
- Patients are referred for biochemical risk assessment if there is ingestion of:
  - ≥**10 g or ≥200 mg/kg** (whichever is less) over a single 24-hour period
  - ≥**12 g or ≥300 mg/kg** (whichever is less) over a single 48-hour period
  - ≥**daily therapeutic dose (4 g/day or 60 mg/kg/day)** for more than 48 hours with associated nausea, vomiting or abdominal pain.
- Patients with significant pre-existing conditions (nutritional, metabolic, genetic) may develop hepatotoxicity even with therapeutic dosing.
- Biochemical risk assessment is based on an untimed serum paracetamol level and ALT at presentation:
  - ALT <50 U/L and paracetamol level <20 mg/L (<132 micromol/L)
    - Low risk for developing significant hepatotoxicity.
    - Further investigation for paracetamol hepatotoxicity is not required.
    - Antidotal therapy with N-acetylcysteine is not indicated.
  - ALT ≥50 U/L or paracetamol level ≥20 mg/L (≥132 micromol/L)
    - Patients at higher risk of developing significant hepatotoxicity.
    - Commence N-acetylcysteine pending further evaluation.
- N-acetylcysteine is a safe and effective antidote. If there is any confusion regarding interpretation of paracetamol levels and a perceived risk of hepatotoxicity, it is always justified to initiate therapy with N-acetylcysteine and monitor the patient's progress.
- **Children:** patients <6 years of age are most at risk of hepatotoxicity from repeated supratherapeutic dosing. Biochemical risk assessment is required if repeated supratherapeutic ingestion is considered possible.

Toxic mechanism

Supratherapeutic doses of paracetamol can result in depletion of hepatic glutathione stores. Once glutathione levels are depleted to below 30% of normal, the same toxicity is observed as following acute paracetamol overdose.

Toxicokinetics

See **Chapter 3.60: Paracetamol: Immediate-release preparations (acute overdose)**.

CLINICAL FEATURES

- Patients who develop hepatic injury following supratherapeutic paracetamol overdose manifest the same clinical features as acute paracetamol poisoning (see **Table 3.60.1**).

INVESTIGATIONS

- Serum paracetamol level and ALT
  - Determine the risk of hepatotoxicity and requirement for N-acetylcysteine.
- Liver function tests, urea and electrolytes, coagulation studies, acid–base status and blood glucose
  - Indicated following initial biochemical risk assessment if hepatotoxicity is confirmed.
  - Monitor the clinical course of those patients with hepatic injury as detailed in **Chapter 3.60: Paracetamol: Immediate-release preparations (acute overdose)**.

MANAGEMENT

Resuscitation, supportive care and monitoring

- Resuscitation is required only in the rare instances of coma due to delayed presentation with established hepatic failure. In such cases, urgent attention to airway, breathing and circulation, plus correction of hypoglycaemia, is required.
- General supportive care and monitoring measures are indicated, as outlined in **Chapter 1.4: Supportive care and monitoring**. A management flow chart for repeated therapeutic ingestion of paracetamol is shown in **Figure 3.62.1**.

Decontamination

- Gastrointestinal decontamination is not indicated.

Enhanced elimination

- Not clinically useful.

Antidotes

- N-acetylcysteine is administered immediately if there are clinical features suggestive of hepatotoxicity and a history of repeated supratherapeutic ingestion of paracetamol.
- In asymptomatic patients, the biochemical risk assessment determines the requirement for N-acetylcysteine (see **Figure 3.62.1**).
- If N-acetylcysteine is started, serum ALT and paracetamol levels are repeated 8 hours after the initial levels. A rise in hepatic transaminase levels (e.g. increasing >50% over 8 hours) is consistent with evolving paracetamol hepatotoxicity (but does not

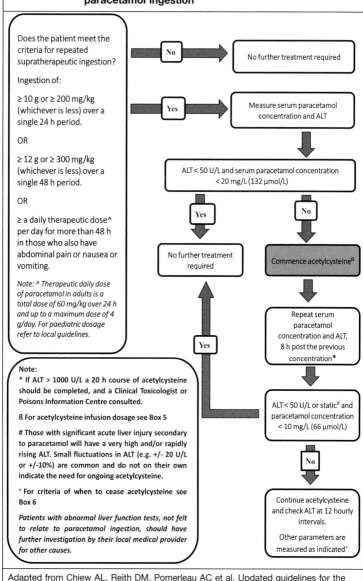

FIGURE 3.62.1 Management flow chart for repeated supratherapeutic paracetamol ingestion

Does the patient meet the criteria for repeated supratherapeutic ingestion?

Ingestion of:

≥ 10 g or ≥ 200 mg/kg (whichever is less) over a single 24 h period.

OR

≥ 12 g or ≥ 300 mg/kg (whichever is less) over a single 48 h period.

OR

≥ a daily therapeutic dose^ per day for more than 48 h in those who also have abdominal pain or nausea or vomiting.

Note: ^ Therapeutic daily dose of paracetamol in adults is a total dose of 60 mg/kg over 24 h and up to a maximum dose of 4 g/day. For paediatric dosage refer to local guidelines.

No → No further treatment required

Yes → Measure serum paracetamol concentration and ALT

ALT < 50 U/L and serum paracetamol concentration < 20 mg/L (132 µmol/L)

Yes → No further treatment required

No → Commence acetylcysteine^ß

Repeat serum paracetamol concentration and ALT, 8 h post the previous concentration*

ALT < 50 U/L or static^# and paracetamol concentration < 10 mg/L (66 µmol/L)

Yes ↑

No → Continue acetylcysteine and check ALT at 12 hourly intervals.

Other parameters are measured as indicated^+

Note:
* If ALT > 1000 U/L a 20 h course of acetylcysteine should be completed, and a Clinical Toxicologist or Poisons Information Centre consulted.

ß For acetylcysteine infusion dosage see Box 5

Those with significant acute liver injury secondary to paracetamol will have a very high and/or rapidly rising ALT. Small fluctuations in ALT (e.g. +/- 20 U/L or +/-10%) are common and do not on their own indicate the need for ongoing acetylcysteine.

+ For criteria of when to cease acetylcysteine see Box 6

Patients with abnormal liver function tests, not felt to relate to paracetamol ingestion, should have further investigation by their local medical provider for other causes.

Adapted from Chiew AL, Reith DM, Pomerleau AC et al. Updated guidelines for the management of paracetamol poisoning in Australia and New Zealand. Medical Journal of Australia 2019; 212(4):175–183.

confirm it) and justifies continuation of N-acetylcysteine until the patient is clinically well and the ALT is falling.

DISPOSITION AND FOLLOW-UP
- Patients with clear evidence of resolving hepatotoxicity (undetectable paracetamol, falling ALT, INR <2 and who are clinically well) do not require further N-acetylcysteine treatment and are fit for medical discharge.
- Patients with fulminant hepatic failure require management in an intensive care unit and referral to a liver transplant service (see **Chapter 3.60: Paracetamol: Immediate-release preparations (acute overdose)** for referral criteria).

HANDY TIPS
- Obtain a full analgesic-use history in all patients presenting with pain conditions.
- Elevation of ALT may be related to other pathologies. In the absence of comparative previous values, N-acetylcysteine is started and continued until it is demonstrated that the ALT is not rising rapidly.

PITFALL
- Failure to consider repeated supratherapeutic ingestion of paracetamol as a cause for hepatotoxicity.

References

Chiew AL, Reith DM, Pomerleau AC et al. Updated guidelines for the management of paracetamol poisoning in Australia and New Zealand. Medical Journal of Australia 2019; 212(4):175–183.

Daly FSS, O'Malley GF, Heard K et al. Prospective evaluation of repeated supratherapeutic acetaminophen (paracetamol) ingestion. Annals of Emergency Medicine 2004; 44(4):393–398.

Dart RC, Erdman AR, Olson KR et al. Acetaminophen poisoning: an evidence-based consensus guideline for out-of-hospital management. Clinical Toxicology 2006; 44:1–18.

3.63 PARAQUAT

Paraquat is a closely regulated herbicide that is highly lethal in overdose. Ingestion of even small amounts can cause corrosive gastrointestinal injury, with rapid onset of fulminant multi-organ failure and death. Severe progressive pulmonary fibrosis is described in patients who survive the initial ingestion. Immediate decontamination is a vital early intervention that may decrease absorption and modify lethal progression.

RISK ASSESSMENT
- Survival after acute paraquat poisoning is related to the dose ingested (see **Table 3.63.1**). This is determined by the

TABLE 3.63.1 Dose-related risk assessment: paraquat

Dose	Effect
<30 mg/kg <10 mL of 20% solution in a 70-kg patient	Corrosive gastrointestinal injury and multi-organ effects Mortality up to 20%
30–150 mg/kg 10–50 mL of 20% solution in a 70-kg patient	Multi-organ failure develops over 2–6 days Pulmonary fibrosis may be prominent Mortality >50%
>150 mg/kg >50 mL of 20% solution in a 70-kg patient	Rapidly progressive respiratory failure, metabolic acidosis and cardiogenic shock Mortality approaches 100%, and death can occur within hours

circumstances of the poisoning (intentional versus accidental) and the concentration of the formulation involved.
— Deliberate self-poisoning with concentrated formulations (20% solution) is invariably fatal.
— Accidental ingestions have better survival rates but death has been reported after unintentional ingestion of <10 mL of paraquat solution.
— Time-critical interventions that may improve prognosis are immediate decontamination and early institution of haemodialysis.
● Inhalational exposures are unlikely to cause significant intoxication.
● Dermal exposure may cause toxicity if there is prolonged skin contact.
● Risk assessment can be refined using urinary and plasma paraquat assays (see **Investigations**).
● **Children:** ingestion of a teaspoonful (5 mL) may be fatal.

Toxic mechanism

Paraquat is a water-soluble quaternary bipyridyl cation. It is directly corrosive to tissues and once it enters cells produces reactive oxygen radicals by redox cycling and depletion of superoxide dismutase. Oxygen free radicals cause lipid peroxidation, with cytotoxic damage to lipid cell membranes, a pronounced inflammatory response and cell death.

Toxicokinetics

Gastrointestinal absorption is rapid but incomplete and the presence of food in the stomach may decrease absorption further. Bioavailability increases with dose and peak blood levels occur within 2–4 hours. It is rapidly distributed to highly vascular tissues such as kidney, liver, lungs, heart and skeletal muscle, and is actively transported into pneumocytes against a concentration gradient. Paraquat is not metabolised and is predominantly excreted by the kidneys.

CLINICAL FEATURES

- Oral burns, central tongue ulceration ('paraquat tongue') and gastrointestinal symptoms are characteristic and occur commonly after ingestion. Corrosive injury may be severe.
- Following large ingestions, multi-system organ failure with severe lactic acidosis, respiratory failure and cardiovascular collapse will lead to death within hours.
- Following accidental ingestion, systemic toxicity may not be evident initially but can develop and progress over 24–48 hours, resulting in multi-organ effects including renal failure and hepatic injury.
- The development of respiratory symptoms at any stage is a significant feature and will likely progress to irreversible pulmonary fibrosis and death.
- A peripheral burning sensation is described in a number of patients and is associated with higher plasma levels and significantly increased mortality.

INVESTIGATIONS

Screening tests in deliberate self-poisoning

- 12-lead ECG, BGL and paracetamol level

Specific investigations

- Lactate and blood gas
  - Lactate >4.4 mmol/L is associated with fatal outcome.
- FBC, EUC, liver function tests
- Chest X-ray
  - Detect lung injury and pulmonary fibrosis.
- Urine paraquat
  - The dithionite spot test is a qualitative colorimetric assay that can be performed on urine by most laboratories.
  - It is most reliable for the presence of paraquat if performed between 6 and 12 hours after ingestion, but may be positive earlier and remain positive for several days following large ingestions.
  - Sodium dithionite reduces paraquat in alkaline solution to a blue-coloured ion. The reaction occurs within 1 minute.
  - A positive test demonstrates that paraquat has been systemically absorbed and the depth of colour gives a semi-quantitative indication of the dose ingested and likely prognosis.
- Plasma paraquat levels (high-performance liquid chromatography)
  - Not readily available within a clinically useful time frame.
  - A number of nomograms attempt to correlate survival with measured paraquat level, but all tend to underestimate mortality (see Senarathna et al. in **References**).
    - Note: The dithionite test can also be performed on plasma and a positive test is associated with mortality.

Resuscitation, supportive care and monitoring

- Paraquat intoxication is a time-critical emergency and patients are managed in an area equipped for cardiorespiratory monitoring and resuscitation.
- Immediate gastrointestinal decontamination takes priority over resuscitation following deliberate or accidental ingestion of paraquat and should be instituted as soon as possible (see **Decontamination**).
- Immediate management of airway, breathing and circulation is rarely required. However, stridor, dysphagia and dysphonia indicate airway injury and potential imminent airway compromise.
- Patients who arrive acutely unwell after deliberate self-poisoning with large ingestions have a lethal prognosis. Decisions regarding intubation or intensive care management should be made in recognition of the expected outcome.
- Supplemental oxygen carries the risk of exacerbating pulmonary and systemic oxidative injury. If required, oxygen administration is targeted to maintain an oxygen saturation of around 90%.
- Supportive care measures are indicated, as outlined in **Chapter 1.4: Supportive care and monitoring**. This may include an early decision to provide palliative care for severely poisoned patients.

Decontamination

- At the scene, administer food or soil to adsorb paraquat and reduce gastrointestinal absorption.
- Administer 50 g of activated charcoal (1 g/kg in children) PO immediately on arrival at hospital.
  - Note: Fuller's earth is a sterilised clay-soil adsorbent that was historically recommended but is now not readily available and offers no advantage over activated charcoal.

Enhanced elimination

- Haemodialysis or haemoperfusion is considered with the greatest urgency in patients who have ingested a dose likely to cause systemic toxicity. The threshold dose is difficult to quantify reliably but can be as little as a mouthful. It is not likely to be indicated for minor exposures (splashes, licks or tastes) and will not prevent fatal outcome following large deliberate self-poisoning ingestions.
- The decision to initiate haemodialysis must be made before the onset of significant clinical features and should not wait for confirmatory laboratory tests or paraquat assays.
- Haemodialysis and haemoperfusion may improve clearance of paraquat if performed early. The time beyond which dialysis is of benefit (due to distribution of paraquat to tissues) is uncertain. Maximal benefit is attained if performed within 2 hours but this intervention may be considered up to 4 hours post ingestion unless signs of severe toxicity are already evident.

Antidotes
- Many adjunctive therapies have been proposed in an attempt to modify acute oxidative and inflammatory injury and decrease the risk of progressive pulmonary fibrosis. Studies to date using N-acetylcysteine, corticosteroids, salicylic acid, vitamins C and E and cyclophosphamide are hypothesis-generating and inconclusive.
- Current recommendations include:
  - N-acetylcysteine at the same dosing regimen as for paracetamol toxicity (see **Chapter 4.17: N-acetylcysteine**).
- High-dose steroid therapy: dexamethasone 8 mg tds initially IV then PO for up to 4 weeks or pulse methylprednisolone with or without a tapering regimen.

DISPOSITION AND FOLLOW-UP
- Patients who are clinically well 12 hours after exposure, without oral burns and with a negative urine dithionite test at least 6 hours after ingestion, do not require further medical management and may be discharged.
- Symptomatic patients should be managed in an intensive care setting.
- Patients with a history of massive ingestion (e.g. >100 mL of 20% paraquat) and early clinical features of intoxication have a hopeless prognosis and decisions regarding intensive care management versus palliation should be made in recognition of the expected outcome.

HANDY TIP
- Immediate pre-hospital gastrointestinal decontamination with anything that is available (food, soil, charcoal) may be life-saving
- Diquat is a herbicide with a similar structure to paraquat. There are less published data regarding diquat toxicity but the risk assessment and management strategies are similar to those for paraquat.

PITFALL
- Routine administration of supplemental oxygen in the absence of hypoxia may exacerbate pulmonary injury.

CONTROVERSIES
- The efficacy of and indications for haemodialysis and the time beyond which it is unlikely to provide any benefit.
- The optimum dose and duration of therapy with steroids and other anti-inflammatory agents is not definitively established.
- The predictive value of the qualitative urinary dithionite test.

Presentations
Paraquat alone: 6.4%, 20%, 24%, 25% w/v
Paraquat concentrate 36% has been discontinued but may still be accessible.
Paraquat–diquat mixtures: 1.25% and 1.25%, 2.5% and 2.5%, 10% and 5%, 10% and 10%, 12.5% and 7.5%, 13.5% and 11.5%
Most products contain colouring (blue-green or red-brown) and stenching agents.

References

Dinis-Oliveira PJ, Duarte JA, Sanchez-Navarro A et al. Paraquat poisonings: mechanisms of lung toxicity, clinical features and treatment. Critical Reviews in Toxicology 2008; 38:13–71.

Eddleston M, Wilks MF, Buckley NA. Prospects for treatment of paraquat-induced lung fibrosis with immunosuppressive drugs and the need for better prediction of outcome: a systematic review. Quarterly Journal of Medicine 2003; 96(11):809–824.

Gao J, Feng S, Wang J et al. Prolonged methylprednisolone therapy after the pulse treatment for patients with moderate-to-severe paraquat poisoning: a retrospective analysis. Medicine 2017; 96(25):e7244.

Gawarammana IB, Buckley NA. Medical management of paraquat ingestion. British Journal of Pharmacology 2011; 5:745–757.

Gawarammana I, Buckley NA, Mohamed F et al. High-dose immunosuppression to prevent death after paraquat self-poisoning – a randomised controlled trial. Clinical Toxicology 2018; 56(7):633–639.

Gawarammana IB, Dawson AH. Peripheral burning sensation: a novel clinical marker of poor prognosis and higher plasma-paraquat concentrations in paraquat poisoning. Clinical Toxicology 2010; 48(4):347–349.

Li S, Zhao D, Li Y et al. Arterial lactate in predicting mortality after paraquat poisoning: a meta-analysis. Medicine 2018; 97(34):e11751.

Senarathna L, Eddleston M, Wilks MF. Prediction of outcome after paraquat poisoning by measurement of the plasma paraquat concentration. Quarterly Journal of Medicine 2009; 102:251–259.

3.64 PHENOTHIAZINES AND BUTYROPHENONES (ANTIPSYCHOTIC AGENTS)

Phenothiazines: Chlorpromazine, Fluphenazine, Pericyazine, Pipotiazine, Prochlorperazine, Thioridazine, Trifluoperazine

Butyrophenones: Droperidol, Haloperidol

These first-generation (typical) antipsychotic agents cause CNS depression, extrapyramidal effects, orthostatic hypotension and anticholinergic toxicity in overdose. Droperidol and haloperidol are commonly used parenteral agents for management of significant behavioural disturbances.

RISK ASSESSMENT

- The toxic dose is not clearly established for all agents. Patients who are drug-naïve are more likely to manifest symptoms at lower doses.
- Extrapyramidal effects are more frequent with prochlorperazine and haloperidol.
- All agents can cause QT prolongation but development of torsades de pointes is uncommon. Thioridazine, which causes QRS and QT prolongation and higher rates of ventricular dysrhythmias, is no longer marketed.
- Seizures are uncommon.
- **Children:** ingestion of even 1 tablet warrants medical assessment. Extrapyramidal effects may develop up to 72 hours post ingestion.

Toxic mechanism

The major therapeutic action of the phenothiazines is mediated via central dopamine (D_2) antagonism. Their adverse effects are secondary to blockade at multiple other receptors, including histamine (H_1), $GABA_A$, muscarinic (M_1), α_1- and α_2-adrenergic and serotonergic (5-HT) receptors. Cardiotoxicity is secondary to sodium and potassium channel blocking effects. The butyrophenones are a separate class of drug but have similar pharmacological and pharmacokinetic properties.

Toxicokinetics

The antipsychotics are rapidly absorbed following oral administration at therapeutic doses and undergo extensive first-pass metabolism with variable bioavailability. Absorption may be slow and erratic following overdose. Antipsychotics are lipid soluble with large volumes of distribution. They undergo extensive hepatic metabolism by cytochrome P450 enzymes. Many have active metabolites and prolonged elimination half-lives.

CLINICAL FEATURES

- Onset of clinical features of intoxication occurs within 2–4 hours of ingestion.
- Sedation, ataxia, orthostatic hypotension and tachycardia are common.
- Fluctuating mental status with intermittent agitated delirium may occur with moderate doses and usually lasts <24 hours.
- Urinary retention is common.
- Coma is uncommon but occasionally occurs following large ingestions.
- Anticholinergic delirium may complicate recovery from coma.
- QT prolongation and torsades de pointes were characteristic of thioridazine overdose but are unlikely to occur with other agents.
- Extrapyramidal effects can be prolonged.

INVESTIGATIONS

Screening tests in deliberate self-poisoning
- 12-lead ECG, BGL and paracetamol level

Specific investigations
- An ECG should be performed on presentation and at 6 hours post ingestion to detect QRS or QT interval prolongation. Further ECGs are only necessary if an abnormality is noted.

MANAGEMENT

Resuscitation, supportive care and monitoring
- Attention to airway, breathing and circulation are paramount. These priorities are managed along conventional lines, as outlined in **Chapter 1.2: Resuscitation**.
- Manage anticholinergic delirium, as outlined in **Chapter 2.6: Anticholinergic toxicity**.
- Monitor for urinary retention with serial bladder scans and insert an indwelling urinary catheter if required.
- General supportive care measures are indicated, as outlined in **Chapter 1.4: Supportive care and monitoring**.

Decontamination
- Activated charcoal is not indicated for patients without coma, as a good outcome is expected with supportive care.

Enhanced elimination
- Not clinically useful.

Antidotes
- Benztropine or benzodiazepine administration is considered in patients with significant extrapyramidal effects.

DISPOSITION AND FOLLOW-UP
- Children are referred for hospital assessment following suspected accidental ingestion of any amount.
- Patients who are clinically well with normal 12-lead ECG (or static pre-existing changes) at 6 hours post ingestion are fit for medical discharge.
- Patients requiring intubation and ventilation are admitted to intensive care. Anticholinergic delirium may predominate as coma resolves, influencing decisions regarding safe extubation.

HANDY TIPS
- Hypotension is usually secondary to peripheral vasodilatation and responds well to infusion of IV crystalloid solution.
- Significant cardiotoxicity is not likely with phenothiazine overdose now that thioridazine is no longer available.
- Inadvertent overdose of depot formulations may result in delayed onset of toxic features.

References
Isbister GK, Balit CR, Kilham HA. Antipsychotic poisoning in young children: a systematic review. Drug Safety 2005; 26(11):1029–1044.

James LP, Abel K, Wilkinson J et al. Phenothiazine, butyrophenone, and other psychotropic medication poisonings in children and adolescents. Clinical Toxicology 2000; 38(6):615–623.

Strachan EM, Kelly CA, Bateman DN. Electrocardiographic and cardiovascular changes in thioridazine and chlorpromazine poisoning. European Journal of Clinical Pharmacology 2004; 60:541–545.

3.65 PHENYTOIN

Phenytoin causes dose-related neurotoxicity, which can occur following acute overdose or due to accumulation in therapeutic dosing. The most significant clinical feature is ataxia, which may require prolonged in-patient management.

RISK ASSESSMENT
- Acute oral overdose results in dose-dependent CNS effects, primarily cerebellar in nature (see **Table 3.65.1**).
- Coma and seizures are rare, even with massive doses.
- Cardiovascular toxicity is not a feature of oral phenytoin ingestion but is reported after rapid intravenous infusion of phenytoin or its water-soluble prodrug fosphenytoin.
- **Children:** accidental ingestion does not require hospital evaluation unless symptoms develop. A dose of >20 mg/kg may cause features of ataxia or drowsiness.

TABLE 3.65.1   Dose-related risk assessment: phenytoin overdose

Dose	Effect
10–15 mg/kg	Standard therapeutic loading dose
>20 mg/kg	Ataxia, dysarthria and nystagmus
>100 mg/kg	Potential for coma and seizures

Toxic mechanism

The primary effect of phenytoin is on the CNS. Phenytoin blocks active sodium channels, increasing the threshold for depolarisation of neuronal tissue and inhibiting the propagation of high-frequency action potentials. In cardiac tissue, phenytoin does not cause QRS widening – it shortens the action potential and increases the refractory period between impulses, leading to the possibility of bradycardia and AV nodal blockade.

Toxicokinetics

Absorption is slow and variable following oral overdose, and peak serum levels may be delayed greater than 48 hours. It is a small molecule with a volume of distribution of 0.6 L/kg and high protein binding (90%). Phenytoin undergoes hepatic hydroxylation by CYP2C9 to form an inactive metabolite. Metabolism is saturable (Michaelis–Menten or zero-order kinetics) and in therapeutic dosing, serum levels and elimination half-life can increase dramatically with small changes in daily dose. Elimination half-lives in poisoned patients may vary greatly due to genetic polymorphism of CYP2C9 and inter-individual variation in elimination rates.

CLINICAL FEATURES

- Neurological toxicity develops slowly over hours following acute overdose. Clinical features of toxicity include nystagmus, dysarthria, ataxia, tremor, dystonia, movement disorders, agitation and sedation.
- Neurological symptoms can persist for several days as serum levels slowly fall.
- Seizures and coma occur rarely and only after massive overdose.
- Prolonged or permanent cerebellar injury is reported after severe intoxication.
- Chronic toxicity presents with gradual onset of ataxia, dysarthria and nystagmus.
- Rapid IV administration of phenytoin is associated with hypotension, bradycardia, ventricular arrhythmias and asystole, in part caused by direct cardiovascular toxicity of the propylene glycol diluent. Fosphenytoin is the water-soluble prodrug of phenytoin, and rapid administration of this agent can also cause cardiovascular toxicity in the absence of propylene glycol.

INVESTIGATIONS

Screening tests in deliberate self-poisoning
- 12-lead ECG, BGL and paracetamol level

Specific investigations
- Serum phenytoin levels
  - Confirm the diagnosis.
  - Correlate with clinical toxicity:
    - Nystagmus is associated with levels >20 mg/L (80 micromol/L).

- Severe ataxia is associated with levels of 30–40 mg/L (120–160 micromol/L).
- Coma is associated with levels >50 mg/L (200 micromol/L).
— Serial phenytoin levels are required in severe toxicity (coma or incapacitating ataxia) to assess response to treatment (see **Enhanced elimination**).

MANAGEMENT

Resuscitation, supportive care and monitoring
- Attention to airway, breathing and circulation are paramount. These priorities are managed along conventional lines, as outlined in **Chapter 1.2: Resuscitation**.
- General supportive care as outlined in **Chapter 1.4: Supportive care and monitoring** ensures a good outcome in the majority of patients.
- Patients are at risk of falls due to ataxia, and ambulation should be supervised while the patient is symptomatic.
- ECG monitoring is not indicated following oral phenytoin overdose or for chronic phenytoin toxicity.

Decontamination
- Give activated charcoal to all cooperative patients following acute phenytoin overdose to reduce drug absorption and length of hospital stay.

Enhanced elimination
- Multiple-dose activated charcoal enhances elimination and should be considered in the setting of prolonged toxicity following acute overdose or chronic poisoning.
- Haemodialysis has been used in cases of massive phenytoin overdose with significant and prolonged elevation in serum levels, particularly in the setting of coma or severe ataxia.

Antidotes
- None available.

DISPOSITION AND FOLLOW-UP
- Children may be observed at home following unintentional exposures. Hospital assessment is required if ataxia or drowsiness develops.
- Patients with nystagmus, ataxia or drowsiness are managed supportively in a ward environment.
- Patients are medically fit for discharge as soon as they are able to walk safely.

HANDY TIPS
- Consider the diagnosis of phenytoin toxicity in any patient on chronic therapy who presents with difficulty walking.
- It may take several days for phenytoin toxicity to resolve.
- Coma can occur in massive phenytoin overdose but other causes should be considered and excluded.

PITFALLS
- Failure to order a phenytoin level in the patient on chronic therapy who presents with ataxia or non-specific symptoms.

- Allowing a patient with phenytoin toxicity to fall during unsupervised attempts at mobilisation.

CONTROVERSY
- The threshold to institute haemodialysis is not clearly defined. The decision to institute this invasive technique is based on an individualised risk–benefit analysis (see **Enhanced elimination**).

Presentations
Phenytoin sodium 30 mg, 100 mg capsules (200)
Phenytoin 50 mg tablets (200)
Phenytoin 30 mg/5 mL suspension (500 mL)
Phenytoin sodium 100 mg/2 mL ampoules (contain propylene glycol diluent)
Phenytoin sodium 250 mg/5 mL ampoules (contain propylene glycol diluent)

References
Anseeuw K, Mowry JB, Burdmann EA et al. Extracorporeal treatment in phenytoin poisoning: systematic review and recommendations from the EXTRIP (Extracorporeal Treatments in Poisoning) workgroup. American Journal of Kidney Disease 2016; 67(2):187–197.

Chan BS, Sellors K, Chiew AL et al. Use of multi-dose activated charcoal in phenytoin toxicity secondary to genetic polymorphism. Clinical Toxicology 2015; 53(2):131–133.

Craig S. Phenytoin poisoning. Neurocritical Care 2005; 3(2):161–170.

Curtis DL, Piibe R, Ellenhorn MJ et al. Phenytoin toxicity: a review of 94 cases. Veterinary and Human Toxicology 1989; 31(92):164–165.

Jones AL, Proudfoot AT. Features and management of poisoning with modern drugs used to treat epilepsy. Quarterly Journal of Medicine 1998; 91:325–332.

Skinner CG, Chang AS, Matthew AR et al. Randomised controlled study on the use of multiple-dose activated charcoal in patients with supratherapeutic phenytoin levels. Clinical Toxicology 2012; 50:764–769.

Wyte CD, Berk WA. Severe oral phenytoin overdose does not cause cardiovascular morbidity. Annals of Emergency Medicine 1991; 20(5):510–512.

3.66 POTASSIUM CHLORIDE

Deliberate self-poisoning by ingestion of potassium chloride is rare but can result in life-threatening hyperkalaemia and cardiac arrest. The principal preparation of concern is slow-release potassium chloride, which is available in bottles of 100 tablets without prescription. A good outcome depends on early risk assessment, gastrointestinal decontamination and haemodialysis where indicated.

RISK ASSESSMENT
- Small ingestions are usually benign in patients with normal renal function.
- Ingestion of >2.5 mmol/kg of potassium can temporarily overwhelm the capacity of the kidneys to excrete potassium and lead to hyperkalaemia.
- The lethal dose of KCl tablets (each containing 8 mmol KCl) in an adult is not well defined.

- Massive ingestion ($>40 \times 600$-mg tablets) prompts early planning for haemodialysis in case severe hyperkalaemia cannot be controlled by other means.
- Patients with renal impairment or cardiac disease may be at higher risk.
- Abdominal X-ray assists risk assessment as slow-release potassium tablets are radio-opaque.
- **Children:** ingestion of three 600-mg KCl tablets may cause significant hyperkalaemia in a 10-kg toddler.

Toxic mechanism

Potassium is the principal intracellular cation. Hyperkalaemia impairs electrical conduction and membrane depolarisation in neuromuscular and cardiac tissue and can result in profound muscle weakness and cardiac arrest. Potassium salts have a direct irritant effect on the gastrointestinal mucosa.

Toxicokinetics

Potassium is rapidly absorbed from the small intestine and distributed primarily to the intracellular compartment. Potassium is excreted in the urine (90–95%), faeces and sweat. Hyperkalaemia develops when the rate of absorption from the gut exceeds the combined rates of redistribution to the intracellular compartment and urinary excretion.

CLINICAL FEATURES

- Following overdose of potassium salts, GI symptoms including abdominal pain, nausea and vomiting are common and occur early. Large GI fluid losses may cause significant hypovolaemia.
- As hyperkalaemia progresses (serum potassium 6–8 mmol/L), lethargy, confusion, weakness, paraesthesia and hyporeflexia develop.
- Paralysis and bradycardia herald cardiac arrest (serum potassium >8 mmol/L).

INVESTIGATIONS

Screening tests in deliberate self-poisoning
- 12-lead ECG, BGL and paracetamol level

Specific investigations
- Serial 12-lead ECGs demonstrate a progression of abnormalities as serum potassium rises: peaked T waves, PR prolongation, loss of P waves, QRS and QT prolongation with eventual progression to sine wave appearance and asystole.
- EUC
- Abdominal X-ray
  - Useful to confirm ingestion of slow-release potassium chloride tablets and can monitor response to decontamination.

MANAGEMENT

Resuscitation, supportive care and monitoring
- Attention to airway, breathing and circulation are paramount. These priorities are managed along conventional lines, as outlined in **Chapter 1.2: Resuscitation**.
- Haemodialysis is potentially life-saving following overdose of potassium salts and should be organised while temporary control of hyperkalaemia is achieved.
- Immediate treatment options for hyperkalaemia include:
  - calcium gluconate 10 mL 10% IV (0.15 mL/kg in children), repeated as indicated

- — insulin 10 U IV and glucose 50 mL 50% IV (insulin 0.1 U/kg and glucose 10 mL/kg 10% IV in children)
- — nebulised salbutamol 10–20 mg (in children: 2.5 mg if <5 years or 5 mg if >5 years)
- — sodium bicarbonate 50–100 mmol slow IV (1 mmol/kg in children) if acidosis is present.
- General supportive care measures including adequate intravenous fluids to maintain urine output are indicated, as outlined in **Chapter 1.4: Supportive care and monitoring**.

Decontamination
- Activated charcoal does not bind potassium chloride and is not indicated.
- Whole bowel irrigation (WBI) can hasten gastrointestinal transit of slow-release potassium chloride tablets. However, decontamination cannot be achieved rapidly enough to prevent lethal hyperkalaemia following large overdoses. Institution of WBI must never delay initiation of haemodialysis if it is required.

Enhanced elimination
- Haemodialysis is the definitive treatment of hyperkalaemia following massive potassium chloride overdose. Initiation of haemodialysis provides immediate control of hyperkalaemia. Haemodialysis must be started before hyperkalaemic cardiac arrest occurs.
- Early planning for haemodialysis is required, based on the initial risk assessment. Indications include:
  - — ingested dose >40 × 600-mg KCl tablets
  - — serum potassium >8.0 mmol/L
  - — rapidly rising serum potassium.
- Serum potassium is monitored closely during haemodialysis and after cessation to ensure that ongoing absorption does not result in recurrent hyperkalaemia.

Antidotes
- None.

DISPOSITION AND FOLLOW-UP
- Patients demonstrating toxicity or having ingested a toxic dose are managed in a critical care area with dialysis facilities.
- Patients are medically fit for discharge once serum potassium normalises on serial measurements.

HANDY TIPS
- Insertion of a haemodialysis catheter may not be required immediately on presentation as long as the serum potassium can be closely monitored in an intensive care setting, and it can be inserted promptly and haemodialysis initiated if the potassium rises to life-threatening levels.
- Cation exchange resins (calcium or sodium polysterene sulfonate) 20–50 g (0.5–1.0 g/kg in children) bind only 1 mmol of potassium per gram. They are not useful following massive slow-release potassium chloride overdose.

- Thresholds for initiation of haemodialysis and whole bowel irrigation.

Presentations
Potassium chloride 600 mg (8 mmol KCl) slow-release tablets (100)

Reference
Su M, Stork C, Ravuri S et al. Sustained-release potassium chloride overdose. Clinical Toxicology 2001; 39(6):641–648.

3.67 PREGABALIN

Pregabalin is prescribed for conditions including neuropathic pain, anxiety and mood disorders. It is increasingly used recreationally for its euphoric effects. The principal toxic effects in overdose are sedation and myoclonus, but coma and seizures can occur.

RISK ASSESSMENT
- Isolated ingestion of pregabalin is unlikely to cause severe toxicity.
- Co-ingestion of other CNS depressants (alcohol, opioids, benzodiazepines) is associated with a greater degree of sedation and is more likely to require intubation and ventilation.
- Seizures are uncommon but can occur at relatively low doses.
- Toxicity may be more significant or prolonged in the presence of renal dysfunction due to decreased clearance of the drug.
- **Children:** ingestions up to 450 mg in children <6 years of age are likely to cause only mild sedation. All symptomatic patients require hospital assessment.

Toxic mechanism
Pregabalin is a gabapentinoid (structural analogue of GABA) that binds to voltage-gated calcium channels in the CNS. Inhibition of calcium influx decreases release of the excitatory neurotransmitters glutamate, noradrenaline and substance P. Additional mechanisms of toxicity in overdose are not clearly defined.

Toxicokinetics
Pregabalin is rapidly and well absorbed, with peak levels occurring within 1–3 hours of ingestion. It is not protein bound, has a small volume of distribution and is excreted largely unchanged in the urine.

CLINICAL FEATURES
- Sedation and altered mental state may progress to coma. Duration of CNS depression in severe cases is usually between 24 and 48 hours.
- Seizures may occur and are generally brief.
- Myoclonus is common and may be misinterpreted as focal seizure activity.
- Nystagmus, ataxia and delirium may occur.

Screening tests in deliberate self-poisoning
- 12-lead ECG, BGL and paracetamol level

Specific investigations
- Pregabalin levels are not readily available and are not useful to guide management.

Resuscitation, supportive care and monitoring
- All patients are managed in an area equipped for cardiopulmonary monitoring and resuscitation.
- Attention to airway, breathing and circulation are paramount. These priorities are managed along conventional lines, as outlined in **Chapter 1.2: Resuscitation**.
- Seizures are managed with titrated intravenous doses of benzodiazepine.

Decontamination
- Activated charcoal is not routinely indicated as a good outcome is likely with supportive care.
- Activated charcoal should be given to all comatose patients following pregabalin overdose once the airway is protected by endotracheal intubation.

Enhanced elimination
- Haemodialysis effectively removes pregabalin but is not routinely indicated even in the presence of coma. It could be considered in cases of severe poisoning in patients with renal dysfunction to shorten the duration of toxicity.

Antidotes
- None available.

- Adult patients with deliberate self-poisoning are observed for 4 hours. If they remain clinically well without sedation, further medical management is not required.
- Patients with clinical features of toxicity can usually be managed in a ward environment for 12–24 hours. They are fit for medical discharge when clinical features resolve.
- Patients with significant sedation require management in an intensive care unit.
- Paediatric patients who are clinically well at 4 hours following accidental ingestion do not require ongoing medical management. Discharge should not occur at night.

References
Cairns R, Schaffer AL, Ryan N et al. Rising pregabalin use and misuse in Australia: trends in utilization and intentional poisonings. Addiction 2019; 114(6):1026–1034.
Isoardi K, Polkinghorne G, Harris K et al. Pregabalin poisoning and rising recreational use: a retrospective observational series. British Journal of Clinical Pharmacology 2020; 86(12):2435–2440.

Wood DM, Berry DJ, Glover G et al. Significant pregabalin toxicity managed with
supportive care alone. Journal of Medical Toxicology 2010; 6:435–437.
Yoo L, Matalon D, Hoffman RS et al. Treatment of pregabalin toxicity in a patient with
kidney failure. American Journal of Kidney Diseases 2009; 54(6):1127–1130.

3.68 QUETIAPINE

**Quetiapine is a widely prescribed second generation (atypical)
antipsychotic agent. Overdose results in characteristic clinical features
– sedation, anticholinergic delirium, tachycardia, hypotension and coma.**

RISK ASSESSMENT

- Quetiapine toxicity is associated with predictable dose-dependent
  CNS depression ranging from sedation to coma (see **Table 3.68.1**).
- Hypotension due to peripheral alpha blockade is characteristic.
- QT prolongation may occur but the risk of torsades de pointes is
  extremely low.
- Co-ingestion of ethanol or other sedative-hypnotic agents
  increases the risk of coma and loss of airway protective reflexes.
- **Children:** accidental ingestion of quetiapine requires hospital
  assessment and observation.

Toxic mechanism

Quetiapine is an antagonist at mesolimbic dopamine (D_2), serotonin (particularly 5-HT$_{2A}$),
histamine (H_1), muscarinic (M_1) and peripheral alpha (α_1) receptors.

Toxicokinetics

Quetiapine is rapidly absorbed and highly protein bound, with a large volume of
distribution (10 L/kg). Peak plasma levels are delayed several hours following ingestion of
modified-release formulations. It is metabolised by hepatic cytochrome P450 3A4 to an
active metabolite, 7-hydroxyquetiapine.

CLINICAL FEATURES

- Onset of toxicity occurs within 2 hours for immediate-release
  formulations and will be delayed with slow-release preparations.
- Sedation and sinus tachycardia are common.
- Anticholinergic features are prominent but may be masked by coma.
- Urinary retention is almost universal.
- Toxicity usually lasts from 12 to 48 hours.

TABLE 3.68.1 Dose-related risk assessment: quetiapine	
Dose	**Effect**
<3 g	Sedation and characteristic sinus tachycardia (frequently >120 beats/minute) Anticholinergic delirium may be prominent
>3 g	Increasing likelihood of coma requiring intubation Significant hypotension can occur

- Hypotension may be profound following large ingestions and is mediated by peripheral alpha blockade. Noradrenaline is the appropriate vasopressor agent.
- QT prolongation can occur; however, torsades de pointes is not reported.
- Seizures occur in <5% of cases.

INVESTIGATIONS
Screening tests in deliberate self-poisoning
- 12-lead ECG, BGL and paracetamol level

MANAGEMENT
Resuscitation, supportive care and monitoring
- Attention to airway, breathing and circulation are paramount. These priorities are managed along conventional lines, as outlined in **Chapter 1.2: Resuscitation**.
- Fluid resuscitation to optimise intravascular volume.
- Noradrenaline is the agent of choice for persistent hypotension.
- Monitor for urinary retention and insert an indwelling urinary catheter if required.
- General supportive care measures are indicated, as outlined in **Chapter 1.4: Supportive care and monitoring**.
- Severe agitated delirium is managed with titrated doses of intravenous benzodiazepine, as outlined in **Chapter 2.4: Approach to delirium**.

Decontamination
- Activated charcoal should be given to all comatose patients following quetiapine overdose once the airway is protected by endotracheal intubation.

Enhanced elimination
- Not clinically useful.

Antidotes
- None available.

DISPOSITION AND FOLLOW-UP
- Children should be observed in hospital following unintentional ingestion of quetiapine. If they remain clinically well without sedation at 4–6 hours (8–12 hours following ingestion of modified-release preparations), they may be discharged. Discharge should not occur at night. Parents are advised that abnormal (extrapyramidal) movements might occur up to 3 days after ingestion.
- Patients who are clinically well with a normal 12-lead ECG at 4 hours (8 hours following ingestion of modified-release preparations) do not require further medical assessment or monitoring.

HANDY TIPS
- Sinus tachycardia exceeding 120 beats/minute is common. No specific intervention is required to control the heart rate.

- Adrenaline infusion may paradoxically exacerbate hypotension caused by quetiapine toxicity due to excessive β_2-mediated vasodilatation. Noradrenaline is the preferred vasopressor agent.
- Untreated urinary retention can exacerbate agitation and requires placement of an indwelling catheter.

CONTROVERSY

- Definitive evidence of clinical benefit following administration of activated charcoal is not available. However, it has been shown to significantly reduce absorption of quetiapine and is indicated for all intubated patients.

Presentations
Quetiapine 25 mg, 200 mg, 300 mg tablets (60)
Quetiapine 100 mg tablets (90)
Quetiapine 50 mg, 150 mg, 200 mg, 400 mg modified-release tablets (60)
Quetiapine 300 mg modified-release tablets (60, 100)

References
Balit CR, Isbister GK, Hackett LP. Quetiapine: a case series. Annals of Emergency Medicine 2003; 42:751–758.

Burns MJ. The pharmacology and toxicology of atypical antipsychotic agents. Journal of Toxicology–Clinical Toxicology 2001; 39(1):1–14.

Hawkins DJ, Unwin P. Paradoxical and severe hypotension in response to adrenaline infusion in massive quetiapine overdose. Critical Care and Resuscitation 2008; 10(4):320–322.

Isbister GK, Balit CR, Kilham HA. Antipsychotic poisoning in young children: a systematic review. Drug Safety 2005; 26(11):1029–1044.

Isbister GK, Duffull SB. Quetiapine overdose: predicting intubation, duration of ventilation, cardiac monitoring and the effect of activated charcoal. International Clinical Psychopharmacology 2009; 24:174–180.

Isbister GK, Friberg LE, Hackett LP et al. Pharmacokinetics of quetiapine in overdose and the effect of activated charcoal. Clinical Pharmacology and Therapeutics 2007; 81(6):821–827.

Ngo A, Ciranni M, Olson KR. Acute quetiapine overdose in adults: a 5-year retrospective case series. Annals of Emergency Medicine 2008; 52:541–547.

Tan HH, Hoppe J, Heard K. A systematic review of cardiovascular effects after atypical antipsychotic medication overdose. American Journal of Emergency Medicine 2009; 27:607–616.

3.69 QUININE

Quinine toxicity is characterised by cinchonism – nausea, vomiting, tinnitus, vertigo and deafness. Larger overdoses may result in life-threatening cardiotoxicity and severe, potentially permanent, retinal toxicity.

RISK ASSESSMENT

- All cases of deliberate self-poisoning should be regarded as having the potential to cause cardiotoxicity and blindness.
- Cinchonism can develop even at therapeutic dosing.
- Cardiotoxicity and visual loss are likely when the ingested dose is >5 g.
- **Children:** ingestion of 1 or 2 tablets by a child is potentially life-threatening.

Toxic mechanism

Quinine is a class 1A antiarrhythmic with sodium- and potassium-channel-blocking effects, causing prolongation of both the QRS and the QT intervals. In overdose, quinine is directly toxic to the retina. Quinine also stimulates pancreatic insulin release in a manner similar to sulfonylureas.

Toxicokinetics

Quinine is rapidly absorbed from the small intestine with a bioavailability of approximately 70%. It is highly protein bound and peak serum levels occur within 2–4 hours. The elimination half-life may be prolonged in patients with renal or hepatic impairment. Elimination is largely via hydroxylation, with approximately 20% being excreted unchanged in the urine. Quinine does not undergo enterohepatic circulation.

CLINICAL FEATURES

- Cinchonism
  - Characterised by nausea, vomiting, tinnitus, vertigo and deafness.
  - Occurs early following overdose.
- Cardiovascular
  - Hypotension, sinus tachycardia, QRS widening and prolongation of the QT and PR intervals.
  - Wide-complex tachycardia and torsades de pointes may occur.
  - These effects usually occur relatively early (within 8 hours) and resolve as blood quinine concentration falls.
- Central nervous system
  - Drowsiness and confusion can occur with larger ingestions.
  - Coma and seizures are rare.
- Ocular
  - Visual disturbance is delayed and becomes apparent 6–8 hours post ingestion. Patients may present the following day with complete blindness.
  - Manifestations include blurred vision, disturbances in colour perception, pupillary dilatation and visual field defects. Complete visual loss develops in severe cases.
  - Improvement in visual deficits usually occurs over days to weeks, although permanent residual deficits do occur. These are more likely in patients who develop complete blindness during the acute phase.
- Metabolic
  - Hypokalaemia
  - Hypoglycaemia.

INVESTIGATIONS

Screening tests in deliberate self-poisoning

- 12-lead ECG and paracetamol level

Specific investigations

- Serial 12-lead ECGs
- EUC, blood glucose levels
- Visual field testing
- Quinine blood levels: these correlate well with toxicity (>10 mg/L at 6 hours is associated with cardiovascular toxicity and visual disturbance) but are not available in a clinically relevant time frame and do not assist clinical decision making.

Resuscitation, supportive care and monitoring

- Quinine overdose is a life-threatening emergency and is managed in an area equipped for cardiorespiratory monitoring and resuscitation.
- Clinical features requiring immediate intervention include:
  - Broad complex tachycardias with haemodynamic compromise
    - Manage initially with bolus IV sodium bicarbonate 1–2 mmol/kg IV, intubation and hyperventilation (see **Chapter 4.24: Sodium bicarbonate**).
      - Note: Multiple doses of sodium bicarbonate can cause significant alkalaemia, exacerbating hypokalaemia and increasing the risk of torsades de pointes.
  - Torsades de pointes
    - Electrical cardioversion may be required for persistent episodes that result in altered mental state or haemodynamic instability.
    - Magnesium 10 mmol IV bolus (0.05 mmol/kg in children) over 1–2 minutes, repeated once if torsades de pointes recurs.
    - Isoprenaline or overdrive electrical pacing are other treatment options to increase the resting heart rate to a target of >100 beats/min.
    - Ensure that all QT-dependent electrolytes (potassium, calcium, magnesium) are at the upper limit of normal (see **Chapter 2.17: The 12-lead ECG in toxicology**).
  - Hypotension
    - Manage initially with appropriate volume resuscitation, but inotropic and vasopressor support may be required. Options include adrenaline, noradrenaline and high-dose insulin therapy, guided by assessment of cardiovascular function (see **Chapter 2.2: Hypotension**).
- General supportive care measures are indicated, as outlined in **Chapter 1.4: Supportive care and monitoring**.

Decontamination

- Administer 50 g activated charcoal to all overdose patients. Antiemetics may aid administration. If there is significant CNS depression or seizures, activated charcoal is only administered by nasogastric tube after the airway is secured by endotracheal intubation.
- Because of the risk of severe retinal toxicity, early intubation to facilitate safe administration of activated charcoal can be justified.

Enhanced elimination

- Multiple-dose activated charcoal enhances the elimination of quinine. This intervention is indicated in any patient who has ingested >5 g of quinine or who has any degree of visual disturbance.

Antidotes

- None available.

DISPOSITION AND FOLLOW-UP

- All children suspected of ingesting quinine must be observed and monitored for 6 hours post ingestion.
- Patients who are asymptomatic and have a normal ECG at 6 hours following ingestion are fit for medical discharge.
- Patients with symptoms or an abnormal ECG must be admitted for ongoing observation and monitoring until symptoms resolve.
- All patients with quinine toxicity need formal ophthalmological review prior to discharge.

HANDY TIPS

- Consider quinine overdose in any patient with deliberate self-poisoning who complains of visual disturbance.
- Anticipate the onset of visual disturbance in any patient who has ingested >5 g of quinine.

PITFALL

- Failure to warn the patient that visual disturbance may develop 6–8 hours later. It is very disturbing for the patient to awake the following morning and unexpectedly discover they are blind.

CONTROVERSIES

- Historically, the visual disturbance was thought to be caused by retinal arterial vasospasm. Treatments such as vasodilators, stellate ganglion blocks and hyperbaric oxygen therapy were used in attempts to prevent blindness. The visual loss is due to direct retinal toxicity and cannot be prevented by any of these interventions. Decontamination and enhanced elimination with multiple-dose activated charcoal offer the best chance of minimising retinal toxicity.
- Excessive IV administration of potassium may lead to rebound hyperkalaemia following resolution of toxicity. In practice, the risk of ventricular dysrhythmias due to hypokalaemia outweighs this potential risk.

References

Boland ME, Roper SM, Henry JA. Complications of quinine poisoning. Lancet 1985; 1(8425):384–385.

Guly U, Driscoll P. The management of quinine-induced blindness. Archives of Emergency Medicine 1992; 9:317–322.

Huston M, Levinson M. Are one or two dangerous? Quinine and quinidine exposure in toddlers. Journal of Emergency Medicine 2006; 31(4):395–401.

Jaeger A. Quinine and chloroquine. Medicine 2012; 40(3):154–155.

Langford NJ, Good AM, Laing WJ et al. Quinine intoxications reported to the Scottish Poisons Information Bureau 1997–2002: a continuing problem. British Journal of Clinical Pharmacology 2003; 56:576–578.

3.70 RISPERIDONE

Deliberate self-poisoning with this second-generation (atypical) antipsychotic agent is relatively benign. Supportive care ensures a good outcome.

RISK ASSESSMENT
- Risperidone causes minimal toxicity in overdose.
- Toxic effects include sinus tachycardia (50%) and acute dystonia (10%).
- Significant CNS depression does not occur following risperidone ingestion.
- **Children:** accidental ingestion of risperidone requires hospital assessment and observation. Acute dystonic reactions are more frequent in paediatric patients and may be delayed in onset.

Toxic mechanism

Risperidone is an antagonist at mesolimbic dopamine (D_2), serotonin (particularly 5-HT$_{2A}$), central alpha (α_2) and peripheral alpha (α_1) receptors. Compared with other antipsychotic agents in its class, it has much lower affinity for histamine (H_1) and muscarinic (M_1) receptors.

Toxicokinetics

Risperidone is rapidly absorbed after oral administration. It is highly protein bound and has a moderate volume of distribution (1.5 L/kg). Risperidone undergoes hepatic metabolism by cytochrome P450 2D6 to the active metabolite 9-hydroxyrisperidone (paliperidone). Renal impairment prolongs the elimination half-life.

CLINICAL FEATURES
- Clinical features of toxicity usually occur within 4 hours.
- Sinus tachycardia is common but active intervention is not required.
- Mild sedation may be observed.
- Acute dystonias occur frequently.
- Significant QT prolongation is not expected.
- Clinical features of toxicity resolve within 6–24 hours.

INVESTIGATIONS
Screening tests in deliberate self-poisoning
- 12-lead ECG, BGL and paracetamol level

MANAGEMENT
Resuscitation, supportive care and monitoring
- Acute resuscitation will not be required for isolated risperidone ingestion.
- General supportive care measures are indicated, as outlined in **Chapter 1.4: Supportive care and monitoring**.

Decontamination
- Activated charcoal is not indicated.

Enhanced elimination
- Not clinically useful.

Antidotes
- Benztropine or benzodiazepines may be required to treat acute dystonia.

DISPOSITION AND FOLLOW-UP
- All paediatric ingestions should be referred for hospital assessment and observation.

- Patients who are clinically well 4–6 hours following ingestion do not require further acute medical management.
- At discharge, parents should be advised that abnormal (extrapyramidal) movements may occur up to 3 days following ingestion.

PITFALL
- Failure to warn parents of the possibility of delayed abnormal (extrapyramidal) movements after unintentional paediatric exposure.

References

Burns MJ. The pharmacology and toxicology of atypical antipsychotic agents. Journal of Toxicology–Clinical Toxicology 2001; 39(1):1–14.

Cobaugh DJ, Erdman AR, Booze LL et al. Atypical antipsychotic medication poisoning: an evidence based consensus guideline for out-of-hospital management. Clinical Toxicology 2007; 45(8):918–942.

Isbister GK, Balit CR, Kilham HA. Antipsychotic poisoning in young children: a systematic review. Drug Safety 2005; 26(11):1029–1044.

Page CB, Calver LA, Isbister GK. Risperidone overdose causes extrapyramidal effects but not cardiac toxicity. Journal of Clinical Psychopharmacology 2010; 30:387–390.

Tan HH, Hoppe J, Heard K. A systematic review of cardiovascular effects after atypical antipsychotic medication overdose. American Journal of Emergency Medicine 2009; 27:607–616.

3.71 SALICYLATES

Acetylsalicylic acid (aspirin), Methyl salicylate

Acute poisoning with salicylates presents with classical symptoms of nausea, vomiting, tinnitus and hyperpnoea. Seizures and coma are late manifestations caused by cerebral oedema and are associated with a high fatality rate. Chronic intoxication has a more insidious presentation and the diagnosis may be missed. Urinary alkalinisation and haemodialysis are highly effective methods of enhancing elimination.

RISK ASSESSMENT
- The severity of clinical features following acute aspirin overdose is dose-related (see **Table 3.71.1**) and progresses over hours.
- Chronic poisoning has an increased risk of an adverse outcome.
- In terms of the salicylate dose, 1 g of methyl salicylate is equivalent to 1.5 g of acetylsalicylate (1 mL of oil of wintergreen (98% methyl salicylate) is equivalent to 1400 mg of aspirin).
- **Children:** rarely ingest a dose of aspirin sufficient to cause toxicity. In contrast, small ingestions of methyl salicylate products (less than a teaspoon of oil of wintergreen) can cause severe toxicity. Chronic salicylate poisoning has been reported after regular use of topical salicylate products in infants.

Toxic mechanism

Salicylates cause irreversible inhibition of cyclooxygenase enzymes, resulting in decreased prostaglandin synthesis. Nausea and vomiting are caused by gastric irritation and stimulation of the chemoreceptor trigger zone. Direct stimulation of the medullary

TABLE 3.71.1	Dose-related risk assessment: acute acetylsalicylic acid (aspirin) overdose
Dose	**Effect**
<150 mg/kg	Minimal symptoms
150–300 mg/kg	Mild-to-moderate intoxication Nausea, vomiting, tinnitus (salicylism) Hyperpnoea (respiratory alkalosis)
>300 mg/kg	Severe intoxication Potential for altered mental state and seizures Progressive metabolic acidosis
>500 mg/kg	Potentially lethal

respiratory centre causes hyperpnoea and respiratory alkalosis. Uncoupling of oxidative phosphorylation in the mitochondria causes lactic acidosis, and ketone production from fatty acid metabolism contributes to the metabolic acidosis. Death is caused by cerebral oedema due to very high salicylate levels in the CNS.

Toxicokinetics

Salicylates are rapidly absorbed following therapeutic administration and highly protein bound, with a small volume of distribution. In overdose, the kinetics change markedly. Absorption is delayed due to pylorospasm and the formation of bezoars within the stomach. Protein binding is saturated, leading to an increase in free salicylate levels. Hepatic metabolism changes from first order to zero order kinetics. As a result, the elimination half-life of 2–4 hours in normal therapeutic dosing increases up to 24 hours.

In an acidic environment, more salicylate is in the uncharged form, favouring movement across cell membranes (blood–brain barrier, renal tubular epithelium). Alkalinisation increases the proportion of salicylate in the charged form, decreasing the movement of salicylate into the CNS and promoting urinary salicylate excretion as it is unable to be reabsorbed across the renal tubular epithelium.

CLINICAL FEATURES

Acute salicylate intoxication

- Onset of clinical features progresses over hours and severe toxicity may not be evident until 6–12 hours following ingestion. Deterioration may then be very rapid.
- Gastrointestinal
  - Nausea, vomiting
- Central nervous system
  - Tinnitus, decreased hearing, vertigo
  - Confusion, agitation, seizures
  - May progress to cerebral oedema and death
- Acid–base disturbance
  - Respiratory alkalosis (initial phase)
  - Mixed acid–base disturbance – respiratory alkalosis and worsening metabolic acidosis
  - The development of acidaemia is an ominous prognostic sign as rapid clinical deterioration can occur
- Other
  - Hyperthermia, hyper/hypoglycaemia, hypokalaemia

Chronic salicylate intoxication
- Difficult to diagnose clinically and often missed.
- Most common in elderly patients.
- Often presents with non-specific symptoms such as confusion, delirium, dehydration, fever and unexplained metabolic acidosis.
- Cerebral and pulmonary oedema are more common than in acute poisoning.

INVESTIGATIONS
Screening tests in deliberate self-poisoning
- 12-lead ECG, BGL and paracetamol level

Specific investigations
- Salicylate level
  - Therapeutic range is 1.1–2.2 mmol/L (15–30 mg/dL, 150–300 mg/L).
  - Serial levels every 2–4 hours are useful to identify ongoing or delayed absorption.
- Blood gases
  - Detect and monitor acid–base disturbances.
- EUC
  - Detect and correct hypokalaemia prior to urinary alkalinisation.

MANAGEMENT
The majority of patients with acute salicylate overdose do not require immediate resuscitation and the mainstays of treatment are decontamination and enhanced elimination. Resuscitation may be required for a minority of patients with acute severe poisoning or chronic poisoning with established toxicity.

Resuscitation, supportive care and monitoring
- Severe salicylate poisoning is a life-threatening emergency managed in an area equipped for cardiorespiratory monitoring and resuscitation.
- Attention to airway and breathing is paramount. In patients maintaining effective ventilation, intubation is to be avoided as even a brief period of apnoea during standard rapid sequence intubation can lead to death.
- If intubation and ventilation is required for coma or ineffective ventilation, it is imperative to maintain adequate hyperventilation to maximise respiratory alkalosis.
- Serum alkalinisation is an immediate priority to prevent further movement of salicylate into the CNS:
  - Administer IV sodium bicarbonate boluses 1–2 mmol/kg guided by serial blood gases and clinical response.
- Immediate haemodialysis is potentially life-saving in severe toxicity and should be organised while resuscitation continues.
- Ensure sufficient fluid replacement with intravenous crystalloid to account for gastrointestinal and insensible losses.

Decontamination
- Activated charcoal should be given to all symptomatic patients and for ingestions >150 mg/kg. Due to delayed and prolonged

absorption, activated charcoal should be given up to at least 8 hours following ingestion, and repeated doses should be considered.

Enhanced elimination
- Urinary alkalinisation is indicated in all patients with symptomatic salicylate poisoning. Further details on the rationale and use of this intervention are provided in **Chapter 1.7: Enhanced elimination** and **Chapter 4.24: Sodium bicarbonate**.
- Haemodialysis effectively removes salicylate but is rarely required if early decontamination and urinary alkalinisation are implemented. Consider this intervention in the following circumstances:
  - urinary alkalinisation not feasible
  - serum salicylate levels rising to >4.4 mmol/L (>60 mg/dL, >600 mg/L) despite decontamination and urinary alkalinisation
  - severe toxicity as evidenced by altered mental status or acidaemia
  - renal failure
  - very high serum salicylate levels:
    - acute poisoning >7.2 mmol/L (>100 mg/dL, >1000 mg/L)
      - Note: The threshold to dialyse in acute poisoning is lower in the elderly (>4.4 mmol/L, >60 mg/dL, >600 mg/L).
    - chronic poisoning >4.4 mmol/L (>60 mg/dL, >600 mg/L).

Antidotes
- None available.

DISPOSITION AND FOLLOW-UP
- All children suspected of ingesting methyl salicylate products should be observed in hospital for signs of salicylate toxicity for at least 6 hours.
- All symptomatic patients require admission for careful monitoring and enhanced elimination techniques. Therapy is ceased when the salicylate level falls to within the normal range (1.1–2.2 mmol/L, 15–30 mg/dL, 150–300 mg/L) and the clinical features and acid–base abnormalities have resolved.
- Patients with significant toxicity are managed in an intensive care unit.

HANDY TIPS
- Urgent haemodialysis is indicated in any patient who requires intubation for salicylate poisoning (but not if intubated because of co-ingestants).
- Consider salicylate toxicity in any elderly patient with altered mental status and metabolic acidosis.
- Although salicylate classically causes an elevated anion gap metabolic acidosis, some blood gas machines may record a normal or low anion gap by mistaking salicylate ions for chloride.

PITFALLS
- Failure to appreciate the potential for ongoing delayed absorption from the gastrointestinal tract.

- Failure to maintain alkalaemia after intubation and ventilation, leading to catastrophic clinical deterioration due to rapid redistribution of salicylate to the CNS.
- Failure to identify oil of wintergreen as methyl salicylate and determine aspirin equivalence when constructing a risk assessment.
- Failure to diagnose chronic aspirin poisoning.
- Confusion between reported units for salicylate concentration, leading to misinterpretation of results.

Presentations

Aspirin 100 mg tablets (30, 90, 112)
Aspirin 100 mg enteric coated tablets (28, 84, 140, 168)
Aspirin 300 mg dispersible tablets (24, 42, 48, 60, 96)
Aspirin 320 mg tablets (20)
Aspirin 500 mg dispersible tablets (16, 120)
Aspirin 650 mg tablets (100)
Aspirin 100 mg/clopidogrel 75 mg tablets (30)
Aspirin 300 mg/codeine 8 mg dispersible tablets (60)
Aspirin 25 mg/dipyridamole 200 mg controlled-release tablets (60)
Methyl salicylate is found in oil of wintergreen (98% methyl salicylate) and various products marketed for topical application, including certain Asian herbal remedies.

References

Davis JE. Are one or two dangerous? Methyl salicylate exposure in toddlers. Journal of Emergency Medicine 2007; 32(1):63–69.

Juurlink DN, Gosselin S, Kielstein JT et al. Extracorporeal treatment for salicylate poisoning: systematic review and recommendations from the EXTRIP workgroup. Annals of Emergency Medicine 2015; 66(2):165–181. doi:10.1016/j.annemergmed.2015.03.031.

O'Malley GF. Management of the salicylate poisoned patient. Emergency Medicine Clinics of North America 2007; 25(2):333–336.

Pearlman BL, Gambhir R. Salicylate intoxication: a clinical review. Postgraduate Medicine 2009; 121(4):162–168.

3.72 SELECTIVE SEROTONIN REUPTAKE INHIBITORS (SSRIs)

Citalopram, Escitalopram, Fluoxetine, Fluvoxamine, Paroxetine, Sertraline

Deliberate self-poisoning with the selective serotonin reuptake inhibitors (SSRIs) is common and usually follows a benign course. Citalopram and escitalopram are notable for their ability to cause dose-dependent QT interval prolongation.

RISK ASSESSMENT

- Mild symptoms of serotonin toxicity occur in less than 20% of patients and usually resolve within 24 hours.
- Seizures occur infrequently but are more common with citalopram overdose.
- Citalopram and escitalopram ingestions are associated with QT prolongation but the incidence of torsades de pointes is very low.
- Exposure to other serotonergic agents, such as monoamine oxidase inhibitors, venlafaxine, tramadol or amphetamines, greatly increases the risk of severe serotonin toxicity.

- **Children:** unintentional paediatric ingestion of up to 3 tablets is benign and referral to hospital is not required unless symptoms develop.

Toxic mechanism
SSRIs enhance central serotonergic neurotransmission by inhibiting serotonin reuptake. They have little affinity for adrenergic, dopaminergic, cholinergic, serotonergic or histamine receptors.

Toxicokinetics
SSRIs are rapidly absorbed following oral administration. In general, they are highly protein bound, have large volumes of distribution and undergo hepatic metabolism to metabolites that are renally excreted. Didesmethylcitalopram is the metabolite of citalopram responsible for QT prolongation. Elimination half-lives are approximately 24 hours.

CLINICAL FEATURES
- Mild serotonin toxicity occurs in fewer than 20% and manifests primarily as anxiety, tremor, tachycardia and mydriasis (see **Chapter 2.5: Serotonin toxicity**).
- Severe serotonin toxicity does not develop unless there is exposure to other serotonergic agents.
- Seizures are usually brief and self-limiting, and may be heralded by increased anxiety, sweating, tremor, tachycardia and mydriasis.
- QT prolongation occurs after citalopram and escitalopram overdose and is dose-dependent. There are rare reports of torsades de pointes following citalopram overdose.

INVESTIGATIONS
Screening tests in deliberate self-poisoning
- 12-lead ECG, BGL and paracetamol level

Specific investigations
- Serial 12-lead ECGs
  - Dose-dependent prolongation of the QT interval is described in citalopram and escitalopram overdose.

MANAGEMENT
Resuscitation, supportive care and monitoring
- Attention to airway, breathing and circulation are paramount (see **Chapter 1.2: Resuscitation**).
- Increasing anxiety, sweating, tremor, tachycardia and mydriasis may herald the onset of seizures.
  - Give titrated doses of intravenous benzodiazepines (midazolam or diazepam 2.5–10 mg IV). Further doses may be required to achieve improvement in agitation and neuromuscular activity.
- Management of serotonin toxicity is discussed in **Chapter 2.5: Serotonin toxicity**.
- Cardiac monitoring is indicated for at least 12 hours following ingestion of:
  - >600 mg citalopram
  - >300 mg escitalopram
    - If the QT nomogram indicates low risk of torsades de pointes at that time, ongoing cardiac monitoring is not required (see **Figure 2.17.4**).

- Management of torsades de pointes:
  - Electrical cardioversion may be required for persistent episodes that result in altered mental state or haemodynamic instability.
  - Magnesium 10 mmol IV bolus (0.05 mmol/kg in children) over 1–2 minutes, repeated once if torsades de pointes recurs.
  - Isoprenaline or overdrive electrical pacing are other treatment options to increase the resting heart rate to a target of >100 beats/min.
  - Ensure that all QT-dependent electrolytes (potassium, calcium, magnesium) are at the upper limit of normal (see **Chapter 2.17: The 12-lead ECG in toxicology**).

Decontamination
- Some authorities recommend that 50 g of activated charcoal should be administered to alert and cooperative patients who have ingested >600 mg citalopram or >300 mg escitalopram if it can be administered within 4 hours after the overdose.
  - The aim is to reduce the duration of QT prolongation and risk of torsades de pointes. However, the risk of seizure following overdose with these agents is greater than that of dysrhythmias, and the risk of aspiration of activated charcoal may outweigh the proposed clinical benefit (see **Controversies**).
- Overdose with other SSRIs has an excellent outcome with minimal supportive care; activated charcoal is not indicated unless warranted by co-ingestants.

Enhanced elimination
- Not clinically useful.

Antidotes
- None available.

DISPOSITION AND FOLLOW-UP
- Paediatric patients may be observed at home following accidental exposure. If significant symptoms occur, referral to hospital for assessment is appropriate.
- Patients who have ingested >600 mg citalopram or >300 mg escitalopram are observed with cardiac monitoring for at least 12 hours. Monitoring should continue if the QT interval is abnormal at this stage (see **Chapter 2.17: The 12-lead ECG in toxicology**).
- All other patients who deliberately self-poison with SSRIs are observed for 6 hours. Asymptomatic patients with a normal ECG are fit for medical discharge.
- Patients with serotonin toxicity require supportive care in a ward environment, usually for no more than 12–24 hours. They are fit for medical discharge as soon as clinical features resolve.
- Patients who develop severe serotonin toxicity require management in an intensive care unit.

HANDY TIP
- Coma is not a typical feature of SSRI poisoning and other causes should be sought.

PITFALL

- Failure to administer benzodiazepines to patients with increasing anxiety, sweating, tremor, tachycardia and mydriasis.

CONTROVERSY

- Activated charcoal reduces citalopram and escitalopram absorption and decreases maximal QT in pharmacokinetic models. However, given that torsades de pointes is extremely rare, the clinical benefit of this intervention to prevent dysrhythmias is not known.

Presentations

Citalopram hydrobromide 10 mg, 20 mg, 40 mg tablets (28)
Escitalopram oxalate 10 mg, 20 mg tablets (28)
Escitalopram oxalate 10 mg/mL oral solution (28 mL)
Fluvoxamine maleate 50 mg, 100 mg tablets (30)
Fluoxetine hydrochloride 20 mg capsules or tablets (28)
Paroxetine hydrochloride 20 mg tablets (30)
Sertraline hydrochloride 50 mg, 100 mg tablets (30)

References

Hayes BD, Klein-Schwartz W, Clark RF et al. Comparison of toxicity of acute overdose with citalopram and escitalopram. Journal of Emergency Medicine 2010; 39(1):44–48.

Isbister GK, Bowe SJ, Dawson A et al. Relative toxicity of selective serotonin reuptake inhibitors (SSRIs) in overdose. Journal of Toxicology–Clinical Toxicology 2004; 42(3):277–285.

Isbister GK, Friberg LE, Duffull SB. Application of pharmacokinetic-pharmacodynamic modelling in the management of QT abnormalities after citalopram overdose. Intensive Care Medicine 2006; 32(7):1060–1065.

Isbister GK, Friberg LE, Stokes B et al. Activated charcoal decreases QT prolongation after citalopram overdose. Annals of Emergency Medicine 2008; 52(1):86–87.

Jimmink A, Caminada K, Hunfeld NG et al. Clinical toxicology of citalopram after acute intoxication with the sole drug or in combination with other drugs: overview of 26 cases. Therapeutic Drug Monitoring 2008; 30(3):365–371.

Kelly CA, Dhaun N, Laing WJ et al. Comparative toxicity of citalopram and the newer antidepressants after overdose. Journal of Toxicology–Clinical Toxicology 2004; 42(1):67–71.

Van Gorp F, Duffull S, Hackett LP et al. Population pharmacokinetics and pharmacodynamics of escitalopram in overdose and the effect of activated charcoal. British Journal of Clinical Pharmacology 2011; 73:402–410.

Van Gorp F, Whyte IM, Isbister GK. Clinical and ECG effects of escitalopram overdose. Annals of Emergency Medicine 2009; 54(3):404–408.

3.73 STRYCHNINE

Strychnine is a plant alkaloid commercially available for pest control or as a component of alternative natural remedies. Strychnine poisoning causes generalised skeletal muscle spasms, leading to tetany. The cause of death is respiratory failure, and intubation, ventilation and neuromuscular paralysis are life-saving.

RISK ASSESSMENT

- Ingestion of as little as 30 mg (1 g of 0.03% powder) by an adult is potentially lethal. Death can occur within 30 minutes.
- Any deliberate ingestion is likely to be rapidly lethal without early intervention.
- Sublethal doses lead to painful generalised muscle spasms and rigidity.
- **Children:** any ingestion is potentially lethal.

Toxic mechanism

Strychnine is a competitive antagonist of the inhibitory neurotransmitter glycine, predominantly at brainstem and spinal receptors. Loss of normal inhibitory tone leads to neuromuscular hyperexcitability with severe, progressive muscle spasms and rigidity. Ventilatory failure occurs secondary to severe muscular spasm.

Toxicokinetics

Strychnine is rapidly and completely absorbed following ingestion or inhalation, but dermal exposure can result in delayed onset of toxicity. It has a large volume of distribution (13 L/ kg), with an elimination half-life of 10–16 hours. It undergoes hepatic metabolism to inactive metabolites, but up to 30% of an ingested dose may be excreted unchanged in the urine.

CLINICAL FEATURES

- Nausea, anxiety, agitation, twitching and muscle spasms occur within minutes of ingestion.
- Generalised painful muscle spasms of voluntary muscles (risus sardonicus, opisthotonos) occur spontaneously or can be precipitated by any external stimulus. In severe cases, this results in hyperthermia, rhabdomyolysis, lactic acidosis and haemodynamic compromise.
- Death results from hypoxia due to ventilatory failure from sustained muscle contractions.
- It is characteristic of strychnine poisoning that the patient remains awake during episodes of tetany. Loss of consciousness does not occur until secondary hypoxia develops.
- Muscle spasms and rigidity resolve within 24 hours if ventilation and oxygenation are maintained.

INVESTIGATIONS

Screening tests in deliberate self-poisoning

- 12-lead ECG, BGL and paracetamol level

Specific investigations

- Serum strychnine levels are not readily available and do not assist management. Serum and urine levels are useful to confirm the diagnosis retrospectively, especially in forensic cases.
- EUC, venous blood gases, lactate and CK.

MANAGEMENT

Resuscitation, supportive care and monitoring

- Strychnine poisoning is a time-critical life-threatening emergency.
- Immediate life-threats are:
  - generalised muscle rigidity
  - respiratory failure.

- Prompt intubation, ventilation and neuromuscular paralysis are life-saving.
- Resuscitation proceeds along conventional lines, as outlined in **Chapter 1.2: Resuscitation**.
- Milder toxicity without generalised spasm or rigidity is treated with titrated IV benzodiazepines to achieve improvement in neuromuscular symptoms.
- It is essential to give adequate sedation and analgesia as consciousness is preserved throughout.

Decontamination
- Activated charcoal is not administered until the airway is secured.

Enhanced elimination
- Not clinically useful.

Antidotes
- None available.

DISPOSITION AND FOLLOW-UP
- Patients who are clinically well without neuromuscular features 4 hours after ingestion of strychnine do not require ongoing medical observation. Patients are advised that dermal exposure may result in the delayed onset of symptoms and they should return for assessment and management if this occurs.
- Patients with clinical features of strychnine poisoning are managed in an intensive care unit.

HANDY TIPS
- Patients with mild symptoms may rapidly develop lethal muscle rigidity requiring immediate intubation, ventilation and paralysis.
- Following deliberate self-poisoning, many patients do not reach hospital alive.

PITFALL
- Failure to institute prompt intubation and paralysis to prevent secondary complications of hyperthermia, lactic acidosis, rhabdomyolysis and hypoxic brain injury.

Presentations
Preparations available to the public contain 0.3% to 0.5% strychnine, but those used by licensed exterminators may contain from 5% to 100% strychnine. Strychnine may be found in natural or alternative medicines, and has been added as an adulterant to illicit drugs such as amphetamines, cocaine and heroin.

References
Edmunds M, Sheehan TM, Van't Hoff W. Strychnine poisoning: clinical and toxicological observations on a non-fatal case. Journal of Toxicology–Clinical Toxicology 1986; 24:245–255.

Makarovsky I, Markel G, Hoffman A et al. Strychnine: a killer from the past. Israeli Medical Association Journal 2008; 10(2):142–145.

Palatnick W, Meatherall R, Sitar D et al. Toxicokinetics of acute strychnine poisoning. Journal of Toxicology–Clinical Toxicology 1997; 35:617–620.

3.74 SULFONYLUREAS

Glibenclamide, Gliclazide, Glimepiride, Glipizide

Sulfonylurea toxicity can result in profound and recurrent hypoglycaemia following overdose or accidental ingestion. It can also occur during therapeutic administration, particularly if there is hepatic or renal dysfunction. Octreotide is the definitive antidote and early administration decreases the occurrence of hypoglycaemic episodes.

RISK ASSESSMENT
- Any ingestion of sulfonylureas can result in severe hypoglycaemia.
- Sulfonylurea-induced hypoglycaemia is likely to recur following initial resolution after intravenous glucose administration, and octreotide is the definitive antidote.
- Elderly patients with hepatic or renal dysfunction are at particular risk of toxicity from therapeutic dosing and may also benefit from treatment with octreotide.
- The onset of hypoglycaemia may be delayed up to 8 hours following overdose, and even longer for modified-release preparations.
- Toxicity may persist for several days, depending on the preparation ingested and the size of the overdose.
- **Children:** ingestion of 1 tablet of any sulfonylurea is sufficient to cause profound and potentially fatal hypoglycaemia in a child. The diagnosis should be considered in any child who presents with hypoglycaemia.

Toxic mechanism
Sulfonylureas bind to the cell membrane of pancreatic beta cells to promote insulin release. Excessive stimulation of endogenous insulin results in a hyperinsulinaemic state.

Toxicokinetics
Sulfonylureas are rapidly and completely absorbed, with peak serum levels occurring within 4–8 hours for immediate-release preparations and longer for modified-release formulations. They are metabolised in the liver to active and inactive metabolites, which undergo renal excretion. Elimination half-life varies between agents and is prolonged following overdose.

CLINICAL FEATURES
- Autonomic and CNS manifestations of hypoglycaemia including:
  - sweating, tachycardia and confusion
  - altered mental status progressing to coma.

INVESTIGATIONS
Screening tests in deliberate self-poisoning
- 12-lead ECG and paracetamol level

Specific investigations
- Serial BGLs
- EUC

Resuscitation, supportive care and monitoring

- Administer concentrated IV glucose solutions as part of the initial resuscitation of the hypoglycaemic patient.
- Give adults 50 mL of 50% glucose IV bolus (2–5 mL/kg of 10% glucose in children).
- Maintain euglycaemia by continued administration of concentrated glucose solution until octreotide can be started (see **Antidotes**).
- BGLs are monitored closely with bedside testing. They should be checked at least hourly in the initial phase of treatment. This frequency can be reduced in the stable patient on octreotide.

Decontamination

- Oral activated charcoal can be given where the patient presents within 1 hour of acute overdose, providing mental state permits. Activated charcoal should be administered up to 4 hours following ingestion of a modified-release preparation.

Enhanced elimination

- Not clinically useful.

Antidotes

- Octreotide is the specific antidote for sulfonylurea-induced hypoglycaemia. Give adults a 50-microgram IV bolus followed by 25 microgram/hour continuous infusion for at least 24 hours. Give children 1 microgram/kg IV followed by 1 microgram/kg/hour continuous infusion (see **Chapter 4.19: Octreotide** for further details).

DISPOSITION AND FOLLOW-UP

- All children with suspected sulfonylurea ingestion require observation in hospital and monitoring of BGLs with bedside testing for at least 18 hours.
- All adult patients with definite or suspected sulfonylurea overdose require observation for clinical features of hypoglycaemia and monitoring of BGLs with bedside testing for at least 8 hours (12 hours for modified-release preparations) from the time of the overdose.
- Patients who remain euglycaemic and clinically well after an appropriate duration of observation may be discharged.
- Symptomatic patients with hypoglycaemia treated with IV glucose and octreotide are admitted. They are medically fit for discharge once they maintain euglycaemia on a normal diet for at least 12 hours from the time of discontinuation of octreotide.
- Patients who develop hypoglycaemia on therapeutic doses of a sulfonylurea always require admission for prolonged observation to exclude recurrent hypoglycaemia. Oral or IV glucose administration, octreotide dosing, treatment of intercurrent medical conditions and re-evaluation of diabetic therapy is required as indicated.

HANDY TIPS

- Early institution of octreotide therapy can prevent the requirement for concentrated glucose infusions and central venous access.
- Octreotide may be administered SC if IV access is not readily available.

- Patients who develop an isolated episode of hypoglycaemia on therapeutic dosing may be treated effectively with a single IV or SC dose of octreotide without requiring an ongoing infusion.
- Non-diabetic patients are at particular risk of hypoglycaemia during weaning of glucose infusions because exogenous glucose administration stimulates endogenous pancreatic insulin release, prolonging the hyperinsulinaemic state.
- IV boluses of 50% glucose are a profound stimulus for endogenous insulin release. Attempts should be made to limit bolus IV glucose therapy in response to borderline hypoglycaemia unless significant clinical features are evident.
- Do not ignore a BGL <4 mmol/L following sulfonylurea overdose. It heralds the onset of profound hypoglycaemia.
- Documentation of hypoglycaemia is essential to confirm the diagnosis of sulfonylurea toxicity. Intravenous glucose or octreotide should not be given until hypoglycaemia is confirmed.

PITFALLS
- Failure to admit a patient on therapeutic sulfonylurea who presents with hypoglycaemia. Prolonged monitoring of blood glucose levels is required to detect and manage recurrent episodes.
- Failure to observe asymptomatic paediatric ingestions for a sufficient period to detect delayed hypoglycaemia.

CONTROVERSIES
- The observation period required for suspected ingestion of modified-release preparations is unknown. Onset of hypoglycaemia could be delayed greater than 24 hours.
- Optimal dose and route for administration of octreotide are yet to be established. A safe approach is suggested in **Chapter 4.19: Octreotide**.
- The role of insulin assays in monitoring response to octreotide therapy.

Presentations
Glibenclamide 5 mg tablets (100)
Glibenclamide 1.25 mg/metformin 250 mg tablets (90)
Glibenclamide 2.5 mg/metformin 500 mg tablets (90)
Glibenclamide 5 mg/metformin 500 mg tablets (90)
Gliclazide 80 mg tablets (100)
Gliclazide 30 mg modified-release tablets (100)
Gliclazide 60 mg modified-release tablets (60)
Glimepiride 1 mg, 2 mg, 3 mg, 4 mg tablets (30)
Glipizide 5 mg tablets (100)

References
Harrigan RA, Nathan MS, Beattie P. Oral agents for the treatment of type 2 diabetes mellitus: pharmacology, toxicity and treatment. Annals of Emergency Medicine 2001; 38:68–78.

Klein-Schwartz W, Stassinos GL, Isbister GK. Treatment of sulfonylurea and insulin overdose. British Journal of Clinical Pharmacology 2016; 81(3):496–504.

Lung DD, Olson KR. Hypoglycemia in pediatric sulfonylurea poisoning: an 8-year poison center retrospective study. Pediatrics 2011; 127(6):e1558–e1564.

Spiller HA, Villalobos D, Krenzelok EP et al. Prospective multicenter study of sulfonylurea ingestion in children. Journal of Pediatrics 1997; 131:141–146.

3.75 THEOPHYLLINE

Theophylline has a narrow therapeutic index and both acute and chronic toxicity can be life-threatening. Seizures and haemodynamic instability require intensive care management and haemodialysis.

RISK ASSESSMENT

- All acute theophylline overdoses develop clinical features of toxicity.
- Ingestion of >50 mg/kg is expected to lead to life-threatening toxicity, manifested by tachydysrhythmias and seizures (see **Table 3.75.1**).
- Chronic theophylline poisoning has an increased risk of an adverse outcome. Patients are often elderly with co-existing medical illnesses.
- **Children:** ingestion of one 200-mg modified-release tablet will produce toxicity in a 10-kg child. Ingestion of multiple tablets can be life-threatening.

Toxic mechanism

Theophylline is a methylxanthine with a structure similar to caffeine. Enhanced release of catecholamines and antagonism of adenosine receptors results in tachydysrhythmias and seizures. Inhibition of phosphodiesterase activity increases cAMP levels, leading to additional adrenergic effects including metabolic disturbances (hypokalaemia, hyperglycaemia).

Toxicokinetics

Theophylline is well-absorbed after oral administration but peak levels may be delayed greater than 12 hours following ingestion of slow-release formulations. It has a small volume of distribution and is metabolised by the cytochrome P450 system, so drug interactions (e.g. macrolide antibiotics, verapamil) can result in significant drug accumulation. The half-life varies dramatically with age – from 30 hours in premature infants to 8 hours in young adults. Across all ages metabolism may be saturable – pharmacokinetics change to zero order and small dose changes can result in rapid increases in serum concentration, prolongation of the elimination phase and the development of toxicity.

Aminophylline is a water-soluble complex of theophylline suitable for intravenous administration. It rapidly dissociates in vivo to release theophylline.

CLINICAL FEATURES

Acute theophylline toxicity

- All acute overdoses present with vomiting, abdominal pain, sinus tachycardia and tremor.

TABLE 3.75.1	Dose-related risk assessment: acute theophylline overdose
Dose	**Effect**
5–10 mg/kg	Therapeutic daily dose
>10 mg/kg	Increasing risk of systemic toxicity Nausea, vomiting, tachycardia, hypotension, seizures
>50 mg/kg	Life-threatening toxicity

- Severe poisoning is associated with:
  - ventricular tachydysrhythmias
  - refractory hypotension
  - seizures
  - metabolic abnormalities:
    - hypokalaemia
    - hypomagnesaemia, hypophosphataemia
    - hyperglycaemia
    - metabolic acidosis.
- Ventricular dysrhythmias and seizures indicate an extremely poor prognosis.

Chronic theophylline toxicity
- Chronic toxicity usually develops in elderly or infant patients related to excessive dosing or drug interactions. Gastrointestinal features and metabolic disturbances are less prominent than with acute overdose, but seizures and dysrhythmias occur frequently and at lower serum theophylline concentrations.

INVESTIGATIONS

Screening tests in deliberate self-poisoning
- 12-lead ECG, BGL and paracetamol level

Specific investigations
- Serial serum theophylline levels:
  - Useful to assess the risk of life-threatening toxicity.
  - In acute overdose, levels correlate well with clinical severity (see **Table 3.75.2**) and are repeated every 2–4 hours until falling.
    - Levels >330 micromol/L (60 mg/L) may be associated with severe toxicity in elderly patients.
  - In chronic intoxication, severe toxicity can occur at levels >220 micromol/L (40 mg/L).
- EUC, venous blood gas, calcium, magnesium, phosphate

MANAGEMENT

Resuscitation, supportive care and monitoring
- Theophylline poisoning is a life-threatening emergency that is managed in an area equipped for cardiorespiratory monitoring and resuscitation.

TABLE 3.75.2	Correlation of serum levels and toxicity: acute theophylline overdose	
Level (micromol/L)	**Level (mg/L)**	**Toxicity**
55–110	10–20	Therapeutic
110–550	20–100	Escalating toxicity
>550	>100	May be fatal without urgent intervention

- The patient who presents with established severe toxicity has a poor prognosis. Immediate resuscitation and control of seizures is required, but supportive care measures may not ensure survival and definitive treatment with haemodialysis is needed.
- Immediate life-threats include:
  - hypotension
  - seizures
  - ventricular tachydysrhythmias.
- Hypotension usually responds to fluid administration, although a noradrenaline infusion may be needed in resistant cases.
- Treat seizures with benzodiazepines, as outlined in **Chapter 2.3: Seizures**.
- Ventricular dysrhythmias may be recurrent and resistant to treatment. Beta-blockers, lidocaine and amiodarone are appropriate treatment options.
- Significant supraventricular tachycardia may benefit from carefully titrated doses of beta-blockers. Metoprolol, labetalol or esmolol can be trialled but may worsen hypotension. Verapamil is an alternative option in the presence of bronchospasm.
- Hypokalaemia (and other metabolic derangements) should be corrected to the upper limit of normal.

Decontamination
- Activated charcoal is indicated following acute overdose even if presentation is delayed, particularly with slow-release preparations. Anti-emetics will be required to control vomiting.

Enhanced elimination
- Haemodialysis is the definitive life-saving intervention in severe theophylline poisoning and highly effective in achieving good clinical outcome if commenced early.
- Haemodialysis or continuous renal replacement therapies are initiated for the following indications:
  - serum theophylline >550 micromol/L (100 mg/L) in the setting of acute overdose
  - serum theophylline >330 micromol/L (60 mg/L) in the setting of chronic toxicity
  - clinical manifestations of severe toxicity – dysrhythmia, hypotension or seizures.
- Multiple-dose activated charcoal enhances the elimination of theophylline by reducing enterohepatic recirculation and may be considered, depending on clinical progress.

Antidotes
- None available.

DISPOSITION AND FOLLOW-UP
- Patients who have acutely ingested immediate-release theophylline preparations and are asymptomatic at 6 hours do not require ongoing medical management.
- Overdose of modified-release tablets requires close observation for 12 hours.
- All symptomatic patients are managed in an intensive care environment.

- If the initial risk assessment indicates potential for severe toxicity, retrieval to a facility with an intensive care unit capable of emergency haemodialysis is undertaken as soon as possible before clinical deterioration occurs.

CONTROVERSIES
- Seizures related to theophylline toxicity may respond poorly to $GABA_A$ receptor blockers such as benzodiazepines. Animal data suggest that anticonvulsants such as levetiracetam may be effective.
- Charcoal haemoperfusion is described as the modality of choice for enhancing theophylline elimination. However, the technique is not widely available and standard haemodialysis or continuous therapies are effective and usually able to be implemented more quickly.

Presentations
Aminophylline 25 mg/mL ampoules (10 mL)
Theophylline 200 mg, 250 mg, 300 mg modified-release tablets (100)
Theophylline 5.32 mg/mL oral liquid (500 mL)

References
Ghannoum M, Wiegand TJ, Liu KD et al. Extracorporeal treatment for theophylline poisoning: systematic review and recommendations from the EXTRIP workgroup. Clinical Toxicology 2015; 53(4):215–229.
Minton NA, Henry JA. Treatment of theophylline overdose. American Journal of Emergency Medicine 1996; 14:606–612.
Shannon M. Life-threatening events after theophylline overdose: a 10-year prospective analysis. Archives of Internal Medicine 1999; 159:989–994.

3.76 THYROXINE

Acute overdose of thyroxine is unlikely to cause significant clinical effects. If symptoms of hyperthyroidism do occur, they are generally mild, delayed in onset and can usually be managed in the outpatient setting.

RISK ASSESSMENT
- The majority of patients with acute thyroxine overdose remain asymptomatic or experience only mild-to-moderate symptoms of hyperthyroidism some 2–7 days later.
- Symptoms are not expected unless >10 mg of thyroxine is ingested.

- The elderly and patients with cardiovascular co-morbidities are at increased risk of complications should hyperthyroid symptoms occur.
- Severe toxicity is more likely to occur following chronic abuse of thyroid hormones.
- **Children:** ingestion of up to 5 mg is associated with minimal symptoms. Severe thyrotoxicosis has not been reported after accidental paediatric ingestion of thyroxine.

Toxic mechanism

Thyroxine (T_4) is converted to tri-iodothyronine (T_3) in the liver and kidney. T_3 binds to the receptors in the cell nucleus and stimulates multiple cardiovascular and metabolic processes.

Toxicokinetics

Thyroxine absorption occurs mainly in the small bowel and bioavailability is highly variable. The peak physiological effect may be delayed up to 1–3 weeks post overdose. Thyroxine is almost completely protein bound and metabolised in the liver by sequential deiodination. Elimination is primarily renal and is shortened from 7 days to 3 days following overdose.

CLINICAL FEATURES

- Following acute ingestion, most patients remain asymptomatic.
- Where symptoms do develop, they are not usually apparent until >24 hours following the ingestion but may then last more than 1 week.
- Signs and symptoms are those of hyperthyroidism and include anxiety, tremor, fever, tachycardia, hypertension and diarrhoea.
- Chronic supratherapeutic ingestion of thyroxine is more likely to cause significant clinical features of hyperthyroidism.

INVESTIGATIONS

Screening tests in deliberate self-poisoning

- 12-lead ECG, BGL and paracetamol level

Specific investigations

- Thyroid function tests after overdose may show marked abnormalities of TSH, T_4 and T_3 but are of no clinical relevance. They do not assist in management following either accidental paediatric ingestion or deliberate self-poisoning and are not indicated.

MANAGEMENT

Resuscitation, supportive care and monitoring

- Resuscitation measures are rarely required.
- General supportive care measures are indicated, as outlined in **Chapter 1.4: Supportive care and monitoring**.
- Beta-blockers rapidly control the adrenergic features of thyroid excess. In symptomatic patients with no contraindications to beta blockade, administer oral propranolol 10–40 mg (0.2–0.5 mg/kg in children) every 6 hours. Metoprolol is an alternative agent that can be given by the oral or intravenous route.
- If beta-blockers are contraindicated, calcium channel blockers (e.g. diltiazem) are a suitable alternative. Administer diltiazem 60–180 mg (1–3 mg/kg in children) every 8 hours.

- Close clinical and physiological monitoring is indicated for patients with severe symptoms.

Decontamination
- Give oral activated charcoal 50 g to cooperative patients who present after acute thyroxine overdose.
- Oral activated charcoal is not indicated in children following accidental ingestion.

Enhanced elimination
- Not clinically useful.

Antidotes
- None available.

DISPOSITION AND FOLLOW-UP
- Children suspected of ingesting up to 5 mg of thyroxine may be observed at home provided they remain asymptomatic.
- Adult patients with acute deliberate self-poisoning rarely require immediate management. If symptoms of hyperthyroidism occur, management with beta-blockers is indicated, usually for a period of 1 week. Thyroxine may be restarted in 1–2 weeks if required.

PITFALLS
- Unnecessary admission for prolonged medical observation.
- Failure to anticipate or recognise the delayed onset of symptoms following large overdoses.

Presentations
Thyroxine 50 microgram, 75 microgram, 100 microgram, 200 microgram tablets (200)

References
Lewander WJ, Lacouture PG, Silva JE et al. Acute thyroxine ingestion in pediatric patients. Pediatrics 1989; 84:262–265.

Litovitz TL, White JD. Levothyroxine ingestions in children: an analysis of 78 cases. American Journal of Emergency Medicine 1985; 3:297–300.

Shilo L, Kovatz S, Hadari R et al. Massive thyroid hormone overdose: clinical manifestations and management. Israeli Medical Association Journal 2002; 4:298–299.

Tunget CL, Clark RF, Turchen SG et al. Raising the decontamination level for thyroid hormone ingestions. American Journal of Emergency Medicine 1995; 13:9–13.

3.77 TRAMADOL AND TAPENTADOL

Tramadol is a synthetic opioid agonist. In overdose, the principal toxic effects of tachycardia and seizures are due to noradrenaline and serotonin re-uptake inhibition. In comparison, tapentadol is less toxic in overdose.

RISK ASSESSMENT
- Tramadol overdose carries a high risk of seizures, which are dose-dependent and may have a significantly delayed onset.

- Opioid effects (sedation and respiratory depression) occur and may require administration of naloxone.
- Serotonin toxicity can occur, particularly if there is co-ingestion of other serotonergic agents.
- Available data for tapentadol suggest that severe toxicity is less likely.
- **Children:** sedation, respiratory depression and seizures can occur with ingestion of a single tablet of either agent. Hospital assessment is recommended following any accidental ingestion.

Toxic mechanism

Tramadol is a partial agonist at mu opioid receptors. It also inhibits noradrenaline and serotonin reuptake in the CNS. Tapentadol has similar opioid and noradrenergic properties but no serotonergic activity.

Toxicokinetics

Tramadol is well absorbed orally and peak levels occur at 2–3 hours after ingestion of standard preparations and 4–12 hours with sustained-release preparations. Peak levels may be further delayed after overdose. It is metabolised in the liver by CYP2D6 to O-desmethyltramadol, a more potent opioid agonist. Tramadol and the active metabolite are renally excreted. In comparison, tapentadol reaches peak levels earlier and has inactive metabolites.

CLINICAL FEATURES

- Noradrenergic effects are prominent and include tachycardia, agitation and seizures.
- Seizures are typically brief and self-limiting but can be recurrent. Onset may be delayed several hours, particularly with slow-release preparations.
- Serotonin toxicity can occur but is unlikely to be severe in isolated tramadol ingestions (see **Chapter 2.5: Serotonin toxicity**).
- Opioid agonist effects include sedation, respiratory depression and miosis.

INVESTIGATIONS

Screening tests in deliberate self-poisoning
- 12-lead ECG, BGL and paracetamol level

MANAGEMENT

Resuscitation, supportive care and monitoring
- Attention to airway, breathing and circulation are paramount. These priorities are managed along conventional lines, as outlined in **Chapter 1.2: Resuscitation**.
- Seizures are treated with titrated doses of IV benzodiazepines, as outlined in **Chapter 2.3: Seizures**.
- Increasing agitation, tachycardia, tremor and myoclonus may herald onset of seizures. Titrated doses of IV benzodiazepines are recommended in an attempt to prevent their occurrence.
- Serotonin toxicity is managed as described in **Chapter 2.5: Serotonin toxicity**.
- General supportive care measures are indicated, as outlined in **Chapter 1.4: Supportive care and monitoring**.

Decontamination
- The decision to administer activated charcoal is based on consideration of the dose ingested, the time since ingestion and the clinical features on presentation. Activated charcoal can be administered to patients who have ingested slow-release formulations who present within 2 hours with minimal symptoms.
- The potential for seizures must be considered when making a risk–benefit analysis of the value of administering activated charcoal.

Enhanced elimination
- Not clinically useful.

Antidotes
- Naloxone may reverse CNS and respiratory depression secondary to opioid effects (see **Chapter 4.18: Naloxone**).

DISPOSITION AND FOLLOW-UP
- Because of the risk of delayed onset of toxicity following tramadol overdose, all patients should be observed for a minimum of 12 hours and until symptom free. Seizures can be delayed up to 24 hours post ingestion in some individuals. Discharge should not occur at night.

PITFALLS
- Failure to anticipate and prepare for delayed symptoms or seizures.
- Administration of activated charcoal shortly before onset of seizures.

CONTROVERSY
- Available evidence suggests that tapentadol is much less toxic than tramadol in overdose. It is reasonable to decrease the observation period following tapentadol overdose if the patient remains clinically well.

Presentations
Tapentadol hydrochloride 50 mg, 75 mg, 100 mg tablets
Tapentadol hydrochloride sustained-release 50 mg, 100 mg, 150 mg, 200 mg, 250 mg tablets (28)
Tramadol hydrochloride 50 mg capsules (20)
Tramadol hydrochloride 50 mg, 150 mg sustained-release tablets (20)
Tramadol hydrochloride 100 mg, 200 mg sustained-release tablets (10, 20)
Tramadol hydrochloride 300 mg sustained-release tablets (10)
Tramadol hydrochloride 100 mg/1 mL oral liquid (10 mL)
Tramadol 50 mg/mL ampoules (2 mL)
Tramadol 37.5 mg/paracetamol 325 mg (20, 50)

References
Ryan NM, Isbister GK. Tramadol overdose causes seizures and respiratory depression but serotonin toxicity appears unlikely. Clinical Toxicology 2015; 53(6):545–550.

Sachdeva DK, Stadnyk JM. Are one or two dangerous? Opioid exposure in toddlers. Journal of Emergency Medicine 2005; 29(1):77–84.

Shadnia S, Soltaninejad K, Heyardi K et al. Tramadol intoxication: a review of 114 cases. Human and Experimental Toxicology 2008; 27:201–205.

Spiller HA, Gorman SE, Villalobos D et al. Prospective multicenter evaluation of tramadol exposure. Journal of Toxicology–Clinical Toxicology 1997; 35(4):361–364.

Amitriptyline, Clomipramine, Dothiepin, Doxepin, Imipramine, Nortriptyline

Tricyclic antidepressant (TCA) poisoning remains a major cause of morbidity and mortality. Deliberate self-poisoning leads to the rapid onset of CNS and cardiovascular toxicity. Sodium bicarbonate administration, prompt intubation and hyperventilation at the first evidence of severe toxicity are life-saving.

RISK ASSESSMENT

- Ingestion of >10 mg/kg is potentially life-threatening (see **Table 3.78.1**).
- Onset of severe toxicity usually occurs within 2 hours of ingestion.
- **Children:** Any child who is suspected of ingesting >2.5 mg/kg is referred to hospital for assessment.

Toxic mechanism

TCAs are noradrenaline and serotonin reuptake inhibitors and $GABA_A$ receptor blockers. Myocardial toxicity is chiefly due to blockade of inactivated fast sodium channels. Other toxic effects are mediated by blockade at muscarinic (M_1), histamine (H_1) and peripheral α_1-adrenergic receptors. TCAs cause reversible inhibition of potassium channels and direct myocardial depression unrelated to conduction abnormalities.

Toxicokinetics

TCAs are rapidly absorbed following therapeutic dosing, with peak levels occurring within 2 hours. However, in overdose, absorption may be prolonged due to anticholinergic effects on gut motility. TCAs are highly protein bound and have large volumes of distribution (5–20 L/kg). TCAs undergo hepatic metabolism by CYP2D6 to active metabolites, and some enterohepatic circulation occurs.

CLINICAL FEATURES

Severe toxicity is characterised by rapid deterioration in clinical status within 2 hours of ingestion. Patients may present alert and orientated,

---

TABLE 3.78.1	**Dose-related risk assessments: tricyclic antidepressants**
Dose	**Effect**
<5 mg/kg	Mild symptoms
5–10 mg/kg	Sedation and anticholinergic effects predominate Significant cardiovascular toxicity not expected
>10 mg/kg	Potential for all major effects (seizures, coma, hypotension, cardiac dysrhythmias) to occur within 2–4 hours of ingestion Anticholinergic delirium often masked by coma
>30 mg/kg	Severe toxicity with pH-dependent cardiotoxicity and coma expected to last >24 hours

only to rapidly develop seizures, coma, hypotension and cardiac dysrhythmias.

- Central nervous system
  - Sedation and anticholinergic delirium are initial signs of toxicity.
  - Seizures may be heralded by myoclonic jerks and can occur early.
  - Coma develops rapidly following onset of seizures.
- Cardiovascular
  - Sinus tachycardia is characteristic
  - Hypotension
  - Broad-complex tachydysrhythmias
  - Broad-complex bradydysrhythmia occurs pre-arrest
- Anticholinergic effects
  - May be evident on presentation or be delayed in onset
  - Agitation and delirium
  - Mydriasis
  - Dry, warm, flushed skin
  - Tachycardia
  - Urinary retention and ileus

INVESTIGATIONS

Screening tests in deliberate self-poisoning

- 12-lead ECG, BGL and paracetamol level

Specific investigations

- Serial ECGs
  - Essential in the management of TCA poisoning (see **Chapter 2.17: The 12-lead ECG in toxicology**).
  - Diagnostic features include:
    - prolongation of QRS interval
    - large terminal R wave in aVR
    - increased R/S ratio (>0.7) in aVR
    - QT prolongation is also noted secondary to potassium channel (hERG) blockade.
  - QRS widening reflects degree of fast sodium channel blockade.
    - QRS >100 ms is predictive of seizures.
    - QRS >160 ms is predictive of ventricular dysrhythmias.

MANAGEMENT

Resuscitation, supportive care and monitoring

- Acute TCA poisoning is a potentially life-threatening emergency managed in an area equipped for cardiorespiratory monitoring and resuscitation.
- Early life-threats that require immediate intervention include:
  - seizures
  - coma
  - cardiac dysrhythmia
  - cardiac arrest.
- The mainstays of treatment for both CNS and cardiovascular toxicity are:
  - administration of IV sodium bicarbonate boluses
  - intubation
  - hyperventilation.

FIGURE 3.78.1 TCA Cardiotoxicity

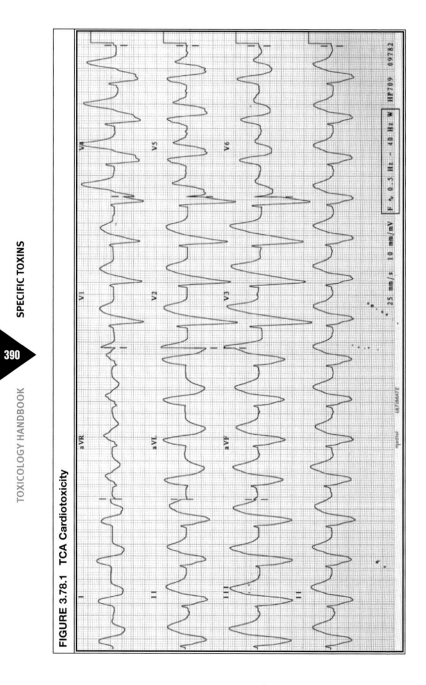

FIGURE 3.78.2 TCA Cardiotoxicity (Post-alkalinisation)

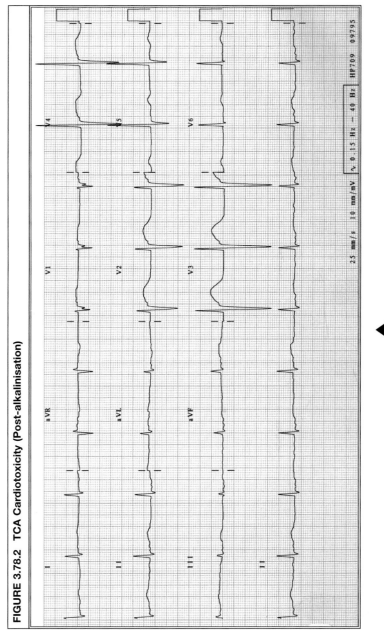

- Administer sodium bicarbonate 1–2 mmol/kg IV repeated every 1–2 minutes until:
  - — restoration of perfusing rhythm
  - — improvement in QRS widening
  - — pH established at 7.5–7.55.
- Intubation and hyperventilation to maintain a therapeutic endpoint of pH 7.5–7.55.
- The majority of TCA poisonings will respond to these interventions with a dynamic improvement in QRS widening and blood pressure.
- The QRS may not return to normal (<100 ms); however, this does not mandate ongoing sodium bicarbonate administration in the presence of haemodynamic stability and a pH maintained at 7.5–7.55 by hyperventilation.
- Hypotension may persist after initial resuscitation with sodium bicarbonate, hyperventilation and IV fluids, and titrated adrenaline or noradrenaline infusions are indicated.
- Rarely patients may remain unstable with broad complex dysrhythmias.
  - — Lidocaine 1–1.5 mg/kg IV can be considered if these continue after the pH is established and maintained at 7.5–7.55.
- Seizures that persist after the pH is maintained at 7.5–7.55 are managed with benzodiazepines, as outlined in **Chapter 2.3: Seizures**.
- General supportive care measures are indicated, as outlined in **Chapter 1.4: Supportive care and monitoring**.

Decontamination
- Activated charcoal should be given to all patients with significant ingestions but is administered only after the airway is secured by endotracheal intubation and after dealing with all resuscitation priorities.

Enhanced elimination
- Not clinically useful.

Antidotes
- Sodium bicarbonate as detailed above; also see **Chapter 4.24: Sodium bicarbonate**.

DISPOSITION AND FOLLOW-UP
- Patients who are clinically well, with normal 12-lead ECG (or static pre-existing changes), normal mental status, no hypotension and no seizures at 6 hours post ingestion do not require further cardiac monitoring or observation and are medically fit for discharge.
- Patients with anticholinergic toxicity or ECG abnormalities require ongoing monitoring until clinically well with a normal ECG.
- Patients with significant toxicity require management in an intensive care unit.

HANDY TIPS
- Resuscitation efforts should not cease until the patient has been treated with sodium bicarbonate, intubated and hyperventilated to

achieve a pH of 7.5–7.55. Numerous reports describe survival with good neurological outcome following cardiac arrest and prolonged resuscitation.

- Seizures will cause a rapid clinical deterioration, due to the acidaemia resulting from lactic acidosis causing increased binding of TCA to CNS and cardiovascular receptors.

PITFALLS
- Insufficient doses of sodium bicarbonate during initial resuscitation of severe TCA poisoning.
- Continued excessive doses of IV sodium bicarbonate after the pH has been established at 7.5–7.55, resulting in life-threatening alkalaemia, pulmonary oedema and cerebral oedema.

Presentations
Amitriptyline hydrochloride 10 mg, 25 mg, 50 mg tablets (50)
Clomipramine hydrochloride 25 mg tablets (50)
Dothiepin hydrochloride 25 mg capsules (50)
Dothiepin hydrochloride 75 mg tablets (30)
Doxepin hydrochloride 10 mg, 25 mg, 50 mg capsules (50)
Imipramine hydrochloride 10 mg, 25 mg tablets (50)
Nortriptyline hydrochloride 10 mg, 25 mg tablets (50)

References
Bateman ND. Tricyclic antidepressant poisoning: central nervous system effects and management. Toxicological Reviews 2005; 24(3):181–186.
Bradberry SM, Thanacoody HKR, Watt BE et al. Management of the cardiovascular complications of tricyclic antidepressant toxicity: role of sodium bicarbonate. Toxicological Reviews 2005; 24(3):195–204.
Heard K, Cain BS, Dart RC et al. Tricyclic antidepressants directly depress human myocardial mechanical function independent of effects on the conduction system. Academic Emergency Medicine 2001; 8(12):1122–1127.
Liebelt EL, Francis PD, Woolf AD. ECG lead aVR versus QRS interval in predicting seizures and arrhythmias in acute tricyclic antidepressant toxicity. Annals of Emergency Medicine 1995; 26(2):195–201.

3.79 VALPROIC ACID (SODIUM VALPROATE)

Valproate overdose causes dose-dependent CNS depression and multi-system organ effects. Early recognition of the likelihood of significant toxicity guides the definitive management decision to intubate, ventilate and institute haemodialysis.

RISK ASSESSMENT
- Most ingestions do not reach the threshold to cause significant CNS depression (see **Table 3.79.1**).
- Increasingly severe multi-system organ effects occur as doses rise above 400 mg/kg.
- Ingestion of >1 g/kg is potentially lethal.
- **Children:** accidental ingestions of <200 mg/kg may be observed at home. Referral to hospital for assessment is indicated if more than this amount has been ingested or if symptoms develop.

TABLE 3.79.1   Dose-related risk assessment: valproic acid

Dose	Effect
<200 mg/kg	Asymptomatic, or mild drowsiness and ataxia only
200–400 mg/kg	Variable CNS depression; intubation unlikely to be required
400–1000 mg/kg	Coma requiring intubation is predicted to develop As doses increase within this range, more severe multi-system toxicity is observed
>1000 mg/kg	Potentially lethal with prolonged coma and cerebral oedema

Toxic mechanism

Valproate increases levels of gamma-aminobutyric acid (GABA), a central inhibitory neurotransmitter. Toxicity is caused by interference with mitochondrial metabolic pathways, particularly the urea cycle, leading to hyperammonaemia and lactic acidosis. Active metabolites may be responsible for the development of cerebral oedema and hepatotoxicity. Other biochemical effects of note include hypernatraemia (related to ingested sodium load) and hypoglycaemia (hepatotoxicity).

Toxicokinetics

Valproate is usually well absorbed following ingestion but absorption may be slow and erratic, particularly with enteric-coated formulations, where peak levels may be delayed up to 18 hours. Valproate is highly protein bound with a small volume of distribution, but the unbound fraction of valproate increases markedly in overdose. It undergoes hepatic metabolism to active metabolites, and the elimination half-life increases from 12 hours at therapeutic dosing to more than 30 hours following overdose.

CLINICAL FEATURES

- Coma is the hallmark of significant valproate toxicity.
- The onset may be delayed several hours and deterioration in conscious state reflects rising serum levels (see below).
- Metabolic and electrolyte abnormalities are characteristic following large ingestions:
  — lactic acidosis with an elevated anion gap
  — hypernatraemia, hypoglycaemia and hypocalcaemia
  — hyperammonaemia
  — other features of systemic toxicity include renal impairment, hepatotoxicity, pancreatitis and bone marrow suppression.
- Hypotension can occur with large ingestions, but cardiac dysrhythmias are not expected.
- Cerebral oedema is the life-threatening complication and is likely related to hyperammonaemia. It may persist for several days even after serum valproate levels return to normal.
  — Note: Hyperammonaemia, cerebral oedema or hepatotoxicity can occur with therapeutic dosing in the absence of acute overdose. These effects may be related to urea cycle abnormalities or congenital metabolic disorders.

TABLE 3.79.2 Correlation of clinical effects with serum valproate level	
Serum valproate	Clinical effects
>500 mg/L (>3500 micromol/L)	Coma is likely Multiple organ-system effects become evident
>1000 mg/L (>7000 micromol/L)	Increased risk of life-threatening cerebral oedema

INVESTIGATIONS

Screening tests in deliberate self-poisoning
- 12-lead ECG, BGL and paracetamol level

Specific investigations
- Serial valproate levels confirm poisoning and are essential to determine the requirement for haemodialysis (see **Table 3.79.2**).
- In the comatose patient, serum valproate levels are repeated every 4–6 hours until normalised.
- Ammonia levels can be performed and may correlate with the severity and duration of coma.
- EUC, FBC, LFT, acid–base status, calcium and lipase to detect and manage multi-system toxicity.

MANAGEMENT

Resuscitation, supportive care and monitoring
- All patients are managed in an area equipped for cardiopulmonary monitoring and resuscitation.
- Attention to airway, breathing and circulation are paramount. These priorities are managed along conventional lines, as outlined in **Chapter 1.2: Resuscitation**.
- The need for intubation is anticipated and performed early in the patient with a declining level of consciousness.
- General supportive care measures are indicated, as outlined in **Chapter 1.4: Supportive care and monitoring**.

Decontamination
- Activated charcoal is recommended for all intentional ingestions of >400 mg/kg sodium valproate that present without established CNS toxicity within 2 hours.
- If there is evidence of CNS toxicity, activated charcoal is only administered after the patient is intubated.

Enhanced elimination
- Haemodialysis removes valproic acid effectively and is indicated when severe systemic toxicity is anticipated or evident:
  - ingestion of >1000 mg/kg
  - serum level >1000 mg/L (7000 micromol/L)
  - severe toxicity with progressive lactic acidosis, cardiovascular instability or evidence of cerebral oedema.
- Haemodialysis is ideally initiated before severe multi-system organ toxicity is established.

- If intermittent haemodialysis is not available, continuous modalities are acceptable, although clearance will be lower.
- Although multiple-dose activated charcoal is not proven to enhance clearance significantly, it is reasonable to administer a repeat dose in intubated patients if bowel sounds remain present.

Antidotes
- None available (see **Controversies**).

DISPOSITION AND FOLLOW-UP
- Patients who ingest >200 mg/kg are observed for 6 hours (immediate-release) or 12 hours (enteric-coated formulation). They are fit for medical discharge if clinically well at this time.

HANDY TIPS
- In the setting of an acute overdose, significant toxicity will not occur without development of coma.
- Consider valproic acid overdose in any patient with unexplained coma, particularly where there is hypernatraemia or lactic acidosis.
- Hyperammonaemia or cerebral oedema may occur with therapeutic dosing in the absence of acute overdose.

PITFALL
- Falsely low valproate levels have been reported in cases where the threshold for the laboratory assay is exceeded. It is essential to ensure that the laboratory performs appropriate dilution of samples in the setting of acute overdose.

CONTROVERSIES
- The threshold valproate level mandating haemodialysis remains debatable. The risks of this invasive intervention are weighed against the likely benefit in improving valproate clearance to decrease the severity and duration of cerebral oedema.
- Carnitine or arginine supplementation have been suggested as treatments for valproate-induced hyperammonaemia or hepatotoxicity. These recommendations are based on small case series and extrapolation from treatment of children with selected inborn errors of metabolism. There is no definitive evidence of benefit but they are considered low-risk interventions.

Presentations
Sodium valproate 100 mg tablets (100)
Sodium valproate 200 mg, 500 mg enteric-coated tablets (100, 200)
Sodium valproate 40 mg/mL oral liquid (300 mL, 600 mL)
Sodium valproate 400 mg, injectable (powder + solvent) (4 mL)

References
Ghannoum M, Laliberté M, Nolin TD et al. Extracorporeal treatment for valproic acid poisoning: systematic review and recommendations from the EXTRIP workgroup. Clinical Toxicology 2015; 53(5):454–465.
Isbister GK, Balit CR, Whyte IM et al. Valproate overdose: a comparative cohort study of self-poisonings. British Journal of Clinical Pharmacology 2003; 55:398–404.

Spiller HA, Krenzelok EP, Klein-Schwartz W et al. Multicenter case series of valproic acid
ingestion: serum concentrations and toxicity. Clinical Toxicology 2000; 38(7):755–760.
Sztajnkrycer MD. Valproic acid toxicity: overview and management. Journal of
Toxicology–Clinical Toxicology 2002; 40(6):789–801.

3.80 VENLAFAXINE AND DESVENLAFAXINE

**Venlafaxine and desvenlafaxine are serotonin and noradrenaline
reuptake inhibitors. Venlafaxine overdose is potentially life-threatening;
it frequently causes seizures, serotonin toxicity and, in very large
ingestions, severe cardiotoxicity. In comparison, desvenlafaxine is less
toxic in overdose and severe cardiotoxicity has not been reported.**

RISK ASSESSMENT

- Venlafaxine overdose carries a high risk of seizures, which are
  dose-dependent and may have a significantly delayed onset.
- Serotonin and noradrenergic toxicity can be severe, especially if
  other serotonergic or stimulant agents are co-ingested.
- Massive ingestions of venlafaxine (greater than 8 g) can cause
  ventricular dysrhythmias, cardiogenic shock and death.
- Desvenlafaxine has a much lower risk of seizures and serotonin
  toxicity.
- **Children:** accidental ingestion of <12.5 mg/kg of venlafaxine is
  unlikely to cause significant symptoms. Referral to hospital is not
  required unless symptoms occur.

Toxic mechanism

Venlafaxine and its metabolite O-desmethylvenlafaxine (desvenlafaxine) are potent
serotonin and noradrenaline reuptake inhibitors (SNRIs). They also exhibit rate-dependent
sodium-channel-blocking activity, with a lesser effect on dopamine reuptake inhibition.
They have no effect on muscarinic, histamine or α_1-adrenergic receptors, and do not
inhibit monoamine oxidase.

Toxicokinetics

Venlafaxine is well absorbed and undergoes extensive first-pass metabolism via CYP2D6
pathways, resulting in bioavailability of only 50%. All currently available preparations are
controlled-release and peak plasma levels occur at 6–8 hours. The elimination half-life is
15 hours and may be increased in hepatic or renal dysfunction. In overdose, CYP2D6
polymorphism may predispose to more severe and prolonged toxicity.

Desvenlafaxine is also well absorbed but does not undergo extensive first-pass
metabolism and has a bioavailability of 80%. Up to 45% of an ingested dose is excreted
unchanged in the urine, with the rest predominantly undergoing glucuronide conjugation.
The elimination half-life is approximately 11 hours.

CLINICAL FEATURES
Venlafaxine

- Onset of significant clinical features of toxicity may be delayed up
  to 6–12 hours following overdose.
- Dysphoria, anxiety, mydriasis, sweating, tremor, clonus,
  tachycardia (up to 160 beats/minute) and hypertension are
  common and may herald the onset of seizures.
- Seizures are generalised, of short duration and self-limiting, but
  may be recurrent. The first seizure may be delayed up to 16 hours.

- Ventricular dysrhythmias, cardiogenic shock and death can occur due to acute catecholamine-induced cardiomyopathy.
- Large venlafaxine overdoses may cause diffuse, severe left ventricular dysfunction.
- Hypoglycaemia, occasionally severe, is reported following venlafaxine and desvenlafaxine overdose, related to stimulation of endogenous insulin release.

Desvenlafaxine
- The toxic effects in overdose can be similarly delayed in onset but are less severe.
- The seizure risk is much lower.
- Severe cardiotoxicity has not been reported.

INVESTIGATIONS
Screening tests in deliberate self-poisoning
- 12-lead ECG, BGL and paracetamol level

Specific investigations
- Serial ECGs
  - Perform a 12-lead ECG on all patients at presentation and repeat as clinically indicated.

MANAGEMENT
Resuscitation, supportive care and monitoring
- Venlafaxine overdose is a life-threatening emergency managed in an area equipped for cardiorespiratory monitoring and resuscitation.
- Attention to airway, breathing and circulation are paramount. These priorities are managed along conventional lines, as outlined in **Chapter 1.2: Resuscitation**.
- Increasing agitation, tachycardia and tremor may herald onset of seizures. Titrated doses of IV benzodiazepines are recommended in an attempt to prevent their occurrence.
- Hyperthermia is a feature of severe serotonin toxicity and must be immediately controlled. Temperature >38.5°C is an indication for continuous core-temperature monitoring, benzodiazepine sedation and IV fluid administration. Temperature >39.5°C requires rapid treatment to prevent multi-organ failure and neurological injury. Intubation, ventilation and paralysis are indicated, as described in **Chapter 2.5: Serotonin toxicity.**
- Cardiotoxicity secondary to acute catecholamine-induced cardiomyopathy may result in progressive tachycardia and hypotension with deterioration to ventricular dysrhythmias.
  - Assessment of cardiac function will guide the choice of inotropic and pressor support (see **Chapter 2.2: Hypotension**).
  - Consider early administration of high-dose insulin therapy in the setting of cardiogenic shock (see **Chapter 4.14: Insulin (high-dose)**).
  - Consider interventions such as extracorporeal membrane oxygenation (ECMO), cardiopulmonary bypass or intra-aortic balloon pump.

- Management options for ventricular dysrhythmias include:
  - standard ACLS protocols
  - bolus sodium bicarbonate 1–2 mmol/kg IV
  - intubation and hyperventilation to a serum pH 7.5–7.55.
    - Note: Multiple doses of sodium bicarbonate can cause significant alkalaemia, exacerbating hypokalaemia and increasing the risk of ventricular dysrhythmias.

Decontamination
- The decision to administer activated charcoal is based on consideration of the dose ingested, the time since ingestion and the clinical features on presentation. Activated charcoal can be administered to patients presenting within 2 hours who have minimal symptoms.
- Following massive overdose of venlafaxine (>8 g), early intubation to facilitate safe administration of activated charcoal can be justified.
- Whole bowel irrigation has been advocated in addition to activated charcoal to decrease venlafaxine absorption. The logistical difficulties involved and lack of clear clinical benefit mean that it is not recommended.

Enhanced elimination
- Not clinically useful.

Antidotes
- None available.

DISPOSITION AND FOLLOW-UP
- Because of the risk of seizures following venlafaxine overdose, all patients should be observed with IV access in place for a minimum of 16 hours and until asymptomatic. Seizures can be delayed up to 24 hours post ingestion in some individuals.
- Patients who ingest >4.5 g require cardiac monitoring and serial ECGs for a period of at least 12 hours post ingestion. ECG monitoring may then cease if the ECG is normal and the patient is clinically well.
- Patients with severe venlafaxine intoxication require management in an intensive care unit.

HANDY TIPS
- Once toxicity develops it may worsen rapidly, and close observation is vital to ensure that clinical deterioration is identified promptly and appropriate intensive care-level management initiated prior to catastrophic haemodynamic collapse.
- Early administration of titrated doses of intravenous benzodiazepines may prevent seizures and limit progression of cardiotoxicity.
- Coma is not secondary to venlafaxine intoxication and indicates co-ingestion or complication.
- Duloxetine and reboxetine are other available serotonin and noradrenaline reuptake inhibitors. Although there are limited published data following overdose, the risk of significant toxicity is considered low and patients can be managed as for desvenlafaxine toxicity.

PITFALLS
- Failure to anticipate and prepare for delayed onset of symptoms and seizures.
- Failure to recognise the significant progression of cardiotoxicity.
- Administration of activated charcoal or initiation of whole bowel irrigation shortly before onset of seizures or cardiovascular toxicity.

CONTROVERSY
- Available evidence suggests that desvenlafaxine is much less toxic in overdose than venlafaxine. It is reasonable to decrease the observation period following desvenlafaxine overdose if the patient remains clinically well.

Presentations
Desvenlafaxine succinate controlled-release tablets 50 mg (7, 28)
Desvenlafaxine succinate controlled-release tablets 100 mg (28)
Venlafaxine controlled-release tablets 37.5 mg, 75 mg, 150 mg (28)

References
Batista M, Dugernier T, Simon M et al. The spectrum of acute heart failure after venlafaxine overdose. Clinical Toxicology 2013; 51(2):92–95.

Howell C, Wilson AD, Waring WS. Cardiovascular toxicity due to venlafaxine poisoning in adults: a review of 235 consecutive cases. British Journal of Clinical Pharmacology 2007; 64(2):192–197.

Isbister GK. Electrocardiogram changes and arrhythmias in venlafaxine overdose. British Journal of Clinical Pharmacology 2009; 67(5):572–576.

Kumar VV, Oscarsson S, Friberg LE et al. The effect of decontamination procedures on the pharmacokinetics of venlafaxine in overdose. Clinical Pharmacology and Therapeutics 2009; 27:911–915.

Vinetti M, Haufroid V, Capron A et al. Severe acute cardiomyopathy associated with venlafaxine overdose and possible role of CYP2D6 and CYP2C19 polymorphisms. Clinical Toxicology 2011; 49(9):865–869.

Whyte IM, Dawson AH, Buckley NA. Relative toxicity of venlafaxine and selective serotonin reuptake inhibitors in overdose compared to tricyclic antidepressants. Quarterly Journal of Medicine 2003; 96(5):369–374.

3.81 WARFARIN

Warfarin poisoning occurs due to intentional overdose or over-anticoagulation during therapeutic administration. Most patients with an acute overdose are asymptomatic at presentation – bleeding is more likely to occur in patients who have become over-anticoagulated on therapeutic dosing. Patients with active bleeding require urgent reversal therapy. In the absence of bleeding, management is determined by the INR level and presence of high-risk factors.

RISK ASSESSMENT
- Acute ingestion <0.5 mg/kg is unlikely to cause a clinically significant increase in INR.
- The risk of bleeding related to the INR has been best studied in the context of therapeutic over-anticoagulation but can be extrapolated to acute overdose.
  - The risk increases progressively as the INR rises above 4.5 and is also influenced by the presence of high-risk factors (see **Table 3.81.1**).

TABLE 3.81.1	High-risk factors for major bleeding related to an elevated INR
Older age	
Recent major bleed (within previous 4 weeks)	
Major surgery (within previous 2 weeks)	
Thrombocytopenia (platelet count $<50 \times 10^9$/L)	
Liver disease	
Concurrent antiplatelet therapy.	

Adapted from Tran HA, Chanilal SD, Harper PL et al. An update of consensus
guidelines for warfarin reversal. Medical Journal of Australia 2013; 198(4):1–7.

- Large intentional ingestions may cause recurrent or prolonged elevation of the INR after initial antidote administration. Doses of Vitamin K recommended in standard guidelines for reversal of therapeutic over-anticoagulation may not be adequate.
- Active bleeding constitutes an emergency and requires urgent reversal therapy (see **Management**).
- **Children:** accidental ingestion of >0.5 mg/kg requires assessment in hospital.

Toxic mechanism
Warfarin inhibits the enzyme vitamin K_1 2,3-epoxide reductase, preventing formation of the active reduced form of vitamin K required as a co-factor for the synthesis of coagulation factors II, VII, IX and X (plus proteins C and S). The 8–12 hour delay before anticoagulation occurs is due to the half-lives of existing vitamin-K-dependent coagulation factors (6, 24, 40 and 60 hours for factors VII, IX, X and II, respectively). An increase in INR may be apparent within 6 hours due to factor VII depletion, but the peak anticoagulant effect occurs up to 72 hours after ingestion.

Toxicokinetics
Warfarin is rapidly absorbed with 100% bioavailability. It has a small volume of distribution (0.2 L/kg) and is 99% protein bound. Warfarin undergoes hepatic metabolism (primarily CYP2C9 enzyme) to form metabolites that undergo enterohepatic recirculation. Genetic polymorphism in vitamin K_1 2,3-epoxide reductase contributes to significant inter-individual variability in response to warfarin, and toxicity in therapeutic dosing is influenced by numerous drug interactions (e.g. antibiotics, inhibitors of CYP2C9) or nutritional status. Warfarin and its metabolites are excreted in urine and faeces with a highly variable elimination half-life of 20–60 hours.

CLINICAL FEATURES
- Patients may remain asymptomatic with a markedly elevated INR.
- Coagulopathy can result in manifestations ranging in severity from purpura, gingival bleeding and epistaxis to haematuria, gastrointestinal bleeding or intracerebral haemorrhage.

INVESTIGATIONS
Screening tests in deliberate self-poisoning
- 12-lead ECG, BGL and paracetamol level

Specific investigations

- INR
  - In patients not previously anticoagulated, the INR may be normal for the first 12–24 hours after accidental or deliberate overdose. A normal INR at 48 hours excludes significant warfarin toxicity.
  - In patients with a requirement for ongoing anticoagulation, the INR is measured at presentation and at 6-hourly intervals thereafter.

MANAGEMENT

Resuscitation, supportive care and monitoring

- In patients with evidence of haemorrhage, attention to airway, breathing and circulation are paramount. These priorities can usually be managed along conventional lines, as outlined in **Chapter 1.2: Resuscitation**.
- If there is active uncontrolled bleeding, administer prothrombin complex concentrate (PCC; 25–50 IU/kg as an initial dose). It is likely that this will provide rapid and adequate immediate reversal of the coagulopathy in most situations (see **Controversy** below).
  - Three-factor PCC contains factors II, IX and X, but only low levels of factor VII.
  - Four-factor PCC has higher levels of factor VII but is not currently available in Australia.
- Fresh frozen plasma (FFP) 150–300 mL as an initial dose provides additional coagulation factors (particularly factor VII). It is recommended in addition to three-factor PCC or if the severity of bleeding is such that all available reversal agents are required.
- If PCC is not available, a higher initial dose of FFP is recommended (10–15 mL/kg).
- Vitamin K 5–10 mg IV is given after consideration of the requirement for ongoing anticoagulation with warfarin (see **Antidotes**). If alternative agents will be used for ongoing therapeutic anticoagulation, full reversal with large doses of vitamin K is appropriate.
- In the absence of active bleeding, the decision to give reversal therapy is determined by the INR level and the presence of high-risk factors for clinically significant bleeding (see **Tables 3.81.1** and **3.81.2**).
- General supportive care measures are indicated, as outlined in **Chapter 1.4: Supportive care and monitoring**.

Decontamination

- Following deliberate self-poisoning, administer 50 g oral activated charcoal to cooperative patients if they present within 2 hours of ingestion.

Enhanced elimination

- Not clinically useful.

Antidotes

- Vitamin K is most widely available as an intravenous formulation but it is also suitable for oral administration.

TABLE 3.81.2	Guidelines for management of warfarin-induced coagulopathy
Significant bleeding Any INR	Three-factor PCC (Australia) 25–50 IU/kg IV FFP 150–300 mL Vitamin K IV 5–10 mg Withhold warfarin (Note: If PCC is unavailable, an increased dose of FFP (10–15 mL/kg) is recommended)

No bleeding
INR >10
	Vitamin K PO or IV 3–5 mg
	If bleeding risk is high:
	     Consider three-factor PCC (Australia) 15–30 IU/kg
	     Withhold warfarin

No bleeding
INR 4.5–10
	If bleeding risk is high:
	     Consider vitamin K 1–2 mg PO or 0.5–1 mg IV
	     Withhold warfarin

INR = international normalised ratio; PCC = prothrombin complex concentrate.

Adapted from Tran HA, Chanilal SD, Harper PL et al. An update of consensus guidelines for warfarin reversal. Medical Journal of Australia 2013; 198(4):1–7.

- In patients with an ongoing therapeutic requirement for anticoagulation with warfarin, vitamin K doses can be titrated as an inpatient in an effort to maintain an INR in the required therapeutic range (see **Chapter 4.27: Vitamin K** for further details).
- Guidelines for management of warfarin-induced coagulopathy, including vitamin K administration, are shown in **Table 3.81.2**.
- Large intentional overdoses (e.g. >100 mg) may result in a pattern of toxicity with rapid, recurrent or prolonged increases in the INR after initial antidote administration. In these cases, the optimal doses of vitamin K are not clearly defined and modification of standard guidelines for reversal of therapeutic over-anticoagulation will be required (see **Handy Tips**).

DISPOSITION AND FOLLOW-UP
Acute overdose
- Children who accidentally ingest >0.5 mg/kg can safely be treated with vitamin K orally (e.g. 10 mg daily for 3 days) without documenting serial INRs, as the risk of developing severe coagulopathy will be very low with this intervention. This will allow early discharge and remove the requirement for serial INR assays. Follow-up INR can be performed >12 hours after the last dose of vitamin K to ensure that no coagulopathy is present if additional reassurance is required.
- Patients with intentional overdose of warfarin but no therapeutic requirement for anticoagulation are admitted for serial INR measurements and titrated doses of vitamin K.
  - It is reasonable to consider treatment with large doses of vitamin K administered orally (e.g. 10 mg twice daily) without serial in-patient INR measurements. Follow-up INR is

indicated at 48–72 hours (including at least one INR >12 hours post dosing with vitamin K) to ensure that coagulopathy has resolved.
- Patients with a therapeutic requirement for anticoagulation are admitted for serial monitoring of INR and receive titrated vitamin K doses, as discussed in **Chapter 4.27: Vitamin K**.

Therapeutic over-anticoagulation
- Therapeutic over-anticoagulation can be managed as either an inpatient or an outpatient based on the INR level and a consideration of bleeding risk (high-risk factors) for the individual patient.

HANDY TIPS
- Patients who have received vitamin K and have an ongoing requirement for anticoagulation may have prolonged warfarin resistance. Alternative agents such as heparin or direct oral anticoagulants are indicated as interim or alternative therapies.
- In large overdoses (e.g. >100 mg), the dose of vitamin K required to reverse coagulopathy or maintain the INR in the therapeutic range is difficult to predict. Early administration of a larger initial dose (e.g. 5–10 mg), or frequent smaller doses, are both reasonable approaches. In all cases, 6-hourly INR monitoring is required to ensure that a severe coagulopathy does not develop.
- Warfarin levels may be useful in cases where paediatric non-accidental injury or occult poisoning is suspected.

PITFALL
- Failure to consider titration of vitamin K dose in patients requiring ongoing therapeutic anticoagulation with warfarin.

CONTROVERSY
- The requirement for FFP in addition to PCC for the effective reversal of warfarin-associated coagulopathy in all patients. A risk–benefit consideration of the severity of bleeding is appropriate to guide this decision (see **References** for Australasian and American guideline recommendations).

Presentations
Warfarin 1 mg, 2 mg, 3 mg, 5 mg tablets (50)

References
Berling I, Mostafa A, Jeffrey E et al. Warfarin poisoning with delayed rebound toxicity. Journal of Emergency Medicine 2017; 52(2):194–196.

Isbister GK, Hackett LP, Whyte IM. Intentional warfarin overdose. Therapeutic Drug Monitoring 2003; 25(6):715–722.

Levine M, Pizon AE, Padilla-Jones A et al. Warfarin overdose: a 25-year experience. Journal of Medical Toxicology 2014; 10:156–164.

Tran HA, Chanilal SD, Harper PL et al. An update of consensus guidelines for warfarin reversal. Medical Journal of Australia 2013; 198(4):1–7.

Witt DM, Nieuwlaat R, Clark NP et al. American Society of Hematology 2018 guidelines for management of venous thromboembolism: optimal management of anticoagulation therapy. Blood Advances 2018; 27(2):3257–3291.

CHAPTER 4
ANTIDOTES

4.1 ATROPINE

Atropine is a competitive muscarinic antagonist used to treat drug-induced bradycardia and poisoning by acetylcholinesterase inhibitors.

Presentations
Atropine sulfate 0.1 mg/mL prefilled syringe (10 mL)
Atropine sulfate 0.4 mg/mL ampoules
Atropine sulfate 0.5 mg/mL ampoules
Atropine sulfate 0.6 mg/mL ampoules
Atropine sulfate 1.2 mg/mL ampoules

TOXICOLOGICAL INDICATIONS
- Poisoning by agents that impair AV conduction such as cardiac glycosides, beta-blockers and calcium channel blockers
- Organophosphate and carbamate poisoning

CONTRAINDICATIONS
- Relative contraindications include:
  - closed angle glaucoma
  - gastrointestinal obstruction
  - obstructive uropathy.

Mechanism of action
Atropine is a competitive antagonist of acetylcholine at muscarinic receptors. It reverses the excessive parasympathetic stimulation that results from inhibition of acetylcholinesterase. It does not act at nicotinic receptors.

Pharmacokinetics
Atropine has a poor oral bioavailability and undergoes hepatic metabolism, with an elimination half-life of 2–4 hours. It crosses the blood–brain and placental barriers. About 50% is excreted unchanged in urine.

ADMINISTRATION
- The patient is managed in a monitored area where equipment, drugs and personnel are available to provide full resuscitative care.

Organophosphate and carbamate poisoning
- Administer an initial IV bolus of 1.2 mg.
- Further doses are given every 2–3 minutes, doubling the dose each time until drying of respiratory secretions is achieved. Heart rate is not a useful end point as tachycardia may persist due to nicotinic effects or respiratory distress.
- Very large doses (up to 100 mg) may be required in severe cases and ongoing atropine administration by infusion may be necessary.

Bradycardia caused by drug-induced AV conduction blockade
- Administer an IV bolus of 0.6 mg.
- Repeat doses of 0.6 mg are given as required up to a maximum of 1.8 mg.

THERAPEUTIC END POINTS
- Drying of respiratory secretions in organophosphate poisoning.
  - Note: The development of anticholinergic features indicates excessive dosing.

ADVERSE DRUG REACTIONS AND THEIR MANAGEMENT

- Excessive atropine administration manifests with clinical features of anticholinergic poisoning, including delirium, tachycardia, mydriasis and urinary retention.
  - No further atropine should be administered while features of anticholinergic poisoning are present.
  - Benzodiazepine sedation may be necessary to control delirium and an indwelling urinary catheter should be inserted because of the risk of urinary retention.

SPECIFIC CONSIDERATIONS

Pregnancy: no restriction on use.
Paediatric: initial paediatric dose is 20 microgram/kg.

HANDY TIP

- Very large doses of atropine may be required to treat organophosphate poisoning – anticipate this need and procure sufficient stocks as soon as possible.

PITFALLS

- Failure to administer sufficient doses of atropine in organophosphate or carbamate poisoning.
- Administration of excessive atropine leading to iatrogenic anticholinergic poisoning.

References

Bardin PG, Van Eeden SF. Organophosphate poisoning: grading the severity and comparing treatment between atropine and glycopyrrolate. Critical Care Medicine 1990; 18(9):956–960.

Eddleston M, Buckley NA, Eyer P et al. Management of acute organophosphorus pesticide poisoning. Lancet 2008; 371:597–607.

4.2 CALCIUM

Calcium is a cation that is essential for normal physiological processes including myocardial conduction and contractility, neuromuscular activity, endocrine function and the clotting cascade.

Presentations

Calcium gluconate 1 g/10 mL vials (0.22 mmol calcium ions/mL)
Calcium gluconate 5 g/50 mL vials (0.22 mmol calcium ions/mL)
Calcium chloride 0.74 g/5 mL ampoules (1.01 mmol calcium ions/mL)
Calcium chloride 1 g/10 mL ampoules (0.68 mmol calcium ions/mL)
Calcium chloride 1 g/10 mL single-use syringe (0.68 mmol calcium ions/mL)

TOXICOLOGICAL INDICATIONS

- Calcium channel blocker poisoning
- Hydrofluoric acid skin exposure
- Hypocalcaemia (systemic fluorosis) following extensive exposure to hydrofluoric acid
- Hypocalcaemia secondary to ethylene glycol poisoning
- Iatrogenic hypermagnesaemia
- Hyperkalaemia

CONTRAINDICATIONS
- Hypercalcaemia
- Digoxin toxicity (controversial)

Mechanism of action
Calcium acts as a physiological antagonist to the effects of hyperkalaemia and hypermagnesaemia on the cardiac conducting system and skeletal muscle. Administration of calcium in hypocalcaemic states restores or maintains ionised calcium at a concentration sufficient to prevent cardiac dysrhythmias. In hydrofluoric acid poisoning, calcium ions bind to fluoride ions and prevent further tissue penetration and injury. Elevation of the ionised calcium concentration may help overcome the negative inotropic and vasodilatory effects of calcium channel blocker poisoning.

Pharmacokinetics
Ninety-nine per cent of the body's calcium is contained within bone. Of the calcium in plasma, about half is ionised and physiologically active while the other half is bound to albumin. Plasma calcium concentration is maintained at close to 2.5 mmol/L by a number of hormonal homeostatic mechanisms.

ADMINISTRATION
- The patient is managed in a monitored area where equipment, drugs and personnel are available to provide full resuscitative care.
- Cardiac monitoring is mandatory during infusion of calcium salts.

Hypocalcaemia/hyperkalaemia/hypermagnesaemia
- Administer 10–20 mL (1–2 g) of calcium gluconate 10% IV over 5–10 minutes and assess clinical and electrocardiographic response. Calcium chloride 10% IV is an alternative option.
- Further administration of calcium salts is guided by serum calcium concentrations, which should not exceed the normal range.

Calcium channel blocker poisoning
- Calcium administration is considered a temporising measure in a severely poisoned patient and is unlikely to provide definitive treatment (see **Chapter 3.21: Calcium channel blockers**).
  - Give 10–20 mL (1–2 g) of calcium gluconate 10% IV over 5–10 minutes and assess haemodynamic response. This may be repeated up to three doses.
  - Calcium chloride 10% IV is an alternative option.

Hydrofluoric acid skin exposure
- Topical 2.5% calcium gel
  - Minor burns.
  - For burns to the hand, put gel in a glove and place hand in the glove.
- Local injection of calcium gluconate 1 g/10 mL
  - Consider if topical application fails to stop pain.
  - Inject 0.5 mL/cm^2 depots intradermally and subcutaneously using a 25 gauge needle to achieve local tissue infiltration.
  - Not suitable for finger exposures.
  - **Do not** inject calcium chloride, as this can cause tissue injury.
- Bier's block (forearm regional intravenous injection)
  - Consider for large HF exposures to fingers, hand or forearm or if gel application to these regions has failed.
  - Insert intravenous line distally in affected forearm.
  - Dilute 10 mL (1 g) calcium gluconate in 40 mL of normal saline.

- — Inject diluted calcium gluconate solution intravenously with pneumatic tourniquet inflated (Bier's block technique).
- — Release cuff after 20 minutes.
- Intra-arterial infusion
  - — Insert arterial line into radial, brachial or femoral artery of affected limb.
  - — Dilute 1 g (10 mL) of calcium gluconate in 40 mL of normal saline.
  - — Infuse diluted calcium gluconate solution over 4 hours and repeat as necessary.

Hydrofluoric acid inhalation injury
- Give nebulised 2.5% calcium gluconate solution.

THERAPEUTIC END POINTS
- Hypocalcaemia/hypermagnesaemia/hyperkalaemia: normalisation of serum calcium and improvement in electrocardiographic features
- Calcium channel blocker poisoning: haemodynamic improvement
- Hydrofluoric acid skin exposure: resolution of pain

ADVERSE DRUG REACTIONS AND THEIR MANAGEMENT
- Vasodilatation, hypotension, dysrhythmias, syncope or cardiac arrest due to over-rapid administration
  - — Interrupt calcium salt administration.
  - — Institute advanced cardiac life support as appropriate.
- Local tissue damage from extravasation of calcium chloride

SPECIFIC CONSIDERATIONS

Pregnancy: no restriction on use.

Paediatric: paediatric dose for hypocalcaemia or calcium channel blocker poisoning is 1.0 mL/kg 10% calcium gluconate solution over 5–10 minutes and repeated after 10–15 minutes if necessary.

HANDY TIPS
- QT duration and clinical features of hypocalcaemia may be a more useful guide to calcium requirements than serum calcium concentrations.
- Calcium gluconate can safely be given via a peripheral line whereas calcium chloride is best given via a central line because of the risk of tissue damage from extravasation. It should not be given in the same intravenous line as sodium bicarbonate.
- 2.5% calcium gluconate gel for treatment of skin exposure to hydrofluoric acid can be prepared by mixing 30 g of amorphous hydrogel wound dressing with 10 mL of calcium gluconate 10% solution. The resultant product will make approximately 40 g of calcium gluconate gel 2.5%.
- Do not use calcium salt solution to irrigate the eye after ocular hydrofluoric acid exposure as it may cause corrosive injury.

- Pain refractory to calcium administration in late-presentation hydrofluoric acid burns may indicate established tissue damage rather than therapeutic failure.
- Very large doses of calcium may be required to maintain eucalcaemia following hydrofluoric acid ingestion.

CONTROVERSIES
- Efficacy and optimal dosing of calcium salts in calcium channel blocker poisoning.
- Most effective route of administration of calcium salts for hydrofluoric acid skin exposures.

References

Graudins A, Burns MJ, Aaron CK. Regional intravenous infusion of calcium gluconate for hydrofluoric acid burns of the upper extremity. Annals of Emergency Medicine 1997; 30:604–607.

Vance MV, Curry SC, Kunkel DB et al. Digital hydrofluoric acid burns: treatment with intraarterial calcium infusion. Annals of Emergency Medicine 1986; 15:890–896.

4.3 CYPROHEPTADINE

Cyproheptadine is a non-selective antihistamine with anticholinergic properties and additional antagonist effects at serotonin receptors. It has been advocated for control of symptoms in mild-to-moderate serotonin toxicity.

Presentations
Cyproheptadine 4 mg tablets (50, 100)

TOXICOLOGICAL INDICATION
- Mild-to-moderate serotonin toxicity

CONTRAINDICATIONS
- Known hypersensitivity
- Acute asthma
- Closed-angle glaucoma
- Bladder neck obstruction

Mechanism of action
Cyproheptadine acts as a competitive antagonist at histamine H_1 and serotonin 5-HT_{1A} and 5-HT_2 receptors. It exerts centrally mediated hormonal effects such as the inhibition of adrenocorticotrophic hormone (ACTH), probably secondary to serotonin antagonism. It also has moderate local anaesthetic action and mild peripheral anticholinergic action.

Pharmacokinetics
Cyproheptadine is well absorbed following oral administration, with peak plasma levels observed after 1–3 hours. Elimination is primarily by hepatic glucuronidation with urinary excretion of metabolites.

ADMINISTRATION
- Administer an initial dose of 12 mg orally and observe for clinical response.
- If a response is observed, continue treatment with 8 mg every 8 hours for 24 hours.

- Therapy should not be required beyond 24 hours, provided agents that may precipitate serotonin toxicity are withheld.
- A longer duration of therapy may be required to treat serotonin toxicity associated with an irreversible monoamine oxidase (MAO) inhibitor.

THERAPEUTIC END POINTS
- Resolution or amelioration of the clinical features associated with serotonin toxicity within 1–2 hours of the initial dose

ADVERSE DRUG REACTIONS AND THEIR MANAGEMENT
- Insignificant adverse effects at therapeutic doses

SPECIFIC CONSIDERATIONS
Pregnancy: no restriction on use.
Paediatric: paediatric dose is not well established. For patients between 7 and 14 years of age, an initial dose of 4 mg followed by 4 mg every 8 hours for 24 hours is suggested.

HANDY TIPS
- Cyproheptadine is not a life-saving antidote. It may ameliorate the symptoms of mild-to-moderate serotonin toxicity, but a good outcome will be achieved in these cases with simple supportive care including mild benzodiazepine sedation.
- Cyproheptadine is not useful in the management of severe serotonin toxicity. Early intubation and neuromuscular paralysis is the key to achieving a good outcome in this circumstance (see **Chapter 2.5: Serotonin toxicity**).

PITFALLS
- Failure to assess clinical response to initial dose.
- Reliance on cyproheptadine to the detriment of good supportive care in the management of serotonin toxicity.

Reference
Graudins A, Stearman A, Chan B. Treatment of the serotonin syndrome with cyproheptadine. Journal of Emergency Medicine 1998; 16(4):615–619.

4.4 DESFERRIOXAMINE

An effective iron chelator that is used to treat systemic iron toxicity or prevent the development of systemic toxicity following acute iron overdose.

Presentations
Desferrioxamine mesylate 500 mg vials (powder for reconstitution)
Desferrioxamine mesylate 2 g vials (powder for reconstitution)

TOXICOLOGICAL INDICATIONS
- Acute iron poisoning

− Established systemic iron toxicity with clinical features of
    severe gastroenteritis, shock, metabolic acidosis and altered
    mental state
  − Significant risk of systemic iron toxicity, as predicted by serum
    iron levels >90 micromol/L or 500 microgram/dL at 4–6 hours
    post ingestion
- Chronic iron overload

CONTRAINDICATIONS
- None

Mechanism of action

Desferrioxamine (DFO) binds avidly to free ferric ion in the plasma to form ferrioxamine.
This stable complex is highly water soluble and is readily excreted in the urine. DFO is
able to remove iron bound to transferrin and haemosiderin, but not from outside the
intravascular compartment. 1000 mg of DFO is able to bind 85 mg of ferric iron.

Pharmacokinetics

The volume of distribution is 1 L/kg and it does not substantially enter tissue
compartments. Steady-state concentrations are achieved at 6–12 hours during
intravenous infusion. DFO undergoes hepatic metabolism, producing multiple
metabolites, one of which is responsible for the drug's toxic effects. Some drug is
excreted unchanged in the urine. The elimination half-life is 3 hours but substantially
increased in renal failure. Ferrioxamine has a smaller volume of distribution than DFO, is
not metabolised but excreted unchanged in the urine, and is dialysable.

ADMINISTRATION
- Cardiac monitoring is mandatory during DFO administration.
- Reconstitute 500 mg of powder with 5 mL sterile water and dilute
  in 100 mL normal saline or 5% glucose.
- Commence IV infusion at an initial dose of 15 mg/kg/hour.
- Reduce the infusion rate if hypotension develops.
- The rate may be increased in life-threatening toxicity up to 40 mg/
  kg/hour, providing significant hypotension does not supervene.
- Continue the infusion until therapeutic end points have been
  achieved but avoid infusions prolonged >24 hours.

THERAPEUTIC END POINTS
- Patient clinically stable
- Serum iron <60 micromol/L (350 microgram/dL)

ADVERSE DRUG REACTIONS AND THEIR MANAGEMENT
- Hypersensitivity reactions
- Hypotension, especially with rapid or high-dose IV infusion
  − Reduce infusion rate if hypotension occurs.
- With prolonged infusions (>24 hours), possible development of
  ARDS
- Toxic retinopathy
- Secondary infections including *Yersinia* sepsis and mucormycosis:
  ferrioxamine complex acts as a siderophore promoting growth of
  these organisms

SPECIFIC CONSIDERATIONS
  Pregnancy: there is no evidence of human teratogenicity with DFO,
  and although it is not known if DFO crosses the placenta, it should

never be withheld in the treatment of pregnant patients with severe iron poisoning.

Paediatric: administration and dose are as for adults.

HANDY TIPS
- DFO is ideally administered before iron moves intracellularly and systemic toxicity develops.
- Intramuscular DFO administration is not indicated in acute iron poisoning.
- Although urine may change to the classical *vin rosé* colour during DFO administration, this is an unreliable sign of effective chelation.
- Six hours of DFO chelation is usually sufficient and it is extremely rare to require therapy beyond 24 hours.

PITFALLS
- Administration of DFO when not clinically indicated.
- Excessive duration of DFO administration.

CONTROVERSIES
- There are no controlled trials or dose–response studies to support the efficacy of DFO chelation for human iron poisoning.
- The optimal indications, dose, route of administration and end points for therapy are not well defined.

References
Howland MA. Risks of parenteral deferoxamine for acute iron poisoning. Journal of Toxicology–Clinical Toxicology 1996; 34(5):491–497.
Tenenbein M. Benefits of parenteral deferoxamine for acute iron poisoning. Journal of Toxicology–Clinical Toxicology 1996; 42(5):485–489.

4.5 DIGOXIN IMMUNE FAB

Digoxin immune Fab is the definitive treatment for digoxin toxicity and is potentially beneficial in poisoning from other cardiac glycosides.

Presentations
Digoxin-specific antibody fragments (Fab) as lyophilised powder 40 mg ampoules

TOXICOLOGICAL INDICATIONS
Cardiac glycoside poisoning where there is an imminent threat to life, or where the risk assessment suggests such a threat, is an absolute indication for immediate administration of digoxin immune Fab. Administration is also justified in any patient whose manifestations of digoxin toxicity are sufficient to warrant inpatient care. Appropriate indications include:
- **Acute digoxin overdose**
  - Cardiac arrest
  - Life-threatening cardiac dysrhythmia
  - Ingested dose >10 mg (adult) or >4 mg (child)
  - Serum digoxin level >15 nmol/L (12 ng/mL)
  - Serum potassium >5.5 mmol/L

- **Chronic digoxin poisoning**
  - Cardiac arrest
  - Life-threatening cardiac dysrhythmia
  - Cardiac dysrhythmia or increased automaticity not likely to be tolerated for a prolonged period
  - Moderate-to-severe gastrointestinal symptoms not attributable to another cause
  - Any symptoms in the presence of impaired renal function
- **Other cardiac glycoside poisoning**
  - Oleander and other plants
  - Bufotoxin (cane toad)

CONTRAINDICATIONS
- None

Mechanism of action

Digoxin immune Fab is an antibody fragment derived from ovine immunoglobulins. One ampoule (40 mg) of Fab binds 0.5 mg of digoxin. Digoxin immune Fab binds directly to free intravascular digoxin with much greater affinity than the Na^+–K^+-ATPase receptor. A concentration gradient is created and digoxin dissociates from tissue membrane receptors and moves to the intravascular space where binding to immune Fab occurs.

Pharmacokinetics

Digoxin immune Fab has a small volume of distribution (0.4 L/kg). Digoxin bound to Fab fragments is excreted in the urine, with an elimination half-life of 16–30 hours, but the half-life is markedly increased in renal failure.

ADMINISTRATION
- The patient is managed in a monitored area where equipment, drugs and personnel are available to provide full resuscitative care. Cardiac monitoring is mandatory during antidote administration and until toxicity has resolved.
- The dose required (see below) is diluted in 100 mL normal saline and administered over 15 minutes, except in cardiac arrest, where it is administered as an IV bolus.

CALCULATION OF DOSE REQUIRED

Historically, dosing was based on a calculated assessment of total body burden of digoxin. Current management recognises that it is not necessary to bind the total digoxin load to treat toxicity. The administration of smaller initial doses of digoxin immune Fab will likely be sufficient to bind all intravascular digoxin, with subsequent doses repeated based on clinical status. This will result in reduced total dosing of Fab without compromising the morbidity and mortality benefits.

- **Acute digoxin overdose**
  - The number of ampoules required to bind the total body burden following a known ingested dose is calculated by:
    - Number of ampoules = ingested dose (mg) × 0.8 (bioavailability) × 2
  - The dose of digoxin immune Fab required to treat toxicity will be less than the calculated dose as the ingested dose is distributed to cardiac and non-cardiac tissue. Digoxin Fab will only bind digoxin in the intravascular compartment – smaller

initial doses are indicated, with repeated doses based on the clinical and biochemical response.
— For haemodynamically unstable patients
  – Initiate treatment with 2–5 ampoules.
  – Titrate subsequent doses based on clinical status, ECG features, serum potassium and free digoxin levels (if available) until resolution of digoxin toxicity has occurred.
- **Chronic digoxin poisoning**
  — Number of ampoules required

  $$= \frac{\text{serum digoxin (ng/mL)} \times \text{body weight (kg)}}{100}$$

  — The calculated dose of digoxin immune Fab required in chronic digoxin toxicity is lower than in acute as the serum digoxin level in chronic toxicity is generally lower than in acute poisoning. This is due to widespread distribution of digoxin to non-cardiac tissue. Administration of 1–2 ampoules of Fab will likely bind all intravascular digoxin in chronic toxicity.
  — For haemodynamically unstable patients
    – Initiate treatment with 1–2 ampoules.
    – Titrate subsequent doses based on clinical status and free digoxin levels (if available) until reversal of digoxin toxicity is achieved.
- **Cardiac arrest**
  — The recommended dose of digoxin immune Fab indicated in the setting of cardiac arrest thought to be due to digoxin poisoning is not well defined.
  — It is reasonable to give 5 ampoules of digoxin immune Fab (or as many as immediately available) by rapid intravenous injection while continuing cardiopulmonary resuscitation. This dose is likely to adequately bind all digoxin in the intravenous compartment. The utility of higher doses in the immediate resuscitation phase is unclear and should be determined by assessment of clinical response and ECG features.
- **Other cardiac glycoside poisoning (e.g. oleander)**
  — The serum digoxin level in these scenarios may not be reliable due to variability in laboratory assays.
  — The spectrum of toxicity following other cardiac glycoside poisoning may not exhibit the same risk of ventricular dysrhythmias as digoxin toxicity – bradycardia or atrioventricular block may respond well to atropine or isoprenaline.
  — For haemodynamically unstable patients
    – Initiate treatment with 2–5 ampoules.
    – Titrate subsequent doses based on clinical status and ECG features until resolution of toxicity has occurred.
    – Patients may have a protracted clinical course.

DURATION OF TREATMENT
- In acute toxicity, an improvement in cardiotoxicity and hyperkalaemia is expected within 30–60 minutes of an initial dose of digoxin immune Fab. Further doses are administered based on clinical, biochemical and ECG monitoring.

- In chronic toxicity, gastrointestinal symptoms, constitutional features and automaticity may resolve promptly after digoxin immune Fab, but bradycardia may persist for longer. This is particularly likely if the patient is on other rate-controlling medications.
- Rarely, digoxin toxicity may recur beyond 24 hours (particularly with renal failure) and necessitate further administration of digoxin immune Fab based on clinical and ECG features, or free digoxin levels, if available.

THERAPEUTIC END POINTS
- Resolution of clinical features attributable to digoxin toxicity

ADVERSE DRUG REACTIONS AND THEIR MANAGEMENT

Digoxin immune Fab is a very safe antidote. Theoretical adverse effects, even if they occur, will be of little clinical significance:
- Hypokalaemia
- Allergy (extremely rare)
- Exacerbation of underlying cardiac failure
- Loss of rate control of pre-existing atrial fibrillation.

SPECIFIC CONSIDERATIONS

Pregnancy: no restriction on use.
Paediatric: no restriction on use.

HANDY TIPS
- A single dose of 1 ampoule may be sufficient to minimise the risk of lethal cardiac dysrhythmias in chronic toxicity.
- Serum digoxin levels following treatment may paradoxically increase because most assays measure both free and Fab-bound digoxin. Some laboratories are able to assay free digoxin levels – these provide better guidance for the subsequent administration of Fab, particularly in the setting of poor renal clearance.
- Hyperkalaemia due to acute digoxin poisoning is treated with Fab, not intravenous calcium, as digoxin causes elevation in intracellular myocardial calcium levels.
- Hyperkalaemia due to acute digoxin poisoning may respond completely to appropriate treatment with digoxin immune Fab, as it is caused by acute inhibition of the $Na^+–K^+$-ATPase. In contrast, hyperkalaemia in the setting of chronic digoxin toxicity is likely multi-factorial and often reflects significant renal impairment and metabolic acidosis.
- Administration of digoxin immune Fab to patients with chronic digoxin toxicity may significantly reduce hospital length of stay.

PITFALL
- Withholding digoxin immune Fab from patients with chronic digoxin poisoning because of concerns about expense of the antidote. The risk of death and cost of prolonged unnecessary admission to a monitored bed may greatly exceed the cost of 1–2 ampoules of digoxin immune Fab.

CONTROVERSIES

- The optimal dosing regimen for digoxin immune Fab is unclear – smaller, repeated doses based on clinical status or an infusion over several hours are pharmacokinetically more appropriate options than single large doses.
- Precise indications for digoxin immune Fab. The threshold for antidotal therapy requires a consideration of the risk of cardiovascular deterioration in an individual patient and the clinician's ability or willingness to manage that risk with or without antidotal therapy.
- The dose of digoxin immune Fab is not well defined in poisoning by other cardiac glycosides, such as those contained in oleander.

References

Antman EM, Wenger TL, Butler VP et al. Treatment of 150 cases of life-threatening digitalis intoxication with digoxin-specific Fab antibody fragments: final report of a multicenter study. Circulation 1990; 81(6):1744–1752.

Bateman DN. Digoxin-specific antibody fragments: how much and when? Toxicological Reviews 2004; 23(3):135–143.

Chan B, Buckley N. Digoxin-specific antibody fragments in the treatment of digoxin toxicity. Clinical Toxicology 2014; 52(8):824–836.

Di Domenico R, Walton S, Sanoski CA et al. Analysis of the use of digoxin Fab for the treatment of non life threatening digoxin toxicity. Journal of Cardiovascular Pharmacology and Therapeutics 2000; 5(2):77–85.

Eddleston M, Rajapakse S, Rajakanthan JS et al. Anti-digoxin Fab fragments in cardiotoxicity induced by ingestion of yellow oleander: a randomised controlled trial. Lancet 2000; 355(9208):967–972.

Roberts DM, Gallapatthy G, Dunuwille A et al. Pharmacological treatment of cardiac glycoside poisoning. British Journal of Clinical Pharmacology 2016; 81(3):488–495.

Woolf AD, Wenger T, Smith TW et al. The use of digoxin-specific Fab fragments for severe digitalis intoxication in children. New England Journal of Medicine 1992; 326:1739–1744.

4.6 DIMERCAPROL

British anti-Lewisite (BAL), 2,3-dimercaptopropanol

This intramuscular chelating agent is used for the treatment of life-threatening poisoning from lead, inorganic arsenic and inorganic mercury. These indications are based on historical usage, and dimercaprol has a significant risk of adverse effects. More recently developed analogues (DMSA and DMPS) may provide similar clinical efficacy, although definitive data are not available.

Presentations

Dimercaprol 300 mg, benzyl benzoate 600 mg, peanut oil 2100 mg in 3 mL ampoules

TOXICOLOGICAL INDICATIONS

- Severe lead poisoning or lead encephalopathy in combination with sodium calcium edetate (EDTA)
- Arsenic poisoning (if oral DMSA or IV DMPS are not available)
- Inorganic mercury poisoning
- Gold intoxication

- **Note:** Based on historical evidence, the recommendation for treatment of severe lead encephalopathy is **combination therapy** with intramuscular dimercaprol (BAL) and sodium calcium edetate for two major reasons (see **Controversies**):
  - Concerns that sodium calcium edetate preferentially mobilises lead bone stores which could re-distribute to the CNS and transiently worsen encephalopathy.
  - The use of two chelating agents increases the rate of urinary excretion of lead.
- Other heavy metal poisoning
  - Dimercaprol has been used to chelate bismuth, antimony, chromium, nickel, tungsten and zinc, but clinical experience is limited.

CONTRAINDICATIONS
- Peanut allergy
- G6PD deficiency
- Hepatotoxicity (excluding acute arsenic-mediated)
- Co-administration of iron supplements (toxicity due to dimercaprol-iron conjugates)
- Organic or elemental mercury poisoning

Pharmacodynamics
Dimercaprol is a dithiol compound containing two sulfhydryl (–SH) groups that bind metal ions in a ring structure to form stable dimercaptide chelates, which are readily excreted in the urine.

Pharmacokinetics
Dimercaprol is poorly water soluble and not absorbed orally. It is formulated in a peanut oil solvent and given by deep intramuscular injection. Blood concentrations peak 30 minutes after IM administration and distribution occurs rapidly. It is metabolised predominantly by glucuronic conjugation and the metabolites are excreted in the urine, with a small proportion of unchanged drug undergoing enterohepatic circulation and faecal elimination. Dimercaprol–metal conjugates can be removed by dialysis if renal failure is present.

ADMINISTRATION
- Therapy is always commenced in an intensive care setting due to the severity of the underlying condition and risk of adverse effects.
- Urinary alkalinisation is recommended prior to administration to reduce risk of nephrotoxicity from dissociation of dimercaprol–metal conjugates in acidic urine (see **Chapter 4.24: Sodium bicarbonate**).

Lead encephalopathy
- Commence dimercaprol 4 hours before commencing sodium calcium edetate.
- Give 3–4 mg/kg every 4 hours for 2–5 days based on clinical response.
- See **Chapter 4.25: Sodium calcium edetate** for further information.

Severe inorganic arsenic or mercury poisoning
- Give 3 mg/kg IM every 4 hours for 48 hours
  then
- Give 3 mg/kg IM every 12 hours for 7–10 days depending on clinical response.

ADVERSE DRUG REACTIONS AND THEIR MANAGEMENT

Dimercaprol is associated with a high incidence of dose-dependent adverse effects, being 1, 14 and 65% for doses of 2.5, 3 and 4 mg/kg, respectively. These include:

- Pain and sterile abscess formation at injection sites
- Fever and myalgia
- Chest pain, hypertension and tachycardia
- Headache, nausea and vomiting
- Peripheral paraesthesias; burning sensation of lips, mouth, throat and eyes
- Lacrimation, rhinorrhoea and excessive salivation
- Risk of intravascular haemolysis in patients with G6PD deficiency
- Nephrotoxicity secondary to the dissociation of dimercaprol–metal complexes in acid urine
- Hypertensive encephalopathy at supratherapeutic doses.
  - Note: If alternative agents (DMSA, DMPS or sodium calcium edetate) are not available and ongoing administration of BAL is considered essential, severe adverse effects require a reduction in dose.

SPECIFIC CONSIDERATIONS

Pregnancy: safety not established. Administration should not be withheld if clinically indicated.
Lactation: safety not established.
Paediatric: dose and administration as for adults.

HANDY TIPS

- Dimercaprol is most effective when administered shortly after the exposure.
- Analogues of dimercaprol (oral DMSA, intravenous DMPS) are better tolerated chelating agents and are preferred for most clinical presentations (excluding severe lead encephalopathy).

PITFALL

- Delaying administration of dimercaprol in the setting of life-threatening toxicity while awaiting confirmatory laboratory levels.

CONTROVERSY

- Based on historical evidence, the recommendation for treatment of severe lead encephalopathy is combination therapy with BAL and sodium calcium edetate (due to concerns that sodium calcium edetate alone preferentially mobilises lead bone stores which may re-distribute to the CNS and transiently worsen encephalopathy). The relative efficacy and clinical benefit of the newer agents (DMSA or DMPS) as monotherapy in this setting has not been definitively studied but case series suggest that the outcomes are similar and may be appropriate alternative regimens (see **References**).

References

Alexander FW, Delves HT. Deaths from acute lead poisoning. Archives of Disease in Childhood 1972; 47:446–448.

Kosnett MJ. The role of chelation in the treatment of arsenic and mercury poisoning. Journal of Medical Toxicology 2013; 9:347–354.

Thurtle N, Greig J, Cooney L et al. Description of 3,180 courses of chelation with dimercaptosuccinic acid in children ≤ 5 y with severe lead poisoning in Zamfara, Northern Nigeria: a retrospective analysis of programme data. PLoS Med 2014; 11(10). doi:10.1371/journal.pmed.1001739 pmed.1001739.

Vilensky JA, Redman K. British anti-lewisite (dimercaprol): an amazing history. Annals of Emergency Medicine 2003; 41:378–383.

4.7 DMSA (SUCCIMER) AND DMPS (UNITHIOL)

DMSA: 2,3-Dimercaptosuccinic acid (Succimer)

DMPS: 2,3-Dimercapto-1-propanesulfonic acid (Unithiol)

DMSA (oral) and DMPS (intravenous) are water-soluble analogues of dimercaprol used in the treatment of lead, arsenic and mercury poisoning.

Presentations
Succimer 100 mg tablets (100), obtained under the Special Access Scheme in Australia
Unithiol 250 mg/5 mL ampoules (5), obtained under the Special Access Scheme in Australia

TOXICOLOGICAL INDICATIONS
- Adult lead poisoning
  - Symptomatic
  - Asymptomatic with blood lead level >70 microgram/dL
- Paediatric lead poisoning
  - Symptomatic
  - Asymptomatic with blood lead level >45 microgram/dL
- Other heavy metal poisoning
  - Has been used to chelate arsenic, mercury, bismuth, antimony and copper, but clinical experience is limited

CONTRAINDICATIONS
- Known hypersensitivity
- Ongoing heavy metal exposure

Mechanism of action
DMSA and DMPS are both dithiol compounds containing two sulfhydrl (–SH) groups. They bind metal ions in a ring structure to form stable dimercaptide chelates, which are readily excreted in the urine.

Pharmacokinetics
Following oral administration, succimer is rapidly absorbed and undergoes rapid metabolism. Metabolites and some unchanged drug are excreted in the urine.

ADMINISTRATION
- Lead poisoning (see **Chapter 3.46: Lead** for indications)
  - DMSA may be administered as an inpatient or outpatient.
  - The recommended dose is 10 mg/kg orally 3 times per day for 5 days.
  - Blood lead levels are followed after completion of this initial course.

- — Further courses are indicated if blood levels rebound in the absence of continued lead exposure.
- — DMPS is given intravenously if parenteral chelation is required (e.g. due to severe gastrointestinal symptoms). The recommended dose is 5 mg/kg IV 6 hourly.
- — For severe poisoning (lead encephalopathy), DMSA is used after initial chelation with parenteral agents (DMPS, BAL, sodium calcium edetate – see **Chapter 4.25: Sodium calcium edetate** and **Chapter 4.6: Dimercaprol**).
- Recommended dosing regimens of DMSA or DMPS for arsenic, mercury and other heavy metal poisonings are the same as for lead poisoning.

ADVERSE DRUG REACTIONS AND THEIR MANAGEMENT
- Hypersensitivity reactions
- Gastrointestinal symptoms are common.
- Transient liver function test abnormalities
- Reversible neutropenia (rare)

SPECIFIC CONSIDERATIONS
Pregnancy: safety is not established. Consideration is given to chelation therapy at lower blood levels because of the susceptibility of the fetal central nervous system to lead.
Paediatric: dose and administration as for adults.

HANDY TIPS
- Oral DMSA is the preferred chelating agent for most clinical presentations (excluding severe lead encephalopathy).
- DMSA can be given on an outpatient basis to compliant patients. It is essential that ongoing exposure to lead is eliminated to prevent enhanced lead absorption during chelation.
- DMSA and DMPS cause minimal loss of other essential elements (zinc, copper, iron) compared to dimercaprol and calcium disodium edetate.

PITFALL
- DMSA and DMPS are only available in Australia under the Special Access Scheme.

CONTROVERSIES
- The threshold blood lead level for DMSA chelation in children is controversial. Although levels <45 microgram/dL have adverse effects on neurodevelopment, current studies do not provide clear evidence of improved neurological outcomes following chelation.
- Based on historical evidence, the recommendation for treatment of severe lead encephalopathy is combination therapy with intramuscular dimercaprol (BAL) and sodium calcium edetate (due to concerns that sodium calcium edetate preferentially mobilises lead bone stores which could re-distribute to the CNS and transiently worsen encephalopathy). The relative efficacies and clinical benefits of the newer agents (DMSA or DMPS) as

monotherapy in this setting have not been definitively studied, but case series suggest that outcomes are similar and they may be appropriate alternative regimens (see **References**).

References

Arnold J, Morgan B. Management of lead encephalopathy with DMSA after exposure to lead-contaminated moonshine. Journal of Medical Toxicology 2015; 11:464–467.

Bradberry S, Vale A. A comparison of sodium calcium edetate (edetate calcium disodium) and succimer (DMSA) in the treatment of inorganic lead poisoning. Clinical Toxicology 2009; 47(9):841–858.

Dietrich KN, Ware HH, Salganik M et al. Effect of chelation on the neuropsychological and behavioral development of lead-exposed children after school entry. Pediatrics 2004; 114:19–26.

Kosnett MJ. Chelation for heavy metals (arsenic, lead, and mercury): protective or perilous? Clinical Pharmacology & Therapeutics 2010; 88(3):412–415.

Thurtle N, Greig J, Cooney L et al. Description of 3,180 courses of chelation with dimercaptosuccinic acid in children ≤ 5 y with severe lead poisoning in Zamfara, Northern Nigeria: a retrospective analysis of programme data. PLoS Med 2014; 11(10). doi:10.1371/journal.pmed.1001739 pmed.1001739.

Treatment guidelines for lead exposure in children: Committee on Drugs. Pediatrics 1995; 96:155–160.

4.8 ETHANOL

Competitively blocks the formation of toxic metabolites in toxic alcohol ingestions due to its higher affinity for the enzyme alcohol dehydrogenase (ADH). Its chief application is in methanol and ethylene glycol ingestions, although it has been used for other toxic alcohol poisonings. Ethanol is now regarded as the second-choice antidote in those countries with access to the specific ADH blocker, fomepizole.

Presentations

Pure ethanol 20 mL ampoule (pharmaceutical grade)

Commercial alcoholic beverages with alcohol content from 5% to 70%

TOXICOLOGICAL INDICATIONS

- Methanol poisoning (confirmed or suspected)
- Ethylene glycol poisoning (confirmed or suspected)
- Other toxic alcohol ingestion

CONTRAINDICATIONS

- Recent ingestion of disulfiram (or drugs that may cause a disulfiram-like reaction)

Mechanism of action

Alcohol dehydrogenase has a much higher affinity (up to 20×) for ethanol than for ethylene glycol or methanol. Ethanol competitively inhibits the conversion of these other alcohols to their toxic metabolites by blocking the receptor sites of ADH. Inhibition is virtually complete at ethanol concentrations greater than 100 mg/dL (22 mmol/L).

Pharmacokinetics

Ethanol is rapidly absorbed after oral administration and distributed throughout the total body water. It rapidly crosses both the placenta and the blood–brain barrier. Elimination is principally by enzymatic oxidation in the liver in a two-step process involving alcohol dehydrogenase and aldehyde dehydrogenase. Metabolic capacity is saturated at relatively low concentrations. The rate of metabolism is extremely variable between individuals.

ADMINISTRATION

- Therapy should be commenced in a monitored area with personnel and equipment available to monitor mental status and blood or breath alcohol levels every 2 hours.
- Ethanol may be administered by the oral, nasogastric or intravenous route to maintain a blood ethanol concentration of 100–150 mg/dL (22–33 mmol/L).

Oral or nasogastric administration

- Loading dose: 2 mL/kg of 40% ethanol, or 3 × 40 mL shots of vodka in a 70-kg adult.
  - Note: Omit the loading dose of ethanol in the already ethanolintoxicated patient.
- Maintenance: 0.2–0.4 mL/kg/hour of 40% ethanol, or a 20–40 mL shot each hour.

Intravenous administration

- Loading dose: 8 mL/kg of 10% ethanol.
- Maintenance infusion rate: 1–2 mL/kg/hour of 10% ethanol.
- Note: A 10% ethanol solution is prepared by adding 100 mL of 100% ethanol to 900 mL of 5% glucose.
  - Remember: the required maintenance dose is extremely variable. The doses outlined above are a guide only and must be adjusted to maintain blood alcohol concentrations in the desired range.
- Continue maintenance ethanol therapy until the toxic alcohol poisoning has been definitively treated with haemodialysis.

ADVERSE DRUG REACTIONS AND THEIR MANAGEMENT

- Local phlebitis from intravenous solutions
- Ethanol intoxication
  - Reduce rate of ethanol administration if blood ethanol concentration exceeds 150 mg/dL (33 mmol/L).
- Hypoglycaemia, especially in children

SPECIFIC CONSIDERATIONS

Pregnancy: ethanol and the toxic alcohols readily cross the placenta. There is no absolute contraindication to ethanol administration in the pregnant woman with toxic alcohol poisoning.

Paediatric: there is no absolute contraindication to ethanol administration in the child with toxic alcohol poisoning, but the child must be carefully monitored for adverse effects such as sedation and hypoglycaemia.

HANDY TIPS

- Ethanol for intravenous therapy is difficult to procure – alcoholic spirits suitable for oral administration are ubiquitous.
- Therapeutic administration of ethanol may be delayed in the patient who already has a high ethanol level.
- Breath ethanol estimations may be substituted for repeated blood ethanol levels during maintenance therapy.

PITFALLS

- Delay in starting therapy.
- Failure to monitor blood ethanol levels closely resulting in sub- or supratherapeutic concentrations.

CONTROVERSIES

- Relative merits of fomepizole over ethanol in the management of toxic alcohol poisoning.
- Clinical efficacy of ethanol in the treatment of poisoning with other toxic alcohols, including glycol ethers, diethylene glycol, triethylene glycol, propylene glycol and butanediol.
- Requirement for ongoing or increased intravenous dosing of ethanol after commencement of dialysis.

References

Barceloux DG, Krenzelok EK, Olson K et al. American Academy of Clinical Toxicology Practice Guidelines on the Treatment of Ethylene Glycol Poisoning. Journal of Toxicology–Clinical Toxicology 1999; 37(5):537–560.

Beatty L, Green K, Magee K et al. A systematic review of ethanol and fomepizole use in toxic alcohol ingestion. Emergency Medicine International 2013; 2013:638–057.

Lepik KJ, Levy AR, Sobolev BG et al. Adverse drug events associated with the antidotes for methanol and ethylene glycol poisoning: a comparison of ethanol and fomepizole. Annals of Emergency Medicine 2009; 53:439–450.

4.9 FLUMAZENIL

Competitive benzodiazepine antagonist with a specific role in the management of benzodiazepine poisoning.

Presentations

Flumazenil 0.5 mg/5 mL ampoules

TOXICOLOGICAL INDICATIONS

- Benzodiazepine overdose
  - Accidental paediatric ingestion with compromised airway and breathing
  - Benzodiazepine ingestion with respiratory compromise in a patient who is not considered a candidate for intubation and ventilation (e.g. elderly patient with significant co-morbidities)
  - Deliberate self-poisoning with compromised airway and breathing, and equipment and skills to intubate and ventilate not readily available
    - Note: Isolated benzodiazepine overdose rarely causes CNS depression sufficient to warrant intervention.
- To confirm diagnosis of benzodiazepine intoxication
  - Useful if it avoids invasive or expensive further investigation to exclude alternative diagnoses
- Reversal of procedural sedation with benzodiazepines

CONTRAINDICATIONS

- Known seizure disorder
- Known or suspected co-ingestion of pro-convulsant drugs
- Known or suspected benzodiazepine dependence
- QRS prolongation on ECG (suggests possibility of co-ingestion of tricyclic antidepressant)

Mechanism of action

Flumazenil is a 1,4-imidazobenzodiazepine structurally similar to midazolam. It acts as a competitive antagonist at the benzodiazepine receptor sites in the CNS. Binding inhibits benzodiazepine activity at the GABA–benzodiazepine complex and reverses the CNS effects of benzodiazepines.

Pharmacokinetics

Flumazenil has a volume of distribution of 1 L/kg at steady state. It undergoes rapid and extensive hepatic metabolism to inactive metabolites. Elimination half-life is 40–80 minutes. These pharmacokinetic properties are unaltered following benzodiazepine overdose.

ADMINISTRATION

- Flumazenil should only be administered in an environment where equipment and personnel are available to manage a seizure.
- Give an initial dose of 0.1–0.2 mg IV and repeat every minute until reversal of sedation is achieved.
- Maximal response should be observed with a dose not exceeding 2 mg.
- Re-sedation is expected and normally occurs at around 90 minutes. If necessary, repeated doses may be given to maintain adequate reversal of benzodiazepine sedation. Occasionally a flumazenil infusion may be of value.
  - Note: Patients must be observed for re-sedation for several hours following the last dose of flumazenil.

ADVERSE DRUG REACTIONS AND THEIR MANAGEMENT

Benzodiazepine withdrawal syndrome

- Manifests as agitation, tachycardia and seizures.
- Mild benzodiazepine withdrawal will be short-lived and does not require specific management.
- Severe withdrawal syndrome requires administration of benzodiazepines in titrated doses.

Seizures

- Most commonly occur in patients with benzodiazepine dependence, co-ingestion of pro-convulsant drugs or an underlying seizure disorder.
- Withhold further flumazenil.
- Repeated or prolonged seizures require administration of benzodiazepines in titrated doses.
- Alternative agents such as barbiturates, and/or intubation and ventilation, may be required in the setting of uncontrolled recurrent seizure activity.

SPECIFIC CONSIDERATIONS

Pregnancy: safety not established. Administration should not be withheld if clinically indicated.

Paediatric: give 0.01–0.02 mg/kg repeated every minute as necessary. Flumazenil administration is extremely safe in children who have ingested benzodiazepines as they are unlikely to be benzodiazepine-dependent.

HANDY TIPS

- Flumazenil may be life-saving if personnel and equipment for definitive airway control are not available.
- Titrated doses of flumazenil minimise the risk of provoking iatrogenic harm in a patient at risk of benzodiazepine withdrawal seizures.

PITFALLS
- Unnecessary administration to patients with mild benzodiazepine poisoning.
- Administration when contraindicated due to risk of seizures.
- Failure to observe for re-sedation.

CONTROVERSY
- Role of flumazenil in management of the undifferentiated overdose patient.

References

Kreshak AA, Cantrell FL, Clark RF et al. A poison center's ten-year experience with flumazenil administration to acutely poisoned adults. Journal of Emergency Medicine 2012; 43:677–682.

Ngo AS, Anthony CR, Samuel M et al. Should a benzodiazepine antagonist be used in unconscious patients presenting to the emergency department? Resuscitation 2007; 74(1):27–37.

Seger D. Flumazenil: treatment or toxin. Journal of Toxicology–Clinical Toxicology 2004; 42(2):209–216.

The Flumazenil in Benzodiazepine Intoxication Multicenter Study Group. Treatment of benzodiazepine overdose with flumazenil. Clinical Therapeutics 1992; 14:978–995.

4.10 FOLINIC ACID

Leucovorin, 5-formyltetrahydrofolic acid

This agent is the active form of folic acid. It is routinely used for 'rescue therapy' in oncology and haematology treatment protocols following administration of high doses of parenteral methotrexate. Its applications in clinical toxicology include methotrexate toxicity and methanol poisoning.

Presentations

Calcium folinate 15 mg tablets (10)
Calcium folinate 15 mg/2 mL ampoules
Calcium folinate 50 mg/5 mL plastic vials and ampoules
Calcium folinate 100 mg/10 mL plastic vials and ampoules
Calcium folinate 300 mg/30 mL plastic vial

TOXICOLOGICAL INDICATIONS
- Supratherapeutic methotrexate ingestion
    - This usually occurs in the context of accidental daily dosing of methotrexate rather than the usual weekly dosing.
    - Folinic acid therapy is indicated if:
        - clinical features of methotrexate toxicity are evident
        or
        - the weekly dose has been administered daily for more than 3 consecutive days.
- Single acute oral methotrexate overdose
    - Methotrexate toxicity is a rare occurrence in the setting of acute overdose.
    - Folinic acid should be given empirically if >500 mg (>5 mg/kg in children) has been ingested, until methotrexate levels are available to more fully assess risk of toxicity.
    - If less than 500 mg of methotrexate is ingested, consider folinic acid if methotrexate levels are not available within 24 hours.

- Adjunctive treatment for methanol poisoning
- Massive pyrimethamine and trimethoprim poisoning

CONTRAINDICATIONS
- Known hypersensitivity

Mechanism of action

Folinic acid is the reduced biologically active form of folic acid and is essential for DNA/RNA synthesis. Methotrexate acts as an antimetabolite, preventing the reduction of folic acid to folinic acid by inhibiting dihydrofolate reductase. Administration of exogenous folinic acid bypasses this inhibition and restores DNA/RNA synthesis. Folates also enhance the elimination of formate in methanol poisoning.

Pharmacokinetics

Oral bioavailability of folinic acid is almost 100% after a 15-mg dose, but falls with higher doses. The active isomer has a volume of distribution of 13.6 L and an elimination half-life of 35 minutes. Elimination is predominantly by metabolism to an active metabolite, 5-methyltetrahydrofolate, which has a volume of distribution of 40 L and an elimination half-life of over 400 minutes.

ADMINISTRATION

Methotrexate overdose
- Give 15 mg PO, IM or IV every 6 hours.
- For single acute methotrexate overdose, therapy may be ceased when methotrexate level is confirmed to be below the threshold for toxicity (see **Table 3.52.1**) for an acute single overdose. It is otherwise continued for at least 3 days and until the clinical and laboratory features (especially haematological abnormalities) have resolved.
- With toxicity from supratherapeutic dosing, therapy is continued until clear resolution of toxicity (especially bone marrow recovery) is documented.

Methanol poisoning
- Give 2 mg/kg IV every 6 hours.
- Continue until poisoning is definitively treated.

ADVERSE DRUG REACTIONS
- Anaphylaxis (rare)
- Seizures (rare)
- Hypercalcaemia with rapid IV administration (>160 mg/minute)

SPECIFIC CONSIDERATIONS
Pregnancy: no restriction on use.
Paediatric: dosing for methotrexate toxicity is the same as for adults.

HANDY TIP
- Folinic acid administration is rarely necessary following acute single methotrexate overdose.

PITFALL
- Administration of folic acid instead of folinic acid (folic acid is not an effective antidote for methotrexate toxicity).

Reference
Bateman DN, Page CB. Antidotes to coumarins, isoniazid, methotrexate and thyroxine, toxins that work via metabolic processes. British Journal of Clinical Pharmacology 2016; 81(3):437-445. https://doi:org/10.1111/bcp.12736.

4.11 FOMEPIZOLE

Alcohol dehydrogenase inhibitor used in the management of methanol and ethylene glycol poisoning. Because it has a favourable adverse effect profile, it is a preferable antidote to the more commonly used alcohol dehydrogenase inhibitor, ethanol. However, it is expensive and not readily available in Australia and New Zealand.

Presentations
Fomepizole 1.5 g/1.5 mL ampoules
Fomepizole sulfate 160 mg/20 mL ampoules (equivalent to 100 mg of fomepizole per 20 mL ampoule)

TOXICOLOGICAL INDICATIONS
- Methanol poisoning (confirmed or suspected)
- Ethylene glycol poisoning (confirmed or suspected)
- Other toxic alcohol poisoning (confirmed or suspected – see **Chapter 3.5: Alcohol: Other toxic alcohols**)
  - Note: May be used alone or in combination with haemodialysis.

CONTRAINDICATIONS
- Known hypersensitivity (not yet reported)

Mechanism of action
Fomepizole is a potent competitive inhibitor of alcohol dehydrogenase. It blocks the first stage in the metabolism of methanol and ethylene glycol to their respective toxic metabolites. The toxic alcohols are then excreted unchanged, primarily in the urine, with a half-life of greater than 48 hours for methanol and a shorter half-life of approximately 20 hours for ethylene glycol. Although there are limited data to support use of fomepizole in rarer cases of diethylene glycol or glycol ether ingestion, it likely exerts a beneficial effect to minimise the production of toxic metabolites by the same mechanism.

Pharmacokinetics
Fomepizole has a small volume of distribution (0.7 L/kg). It undergoes hepatic metabolism to form an inactive metabolite, 4-carboxypyrazole. Metabolism is saturable at therapeutic doses. Fomepizole induces its own metabolism when administered for more than 48 hours and is dialysable.

ADMINISTRATION
- Intravenous
  - Loading dose: 15 mg/kg in 100 mL of normal saline or 5% glucose IV over 30 minutes.
  - Maintenance dose: 10 mg/kg in 100 mL of normal saline or 5% glucose IV over 30 minutes every 12 hours for 48 hours.

- Note: If administration for more than 48 hours is required, increase to 15 mg/kg every 12 hours to compensate for induction of metabolism.
- Monitoring of fomepizole concentrations is not necessary.
- If haemodialysis is undertaken, fomepizole should be given every 4–8 hours rather than every 12 hours or, alternatively, as a continuous infusion at 0.5–1 mg/kg/hour for the entire duration of haemodialysis.
- Oral dosing: fomepizole can be administered orally at the same dosing as the intermittent IV regimen.

THERAPEUTIC END POINTS
- Treatment continues until ethylene glycol or methanol levels are <20 mg/dL, in combination with other favourable biochemical and clinical parameters.

ADVERSE DRUG REACTIONS AND THEIR MANAGEMENT
- The adverse effect profile is benign. The most common adverse effect is discomfort at the infusion site. Minor symptoms such as headache, nausea or dizziness may occur.

SPECIFIC CONSIDERATIONS
Pregnancy: safety not established. Ethanol should be considered as an alternative.
Paediatric: no restriction on use.

CONTROVERSIES
- The appropriate threshold concentration of ethylene glycol or methanol at which an alcohol dehydrogenase inhibitor should be started is not established. The currently recommended concentration of 20 mg/dL is undoubtedly conservative.
- The superiority of fomepizole over ethanol as an alcohol dehydrogenase inhibitor. Potential advantages of fomepizole include ease of administration, more predictable pharmacokinetics, improved adverse effect profile, easier monitoring of therapy and potentially reduced need for haemodialysis. The principal disadvantages are availability and higher cost.
- Whether prolonged antidotal therapy with fomepizole is justified to avoid the use of haemodialysis in the setting of methanol poisoning (see **Chapter 3.4: Alcohol: Methanol**).
- Fomepizole is the preferred antidotal therapy for paediatric poisoning with toxic alcohols due to the risk of serious adverse effects from ethanol administration in this population and the logistical difficulties inherent in instituting haemodialysis in paediatric patients.

References
Barceloux DG, Krenzelok EP, Olson K et al. American Academy of Clinical Toxicology Practice Guidelines on the Treatment of Ethylene Glycol Poisoning. Ad Hoc Committee. Journal of Toxicology–Clinical Toxicology 1999; 37(5):537–560. doi:10.1081/clt-100102445.
Beatty L, Green K, Magee K et al. A systematic review of ethanol and fomepizole use in toxic alcohol ingestion. Emergency Medicine International 2013; 2013:638–057.
Brent J. Fomepizole for the treatment of pediatric ethylene and diethylene glycol, butoxyethanol, and methanol poisonings. Clinical Toxicology 2010; 48(5):401–406.

Brent J, McMartin K, Phillips SP et al. Fomepizole for the treatment of ethylene glycol poisoning. New England Journal of Medicine 1999; 340:832–838.

Brent J, McMartin K, Phillips SP et al. Fomepizole for the treatment of methanol poisoning. New England Journal of Medicine 2001; 344:424–429.

Hassanian-Moghaddam H, Zamani N, Roberts DM et al. Consensus statements on the approach to patients in a methanol poisoning outbreak. Clinical Toxicology 2019; 57(12):1129–1136.

Lepik KJ, Levy AR, Sobolev BG et al. Adverse drug events associated with the antidotes for methanol and ethylene glycol poisoning: a comparison of ethanol and fomepizole. Annals of Emergency Medicine 2009; 53:439–450.

Mégarbane B. Treatment of patients with ethylene glycol or methanol poisoning: focus on fomepizole 2010; 2:67–75.https://doi.org/10.2147/OAEM.S5346.

Marraffa J, Forrest A, Grant W et al. Oral administration of fomepizole produces similar blood levels as identical intravenous dose. Clinical Toxicology 2008; 46(3):181–186.

McMartin K, Jacobsen D, Hovda KE. Antidotes for poisoning by alcohols that form toxic metabolites. British Journal of Clinical Pharmacology 2015; 81(2):505–515.

4.12 GLUCOSE

Symptomatic hypoglycaemia resulting from toxic exposures must be immediately corrected by administration of glucose. In all but the mildest of cases this is achieved with an intravenous bolus of hypertonic glucose solution.

Presentations
Multiple formulations of IV glucose in the range of 5–70% solutions

TOXICOLOGICAL INDICATIONS
- Correction of hypoglycaemia caused by the following agents:
  — Ethanol ingestion (especially children)
  — Insulin
  — Propranolol
  — Quinine, chloroquine or hydroxychloroquine
  — Paracetamol or other hepatotoxic agents
  — Salicylate
  — Sulfonylurea
  — Valproate
  — Venlafaxine or desvenlafaxine.
- Combined with high-dose insulin (used as an inotropic agent) to maintain euglycaemia (see **Chapter 4.14: Insulin (high-dose)**):
  — Diltiazem or verapamil poisoning
  — Beta-blocker poisoning
  — Acute stress-induced (sympathomimetic) cardiotoxicity.

CONTRAINDICATIONS
- No absolute contraindications

Mechanism of action
Parenteral administration of glucose solutions rapidly corrects hypoglycaemia. However, the effect will be of relatively short duration in hyperinsulinaemic states. When insulin is used therapeutically in the management of calcium channel and beta-blocker toxicity, or to control hyperkalaemia, concomitant administration of glucose is required to maintain euglycaemia.

Pharmacokinetics

Under normal conditions, blood glucose concentration is maintained within a relatively narrow range by a variety of homeostatic mechanisms. Toxic hypoglycaemia is usually a result of a hyperinsulinaemic state.

ADMINISTRATION

- The patient is managed in a monitored area where equipment and personnel are available to frequently monitor blood glucose levels and observe for clinical features of hypoglycaemia.
- **Initial correction of symptomatic hypoglycaemia**
  - Adult – initial bolus of 50 mL of 50% glucose IV; repeat if no immediate clinical improvement
  - Child – 2–5 mL/kg bolus of 10% glucose IV; repeat if no immediate clinical improvement.
- **Deliberate self-poisoning with insulin**
  - Ongoing glucose infusion will be necessary, as the glucose requirement may be massive; the infusion rate is titrated to maintain euglycaemia or mild hyperglycaemia. Concentrated glucose solutions (50% glucose) are often required in order to prevent administration of excessive fluid volumes with less concentrated solutions (10% glucose)
    - Note: A central line is usually necessary to allow infusion of concentrated solutions (50% glucose) in order to minimise pain and severe phlebitis.
- **Deliberate self-poisoning with sulfonylureas**
  - Patients require infusion of large volumes of concentrated glucose solution, until such time as the hyperinsulinaemic state is controlled by administration of octreotide (see **Chapter 4.19: Octreotide**).
- **Hypoglycaemia from other causes**
  - Usually have a much lower ongoing glucose requirement (e.g. therapeutic sulfonylurea toxicity)
  - Oral supplementation may suffice, but admission to hospital for ongoing monitoring is essential.

THERAPEUTIC END POINTS

- Euglycaemia or mild hyperglycaemia

ADVERSE DRUG REACTIONS AND THEIR MANAGEMENT

- Hyperglycaemia
- Hypokalaemia secondary to insulin-mediated intracellular shift of potassium
- Hyponatraemia
- Hyperosmolality
- Local thrombophlebitis
- Rebound hypoglycaemia due to further stimulation of insulin secretion (especially in sulfonylurea overdose)
  - Attempts should be made to limit bolus IV glucose therapy in response to borderline hypoglycaemia unless significant clinical features are evident.

SPECIFIC CONSIDERATIONS

Pregnancy: no restriction on use.

HANDY TIPS
- Anticipate the need for large ongoing glucose requirement following deliberate self-poisoning with insulin and consider insertion of a central line to commence 50% glucose solution.
- Start octreotide after initial correction of hypoglycaemia in a patient with sulfonylurea overdose.
- Serum potassium replacement is necessary with glucose infusions.

PITFALLS
- Failure to anticipate ongoing glucose requirement in a patient with deliberate self-poisoning with insulin.
- Failure to start octreotide after initial treatment with glucose in the patient with deliberate self-poisoning with a sulfonylurea.

4.13 HYDROXOCOBALAMIN

Vitamin B12a

Hydroxocobalamin is a vitamin B12 (cyanocobalamin) precursor. In high doses, it is an effective chelator of cyanide.

Presentations
Kits containing 2 vials of hydroxocobalamin 2.5 g as lyophilised powder and 2 vials of 100 mL normal saline for reconstitution (Cyanokit®)
Hydroxocobalamin chloride 1 mg/mL ampoules

TOXICOLOGICAL INDICATIONS
- Known cyanide poisoning with serious clinical effects (altered mental status, seizures, hypotension, significant lactic acidosis in context of relatively normal oxygen saturation)
- Suspected cyanide poisoning with serious clinical effects
  - It is the preferred cyanide antidote in this situation because of its relatively benign adverse effects even if administered to a patient without cyanide poisoning.

CONTRAINDICATIONS
- Known hypersensitivity

Mechanism of action
Hydroxocobalamin has a complex molecular structure with a cobalt ion bound to a hydroxyl group at its centre, and it has a high affinity for cyanide. Cyanide binds to the central cobalt ion and displaces the hydroxyl group, forming cyanocobalamin, which is relatively non-toxic even in high concentrations and is excreted in the urine.
Hydroxocobalamin prevents cyanide from entering tissues and binding to cytochrome oxidase and also enhances reactivation of inhibited cytochrome oxidase by promoting removal of cyanide from the intracellular space.

Pharmacokinetics
Hydroxocobalamin has a small volume of distribution of 0.1–0.5 L/kg. It is largely excreted unchanged in the urine, with an elimination half-life from 1.5 to 26 hours.

Cyanocobalamin is also excreted in the urine, with an elimination half-life of approximately 9 hours.

ADMINISTRATION
- The patient is managed in a monitored area where equipment, drugs and personnel are available to provide full resuscitative care.
- Reconstitute hydroxocobalamin 2.5 g (1 ampoule) with 100 mL normal saline provided in the kit. Administer reconstituted solution IV over 15 minutes.
- Repeat the process with second vial in the kit to give a total dose of 5 g.
- This dose should be sufficient to bind 100 mg of cyanide; however, if the ingested dose is known to be greater than this, a larger initial dose could be administered.
- For patients in cardiac arrest from cyanide poisoning, hydroxocobalamin 5 g IV should be given more rapidly while resuscitation efforts continue.
- If there is no improvement within 15 minutes, repeat administration of hydroxocobalamin should be considered.
- Sodium thiosulfate promotes additional detoxification of cyanide by the enzyme rhodanese and administration is indicated if it is available (see **Chapter 4.26: Sodium thiosulfate**).

THERAPEUTIC END POINTS
- Improvement in conscious state
- Haemodynamic stability
- Improvement in metabolic acidosis

ADVERSE DRUG REACTIONS AND THEIR MANAGEMENT
- Minor hypertension, bradycardia and tachycardia have been occasionally reported, but are unlikely to require specific treatment.
- Orange-red discolouration of the skin, mucous membranes, urine, plasma and other bodily fluids occurs and lasts for 12–48 hours, but is not consequential.
- Acute allergic reactions have not been reported following single high-dose therapy in poisoned patients.

SPECIFIC CONSIDERATIONS
Pregnancy: no restriction on use.
Paediatric: the paediatric dose has not been determined, but it is reasonable to commence with 50 mg/kg.

HANDY TIPS
- Only the Cyanokit® provides a dose of hydroxocobalamin sufficient to treat cyanide poisoning. It is expensive, not widely available and only available in Australia if imported under the Special Access Scheme. The alternative preparation, used to treat pernicious anaemia, contains only 1 mg of hydroxocobalamin. 5000 ampoules and a volume of 5 L would be necessary to obtain the dose necessary to treat one case of cyanide poisoning.
- Failure to improve after the first dose of hydroxocobalamin prompts reconsideration of the diagnosis in suspected cyanide poisoning.

- Hydroxocobalamin and sodium thiosulfate must not be mixed in the same infusion as hydroxocobalamin complexes will result.
- The discolouration of bodily fluids that occurs may interfere with laboratory analyses that use colorimetric methods, including liver enzymes, bilirubin, creatinine, creatine kinase, phosphorus, glucose, magnesium and iron. It is important to recognise the possibility of falsely high or low results.

PITFALLS
- Failure to stock the appropriate preparation.
- Failure to administer an adequate dose.

CONTROVERSIES
- This expensive antidote is rarely required but must be immediately available if it is to be useful. It is appropriate to stock in locations where there is a risk of being confronted with a case of cyanide poisoning.
- Relative efficacy of hydroxocobalamin compared with supportive care and with other cyanide antidotes.
- The requirement for and additional benefit of sodium thiosulfate following hydroxocobalamin administration in cases of cyanide poisoning.

References

Borron SW, Baud FJ, Megarbane B et al. Hydroxocobalamin for severe acute cyanide poisoning by ingestion or inhalation. American Journal of Emergency Medicine 2007; 25:551–558.

Fortin JL, Giocanti JP, Ruttimann M et al. Prehospital administration of hydroxocobalamin for smoke inhalation-associated cyanide poisoning: 8 years of experience in the Paris Fire Brigade. Clinical Toxicology 2006; 44(Supp 1):37–44. doi:10.1080/15563650600811870.

Hall AH, Dart R, Bogdan G. Sodium thiosulfate or hydroxocobalamin for empiric treatment of cyanide poisoning? Annals of Emergency Medicine 2007; 49:806–813.

Reade MC, Davies SR, Morley PT et al. Review article: management of cyanide poisoning. Emergency Medicine Australasia 2012; 24:225–238.

Thompson JP, Marrs TC. Hydroxocobalamin in cyanide poisoning. Clinical Toxicology 2012; 50:875–885.

4.14 INSULIN (HIGH-DOSE)

High-dose insulin (HDI) therapy is the mainstay of treatment in diltiazem and verapamil poisoning and should be started as soon as toxicity is evident. It is also a therapeutic option in severe cardiogenic shock from other toxicological or toxinological causes.

TOXICOLOGICAL INDICATIONS
- Diltiazem and verapamil poisoning
- Beta-blocker poisoning with impaired cardiac contractility unresponsive to catecholamine infusion (see **Chapter 3.18: Beta-blockers**)
- Cardiogenic shock from other causes including:

- Amphetamines and amphetamine-like substances
- Serotonin and noradrenaline reuptake inhibitors (SNRIs)
- Cocaine
- Envenomings
  - Irukandji jellyfish
  - Funnel-web spiders

CONTRAINDICATIONS
- Vasodilatory shock with preserved cardiac contractility.

Mechanism of action

Insulin has a well-established inotropic effect in the setting of toxic cardiogenic shock. Administration of high doses of insulin intravenously overcomes insulin resistance, enhances lactate conversion to pyruvate, reverses anaerobic metabolism and improves glucose utilisation, restoring efficient ATP generation and improving myocardial contractility.

Glucose is given concurrently with insulin to maintain euglycaemia. HDI promotes peripheral vascular dilatation by the generation of endothelial nitric oxide and therefore is not indicated in vasodilatory shock.

ADMINISTRATION
- High-dose insulin is administered under close haemodynamic and biochemical monitoring. Particular attention to blood sugar and serum potassium concentrations is essential during therapy.
- Commence therapy by administering:
  - Glucose 25 g (50 mL of 50% solution) IV bolus
- then
  - Short-acting insulin 1 U/kg IV bolus.
- Continue therapy with:
  - Glucose 25 g/hour IV infusion via a central line
  - Short-acting insulin 1 U/kg/hr IV infusion.
- The glucose infusion is titrated to maintain euglycaemia.
- The insulin infusion may be increased to 4 U/kg/hour depending on haemodynamic response.
- Doses in excess of 4 U/kg/hr have been used, up to a maximum of 10 U/kg/hr. The incremental benefit and requirement for such massive doses is not established.

THERAPEUTIC END POINTS
- Therapy is weaned as cardiovascular toxicity resolves.

ADVERSE DRUG REACTIONS AND THEIR MANAGEMENT
- Hypoglycaemia
  - Glucose infusion is titrated to maintain euglycaemia.
  - Bedside BGL should be checked every 15–30 minutes during initiation and titration of insulin.
  - BGL should be checked every hour once the insulin dose is stable.
- Hypokalaemia
  - Potassium supplementation is required based on serial monitoring.
  - Total body stores are not depleted and potassium will shift back extracellularly once the insulin infusion is stopped.

- Serum potassium concentration should be checked hourly during initiation and titration of insulin.
- Serum potassium concentration should be checked every 6 hours once insulin dose is stable.
- Hypomagnesaemia, hypophosphataemia
  - Magnesium and phosphate levels are optimised based on serial monitoring.

SPECIFIC CONSIDERATIONS
Pregnancy: no restriction on use.
Paediatric: no restriction on use.

HANDY TIPS
- HDI is most effective if commenced as soon as impaired cardiac contractility is identified rather than initiated after failure of escalating dosing of standard catecholamine infusions.
- Because the inotropic effect of HDI is mediated by intracellular biochemical processes, there is a delay of up to an hour before a clinical response is expected or seen.
- Glucose supplementation may be required for up to 24 hours following withdrawal of HDI due to the persistent and prolonged hyperinsulinaemic state.

PITFALL
- Failure to initiate therapy sufficiently early in life-threatening calcium channel blocker (CCB) diltiazem or verapamil toxicity.

CONTROVERSIES
- The use of HDI in severe CCB and beta-blocker poisoning is supported by animal studies and case reports but there are no randomised controlled trials in humans.
- Doses in excess of 4 U/kg/hr have been used, up to a maximum of 10 U/kg/hr. The requirement for and incremental benefit of such massive doses are not established.
- HDI is advocated in cardiogenic shock from other toxicological and toxinological causes, but clinical experience is limited.

References

Engebretsen KM, Kaczmarek KM, Morgan J et al. High-dose insulin therapy in beta-blocker and calcium channel-blocker poisoning. Clinical Toxicology 2011; 49:277–283.

Lheureux PE, Zahir S, Gris M et al. Bench-to-bedside review: hyperinsulinaemia/euglycaemia therapy in the management of overdose of calcium-channel blockers. Critical Care 2006; 10:212.

Megarbane B, Karyo S, Baud FJ. The role of insulin and glucose (hyperinsulinaemia/euglycaemia) therapy in acute calcium channel antagonist and beta-blocker poisoning. Toxicological Reviews 2004; 23(4):215–222.

Yuan TH, Kerns WP, Tomaszewski CA et al. Insulin–glucose as adjunctive therapy for severe calcium channel antagonist poisoning. Journal of Toxicology–Clinical Toxicology 1999; 37(4):463–474.

4.15 INTRAVENOUS LIPID EMULSION

Intravenous lipid emulsion (ILE) is a sterile emulsion of soya bean oil in water, used primarily in parenteral nutrition. It has a clearly defined role in the resuscitation of patients with severe toxicity induced by local anaesthetic agents, but the evidence for benefit in poisonings from other agents is less strong.

Presentations
Intravenous lipid emulsion 10%, 500 mL
Intravenous lipid emulsion 20%, 100 mL, 500 mL
Intravenous lipid emulsion 30%, 250 mL

TOXICOLOGICAL INDICATIONS
- Local anaesthetic-induced cardiovascular collapse, resistant to standard resuscitation protocols
- Considered in cases of refractory cardiac instability or arrest in the context of acute poisoning with other highly lipid soluble agents, including propranolol, tricyclic antidepressants and verapamil

CONTRAINDICATIONS
- Inadequate standard resuscitative efforts
- Hypersensitivity to egg, soya or peanut protein

Mechanism of action
The mechanism of action is not clearly defined and multiple theories are proposed, including creation of an intravascular phase ('lipid sink') that sequesters lipid-soluble drug; promotion of redistribution of drug from cardiac and neural tissue to other organs (e.g. liver, skeletal muscle); increased myocardial ATP generation due to improved fatty acid delivery to mitochondria; and restoration of myocyte function by activation of calcium and potassium channels and an increase in intracellular calcium.

ADMINISTRATION
- Continue standard resuscitation protocols during administration.
- Give 1–1.5 mL/kg ILE 20% as an IV bolus over 1 minute.
- Repeat bolus once or twice at 3–5 minute intervals based on clinical response
  then
- Infuse ILE 0.25 mL/kg/minute until haemodynamic stability is restored.
- Increase to 0.5 mL/kg/minute if hypotension persists.
- Increasing the total dose above 8 mL/kg is unlikely to be beneficial.

THERAPEUTIC END POINTS
- Return of spontaneous circulation with stabilisation of haemodynamic parameters. Infusion may be restarted if hypotension recurs on cessation.

ADVERSE DRUG REACTIONS AND THEIR MANAGEMENT
- Immediate: allergy and anaphylaxis.
- Acute lung injury (lipoid pneumonitis), pulmonary hypertension, haematuria, hypertriglyceridaemia and pancreatitis have been described. Management is supportive.

SPECIFIC CONSIDERATIONS
Pregnancy: safety is not established. Administration should not be withheld if clinically indicated.
Paediatric: there are no reports of paediatric administration, but administration should not be withheld if clinically indicated.

HANDY TIP
- A suitable dosing regimen of ILE 20% for resuscitating a 70-kg adult would be an IV bolus of 100 mL followed by an infusion of 400 mL over 20 minutes while continuing advanced life support. If no response, repeat boluses twice more while giving further adrenaline. If hypotension persists, increase infusion rate to 400 mL over 10 minutes.

CONTROVERSIES
- Optimum dosing regimens of ILE are yet to be established.
- Short- and long-term adverse effects of ILE require further study.
- Role of ILE in poisoning other than that by local anaesthetic agents requires further study.
  - Published human case reports are of variable quality and interpretation of possible benefit is subject to significant publication bias.
- Proprietary formulations of ILE generally have an alkaline pH, and the contribution of pH to any observed antidotal effect requires further study.

References
Felice KL, Schumann HM. Intravenous lipid emulsion for local anaesthetic toxicity: a review of the literature. Journal of Medical Toxicology 2008; 4(3):184–191.

Hoegberg LCG, Bania TC, Lavergne V et al. Systematic review of the effect of intravenous lipid emulsion therapy for local anesthetic toxicity. Clinical Toxicology 2016; 54(3):167–193.

Levine M, Skolnik AB, Ruha A-M et al. Complications following antidotal use of intravenous lipid emulsion therapy. Journal of Medical Toxicology 2014; 10:10–14.

The Association of Anaesthetists of Great Britain and Ireland. Guidelines for the management of severe local anaesthetic toxicity 2010; https://anaesthetists.org/Home/Resources-publications/Guidelines/Management-of-severe-local-anaesthetic-toxicity.

Turner-Lawrence DE, Kerns W. Intravenous fat emulsion: a potential novel antidote. Journal of Medical Toxicology 2008; 4(2):109–114.

Weinberg G. Lipid rescue resuscitation from local anaesthetic cardiac toxicity. Toxicological Reviews 2006; 25(3):139–145.

4.16 METHYLENE BLUE

Methylene blue is the treatment of choice for drug-induced methaemoglobinaemia. It has also been proposed as a potential treatment for severe vasoplegic shock; however, evidence for benefit is limited.

Presentations
Methylene blue trihydrate 50 mg/5 mL ampoules

TOXICOLOGICAL INDICATIONS
- Symptomatic drug-induced methaemoglobinaemia with features of hypoxaemia (e.g. chest pain, dyspnoea or confusion)
- Consider in asymptomatic patients with methaemoglobin (MetHb) levels >20%
- Methylene blue has also been used in anaphylactic and toxic shock states where hypotension persists despite vasopressor administration

CONTRAINDICATIONS
- G6PD deficiency: lack of NADPH in this condition causes methylene blue to be ineffective as it cannot be reduced to leucomethylene blue. Haemolysis may also occur.
- Renal impairment: dose needs to be reduced.
- Methaemoglobinaemia reductase deficiency.
- Known hypersensitivity.

Mechanism of action
Methylene blue dramatically increases the natural rate of reduction of MetHb to haemoglobin. Methylene blue is reduced to leucomethylene blue by methaemoglobin reductase in the presence of NADPH. Leucomethylene blue then reduces MetHb to haemoglobin.

Methylene blue inhibits nitric oxide synthase and guanylate cyclase and scavenges endothelial nitric oxide. In shock states, it appears to have both vasoconstrictive and positive inotropic effects.

Pharmacokinetics
Methylene blue is rapidly reduced to leucomethylene blue, which is predominantly excreted in the urine as a salt complex.

ADMINISTRATION
- Administer 1–2 mg/kg (0.1–0.2 mL/kg of 1% solution) IV slowly over 5 minutes. Follow with a normal saline flush to minimise venous irritation.
- MetHb levels should be measured hourly until a consistent fall is documented.
- Methaemoglobinaemia usually responds to a single dose. However, a further dose of 1–2 mg/kg may be repeated if the initial response is inadequate.
- In rare instances, such as dapsone poisoning, when methaemoglobin formation may continue for days, repeat dosing every 6–8 hours may be necessary for several days.
- A single dose of 1–2 mg/kg has been suggested as adjunctive therapy in vasodilatory shock, but data on clinical benefit are limited.

THERAPEUTIC END POINTS
- Resolution of symptoms of hypoxaemia
- Response is confirmed by repeat MetHb estimations.
- Stabilisation of haemodynamic parameters.

ADVERSE DRUG REACTIONS AND THEIR MANAGEMENT
- Local pain and irritation commonly occur at site of administration and extravasation can result in local tissue necrosis.
- Common non-specific adverse effects include headache, dizziness, restlessness, nausea, vomiting, chest discomfort and shortness of breath.
- Blue discolouration of mucous membranes which mimics cyanosis.
- Methylene blue may paradoxically cause methaemoglobinaemia when given in high doses (>7 mg/kg) secondary to a direct oxidative effect on haemoglobin.
- Acute haemolytic anaemia may occur in G6PD-deficient individuals and with very large doses of methylene blue (>15 mg/kg).

SPECIFIC CONSIDERATIONS
    Pregnancy: no restrictions on use.
    Lactation: no restrictions on use.
    Paediatric: Initial paediatric dose is 1 mg/kg.

HANDY TIPS
- Patients with pre-existing conditions affecting tissue oxygenation, such as anaemia or coronary artery disease, may require methylene blue administration at MetHb concentrations as low as 10%.
- Standard pulse oximetry is unreliable in these clinical presentations as MetHb and methylene blue both interfere with the readings.
  - Methaemoglobinaemia causes cyanosis and blue discoloration of skin, and oximetry readings characteristically show a reading of around 85%.
  - Methylene blue also causes interference with pulse oximetry and readings may worsen after administration, even when methaemoglobinaemia has resolved and the patient's clinical features have improved.
- Consider the following problems if MetHb levels are not falling after 2 doses of methylene blue:
  - Massive ongoing exposure to oxidising agent
  - Sulfhaemoglobinaemia (e.g. by sulfonamides)
  - G6PD deficiency
  - Methaemoglobin reductase deficiency
  - Haemoglobinopathies
  - Excessive methylene blue administration.
- If methaemoglobinaemia persists despite methylene blue administration, consider exchange transfusion or hyperbaric oxygen therapy.

- The MetHb concentration mandating methylene blue treatment. It may be reasonable to monitor asymptomatic patients with elevated levels even >20% and not treat unless features of hypoxaemia develop.
- The indications for and clinical benefits of methylene blue in refractory vasodilatory shock states require further study.

References
Clifton J, Leiken JB. Methylene blue. American Journal of Therapeutics 2003; 10:289–291.

Lo JCY, Darracq MA, Clark RF. A review of methylene blue treatment for cardiovascular collapse. Journal of Emergency Medicine 2014; 46:670–679.

4.17 N-ACETYLCYSTEINE

N-acetylcysteine (NAC) is a sulfhydryl donor used as the antidote for paracetamol poisoning. It is almost completely protective against paracetamol-induced hepatotoxicity when administered within 8 hours of an overdose. It is an extremely safe antidote and adverse effects are limited to mild anaphylactoid reactions. The currently recommended treatment regimen consists of two infusions administered over a total of 20 hours, and has a decreased incidence of anaphylactoid reactions compared to the historical three-bag regimen.

Presentations
200 mg/mL injectable (10 mL, 30 mL)

TOXICOLOGICAL INDICATIONS
- Acute paracetamol overdose
- Repeated supratherapeutic paracetamol ingestion
- Established paracetamol-induced hepatotoxicity
  - Note: The risk assessment for paracetamol-induced hepatotoxicity is based on the dose ingested and serum paracetamol and hepatic transaminase levels, and is discussed in detail in **Chapter 3.60: Paracetamol: Immediate-release preparations (acute overdose), Chapter 3.61: Paracetamol: Modified-release formulations** and **Chapter 3.62: Paracetamol: Repeated supratherapeutic ingestion**
- NAC is indicated for its antioxidant properties for use in poisonings by a variety of other agents, including paraquat, acrylonitrile, cyclophosphamide, amanita mushrooms and hydrocarbons including carbon tetrachloride, chloroform and essential oils

CONTRAINDICATIONS
- None

Mechanism of action
NAC prevents N-acetyl-p-benzoquinone imine (NAPQI)-induced hepatotoxicity when given within 8 hours of an acute paracetamol overdose. It ameliorates the clinical course

of toxicity when given after that time or following repeated supratherapeutic ingestion. Four possible mechanisms contribute to this action:

1 increased glutathione availability
2 direct binding to NAPQI
3 provision of inorganic sulfate
4 reduction of NAPQI back to paracetamol.

The antioxidant properties of NAC may offer benefit in a number of other poisonings in which oxidative stress is an important toxic mechanism and may also explain its beneficial effects in liver failure of any cause.

Pharmacokinetics
NAC metabolism is complex, with a variety of sulfur-containing compounds being produced. Plasma half-life following IV administration is 6 hours and 30% is eliminated unchanged in the urine.

ADMINISTRATION
- Patients are monitored for an anaphylactoid reaction during and after the initial dose of NAC. Cardiac monitoring is not required after that time.
- Give 200 mg/kg NAC (1 mL/kg of 200 mg/mL NAC solution) in 500 mL 5% glucose IV over 4 hours
  followed by
- 100 mg/kg NAC (0.5 mL/kg of 200 mg/mL NAC solution) in 1000 mL 5% glucose over 16 hours.
- The standard treatment duration is 20 hours; however, it may be stopped earlier if the risk of hepatotoxicity is excluded.
- NAC should be continued beyond 20 hours in patients if paracetamol remains detectable at the end of the infusion or if there is biochemical evidence of hepatotoxicity.
  — Repeat the final dose of 100 mg/kg NAC in 1000 mL of 5% glucose IV over 16 hours until paracetamol is undetectable, transaminases stabilise or improve and the patient is clinically well.

THERAPEUTIC END POINTS
- Absent or resolving hepatotoxicity as determined by monitoring of transaminase levels

---

ADVERSE DRUG REACTIONS AND THEIR MANAGEMENT
- Anaphylactoid reactions (resulting from direct histamine release or complement activation, in contrast to IgE-mediated anaphylaxis) occur in up to 10% of patients. Clinical features can be cutaneous (erythema, rash or angiodema) or systemic (hypotension or wheeze). These usually occur during or shortly after the initial infusion and are generally mild.
  — The infusion should be temporarily ceased.
  — Oral antihistamines, intravenous fluids and inhaled bronchodilators are given as clinically indicated.
  — Progression to severe anaphylaxis is not expected and adrenaline is not routinely indicated.
  — The infusion may be restarted when symptoms have improved.

SPECIFIC CONSIDERATIONS

Pregnancy: NAC crosses the placenta. When indicated, it is beneficial for both mother and fetus.

Paediatric: the dose of NAC is the same as for adults. However, it should be infused in smaller volumes of 5% glucose (use 0.45% sodium chloride with 5% glucose if there are concerns about development of hyponatraemia).

- Children <20 kg body weight:
  - 200 mg/kg NAC (1 mL/kg of 200 mg/mL NAC solution) in 100 mL 5% glucose IV over 4 hours

    followed by
  - 100 mg/kg NAC (0.5 mL/kg of 200 mg/mL NAC solution) in 250 mL 5% glucose over 16 hours.
- Children 20–50 kg body weight:
  - 200 mg/kg NAC (1 mL/kg of 200 mg/mL NAC solution) in 250 mL 5% glucose IV over 4 hours

    followed by
  - 100 mg/kg NAC (1 mL/kg of 200 mg/mL NAC solution) in 500 mL 5% glucose IV over 4 hours.

HANDY TIPS

- Always prescribe NAC infusions using a preformatted chart which indicates both the volume of NAC solution and the mg/kg dose. This practice reduces the chance of a dosing error. An example of a dosing chart is shown in **Appendix 3: N-acetylcysteine (NAC) IV infusion for paracetamol poisoning**.
- A previously documented anaphylactoid reaction during NAC administration is not a contraindication to this potentially life-saving treatment. Pre-treatment with an oral antihistamine or bronchodilators is indicated prior to NAC administration.

PITFALLS

- Failure to initiate NAC empirically in the patient who presents more than 8 hours following a paracetamol overdose of ≥200 mg/kg.
- Failure to warn patient and staff of the possibility of a mild anaphylactoid reaction occurring early in treatment.

CONTROVERSIES

- The optimal regimen for administration of NAC is not clearly defined for all presentations. Multiple protocols exist including a number of regimens of shorter duration.
- The two-bag regimen has clear benefit in decreasing the incidence of anaphylactoid reactions and for ease of administration, but is not proven to be superior to the historical three-bag regimen in the prevention of hepatotoxicity.
- Use of increased doses of NAC has been advocated following massive ingestions and a paracetamol level > double the nomogram line (see **Chapter 3.60: Paracetamol: Immediate-release preparations (acute overdose)** and **Chapter 3.61: Paracetamol: Modified-release formulations**).

References

Bateman DN, Dear JW, Christensen MB et al. Reduction of adverse effects from intravenous acetylcysteine treatment for paracetamol poisoning: a randomized controlled trial. Lancet 2014; 383:697–704.

Chiew A, Dalhoff KP, Pomerleau AC et al. Updated guidelines for the management of paracetamol poisoning in Australia and New Zealand. Medical Journal of Australia 2019; 212(4):175–183.

Daoud FSS, Fountain JS, Murray L et al. Two-bag intravenous N-acetylcysteine, antihistamine pretreatment and high plasma paracetamol levels are associated with a lower incidence of anaphylactoid reactions to N-acetylcysteine. Clinical Toxicology 2020; 58(7):698–704. doi:10.1080/15563650.2019.1675886.

Kerr F, Dawson A, Whyte IM et al. The Australasian Clinical Toxicology Investigators Collaboration randomized trial of different loading infusion rates of N-acetylcysteine. Annals of Emergency Medicine 2005; 45:409–413.

Prescott LF, Illingworth RN, Critchley JA. Intravenous N-acetylcysteine: the treatment of choice for paracetamol poisoning. British Medical Journal 1979; 2:1097.

Rumack BH, Bateman DH. Acetaminophen and acetylcysteine dose and duration: past, present and future. Clinical Toxicology 2012; 50:91–98.

Schmidt LE, Rasmussen DN, Petersen TS et al. Fewer adverse effects associated with a modified two-bag intravenous acetylcysteine protocol compared to traditional three-bag regimen in paracetamol overdose. Clinical Toxicology 2018; 56(11):1128–1134. doi:10.1080/15563650.2018.1475672.

4.18 NALOXONE

Naloxone is a competitive opioid antagonist used as a resuscitation antidote in opioid intoxication.

Presentations

Naloxone hydrochloride 400 microgram/1 mL ampoules
Naloxone hydrochloride 800 microgram/2 mL pre-filled syringe
Naloxone hydrochloride 2 mg/5 mL pre-filled syringe
Naloxone hydrochloride 1.8 mg/0.1 mL nasal spray

TOXICOLOGICAL INDICATIONS
- Reversal of CNS and respiratory depression caused by opioid toxicity
- Reversal of CNS and respiratory depression caused by clonidine toxicity

CONTRAINDICATIONS
- None

Mechanism of action

Naloxone is a pure competitive opioid antagonist at mu, kappa and delta receptors. It reverses opioid effects, including effects of sedation and respiratory depression.

Pharmacokinetics

Onset of action is rapid after IV or IM administration, but there is poor oral bioavailability with an extensive first-pass effect. It is metabolised by the liver, with an elimination half-life of 60–90 minutes. Duration of effect depends on the dose given and the rate of elimination of the opioid agonist, but is usually from 30 to 120 minutes.

ADMINISTRATION
- Treatment dose is variable and the response depends on the amount and type of opioid agonist present.

- **Opioids**
  - Give an initial bolus dose of 100 micrograms IV or 200–400 micrograms IM or SC if IV access cannot be established. Larger initial doses may safely be used where the patient is not opioid dependent.
  - Repeated doses of 100 micrograms IV every 30–60 seconds may be given until adequate spontaneous respiration is re-established.
  - Doses >400 micrograms are rarely required following heroin overdose; however, much larger doses may be required in overdose from partial opioid agonists (e.g. buprenorphine) or fentanyl analogues.
- **Clonidine**
  - Very large doses of naloxone are indicated for reversal of clonidine-induced sedation, respiratory depression and hypotension, particularly in children.
  - Give an initial bolus dose of 2–5 mg IV, repeated every 1–2 minutes up to a maximum dose of 10 mg.
- The dose of naloxone and duration of treatment required is variable and dependent on the receptor affinity of the opioid agonist as well as the absorption and elimination kinetics.
- Clinically significant re-sedation is unlikely following heroin overdose. However, following overdose with other agents (e.g. controlled-release morphine, oxycodone or methadone), re-sedation is expected and a naloxone infusion may be necessary.
  - Commence the naloxone infusion rate at two-thirds of the initial dose required/hour. Administration of 100 microgram/hour can be obtained by diluting 2 mg of naloxone in 100 mL normal saline and running at 5 mL/hour.
  - Monitor the patient for evidence of opioid withdrawal and titrate the infusion according to clinical response.

THERAPEUTIC END POINTS
- In the non-opioid-dependent individual, naloxone may be given in a dose sufficient to achieve and maintain a normal mental status.
- In the opioid-dependent individual, naloxone dose should be sufficient to permit maintenance of an adequate airway and respiratory rate in a patient who is rousable, without precipitating acute withdrawal.
- All patients given naloxone should be observed for re-sedation for at least 2 hours after the last dose.

ADVERSE DRUG REACTIONS AND THEIR MANAGEMENT
- In non-opioid-dependent individuals, naloxone does not cause significant adverse effects, even in very large doses.
- In opioid-tolerant patients, acute withdrawal can occur.
- If a withdrawal syndrome is inadvertently produced, immediately cease further administration of naloxone. Physical and chemical control of the symptomatic patient may be necessary if reassurance fails. Avoid long-acting chemical sedation as the duration of naloxone-induced withdrawal is short (usually <90 minutes).

SPECIFIC CONSIDERATIONS

Pregnancy: safety not established. Administration should not be withheld if clinically indicated.

Paediatric: naloxone can usually be given with impunity to suspected cases of paediatric opioid intoxication as children are unlikely to be opioid-dependent. Give a 400-microgram bolus IV to exclude or confirm the diagnosis of opioid intoxication.

HANDY TIPS

- Do not completely reverse opioid intoxication in opioid-dependent patients as acute withdrawal will render assessment and management more difficult.
- IV administration is preferred to IM as it allows more exact titration of dose.
- Anticipate the need for ongoing naloxone administration following overdose of methadone, oxycodone or controlled-release oral morphine.
- Monitor patients on naloxone infusion for both re-sedation and withdrawal and adjust the rate of infusion accordingly.

PITFALLS

- Precipitating severe acute withdrawal syndrome in opioid-dependent patients.
- Failure to detect and correct re-sedation following initial response to naloxone.

CONTROVERSIES

- Intranasal naloxone is an effective route of administration for opioid reversal and has an important role particularly in the pre-hospital setting.
- The dose of naloxone recommended for reversal of clonidine-induced sedation and respiratory depression is markedly higher than for standard opioid reversal. Published evidence supports this as a safe and effective treatment that can prevent the requirement for intubation, particularly in children.

References

Ashton H, Hassan Z. Best evidence topic report: intranasal naloxone in suspected opioid overdose. Emergency Medicine Journal 2006; 23:221–223.

Lynn RR, Galinkin JL. Naloxone dosage for opioid reversal: current evidence and clinical implications. Therapeutic Advances in Drug Safety 2018; 9(1):63–88.

Seger DL, Loden JK. Naloxone reversal of clonidine toxicity: dose, dose, dose. Clinical Toxicology 2018; 56(10):873–879.

4.19 OCTREOTIDE

Long-acting synthetic octapeptide analogue of somatostatin indicated for the management of sulfonylurea-induced hypoglycaemia.

Presentations

Octreotide 50 microgram/mL injectable (1 mL)
Octreotide 100 microgram/mL injectable (1 mL)

Octreotide 200 microgram/mL injectable (1 mL)
Octreotide 10 mg, 20 mg, 30 mg injectable (powder and solvent)

TOXICOLOGICAL INDICATIONS
- Drug-induced hyperinsulinaemic states resulting in persistent hypoglycaemia (blood glucose <4 mmol/L) including:
  — Intentional sulfonylurea overdose
  — Therapeutic sulfonylurea-induced hypoglycaemia
  — Quinine-induced hypoglycaemia

CONTRAINDICATIONS
- None

Mechanism of action
Octreotide binds to somatostatin receptors on pancreatic beta cells, closing calcium channels, inhibiting calcium influx and subsequent insulin release. It is particularly effective in sulfonylurea-induced hypoglycaemia because it acts 'downstream' from the sulfonylurea receptor site to reduce insulin secretion.

Pharmacokinetics
Octreotide has a bioavailability of 100% following SC administration. Peak levels are achieved within 30 minutes, but are only half those achieved following IV administration. About 30% is excreted unchanged by the kidney, with an elimination half-life of 90 minutes.

ADMINISTRATION
- The patient is managed in a monitored area where equipment and personnel are available to frequently monitor blood glucose levels and observe for clinical features of hypoglycaemia.
- Documentation of hypoglycaemia and immediate management (IV glucose) is required prior to initiation of octreotide therapy.
- **Sulfonylurea overdose**
  — Give adults 50 microgram IV bolus followed by 25 microgram/ hour continuous infusion (1 microgram/kg IV followed by 1 microgram/kg/hour continuous infusion in children).
  — An infusion of 25 microgram/hour can be given by diluting 500 micrograms of octreotide in 500 mL of normal saline and running at 25 mL/hour.
  — An alternative to IV infusion is 100 micrograms SC or IM every 6 hours. Breakthrough hypoglycaemia may occur between doses.
  — Normoglycaemia is usually maintained without requirement for IV glucose supplementation once the octreotide infusion is commenced. If hypoglycaemia recurs, it should be corrected with 50% glucose IV and the octreotide infusion rate doubled.
- **Sulfonylurea-induced hypoglycaemia during therapeutic dosing**
  — A single dose of octreotide 50–100 micrograms IV or SC may be adequate to prevent subsequent episodes of hypoglycaemia, without requirement for an infusion. Close monitoring of glucose levels is essential.

THERAPEUTIC END POINTS
- Normoglycaemia must be maintained for 12 hours off octreotide and on a normal diet before the patient is medically fit for discharge.

ADVERSE DRUG REACTIONS AND THEIR MANAGEMENT
- Minor nausea only.

SPECIFIC CONSIDERATIONS
Pregnancy: safety is not established. Administration should not be withheld if clinically indicated.

Paediatric: the optimal dose in children is unknown. Given the absence of significant adverse effects, commence therapy with an initial bolus of 1 microgram/kg IV or SC followed by an intravenous infusion of 1 microgram/kg/hour.

HANDY TIP
- Initiation of therapy with a bolus of 100 micrograms SC is effective in stabilising a patient in a remote location prior to transfer to the place of definitive care. This dose may be brought in by a retrieval team if unavailable on site.

PITFALL
- Failure to start therapy when hypoglycaemia first develops following sulfonylurea overdose.

CONTROVERSIES
- Intravenous versus subcutaneous administration and optimal dosing regimens.

References

Boyle PJ, Justice K, Krentz AJ et al. Octreotide reverses hyperinsulinemia and prevents hypoglycaemia induced by sulfonylurea overdoses. Journal of Clinical Endocrinology and Metabolism 1993; 77:752–756.

Dougherty PP, Klein-Schwartz W. Octreotide's role in the management of sulfonylurea-induced hypoglycemia. Journal of Medical Toxicology 2010; 6(2):199–206. https://doi.org/10.1007/s13181-010-0064-z.

Fasano CJ, O'Malley G, Dominici P et al. Comparison of octreotide and standard therapy versus standard therapy alone for the treatment of sulfonylurea-induced hypoglycemia. Annals of Emergency Medicine 2008; 51:400–406.

Glatstein M, Scolnik D, Bentur Y. Octreotide for the treatment of sulfonylurea poisoning. Clinical Toxicology 2012; 50(9):795–804. doi:10.3109/15563650.2012.734626.

McLaughlin SA, Crandall CS, McKinney PE. Octreotide: an antidote for sulfonylurea induced hypoglycaemia. Annals of Emergency Medicine 2000; 36:133–138.

4.20 PENICILLAMINE

An oral chelating agent for a broad range of heavy metals. It is the agent of choice in very few scenarios due to a poor side-effect profile and the existence of better tolerated and more efficacious agents.

Presentations
Penicillamine 125 mg, 250 mg tablets (100)

TOXICOLOGICAL INDICATIONS
- Copper toxicity (Wilson's disease)

- Second-line drug for chelation of other heavy metals, including arsenic, iron, lead, mercury and zinc

CONTRAINDICATIONS
- Penicillin allergy
- Pregnancy
- Renal failure (unable to excrete chelates)

Mechanism of action
Penicillamine is an orally administered chelating agent. It is a penicillin derivative without antibiotic activity. It binds to heavy metals with varying degrees of efficacy. The penicillamine–metal chelate is soluble and eliminated by renal excretion.

Pharmacokinetics
Penicillamine is well absorbed following oral administration with peak concentrations occurring within hours. It is distributed throughout the body water. Elimination is urinary mainly as sulfide conjugates. Elimination half-life is up to 90 hours.

ADMINISTRATION
- Administer 4–7 mg/kg orally four times a day.
- Maximum adult daily dose is 2 g.
- Monitor closely for adverse effects:
  - Second weekly full blood count and urinalysis
  - Weekly urine and/or blood testing for target heavy metal.
- Commencing therapy in the lower dose range may minimise adverse effects.
- Duration of therapy depends upon ability to tolerate the antidote and the rate of elimination of the target metal. Months of therapy may be required.

THERAPEUTIC END POINTS
- Blood metal concentrations in desired range

ADVERSE DRUG REACTIONS AND THEIR MANAGEMENT
- Drug reactions are multiple and frequent, especially in the higher dose range. They are commonly responsible for cessation of therapy and include:
  - Cutaneous hypersensitivity: erythematous skin reactions
  - Systemic hypersensitivity: fever, proteinuria, haematuria, erythema multiforme
  - Haematological: bone marrow hypoplasia with varying degrees of thrombocytopenia, leucopenia and fatal agranulocytosis
  - Neurological: myasthenia gravis, peripheral neuropathy
  - Nephrotoxicity: nephrotic syndrome, glomerulonephritis
  - Other: Goodpasture's syndrome, hepatotoxicity, pancreatitis.
- Therapy should be ceased if significant cutaneous reactions, abnormal urinalysis or falling white cell or platelet counts occur.

SPECIFIC CONSIDERATIONS
Pregnancy: this drug is teratogenic and is avoided in pregnancy.
Paediatrics: dose as for adults. Lower doses will minimise adverse effects.

- Should only be prescribed by clinicians experienced with its use and adverse effects.

- Lower dose regimens may achieve comparable clinical efficacy with improved adverse effect profile.

References

Liebelt EL, Shannon MW. Oral chelators for childhood lead poisoning. Pediatric Annals 1994; 23(11):616–619, 623–626.

Shannon MW, Townsend MK. Adverse effects of reduced-dose D-penicillamine in children with mild-to-moderate lead poisoning. Annals of Pharmacotherapy 2000; 34(1):15–18.

4.21 PHYSOSTIGMINE

A competitive acetylcholinesterase inhibitor indicated for the treatment of central anticholinergic delirium. However, it is not readily available in Australia and New Zealand due to difficulties in acquisition.

Presentations

Physostigmine 1 mg/2 mL ampoules

TOXICOLOGICAL INDICATIONS
- Central antimuscarinic manifestations (agitated delirium) not easily controlled with benzodiazepine sedation
- Isolated anticholinergic agent poisoning (i.e. atropine, benztropine)

CONTRAINDICATIONS
- Bradydysrhythmias
- Intraventricular cardiac conduction block (QRS >100 ms)
- AV block
- Bronchospasm

Mechanism of action

Physostigmine is a carbamate with a tertiary amine structure. It produces reversible inhibition of acetylcholinesterase and accumulation of acetylcholine. The increased concentration of acetylcholine overcomes the postsynaptic muscarinic receptor blockade produced by anticholinergic agents.

Pharmacokinetics

Physostigmine is only given by titrated intravenous dosing due to poor oral bioavailability. Because of its tertiary amine structure (uncharged), it is able to cross the blood–brain barrier to exert its central effects. It is rapidly metabolised by cholinesterase, with an elimination half-life of about 20 minutes.

ADMINISTRATION
- The patient is managed in a monitored area where equipment, drugs and personnel are available to provide full resuscitative care.
- Confirm absence of conduction defects on 12-lead ECG.

- Administer 0.5–1 mg as a slow IV push over 5 minutes and repeat every 10 minutes until the desired clinical effect is observed.
- It is rare for a total dose of more than 2 mg to be required.
- The duration of action of physostigmine is short and anticholinergic delirium may recur within 2 hours. Further titrated doses of physostigmine may be required.

THERAPEUTIC END POINTS
- Resolution of delirium

ADVERSE DRUG REACTIONS AND THEIR MANAGEMENT
- Excessive doses of physostigmine produce clinical features of cholinergic stimulation including:
  - Seizures, usually seen following rapid administration
  - Bradycardia and variable degrees of heart block
  - Bronchospasm and bronchorrhoea
  - Nausea, vomiting and diarrhoea.
- The cholinergic manifestations of physostigmine overdose should be managed with good supportive care and, if necessary, administration of titrated doses of atropine until there is resolution of bradycardia and drying of respiratory secretions.
- Physostigmine may also prolong the effect of suxamethonium or inhibit the action of non-depolarising neuromuscular blockers.

SPECIFIC CONSIDERATIONS
Pregnancy: safety not established. Alternative agents should be considered.
Paediatric: initial paediatric dose is 0.02 mg/kg to a maximum of 0.5 mg.

HANDY TIPS
- Administration of physostigmine is particularly useful to confirm or exclude the diagnosis of anticholinergic delirium and avoid the need for further investigation to exclude alternative diagnoses.
  - The response to physostigmine administration can be immediate and dramatic, completely resolving the delirium and simplifying patient management.
- Although the duration of action of physostigmine is relatively short (about 2 hours), repeat doses are not always required after initial reversal of delirium.
- Use of physostigmine may prevent the need to administer large doses of benzodiazepine to the delirious patient and thus reduce the likelihood of excessive sedation and pulmonary aspiration.
- Do not give physostigmine as an intravenous infusion – it is likely to precipitate a cholinergic crisis.
- Neostigmine is not a substitute for physostigmine as it does not cross the blood–brain barrier.

PITFALL
- Inadequate or excessive doses of physostigmine. This can usually be avoided by careful titration of dose to clinical effect.

CONTROVERSIES

- Physostigmine fell out of favour in the treatment of anticholinergic poisoning in the 1970s following a number of reports of bradydysrhythmias and asystole in patients with pre-existing or drug-induced cardiac conduction abnormalities. The risk of such adverse effects is minimised by detailed evaluation of the ECG and careful dose titration.
- Other centrally acting cholinesterase inhibitors such as rivastigmine have been suggested as alternative agents in the treatment of anticholinergic delirium but are not available as IV formulations. Oral or transdermal administration have a much slower onset of action and clinical benefit is not well established.

References

Boley SP, Olives TD, Bangh SA et al. Physostigmine is superior to non-antidote therapy in the management of antimuscarinic delirium: a prospective study from a regional poison center. Clinical Toxicology 2019; 57(1):50–55. doi:10.1080/15563650.2018.1485154.

Burns MJ, Linden CH, Graudins A et al. A comparison of physostigmine and benzodiazepines for the treatment of anticholinergic poisoning. Annals of Emergency Medicine 2000; 35:374–381.

Dawson AH, Buckley NA. Pharmacological management of anticholinergic delirium – theory, evidence and practice. British Journal of Clinical Pharmacology 2016; 81(3):516–524. doi:10.1111/bcp.12839.

Suchard JR. Assessing physostigmine's contraindication in cyclic antidepressant ingestions. Journal of Emergency Medicine 2003; 25(2):185–191.

4.22 PRALIDOXIME

This is the agent available in Australasia to reactivate acetylcholinesterase enzymes following organophosphate poisoning.

Presentations

Pralidoxime iodide 500 mg/20 mL vials

TOXICOLOGICAL INDICATIONS

- Organophosphate (OP) poisoning
- Carbamate poisoning
  - Although not usually required for carbamates, it should not be withheld in severe poisoning or if there is any doubt regarding the nature of the agent.
- Nerve agent poisoning

CONTRAINDICATIONS

- Known hypersensitivity

Mechanism of action

Pralidoxime reactivates acetylcholinesterase that has been inhibited by binding to OP or carbamate pesticides. It is only effective if given before irreversible binding or 'ageing' takes place. Re-establishment of enzymatic function rapidly reverses the nicotinic and muscarinic effects of OP poisoning. Atropine is usually administered prior to pralidoxime and the effect at muscarinic receptors is synergistic, but atropine is not effective at nicotinic receptors. An improvement in muscle strength may be observed within 10–40 minutes of administration of pralidoxime.

Pharmacokinetics
Following IV administration, pralidoxime has a volume of distribution of 0.8 L/kg. Over 80% of an administered dose is excreted unchanged by the kidney, with an elimination half-life of 75 minutes. These volumes of distribution and elimination half-lives increase in poisoned patients and during continuous IV infusion. An infusion of 500 mg/hour achieves levels of >4 microgram/mL (postulated target concentration) within 15 minutes and maintains them for the duration of the infusion.

ADMINISTRATION
- The patient with confirmed organophosphate poisoning has a life-threatening illness and is managed in a critical care environment with full monitoring and resuscitation facilities available.
- Administer the initial dose of 2 g pralidoxime in 100 mL of normal saline IV over 15 minutes
  then
- Commence pralidoxime infusion at 500 mg/hour (pralidoxime 6 g in 500 mL of normal saline at 42 mL/hour).
- Higher infusion rates are rarely indicated but may be considered if clinical response is poor.
- The infusion may be discontinued after 24 hours provided the patient is clinically well; the time of cessation is within daylight hours and the patient remains under close observation for a further 24 hours. If clinical evidence of OP poisoning recurs, the infusion is recommenced for a further 24 hours.
- When facilities are available to perform rapid red cell anticholinesterase activity assays, these should be done before the infusion is ceased and then repeated after 4–6 hours. If activity is maintained, further administration of pralidoxime is unlikely to be required.

ADVERSE DRUG REACTIONS
- Usually minimal or mild.
- Non-specific adverse effects include nausea, headache, dizziness, drowsiness, blurred vision and hyperventilation.
- Rapid administration can cause tachycardia, laryngospasm, muscle rigidity, hypertension and transient neuromuscular blockade.

SPECIFIC CONSIDERATIONS
Pregnancy: safety not established. Administration should not be withheld if clinically indicated.
Paediatric: children are treated with an initial dose of 25–50 mg/kg followed by an infusion of 10–20 mg/kg/hour.

HANDY TIPS
- Administration beyond 24 hours after OP ingestion is unlikely to be effective, but a therapeutic trial may still be warranted.
- Poisoning from certain OPs may be less responsive to pralidoxime than others.

- Failure to administer an appropriate dose.
- Inadequate duration of treatment.
- Late initiation of treatment.

CONTROVERSIES
- The value of pralidoxime in improving clinical outcome from OP poisoning is disputed. Although pralidoxime has been shown to reactivate red cell acetylcholinesterase in OP-poisoned patients, it has not been shown to improve survival or reduce the need for intubation. Some clinical trials associate poorer clinical outcome with oxime therapy.
- Optimal dosing and duration of pralidoxime is not established and almost certainly varies with different OPs. It may be that currently recommended doses are not optimal and this may contribute to the poor response to oximes observed in clinical trials.
- The role of pralidoxime in carbamate poisoning.

References
Buckley NA, Eddleston M, Li Y et al. Oximes for acute organophosphate poisoning. Cochrane Database of Systematic Reviews 2011; 2.
Eddleston M, Eyer P, Worek F et al. Pralidoxime in acute organophosphorus insecticide poisoning – a randomised controlled trial. PLoS Medicine 2009; 6(6):e1000104 June.

4.23 PYRIDOXINE

Vitamin B6

Intravenous pyridoxine is used in high doses to treat the seizures and metabolic acidosis associated with isoniazid overdose and poisoning from other hydrazine compounds.

Presentations
Pyridoxine hydrochloride 50 mg/mL vials
Pyridoxine hydrochloride 250 mg/mL vials, obtained under the Special Access Scheme in Australia

TOXICOLOGICAL INDICATIONS
- Metabolic acidosis and seizures induced by hydrazine compounds (includes isoniazid, *Gyromitra* mushrooms and hydrazine, a component of jet and rocket fuels)
- Adjunct in the treatment of ethylene glycol toxicity

CONTRAINDICATIONS
- Known hypersensitivity

Mechanism of action
The active form of pyridoxine, pyridoxal 5-phosphate (P5P), is known as vitamin B6. It is an important cofactor in over 100 enzymatic reactions involving amino acid metabolism. P5P is an essential coenzyme in the conversion of L-glutamic acid to GABA. The hydrazines, including isoniazid, inhibit the formation of P5P, bind to and inactivate existing P5P and enhance elimination of P5P, thereby producing a state of GABA

depletion leading to CNS excitation and seizures. Large doses of pyridoxine overcome this inhibition and restore normal GABA concentration and activity.

Pharmacokinetics
Pyridoxine has an oral bioavailability of about 50% and a volume of distribution of 0.6 L/kg. It is rapidly metabolised at extrahepatic sites to the active phosphate ester and other compounds.

ADMINISTRATION
- The patient is managed in a monitored area where equipment, drugs and personnel are available to provide full resuscitative care.
- EEG monitoring is mandatory during pyridoxine administration if the patient is intubated and paralysed.
- Isoniazid overdose
  - Administer an initial dose of 1 g pyridoxine for each gram of isoniazid ingested up to a maximum dose of 5 g (70 mg/kg in children).
  - Give this dose as a slow IV infusion at 0.5 g/minute until seizures stop or infusion is complete. The remainder of the dose may then be infused over 4 hours.
  - If the ingested dose of isoniazid is unknown, give 5 g of pyridoxine empirically.
  - Benzodiazepines are given concomitantly as they have a synergistic effect in seizure management.
- Hydrazine or monomethylhydrazine poisoning
  - Administer an initial bolus of 25 mg/kg intravenously.
- Ethylene glycol poisoning
  - Give 50 mg IV every 6 hours.

THERAPEUTIC END POINTS
- Control of seizures

ADVERSE DRUG REACTIONS AND THEIR MANAGEMENT
- Chronic high oral pyridoxine dosing is associated with peripheral neuropathy, but this does not occur with acute dosing for isoniazid overdose.

SPECIFIC CONSIDERATIONS
Pregnancy: no restriction on use.
Paediatric: no restriction on use.

HANDY TIPS
- Pyridoxine is readily available only in 50 mg vials. Large numbers (100) of these will need to be procured to treat a single case of isoniazid poisoning. If the recommended dose cannot be immediately obtained, all available pyridoxine, together with high-dose benzodiazepines, should be administered as an interim measure.
- Always administer benzodiazepines in addition to pyridoxine because of the likely synergistic effect on seizure control.

PITFALL
- Failure to administer benzodiazepines concurrently.

CONTROVERSIES

- Human experience with pyridoxine in isoniazid poisoning is confined to case reports. It may be that severe isoniazid toxicity can be successfully managed using supportive care and high-dose benzodiazepine therapy alone.
- Utility of pyridoxine in ethylene glycol poisoning.

Reference

Lheureux P, Penaloza A, Gris M. Pyridoxine in clinical toxicology: a review. European Journal of Emergency Medicine 2005; 12:78–85.

4.24 SODIUM BICARBONATE

Sodium bicarbonate is used in clinical toxicology primarily as an antidote for agents causing sodium channel blockade and as an alkalinising agent to modify drug distribution and excretion.

Presentations

Sodium bicarbonate 8.4% 100 mmol/100 mL vial

TOXICOLOGICAL INDICATIONS

- Cardiotoxicity secondary to fast sodium channel blockade
  - Tricyclic antidepressants
  - Bupropion
  - Chloroquine/hydroxychloroquine
  - Dextropropoxyphene
  - Propranolol
  - Local anaesthetic agents
  - Flecainide, quinidine, quinine
- Prevention of redistribution of drug to the CNS
  - Severe salicylate poisoning
- Immediate correction of profound life-threatening metabolic acidosis
  - Toxic alcohol poisoning (ethylene glycol, methanol and other toxic alcohols)
  - Cyanide poisoning
  - Metformin-associated lactic acidosis
- Enhanced urinary drug elimination
  - Salicylate poisoning
  - Phenobarbitone poisoning
- Increased urinary solubility
  - Methotrexate toxicity
  - Drug-induced rhabdomyolysis

CONTRAINDICATIONS

- Acute pulmonary oedema
- Hypokalaemia
- Metabolic or respiratory alkalosis
- Severe hypernatraemia

Mechanism of action

Administration of intravenous hypertonic sodium bicarbonate provides a sodium component that increases extracellular sodium concentration and increases plasma bicarbonate concentration, raising serum pH. It also results in urinary bicarbonate excretion, increasing urinary pH. The mechanism by which sodium bicarbonate reverses sodium channel blockade is not fully understood. The increase in sodium concentration, the change in pH, or a combination of both may be responsible for this beneficial effect. Sodium bicarbonate modifies drug distribution and excretion by production of an alkaline pH in plasma or urine, thereby decreasing the toxicity of specific agents by preventing entry into cells.

These properties allow sodium bicarbonate to be used with benefit in a number of situations in clinical toxicology.

Elevation of serum pH
- Improved fast sodium channel function
  - A number of drugs cause cardiotoxicity by impairing sodium flux through the fast sodium channels of the cardiac conducting system during depolarisation.
  - Raising the serum pH improves fast sodium channel function and mitigates this toxic effect. Any increase from baseline pH is beneficial but the effect is maximal at pH 7.50–7.55.
  - The sodium load provided by sodium bicarbonate administration has a separate and additive positive effect on sodium channel function.
- Alteration of drug distribution
  - Elevation of serum pH can reduce the proportion of drug in uncharged form, reduce its ability to cross cell membranes and hence reduce the proportion of drug that distributes to tissue compartments (especially the CNS).
- Immediate correction of severe life-threatening metabolic acidosis
  - Profound metabolic acidosis has negative effects on cardiovascular function and may be life-threatening at pH approaching 6.7, irrespective of the underlying toxic cause.

Alkalinisation of urine
- 'Ion trapping' and enhanced urinary elimination
  - An alkaline urinary pH results in some drugs being predominantly in the charged form and unable to be reabsorbed across the tubular epithelium.
- Increased solubility
  - An alkaline urinary pH promotes water solubility of some drugs and of myoglobin, thus limiting tubular precipitation and secondary renal injury in addition to promoting urinary excretion.

Pharmacokinetics
Sodium bicarbonate ($NaHCO_3$) dissociates in water to provide sodium (Na^+) and bicarbonate (HCO_3^-) ions. Sodium is the principal cation in the extracellular fluid. Bicarbonate is a normal constituent of body fluids and plasma concentration is regulated. Under normal conditions, very little bicarbonate is excreted in the urine. Bicarbonate combines with hydrogen ions to form carbonic acid, which dissociates to form H_2O and CO_2.

Administration
Cardiotoxicity secondary to fast sodium channel blockade
- **Resuscitation from severe cardiotoxicity (cardiac arrest, ventricular dysrhythmias and hypotension)**
  - Sodium bicarbonate administration occurs in concert with advanced cardiac life support, including establishment of an airway, hyperventilation and administration of IV fluid boluses.

- Administer sodium bicarbonate 1–2 mmol/kg IV repeated every 1–2 minutes until:
  - restoration of perfusing rhythm
  - improvement in QRS widening
  - pH established at 7.5–7.55.
- Following clinical stabilisation, further administration of sodium bicarbonate is guided by repeated blood gas estimations.
- The QRS may not return to normal (<100 ms). However, this does not mandate ongoing sodium bicarbonate administration in the presence of haemodynamic stability and a pH maintained at 7.5–7.55 by hyperventilation.

- **Maintenance of serum alkalinisation in severe cardiotoxicity**
  - Should be considered following resuscitation in the presence of ongoing ventricular dysrhythmias, hypotension and a prolonged QRS if the pH is not maintained at 7.5–7.55 by hyperventilation alone.
  - Commence an infusion of 150 mmol sodium bicarbonate diluted in 850 mL 5% glucose at 250 mL/hour.
  - Check blood gases hourly and maintain serum pH in the range of 7.50–7.55.
  - Cease infusion following resolution of cardiovascular toxicity as determined by clinical and ECG criteria.
    - Note: In practice, it is far easier and safer, and of comparable efficacy, to maintain serum alkalinisation with hyperventilation in the intubated patient.

Prevention of redistribution of salicylate to CNS
- Serum alkalinisation is an immediate priority to prevent movement of salicylate into the CNS in severe salicylate poisoning.
- The pH should be maintained at 7.5–7.55 at all times.
- Administer IV sodium bicarbonate boluses 1–2 mmol/kg.
- Commence infusion of 150 mmol sodium bicarbonate in 850 mL 5% glucose at 250 mL/hour.
- Further IV boluses are determined by serial blood gases and clinical response.
- Serum alkalinisation is maintained until definitive care with haemodialysis.

Urinary alkalinisation
- Correct hypokalaemia if present (it is difficult to alkalinise the urine in the presence of systemic hypokalaemia).
- Give 1–2 mmol/kg sodium bicarbonate IV bolus.
- Commence infusion of 150 mmol sodium bicarbonate in 850 mL 5% glucose at 250 mL/hour.
- 20 mmol of KCl may be added to the infusion to maintain normokalaemia.
- Monitor serum pH, bicarbonate and potassium at least every 4 hours.
- Regularly dipstick urine and aim for urinary pH >7.5.
- Continue until clinical and laboratory evidence of toxicity is resolving.
  - Note: Sodium bicarbonate ($NaHCO_3$) should not be administered through an intravenous line running fluids containing calcium or magnesium.

ADVERSE DRUG REACTIONS
- Alkalosis (serum pH >7.6 is detrimental to cardiovascular function)
- Hypernatraemia and hyperosmolarity
- Fluid overload and acute pulmonary oedema
- Hypokalaemia
- Local tissue inflammation secondary to extravasation

SPECIFIC CONSIDERATIONS
Pregnancy: no restriction on use.
Lactation: no restriction on use.
Paediatric: in children, the dosing of sodium bicarbonate uses the same formulations as for adults, with the same endpoints of a serum pH of 7.5–7.55 and a urinary pH of >7.5.
- sodium bicarbonate IV bolus: 1–2 mmol/kg of sodium bicarbonate 8.4%.
- sodium bicarbonate infusion: 150 mmol sodium bicarbonate 8.4% in 850 mL 5% glucose administered at 1.5 times the hourly rate of maintenance fluids.

HANDY TIP
- Close clinical and biochemical monitoring is essential during sodium bicarbonate administration to prevent development of complications resulting from volume overload and osmotic shifts.

PITFALLS
- Inadequate doses of sodium bicarbonate during resuscitation of severe tricyclic antidepressant poisoning.
- Failure to correct hypokalaemia when attempting urinary alkalinisation.
- Failure to recognise and rapidly treat acidaemia in the patient with severe salicylate poisoning.
- Continued, excessive doses of IV sodium bicarbonate once the pH is established at 7.5–7.55, resulting in life-threatening alkalaemia, pulmonary oedema and cerebral oedema.

CONTROVERSIES
- Utility of and indications for urinary alkalinisation in toxic rhabdomyolysis.
- Relative efficacy of hyperventilation versus administration of sodium bicarbonate in the management of tricyclic antidepressant toxicity.
- Precise mechanism by which urinary alkalinisation enhances salicylate elimination.

References
Bradberry SM, Thanacoody HK, Watt BE et al. Management of the cardiovascular complications of tricyclic antidepressant poisoning: role of sodium bicarbonate. Toxicological Reviews 2005; 24(3):195–204.
Bruccoleri RE, Burns MM. A literature review of the use of sodium bicarbonate for the treatment of QRS widening. Journal of Medical Toxicology 2016; 12:121–129.
Proudfoot AT, Krenzelok EP, Brent J et al. Does urine alkalinization increase salicylate elimination? If so, why? Toxicological Reviews 2003; 22(3):129–136.

4.25 SODIUM CALCIUM EDETATE

Calcium disodium edetate, calcium disodium versenate, calcium disodium ethylenediaminetetraacetic acid (EDTA)

An intravenous heavy metal chelating agent primarily used in the treatment of severe lead poisoning, including lead encephalopathy.

Presentations
Sodium calcium edetate 1 g/5 mL ampoules

TOXICOLOGICAL INDICATIONS
- Lead encephalopathy
- Second-line chelating agent when DMSA or DMPS is either not available or not tolerated (see **Chapter 4.7: DMSA (succimer) and DMPS (unithiol)**)
- Other heavy metal poisoning (efficacy unknown)
  - **Note:** Based on historical evidence, the recommendation for treatment of severe lead encephalopathy is **combination therapy** with intramuscular dimercaprol (BAL) and sodium calcium edetate for two major reasons (see **Controversies**):
    - Concerns that sodium calcium edetate preferentially mobilises lead bone stores which could re-distribute to the CNS and transiently worsen encephalopathy.
    - The use of two chelating agents increases the rate of urinary excretion of lead.

CONTRAINDICATIONS
- Relative contraindication: anuric renal failure

Mechanism of action
Sodium calcium edetate binds to divalent and trivalent metals, the calcium component of sodium calcium edetate is displaced and a stable water-soluble metal complex is formed, which is readily excreted in the urine.

Pharmacokinetics
Absorption of sodium calcium edetate is incomplete following oral administration and this antidote is only administered by the intravenous route. The volume of distribution is small and approximates that of the extracellular fluid compartment. It is not metabolised and is renally excreted, with an elimination half-life of 20–60 minutes in the setting of normal renal function.

ADMINISTRATION
- **Lead encephalopathy**
  - Therapy is always commenced in an intensive care setting due to the severity of the underlying condition.
  - Commence dimercaprol (BAL) 3–4 mg/kg **4 hours** before commencing sodium calcium edetate and continue every 4 hours for 2–5 days based on clinical response (see **Chapter 4.6: Dimercaprol**).
  - Dilute sodium calcium edetate 50–75 mg/kg in 500 mL of normal saline or 5% glucose and infuse over 24 hours starting 4 hours after first dose of dimercaprol.

- **Lead poisoning *without* encephalopathy**
  - Oral DMSA is the preferred chelating agent for most clinical presentations (excluding severe lead encephalopathy).
  - Intravenous sodium calcium edetate can be used as a sole chelating agent in this setting if DMSA or DMPS are unavailable or not tolerated.
  - Dilute sodium calcium edetate 25–50 mg/kg in 500 mL of normal saline or 5% glucose and infuse over 24 hours.
- In the setting of encephalopathy, sodium calcium edetate (and dimercaprol) should be continued until the patient is clinically stable.
- Once clinically improved, chelation should be changed to oral DMSA.
- The optimal duration of chelation therapy is best determined by consideration of the individual patient's response, based on clinical features, improvement in blood lead levels and (ideally) assessment of urinary lead excretion. The minimum effective duration appears to be 5 days, but repeated courses may be indicated.

ADVERSE DRUG REACTIONS AND THEIR MANAGEMENT
- Local pain and thrombophlebitis due to rapid IV administration. Local phlebitis may be minimised by:
  - Infusing dilute solution
- General systemic
  - Malaise, fever, myalgia, headache, nausea and vomiting
  - Histamine-release reactions (anaphylactoid)
- Nephrotoxicity secondary to the dissociation of sodium calcium edetate–metal complexes in acidic urine. The risk of nephrotoxicity during therapy is reduced by:
  - Ensuring adequate hydration and urine flow of 1–2 mL/kg/hour
  - Limiting daily dose to 2 g (1 g in children)
  - Urinary alkalinisation is recommended prior to administration to minimise dissociation of sodium calcium edetate–metal complexes in acidic urine (see **Chapter 4.24: Sodium bicarbonate**).

SPECIFIC CONSIDERATIONS
Pregnancy: safety is not established. Administration should not be withheld if clinically indicated.
Paediatric: the doses of sodium calcium edetate are the same for children but may be diluted in a smaller volume of fluid. Oral DMSA is preferred as a chelation agent whenever possible.

HANDY TIP
- Sodium calcium edetate causes increased loss of other essential elements (zinc, copper, iron) compared to DMSA and DMPS.

PITFALLS
- Inadvertent or mistaken administration of dicobalt edetate, an antidote used in the treatment of cyanide poisoning.

- Use of disodium EDTA (a historical lead chelation agent), which can cause life-threatening hypocalcemia.

CONTROVERSY
- Based on historical evidence, the recommendation for treatment of severe lead encephalopathy is combination therapy with intramuscular dimercaprol (BAL) and sodium calcium edetate (due to concerns that sodium calcium edetate preferentially mobilises lead bone stores which could re-distribute to the CNS and transiently worsen encephalopathy). The relative efficacies and clinical benefits of the newer agents (DMSA or DMPS) as monotherapy in this setting have not been definitively studied, but case series suggest that the outcomes are similar and they may be appropriate alternative regimens (see **References**).

References
Alexander FW, Delves HT. Deaths from acute lead poisoning. Archives of Disease in Childhood 1972; 47:446–448.

Arnold J, Morgan B. Management of lead encephalopathy with DMSA after exposure to lead-contaminated moonshine. Journal of Medical Toxicology 2015; 11:464–467.

Bradberry S, Vale A. A comparison of sodium calcium edetate (edetate calcium disodium) and succimer (DMSA) in the treatment of inorganic lead poisoning. Clinical Toxicology 2009; 47:841–858.

4.26 SODIUM THIOSULFATE

Sodium thiosulfate enhances the endogenous cyanide detoxification capacity of the body. It is suitable to use alone in the treatment of mild to moderately severe cases of cyanide poisoning, but should be used in conjunction with other antidotes in severe cyanide toxicity.

Presentations
Sodium thiosulfate 12.5 g/50 mL vials

TOXICOLOGICAL INDICATIONS
- Reasonable suspicion of cyanide poisoning
- May also be useful in poisoning from other agents including:
    - chlorate
    - cisplatin
    - bromate
    - bromine
    - iodine
    - mustard gas
    - nitrogen mustard.

CONTRAINDICATIONS
- None: sodium thiosulfate has little toxicity at the recommended doses

Mechanism of action
The major route for detoxification of cyanide is by conversion to thiocyanate. This conversion is catalysed by the enzyme rhodanese. The capacity of rhodanese is limited by the availability of suitable sulfur donors. Sodium thiosulfate acts as a sulfur donor for

rhodanese and greatly enhances the endogenous cyanide elimination capacity of the body.

Pharmacokinetics

Thiosulfate is rapidly distributed throughout the extracellular space following intravenous injection. Distribution into the brain is limited. Most is eliminated unchanged by renal excretion, with an elimination half-life of 0.5–3 hours. A small amount is oxidised to sulfate via a two-step hepatic process.

ADMINISTRATION

- The patient is managed in a monitored area where equipment, drugs and personnel are available to provide full resuscitative care.
- Administer 12.5 g sodium thiosulfate (50 mL of 25% solution) IV over 10 minutes or 200 mg/kg IV over 10 minutes.
- Repeat after 30 minutes if clinical features of cyanide toxicity persist.

THERAPEUTIC END POINTS

- Improvement in conscious state
- Haemodynamic stability
- Improvement in metabolic acidosis

ADVERSE DRUG REACTIONS

- Adverse effects are mild and of minor importance compared with the risks associated with cyanide poisoning.
- Rapid injection may be associated with nausea and vomiting.
- Other minor adverse effects associated with thiocyanate production are hypotension, nausea, headache, abdominal pain and disorientation.

SPECIFIC CONSIDERATIONS

Pregnancy: safety is not established. Administration should not be withheld if clinically indicated.

Paediatric: the recommended dose of 400 mg/kg is relatively higher than for adults.

HANDY TIPS

- Collect blood for cyanide level before antidote administration.
- The combination of sodium thiosulfate, oxygen and supportive therapy is probably sufficient to treat mild to moderately severe cases of cyanide toxicity.
- Sodium thiosulfate is valuable in doubtful cases of poisoning, such as smoke inhalation, where it may have both therapeutic and diagnostic value.
- In severe poisoning, sodium thiosulfate should be given together with other antidotes, with which it acts synergistically.

CONTROVERSY

- There are no clinical trials that assess the efficacy of thiosulfate in humans. It has a relatively slow onset of action and should probably be regarded as a second-line antidote for acute cyanide poisoning.

References

Hall AH, Dart R, Bogdan G. Sodium thiosulfate or hydroxocobalamin for empiric treatment of cyanide poisoning? Annals of Emergency Medicine 2007; 49:806–813.

Reade MC, Davies SR, Morley PT et al. Review article: management of cyanide poisoning. Emergency Medicine Australasia 2012; 24:225–238.

4.27 VITAMIN K

Vitamin K_1, Phytomenadione, Phytonadione (alternative spelling)

Vitamin K_1 is an essential cofactor in the synthesis of clotting factors II, VII, IX and X. It is used for the reversal of coumarin-induced coagulopathy.

Presentations

Phytomenadione 2 mg/0.2 mL ampoules
Phytomenadione 10 mg/1 mL ampoules
Note: The injectable formulation of vitamin K is suitable for oral administration.

TOXICOLOGICAL INDICATIONS

- Significant coumarin-induced coagulopathy
  — Therapeutic over-warfarinisation
  — Intentional warfarin overdose
  — Ingestion of long-acting anticoagulant rodenticides (e.g. brodifacoum)

CONTRAINDICATIONS

- Known hypersensitivity

Mechanism of action

Phytomenadione is a synthetic fat-soluble analogue of naturally occurring vitamin K_1, an essential cofactor in the synthesis of clotting factors II, VII, IX and X. The coumarin anticoagulants inhibit vitamin K_1 2,3-epoxide reductase, thus preventing the formation of vitamin K hydroxyquinone, the active form of vitamin K. This leads to impaired formation of clotting factors. Administration of high doses of vitamin K overcomes this effect, restoring normal function of the reductase enzyme and allowing production of clotting factors.

Pharmacokinetics

Oral bioavailability is variable and dependent on bile salts but is usually about 50%. It is rapidly metabolised by the liver, with an elimination half-life of about 2 hours. The increase in blood coagulation factors occurs 3–6 hours after an IV dose and 6–12 hours after an oral dose. The short half-life of vitamin K compared to warfarin and long-acting anticoagulant rodenticides means that repeated doses will be required in the setting of large overdoses with established toxicity.

ADMINISTRATION

The administration and dosing of vitamin K is determined by the clinical scenario and requirement for ongoing anticoagulation with warfarin.

Therapeutic over-warfarinisation
- See **Chapter 3.81: Warfarin.**

Warfarin overdose
- No therapeutic requirement for warfarin anticoagulation (patient took someone else's warfarin)
    - Admit for serial INR measurements and titrated doses of vitamin K.
    - Consider treatment with large doses of vitamin K administered orally (e.g. 10 mg twice daily) without serial in-patient INR measurements. Follow-up INR is indicated at 48–72 hours (including at least one INR >12 hours post dosing with vitamin K) to ensure that coagulopathy has resolved.
- Therapeutic requirement for warfarin anticoagulation
    - The dose of vitamin K is guided by the risk assessment and the level of the INR (see **Chapter 3.81: Warfarin**).
    - In large overdoses (e.g. >100 mg), the dose of vitamin K required to reverse coagulopathy or maintain the INR in the therapeutic range is difficult to predict.
        - Early administration of a larger initial dose (e.g. 5–10 mg), or frequent smaller doses, are both reasonable approaches.
    - In all cases, 6-hourly INR monitoring is required to ensure that a severe coagulopathy does not develop.
    - At least one INR >12 hours post dosing with vitamin K is required to ensure that coagulopathy has resolved.

Ingestion of long-acting anticoagulant rodenticide
- Very large daily doses of oral vitamin K are required for a period of weeks to months if anticoagulation develops.
- Initial daily dose is variable and determined under close medical supervision with repeated INR estimations.
- Close medical supervision is also necessary during treatment to ensure compliance and safe cessation of vitamin K therapy.

ADVERSE DRUG REACTIONS AND THEIR MANAGEMENT
- Minor facial flushing, chest tightness, dyspnoea or dizziness with IV administration
- Anaphylaxis following IV administration (rare)
- Intramuscular administration is contraindicated in a coagulopathic patient due to the risk of haematoma formation.

SPECIFIC CONSIDERATIONS

Pregnancy: no restriction on use.

Paediatric: children who accidentally ingest >0.5 mg/kg of warfarin can safely be treated with vitamin K orally (e.g. 10 mg daily for 3 days) without documenting serial INRs, as the risk of developing severe coagulopathy will be very low with this intervention. This will allow early discharge and remove the requirement for serial INR assays. Follow-up INR can be performed >12 hours after the last dose of vitamin K to ensure that no coagulopathy is present if additional reassurance is required.

HANDY TIPS
- Administration of vitamin K may be required for several days in deliberate self-poisoning with warfarin as the half-life of warfarin is significantly longer than for vitamin K.

- The injectable formulation of vitamin K is suitable for oral administration.
- Single unintentional acute ingestion of an anticoagulant rodenticide by a child does not involve a sufficient dose to cause anticoagulation. Neither medical assessment nor vitamin K therapy is necessary.

PITFALLS

- Administration of excessive doses of vitamin K to patients with an ongoing requirement for anticoagulation may result in prolonged warfarin resistance. Alternative agents such as heparin or direct oral anticoagulants are indicated as interim or alternative therapies.
- Administration of vitamin K prior to demonstration of anticoagulant effect in adults who self-poison with long-acting anticoagulant rodenticides.

CONTROVERSY

- The threshold INR for vitamin K administration following therapeutic over-warfarinisation or warfarin overdose. A risk-benefit consideration of the severity of bleeding is appropriate to guide this decision (see **References** for Australasian and American guideline recommendations).

References

Bruno GR, Howland MA, McMeeking A et al. Long-acting anticoagulant overdose: brodifacoum kinetics and optimal vitamin K dosing. Annals of Emergency Medicine 2000; 36(3):262–267.

Dentali F, Ageno W, Crowther M. Treatment of coumarin-associated coagulopathy: a systematic review and proposed treatment algorithms. Journal of Thrombosis and Haemostasis 2006; 4:1853–1863.

Isbister GK, Hackett LP, Whyte IM. Intentional warfarin overdose. Therapeutic Drug Monitoring 2003; 25(6):715–722.

Tran HA, Chanial SD, Harper PL et al. An update of consensus guidelines for warfarin reversal. Medical Journal of Australia 2013; 198(4):1–7.

Witt DM, Nieuwlaat R, Clark NP et al. American Society of Hematology 2018 guidelines for management of venous thromboembolism: optimal management of anticoagulation therapy. Blood Advances 2018; 27(2):3257–3291.

CHAPTER 5
ENVENOMINGS

5.1 APPROACH TO SNAKEBITE

See also specific sections in **Chapter 5: Black snake, Brown snake, Death adder, Tiger snake group, Taipan, Sea snake.**

Definite or suspected snakebite is a regular presentation to emergency departments in most parts of Australia. However, few clinicians encounter enough cases to develop sufficient clinical experience to feel comfortable managing envenoming.

Snakebite is a time-critical emergency presentation and a simple, standardised approach is required to ensure that appropriate patient management occurs (see **Table 5.1.1**).

The clinical effects of the medically important Australian snakes are summarised in **Table 5.1.2**.

RISK ASSESSMENT

Once it is determined that snakebite is a possibility, the risk assessment is straightforward: there is a risk of life-threatening envenoming and a formal process must be completed to assess that possibility. However, in patients with objective clinical evidence of

TABLE 5.1.1   Treatment approach to snakebite
PRE-HOSPITAL

First aid
    Pressure bandage with immobilisation (PBI)
Determine if there is clinical evidence of envenoming
    Patients with objective evidence of envenoming require antivenom as early as possible
Transport
    The patient is transported as soon as possible to a hospital that meets all the following criteria:
        Doctor able to manage snakebite
        Laboratory facilities available at all hours
        Adequate antivenom for definitive treatment

HOSPITAL

Resuscitation
Determine if the patient is envenomed – assessment is performed serially over at least 12 hours and is based on:
    History
    Physical examination
    Laboratory investigations
Determine the type of antivenom required
    Geographical area (prevalent indigenous snakes)
    Clinical and laboratory features
Administer antivenom if indicated
Supportive treatment

TABLE 5.1.2 Clinical effects of Australian Elapidae snakes

Category (genus)	Venom-induced consumptive coagulopathy (VICC)	Anticoagulant coagulopathy	Neurotoxicity	Myotoxicity	Other effects
Brown (*Pseudonaja*)	Complete VICC in 80% Partial VICC in 20%	Not present	Rare and mild	Not present	Early collapse (33%) or cardiac arrest (5%) Systemic symptoms frequently absent* (50%) Thrombotic microangiopathy (15%)
Tiger group (*Notechis, Hoplocephalus, Austrelaps, Tropidechis* spp.)	Complete VICC in 80% Partial VICC in 20%	Not present	Common Onset over hours	Common Onset over hours	Systemic symptoms common* Thrombotic microangiopathy (5%)
Death adders (*Acanthophis*)	Not present	Not present	Common Onset over hours	Common and mild	Systemic symptoms common* Local bite site pain often present

Continued

TABLE 5.1.2 Clinical effects of Australian Elapidae snakes—cont'd

Category (genus)	Venom-induced consumptive coagulopathy (VICC)	Anticoagulant coagulopathy	Neurotoxicity	Myotoxicity	Other effects
Black snakes Mulga (Pseudechis australis) Red-bellied black snake (Pseudechis porphyriacus)	Not present	Common	Not present	Common Onset over hours	Systemic symptoms common* Bite site pain and swelling
Taipan (Oxyuranus)	Complete 50% Partial 50%	Not present	Common Rapid in onset	Common	Systemic symptoms common* Thrombotic microangiopathy (25%)
Sea snakes (Hydrophiidae)	Not present	Not present	Common	Common	Systemic symptoms common*

*Non-specific systemic symptoms: nausea, vomiting, abdominal pain, sweating, diarrhoea.

envenoming (e.g. definite history of a bite with collapse, or clinical evidence of bleeding or neurotoxicity), antivenom treatment is started immediately without waiting for confirmatory investigations.

It is not possible to exclude envenoming without laboratory investigations. Patients with no visible bite mark and who are asymptomatic may still be envenomed. As a result, and for valid reason, many patients each year who are not envenomed are transferred to larger centres for definitive assessment.

It is unusual that a snake is identified with sufficient reliability to preclude further observation or investigation, and there are numerous reports of misidentification of snakes leading to incorrect management decisions. The two venomous snakes that are most reliably identifiable are the death adder and the red-bellied black snake, due to their characteristic appearances.

PRE-HOSPITAL CARE
Resuscitation
In the pre-hospital setting, resuscitation of a snakebite victim is performed according to standard resuscitation guidelines while immediate transport to a medical facility occurs.

First aid
First aid is intended to prevent lymphatic spread of venom from the bite site and delay the onset of systemic effects until the patient is in a facility that can administer adequate doses of antivenom if required.
- Keep the patient as calm and still as possible.
- Do not attempt ineffective or harmful techniques such as tourniquets, ice, cutting, sucking or washing of the bite site.
- Apply a **pressure bandage with immobilisation (PBI)**:
    — broad (15 cm) elasticised pressure bandage over the entire limb starting distally and extending proximally. The pressure should be as for a sprained ankle, but not so tight as to compromise circulation
    — immobilisation of limb
    — immobilisation of the whole patient.
- If the bite is on the torso, apply local pressure over the site and immobilise the patient.
- PBI may be left on for many hours while subsequent management steps are completed. There are multiple reports of sudden deterioration upon removal of the bandage several hours after the bite.
- The PBI is not removed until:
    — the patient has been assessed in an appropriate hospital and there is no objective evidence of envenoming (normal initial physical examination and laboratory investigations)
    or
    — antivenom administration has commenced.

Transport
All patients should be transported to a hospital that meets the following criteria:

1 Doctor is willing to manage the patient.
2 Laboratory facilities are available at all hours.

3 Antivenom is available for definitive treatment of severe envenoming by all snakes indigenous to that geographical area.

If the initial receiving hospital does not meet these criteria, the patient is transferred or retrieved to a hospital that does.

If there is objective clinical evidence of envenoming, antivenom (available on-site or brought in by the retrieval service) is started immediately without waiting for confirmatory investigations.

HOSPITAL MANAGEMENT
Resuscitation
- Most patients presenting with a history of either definite or possible bite and do not require immediate resuscitation.
- Until early envenoming is excluded, patients should be assessed and managed in an area equipped for cardiorespiratory monitoring and resuscitation.
- Rarely, management of immediate threats to airway, breathing and circulation or control of seizures is required. Resuscitation proceeds along conventional lines as outlined in **Chapter 1.2**.
- Early life-threats associated with Australian terrestrial snake envenoming include:
  - cardiac arrest
  - sudden collapse (hypotension)
  - respiratory failure secondary to paralysis
  - seizures
  - uncontrolled haemorrhage secondary to severe venom-induced consumptive coagulopathy (VICC).

Determine whether the patient is envenomed
Seek objective evidence of envenoming based on history, physical examination and laboratory data (see **Table 5.1.3**). Serial physical examinations (looking for bleeding or neurotoxicity) and investigations (FBE, EUC, CK, INR, aPTT, fibrinogen and D-dimer) are performed until envenoming is diagnosed or at least 12 hours following bandage removal.

Point-of-care INR or D-dimer testing should never be used to diagnose envenoming as they are inaccurate and unvalidated in this setting.

Abnormalities on initial physical examination or laboratory studies consistent with snake envenoming prompt immediate antivenom therapy as outlined below.

If the patient remains clinically well and initial laboratory studies are normal, the PBI is removed. If there is sudden clinical deterioration, it is immediately reapplied, antivenom administered and laboratory studies repeated.

If there is no deterioration upon removal of the PBI, the patient is observed and physical examination and laboratory studies repeated serially at 1, 6 and 12 hours following bandage removal. If at any time clinical examination or laboratory results indicate envenoming, appropriate antivenom is administered.

If there is no evidence of envenoming at 12 hours after PBI removal, the patient can be discharged.

TABLE 5.1.3　Assessment of snakebite

History	Physical examination	Laboratory investigations
Geographical area of bite Appearance of snake (usually only useful for death adders and red-bellied black snakes) Anatomical site of bite Number of strikes Use of PBI Early symptoms (e.g. collapse, nausea, vomiting, bleeding, weakness) Pre-hospital course (e.g. hypotension, bleeding from IV sites, urine output)	Vital signs Mental status Evidence of bite (lack of evidence does not exclude envenoming) Lymphadenitis Evidence of abnormal bleeding (especially bite site, gingival margins) Evidence of symmetrical descending flaccid paralysis (ocular, small muscles of face and bulbar function affected first) Respiratory function (e.g. PEFR)	Coagulation profile (INR and aPTT essential; fibrinogen and D-dimer desirable) Full blood count Creatine kinase (CK) Renal function Urinalysis (haematuria/ myoglobinuria) Lactate dehydrogenase (LDH)

Note: Point-of-care INR and D-dimer are inaccurate in VICC and should never be used.

Determine the type of monovalent antivenom required

Monovalent antivenom is recommended in preference to polyvalent antivenom as it is more specific, cheaper and safer to administer – particularly for lower volume antivenoms such as brown and tiger.

Polyvalent antivenom contains the equivalent of 1 ampoule of each terrestrial monovalent antivenom. It has larger volume and is associated with an increased risk of anaphylaxis. It is used to treat black snake, death adder or taipan envenoming where the specific monovalent antivenom is not readily available.

The choice of monovalent antivenom is based upon:
- knowledge of snakes found in the area
- clinical presentation and laboratory abnormalities.

Snake identification may be useful in select cases. This should only be performed by an expert herpetologist.

The snake venom detection kit is no longer recommended for the assessment of snake bite in Australia as it is inaccurate and unreliable.

In many regions, particularly in the south-west and south-east parts of Australia, 1 vial each of brown snake and tiger snake monovalent antivenom will cover the clinically important snakes based on the clinical envenoming syndrome, particularly in the presence of VICC. In areas where taipan, tiger and brown snakes co-exist, patients with VICC are treated with 1 ampoule of polyvalent antivenom.

Administer antivenom
- One vial of the relevant snake monovalent antivenom is sufficient for the majority of snake envenomings, in both adults and children. It is given by intravenous infusion diluted in normal saline.
- The use of more than 1 vial or repeat dose of antivenom should be considered, particularly in the setting of a critically unwell patient or one with rapidly progressive toxicity (e.g. neurotoxicity or myotoxicity).
- Further details on specific monovalent antivenoms and their administration are available in **Chapter 6**.
- The treating doctor administering antivenom must be prepared to manage anaphylaxis (see **Chapter 6.12: Allergic reactions to antivenom**).
- Premedication with adrenaline or antihistamines is not routinely indicated for Australian antivenoms.
- Following the administration of antivenom, the patient's clinical status is monitored and laboratory investigations repeated after 6 and 12 hours and until normalised.
- Even with adequate antivenom administration, it may take from 10 to 20 hours for coagulation studies to begin to improve in patients with VICC and up to 36 hours to return to normal. Resolution of VICC is dependent on synthesis of new clotting factors and administration of further doses of antivenom does not assist this process.

Supportive therapy
General wound care and administration of tetanus prophylaxis may be required.

The benefit of clotting factor replacement in treating VICC is controversial and definitive data are not available. It is reasonable to administer fresh frozen plasma (FFP) following antivenom administration to patients who have active and potentially life-threatening bleeding. Blood products hasten the recovery of INR in some patients but will prolong coagulopathy in others, especially when given early. Their administration is not associated with earlier discharge from hospital.

Complications of snakebite such as neuromuscular paralysis, myotoxicity or thrombotic microangiopathy with acute renal failure require ongoing appropriate supportive care in a high-dependency or intensive care unit in a tertiary hospital.

Serum sickness is unlikely after administration of 1 or 2 ampoules of monovalent antivenom. Prednisolone 25–50 mg/day (1 mg/kg/day for children) for 5 days is indicated if serum sickness develops.

References
Isbister GK, Brown SGA, McCoubrie DL et al. Snakebite in Australia: a practical approach to diagnosis and treatment. Medical Journal of Australia 2013; 199:763–768.
Ryan N, Renai T, Kearney RT et al. Incidence of serum sickness after the administration of Australian snake antivenom (ASP-22). Clinical Toxicology 2016; 54(1):27–33. doi: 10.3109/15563650.2015.1101771.

5.2 BLACK SNAKE

There are many species of black snake found throughout Australia, but the majority of bites occur from:

- *Pseudechis australis*: mulga or 'king brown' snake.
- *Pseudechis porphyriacus*: red-bellied black snake.

Mulga snakes are large, aggressive snakes found throughout inland and northern Australia. They usually inflict a large, painful bite and have the largest venom yield of any Australian snake. Red-bellied black snakes are found throughout the south-eastern coastal and mountainous areas, and the envenoming syndrome is usually less severe than from the mulga.

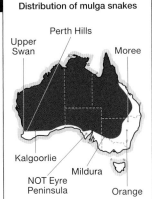

Distribution of mulga snakes

Perth Hills
Upper Swan
Moree
Kalgoorlie
Mildura
NOT Eyre Peninsula
Orange

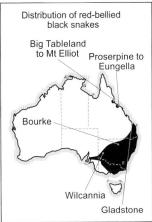

Distribution of red-bellied black snakes

Big Tableland to Mt Elliot
Proserpine to Eungella
Bourke
Wilcannia
Gladstone

TOXINS

Mulga snake venom contains potent myotoxins and less clinically relevant haemotoxins and neurotoxins. The anticoagulant toxins have a mild heparin-like effect and do not cause severe procoagulant defibrination.

Red-bellied black snake venom has similar toxins but the clinical effects are generally less severe.

CLINICAL PRESENTATION AND COURSE
Mulga snake

- The bite is characteristically large and painful, with significant local tissue swelling and possible necrosis. Regional lymphadenitis may occur.
- Systemic features including headache, abdominal pain, nausea or vomiting are prominent and occur in almost all envenomed patients soon after the bite.
- Myotoxicity is common and may progress to severe rhabdomyolysis.
- Anticoagulant coagulopathy is mild and clinically significant bleeding does not occur.
- Acute haemolysis may occur and result in anaemia, although rarely of sufficient magnitude as to require a blood transfusion.
- Long-term neurological effects such as anosmia or numbness, paraesthesia and pain in the region of the bite site are reported.

Red-bellied black snakes
- Envenoming by the red-bellied black snake is usually associated with local pain and systemic symptoms including nausea, vomiting and abdominal pain.
- Myotoxicity occurs, but severe rhabdomyolysis is generally less common than following mulga envenoming.
- Anticoagulant coagulopathy is mild and clinically significant bleeding does not occur.
- Persistent clinical features of anosmia or regional bite-site neurological symptoms can also occur.

MANAGEMENT

See **Chapter 5.1: Approach to snakebite** for a guide to the principles of snakebite management.

Pre-hospital
- Apply a pressure bandage with immobilisation (PBI).
- Transport to a hospital capable of providing definitive care.

Hospital
Resuscitation and supportive care
- Black snake envenoming is rarely an immediate life-threatening emergency. However, patients should be managed in an area capable of cardiorespiratory monitoring and resuscitation.

Antivenom
Mulga snake
- Black snake monovalent antivenom or polyvalent antivenom (see **Chapters 6.1** and **6.7**) can be used to treat envenoming by mulga snakes.
- The majority of mulga snake envenomings can safely be treated with 1 ampoule of black snake monovalent antivenom.
- If black snake antivenom is not available, 1 ampoule of polyvalent antivenom is indicated.
- Administration of antivenom is indicated for patients with any of the following features:
  - systemic symptoms of envenoming
  - laboratory evidence of anticoagulant coagulopathy
  - laboratory evidence of myotoxicity.

Red-bellied black snake
- Tiger snake monovalent antivenom (see **Chapter 6.4**) is used to treat envenoming by red-bellied black snakes.
- Administration of 1 ampoule of tiger antivenom is indicated for patients with any of the following features:
  - systemic symptoms of envenoming
  - laboratory evidence of anticoagulant coagulopathy
  - laboratory evidence of myotoxicity.

INVESTIGATIONS
- The diagnosis of envenoming is based on the combination of history, clinical features and laboratory data.
- Serial laboratory investigations following snakebite include: FBC, EUC, CK and coagulation profile (INR, aPTT, fibrinogen, D-dimer) at presentation and at intervals thereafter (see **Chapter 5.1: Approach to snakebite**).

- The CK rise in myotoxicity is variable and may be prolonged over several days. Severe envenomings can lead to CK levels >100 000, resulting in renal impairment.
- The anticoagulant coagulopathy of black snake envenoming is characterised by:
  - elevated aPTT and INR (usually mild)
  - normal fibrinogen
  - normal D-dimer and fibrin degradation products
  - normal platelet count.

DIFFERENTIAL DIAGNOSIS
- Myotoxicity occurs in taipan, death adder and tiger snake envenoming.

DISPOSITION AND FOLLOW-UP
- All patients must be assessed in a hospital capable of providing definitive care (see **Chapter 5.1: Approach to snakebite**).
- Envenoming is excluded if patients are clinically well with no features of neurotoxicity and normal laboratory parameters at least 12 hours after the bite (and preferably 12 hours after the PBI removal). Discharge should not occur at night.
- Envenomed patients may be discharged following antivenom administration if they are clinically well and the relevant laboratory abnormalities are resolving on serial measurements:
  - resolving anticoagulant coagulopathy
  - decreasing CK
  - normal renal function.

HANDY TIPS
- The mulga snake is sometimes referred to as the 'king brown' snake, leading to confusion regarding the genus of snake and administration of incorrect antivenom.
- Envenoming by the red-bellied black snake is frequently mild and unlikely to be life-threatening, and antivenom may not be required. It is reasonable to consider the risk–benefit analysis prior to administration, particularly if the patient is a snake-handler or at increased risk of anaphylaxis to antivenom.
- A bite from an Australian snake associated with local pain, headache, nausea and vomiting, and a mild anticoagulant coagulopathy is consistent with black snake envenoming.
- The characteristic markings of the red-bellied black snake make visual identification more reliable than for most other terrestrial snakes.

PITFALLS
- Failure to consider that snakebite has occurred.
- Failure to follow the recommended approach for evaluation of snakebite.

CONTROVERSY
- Early administration of antivenom is recommended to limit the severity of myotoxicity. It is not known whether late antivenom

administration alters the clinical course, but antivenom should not be withheld in the setting of significant myotoxicity.

References

Churchman A, O'Leary MA, Buckley NA et al. Clinical effects of red-bellied black snake (*Pseudechis porphyriacus*) envenoming and correlation with venom concentrations: Australian Snakebite Project (ASP-11). Medical Journal of Australia 2010; 193:696–700.

Currie BJ. Snakebite in tropical Australia: a prospective study in the 'Top End' of the Northern Territory. Medical Journal of Australia 2004; 181:693–697.

Johnston CI, Brown SGA, O'Leary MA et al. Mulga snake (*Pseudechis australis*) envenoming: a spectrum of myotoxicity, anticoagulant coagulopathy, haemolysis and the role of early antivenom therapy – Australian Snakebite Project (ASP-19). Clinical Toxicology 2013; 51:417–424.

5.3 BROWN SNAKE

Distribution of brown snakes

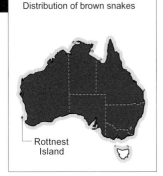

There are many species of brown snakes found throughout Australia, but the most commonly encountered are:
- *Pseudonaja affinis*: dugite
- *Pseudonaja mengdeni*: western brown snake or gwardar
- *Pseudonaja textilis*: eastern brown snake.

Brown snakes are the most common cause of death from snakebite in Australia. The most important manifestation of envenoming is venom-induced consumptive coagulopathy (VICC).

Rottnest Island

TOXINS

The venom contains potent procoagulants, cardiotoxins and a neurotoxin (textilotoxin).

CLINICAL PRESENTATION AND COURSE
- Envenomed patients may present completely asymptomatic with no obvious bite marks.
- Non-specific systemic features of envenoming include headache, nausea, vomiting and abdominal pain.
- The first sign of envenoming may be pre-syncope or sudden collapse.
- Early death from cardiac arrest can occur, secondary to direct cardiotoxicity or vasodilatation.
- The hallmark of brown snake envenoming is VICC. This can develop rapidly after the bite and may be complete or partial. The clinical features of coagulopathy can range from persistent bleeding at venesection sites or gingival margins to catastrophic intracerebral haemorrhage. Partial VICC occurs in about 20% of envenomings and is less likely to cause clinically significant bleeding.

- Thrombotic microangiopathy, characterised by thrombocytopenia, microangiopathic haemolytic anaemia (MAHA) and acute renal failure, occurs in about 15% of brown snake envenomings. Oliguria may be present from the time of envenoming.
- Neurotoxicity is rare, despite the presence of a potent neurotoxin in the venom. Mild diplopia and ptosis are observed occasionally.
- Myotoxicity does not occur.

MANAGEMENT

See **Chapter 5.1: Approach to snakebite** for a guide to the principles of snakebite management.

Pre-hospital
- Apply a pressure bandage with immobilisation (PBI).
- Transport to a hospital capable of providing definitive care.

Hospital
Resuscitation and supportive care
- Brown snake envenoming is a potentially life-threatening emergency and patients should be managed in an area capable of cardiorespiratory monitoring and resuscitation.
- Early life-threats that require immediate intervention include:
  - cardiovascular collapse (hypotension, cardiac arrest)
  - VICC with uncontrolled haemorrhage.
- In cardiac arrest secondary to brown snake envenoming, undiluted antivenom administered as a rapid IV push is indicated in addition to standard cardiopulmonary resuscitation.
- For life-threatening haemorrhage, clotting factor replacement fresh frozen plasma (FFP) is required once adequate antivenom has been given.
- In the absence of severe haemorrhage, administration of FFP, particularly within 6 hours of envenoming, may worsen coagulopathy and is not routinely indicated.

Antivenom
- The majority of brown snake envenomings can safely be treated with 1 ampoule of brown snake antivenom. However, in patients with severe envenoming syndromes or rapidly progressive complications, a second ampoule of brown antivenom may be indicated.

INVESTIGATIONS
- The diagnosis of envenoming is based on the combination of history, clinical features and laboratory data.
- Envenoming is diagnosed if there is a history of collapse, objective clinical evidence of VICC or laboratory abnormalities consistent with brown snake envenoming during 12 hours of observation.
- Serial laboratory investigations following snakebite include: FBC, EUC, CK and coagulation profile (INR, aPTT, fibrinogen, D-dimer) at presentation and at intervals thereafter (see **Chapter 5.1: Approach to snakebite**).
- Complete VICC is defined as:
  - elevated INR (at least >3 but usually unrecordable)
  - undetectable fibrinogen
  - markedly elevated D-dimer.

- Partial VICC is defined as:
  - INR abnormal but <3
  - low but detectable fibrinogen
  - elevated D-dimer.
- Recovery from VICC (INR returning to <2) usually occurs between 10 and 20 hours after the bite.
- Thrombocytopenia may develop.
- Monitor for deteriorating renal function and evidence of MAHA, indicated by raised lactate dehydrogenase (LDH) and fragmented red blood cells on blood film.

DIFFERENTIAL DIAGNOSIS

- Tiger snake and brown snake envenoming may be indistinguishable early in the course as both feature VICC and may present with early collapse. However, in tiger snake envenoming, evidence of neurotoxicity and myotoxicity may develop over the ensuing hours.
- Taipan envenoming also features VICC but it is usually associated with early neurotoxicity and myotoxicity.
- Black snake envenoming is associated with a mild anticoagulant coagulopathy, normal fibrinogen levels and myotoxicity.

DISPOSITION AND FOLLOW-UP

- All patients must be admitted for assessment in a hospital capable of providing definitive care (see **Chapter 5.1: Approach to snakebite**).
- Envenoming is excluded if patients are clinically well with no features of neurotoxicity and normal laboratory parameters at least 12 hours after the bite (and preferably 12 hours after the PBI removal). Discharge should not occur at night.
- Envenomed patients may be discharged following antivenom administration if they are clinically well and the relevant laboratory parameters are resolving on serial measurements:
  - INR <2
  - no evidence of thrombotic microangiopathy (haemoglobin, platelets, creatinine).
- Patients who develop thrombotic microangiopathy require a more prolonged admission for management of acute renal failure and MAHA. Dialysis may be required for standard indications.

HANDY TIPS

- A significant proportion of patients bitten by brown snakes do not become envenomed.
- In the early stages, brown snake envenoming may be indistinguishable from tiger snake envenoming.
- Early collapse after a brown snakebite is strongly suggestive of envenoming.
- Point-of-care INR and D-dimer testing should never be used in suspected snakebite cases as the tests are inaccurate and unvalidated in this setting.

PITFALLS

- Failure to consider that snakebite has occurred.
- Failure to follow the recommended approach for evaluation of snakebite.

CONTROVERSIES

- Published data indicate that administration of antivenom does not hasten recovery from VICC. However, it may reverse or prevent other manifestations of envenoming.
- Administration of clotting factors (FFP or cryoprecipitate) after antivenom administration is associated with earlier recovery from VICC but not with earlier discharge from hospital.
- The efficacy, safety and indications for clotting factor replacement after venom neutralisation in VICC are not yet well defined.
- Plasmapheresis has been used to treat thrombotic microangiopathy but its role remains undefined.

References

Allen GE, Brown SCA, Buckley NA et al. Clinical effects and antivenom dosing in brown snake (*Pseudonaja* spp.) envenoming – Australian Snakebite Project (ASP-14). PLoS ONE 2012; 7(12):e53188.

Brown SG, Caruso N, Borland M et al. Clotting factor replacement and recovery from snake venom-induced consumptive coagulopathy. Intensive Care Medicine 2009; 35(9):1532–1538.

Isbister GK, Buckley NA, Page CB et al. A randomized controlled trial of fresh frozen plasma for treating venom-induced consumption coagulopathy in cases of Australian snakebite (ASP-18). Journal of Thrombosis and Haemostasis 2013; 11:1310–1318.

Isbister GK, Duffull SB, Brown SGA. Failure of antivenom to improve recovery in Australian snakebite coagulopathy. Quarterly Journal of Medicine 2009; 102(8):563–568.

Isbister GK, Little M, Cull G et al. Thrombotic microangiopathy from Australian brown snake (*Pseudonaja*) envenoming. Internal Medicine Journal 2007; 37(8):523–528.

Sutherland SK, Tibballs J. Australian animal toxins: the creatures, their toxins and care of the poisoned patient. South Melbourne: Oxford University Press; 2001.

5.4 DEATH ADDER

There are several species of death adder (*Acanthophis* spp.) found throughout mainland Australia (excluding southern regions) and Papua New Guinea. The most common is:

- *Acanthophis antarcticus*: common death adder.

Death adders are found throughout most of mainland Australia and Papua New Guinea, but cases of envenoming are rare.

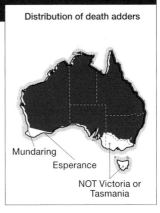

Distribution of death adders

Mundaring
Esperance

NOT Victoria or Tasmania

TOXINS

The venom contains a number of pre-synaptic and post-synaptic neurotoxins. Venom components identified in some species include myotoxins, pro-coagulants and anticoagulants.

- The bite site is usually painful, with evidence of tissue swelling and bruising.
- Systemic envenoming is characterised by a progressive symmetrical descending flaccid paralysis, which usually manifests within 6 hours.
  - Early signs include ptosis, blurred vision, diplopia and difficulty swallowing.
  - In more severe cases, there is progression to generalised paralysis and respiratory failure requiring intubation and ventilation.
- Non-specific symptoms, principally nausea and vomiting, are common.
- Myotoxicity can occur but is not usually severe.

MANAGEMENT

See **Chapter 5.1: Approach to snakebite** for a general guide to the principles of snakebite management.

Pre-hospital
- Apply a pressure bandage with immobilisation (PBI).
- Transport to a hospital capable of providing definitive care.

Hospital
Resuscitation and supportive care
- Death adder envenoming is a potentially life-threatening emergency and patients are managed in an area capable of cardiorespiratory monitoring and resuscitation.
- Early life-threats that require immediate intervention include:
  - descending flaccid paralysis with respiratory failure.
- If respiratory failure is present and antivenom is not available, intubation and ventilation are life-saving.

Antivenom
- Death adder antivenom (see **Chapter 6.3**) is the specific treatment for envenoming. Systemic envenoming, with objective evidence of paralysis, is treated with a dose of 1 ampoule.

INVESTIGATIONS
- The diagnosis of envenoming is based on the correlation of history, clinical features and laboratory data.
- Serial laboratory investigations following snakebite include: FBC, EUC, CK and coagulation profile (INR, aPTT, fibrinogen, D-dimer) at presentation and at intervals thereafter (see **Chapter 5.1: Approach to snakebite**). These investigations are usually normal in death adder envenoming.
- Spirometry or peak flow measurements provide a surrogate method of monitoring respiratory muscle strength and respiratory function.

DIFFERENTIAL DIAGNOSIS
- Envenoming by taipan and tiger snakes causes neurotoxicity. However, envenoming by these snakes is also associated with venom-induced consumptive coagulopathy (VICC).

DISPOSITION AND FOLLOW-UP
- All patients must be admitted for observation to a hospital capable of providing definitive care (see **Chapter 5.1: Approach to snakebite**).
- Severe paralysis requiring intubation and ventilation usually resolves over several days.
- Envenomed patients may be discharged following antivenom administration if they are clinically well with resolution of neurotoxicity and the relevant laboratory parameters are improving on serial measurements:
  - decreasing CK.

HANDY TIPS
- Death adders are nocturnal ambush predators. A common scenario is that the victim is bitten on the lower limb after treading on the snake while walking outside at night. The victim may feel little more than a sting and not see the snake.
- A painful bite site associated with a symmetrical descending flaccid paralysis, but normal blood tests, is characteristic of death adder envenoming.
- Basic resuscitation with maintenance of airway and breathing is life-saving.
- The characteristic appearance of the death adder (diamond-shaped head, tapering tail) makes visual identification more reliable than for most other terrestrial snakes.

PITFALLS
- Failure to consider that snakebite has occurred.
- Failure to follow the recommended approach for evaluation of snakebite.
- Failure to recognise the clinical signs of early neurotoxicity.

CONTROVERSY
- Early administration of antivenom is recommended to prevent the progression of paralysis. It is not known whether late antivenom administration alters the clinical course, but antivenom should not be withheld in the presence of neurotoxicity.

References
Currie BJ. Snakebite in tropical Australia: a prospective study in the 'Top End' of the Northern Territory. Medical Journal of Australia 2004; 181:693–697.

Johnston CI, O'Leary MA, Brown SCA et al. Death adder envenoming causes neurotoxicity not reversed by antivenom – Australian Snakebite Project (ASP-16). PLoS Neglected Tropical Diseases 2012; 6(9):e1841.

Lalloo DG, Trevett AJ, Black J et al. Neurotoxicity, anticoagulant activity and evidence of rhabdomyolysis in patients bitten by death adders (*Acanthophis* sp.) in southern Papua New Guinea. Quarterly Journal of Medicine 1996; 89:25–35.

5.5 TIGER SNAKE GROUP

Distribution of tiger snakes

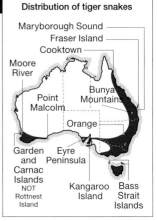

A number of venomous snakes are included within the tiger snake group due to similarities in their envenoming syndromes and management.

Recent re-classification of tiger snakes has shown a single, genetically similar, wide-ranging species (*Notechis scutatus*) across southern Australia (including Tasmania and Western Australia); however, older classifications (eastern or western tiger snake) are still commonly used.

Other genera included here are:
- *Austrelaps* spp.: copperhead snake
- *Hoplocephalus* spp.: pale-headed, broad-headed, Stephen's banded snakes
- *Tropidechis carinatus*: rough-scaled snake.

Tiger snakes (*Notechis scutatus*) are widely distributed within two broad areas – south-eastern (including Tasmania) and south-western Australia. They co-exist with brown snakes in most areas and early clinical features of envenoming are similar. The other genera mentioned inhabit smaller geographical regions in south-eastern Australia and are less commonly encountered.

TOXINS

Tiger snake venom contains pre- and post-synaptic neurotoxins, procoagulants and myotoxins. Envenoming is classically associated with a venom-induced consumptive coagulopathy (VICC), myotoxicity and neurotoxicity.

CLINICAL PRESENTATION AND COURSE

- Systemic envenoming may be heralded by sudden collapse and early death secondary to cardiac arrest.
- Local pain occurs in most cases of envenoming and associated bruising or swelling may be evident.
- Non-specific systemic features of envenoming occur in a majority of patients and include headache, nausea, vomiting and abdominal pain. These symptoms are usually present early in the clinical course.
- VICC occurs rapidly and in almost all cases of envenoming by tiger snakes, and can be complete or partial. The clinical features of coagulopathy can range from persistent bleeding at venesection sites or gingival margins to catastrophic intracerebral haemorrhage. Partial VICC is less likely to cause clinically significant bleeding.
- Neurotoxicity develops in a quarter of envenomings and is a symmetrical descending flaccid paralysis. Characteristic clinical signs of diplopia, ptosis and blurred vision can occur early and

may progress over several hours to bulbar and respiratory weakness requiring intubation and ventilation.

- Myotoxicity develops in a third of patients. Rhabdomyolysis may be severe and lead to significant renal impairment.
- Thrombotic microangiopathy, characterised by thrombocytopenia, microangiopathic haemolytic anaemia (MAHA) and acute renal failure, is reported, but less commonly than with brown snake envenoming.
- Envenoming by the rough-scaled snake is similar to that of tiger snakes.
- Copperhead snakes have neurotoxins and myotoxins, but envenoming is usually mild and coagulopathy uncommon.
- *Hoplocephalus* species produce VICC but not significant paralysis or myotoxicity.

MANAGEMENT

See **Chapter 5.1: Approach to snakebite** for a guide to the principles of snakebite management.

Pre-hospital
- Apply a pressure bandage with immobilisation (PBI).
- Maintenance of an airway and ventilatory support may be life-saving in the pre-hospital setting.
- Transport to a hospital capable of providing definitive care.

Hospital
Resuscitation and supportive care
- Tiger snake envenoming is a potentially life-threatening emergency and patients are managed in an area capable of cardiorespiratory monitoring and resuscitation.
- Early life-threats that require immediate intervention include:
  — cardiovascular collapse (hypotension, cardiac arrest)
  — VICC with uncontrolled haemorrhage
  — paralysis with respiratory failure.
- In cardiac arrest secondary to tiger snake envenoming, undiluted antivenom administered as a rapid IV push is indicated in addition to standard cardiopulmonary resuscitation.
- For life-threatening haemorrhage, clotting factor replacement with fresh frozen plasma (FFP) is required once adequate antivenom has been given.
- In the absence of severe haemorrhage, administration of FFP, particularly within 6 hours of envenoming, may worsen coagulopathy and is not routinely indicated.
- Clinical evidence of neurotoxicity is an indication for antivenom. Tiger snake antivenom does not reverse established paralysis but likely halts progression.

Antivenom
- The majority of tiger snake envenomings can safely be treated with 1 ampoule of tiger snake antivenom. However, in patients with severe envenoming syndromes or rapidly progressive complications, a second ampoule of tiger antivenom is required.
- Note: Tiger snake and brown snake envenoming may have similar clinical presentations as both can cause cardiovascular collapse

or VICC. Administration of 1 ampoule each of both tiger and
brown snake antivenom is recommended in this setting.
- In areas where tiger, brown and taipan co-exist, patients with
VICC are treated with 1 ampoule of polyvalent antivenom to cover
all possibilities.

INVESTIGATIONS
- The diagnosis of tiger snake envenoming is based on the
combination of history, geographical location, clinical features and
laboratory data.
- Envenoming is diagnosed if there is a history of collapse,
objective clinical evidence of coagulopathy or neurotoxicity, or
laboratory abnormalities consistent with tiger snake envenoming
during 12 hours of observation.
- Serial laboratory investigations following snakebite include: FBC,
EUC, CK and coagulation profile (INR, aPTT, fibrinogen, D-dimer)
at presentation and at intervals thereafter (see **Chapter 5.1:
Approach to snakebite**).
- Complete VICC is defined as:
  - elevated INR (at least >3 but usually unrecordable)
  - undetectable fibrinogen
  - markedly elevated D-dimer.
- Partial VICC is defined as:
  - INR abnormal but <3
  - low but detectable fibrinogen
  - elevated D-dimer.
- Recovery from VICC (INR returning to <2) usually occurs between
10 and 20 hours after the bite.
- The D-dimer will remain elevated for several days, and as such, is
not a useful marker of recovery.

DIFFERENTIAL DIAGNOSIS
- Tiger snake and brown snake envenoming may have similar
presentations as both can cause VICC. Neurotoxicity is rare in
brown snake envenoming.
- Taipan envenoming has all the features of tiger snake envenoming.
Differentiation between these two snakes may be possible based
on the geographical location where the snakebite occurs.
- Black snake envenoming causes myotoxicity and a mild
anticoagulant coagulopathy.
- Death adder envenoming causes neurotoxicity but does not cause
coagulopathy or severe myotoxicity.

DISPOSITION AND FOLLOW-UP
- All patients must be assessed in a hospital capable of providing
definitive care (see **Chapter 5.1: Approach to snakebite**).
- Envenoming is excluded if patients are clinically well with no
features of neurotoxicity and normal laboratory parameters at
least 12 hours after the bite (and preferably 12 hours after the PBI
removal). Discharge should not occur at night.
- Envenomed patients may be discharged following antivenom
administration if they are clinically well with complete reversal of

paralysis and the relevant laboratory parameters are resolving on serial measurements:

— INR <2
— decreasing CK
— no evidence of thrombotic microangiopathy (haemoglobin, platelets, creatinine).

- Patients who develop thrombotic microangiopathy require a more prolonged admission for management of acute renal failure and MAHA. Dialysis may be required for standard indications.

HANDY TIPS

- Tiger snake envenoming should be considered in the differential diagnosis of collapse, paralysis or coagulopathy (VICC).
- All patients with partial VICC require treatment with antivenom as there is a significant risk of development of complete VICC, neurotoxicity, myotoxicity and thrombotic microangiopathy.
- Monovalent antivenom is the preferred treatment for envenoming. In geographical regions where tiger and brown snakes co-exist, patients with VICC are treated with 1 ampoule of each monovalent antivenom. In areas where tiger, brown and taipan co-exist, patients are treated with 1 ampoule of polyvalent antivenom.
- Point-of-care INR and D-dimer testing should never be used in suspected snakebite cases as the tests are inaccurate and unvalidated in this setting.

PITFALLS

- Failure to consider that snakebite has occurred.
- Failure to follow the recommended approach for evaluation of snakebite.

CONTROVERSIES

- The definitive dose of antivenom required to treat all tiger snake envenomings is not clearly established. More than 1 ampoule of antivenom is justified, particularly in the setting of severe envenoming.
- Administration of clotting factors (FFP or cryoprecipitate) after antivenom administration can result in earlier recovery from VICC but there is not evidence of benefit for clinical outcomes.
- The efficacy, safety and indications for clotting factor replacement after venom neutralisation in VICC are not yet well defined.

References

Brown SG, Caruso N, Borland M et al. Clotting factor replacement and recovery from snake venom-induced consumptive coagulopathy. Intensive Care Medicine 2009; 35(9):1532–1538.

Gan M, O'Leary MA, Brown SG et al. Envenoming by the rough-scaled snake (*Tropidectis carinatus*): a series of confirmed cases. Medical Journal of Australia 2009; 191(3):183–186.

Isbister GK, Buckley NA, Page CB et al. A randomized controlled trial of fresh frozen plasma for treating venom-induced consumption coagulopathy in cases of Australian snakebite (ASP-18). Journal of Thrombosis and Haemostasis 2013; 11:1310–1318.

Isbister GK, Duffull SB, Brown SGA. Failure of antivenom to improve recovery in Australian snakebite coagulopathy. Quarterly Journal of Medicine 2009; 102(8): 563–568.

Isbister GK, O'Leary MA, Eliott M et al. Tiger snake (*Notechis* spp) envenoming: Australian Snakebite Project (ASP-13). Medical Journal of Australia 2012; 197(3):173–177.

Isbister GK, White J, Currie BJ et al. Clinical effects and treatment of envenoming by *Hoplocephalus* spp. snakes in Australia: Australian Snakebite Project (ASP-12). Toxicon 2011; 58:634–640.

Scop J, Little M, Jelinek GA et al. Sixteen years of severe tiger snake (*Notechis*) envenoming in Perth, Western Australia. Anaesthesia and Intensive Care 2009; 37:613–618.

5.6 TAIPAN

- *Oxyuranus microlepidotus*: inland taipan, small-scaled or fierce snake
- *Oxyuranus scutellatus canni*: Papuan taipan
- *Oxyuranus scutellatus*: coastal taipan
- *Oxyuranus temporalis*: central ranges taipan

Taipans are highly venomous snakes found in tropical coastal regions of north-eastern Australia and in isolated inland areas. Envenoming is characterised by rapid onset of venom-induced consumptive coagulopathy (VICC), neurotoxicity and myotoxicity. The Papuan taipan is one of the most medically important snakes in Papua New Guinea.

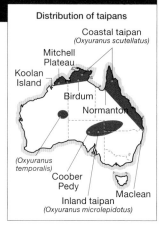

Distribution of taipans

Coastal taipan
(*Oxyuranus scutellatus*)

Mitchell Plateau

Koolan Island

Birdum

Normanton

(*Oxyuranus temporalis*)

Coober Pedy

Inland taipan
(*Oxyuranus microlepidotus*)

Maclean

ENVENOMINGS

488

TOXICOLOGY HANDBOOK

TOXINS

Taipan venom contains potent pre- and post-synaptic neurotoxins, myotoxins and procoagulants.

CLINICAL PRESENTATION AND COURSE

- Bite sites may have minimal or no symptoms apart from visible puncture marks.
- Non-specific systemic features of envenoming include headache, nausea and vomiting.
- The first sign of envenoming may be sudden collapse.
- Neurotoxicity can develop rapidly:
  - Early signs of paralysis include ptosis, blurred vision, diplopia and difficulty swallowing.
- VICC can develop soon after the bite and may be complete or partial. The clinical features of coagulopathy can range from persistent bleeding at venesection sites or gingival margins to catastrophic intracerebral haemorrhage. Partial VICC occurs in up to half of envenomings and is less likely to cause clinically significant bleeding.

- Thrombotic microangiopathy characterised by thrombocytopenia, microangiopathic haemolytic anaemia (MAHA) and acute renal failure is a frequent occurrence in patients with VICC.
- Myotoxicity can occur but is not usually severe.

MANAGEMENT

See **Chapter 5.1: Approach to snakebite** for a general guide to the principles of snakebite management.

Pre-hospital
- Apply a pressure bandage with immobilisation (PBI).
- Transport to a hospital capable of providing definitive care.

Hospital
Resuscitation and supportive care
- Taipan envenoming is a time-critical and life-threatening emergency and patients are managed in an area capable of cardiorespiratory monitoring and resuscitation.
- Early life-threats that require immediate intervention include:
  - cardiovascular collapse (hypotension, cardiac arrest)
  - rapid onset paralysis with secondary respiratory failure
  - VICC with uncontrolled haemorrhage.
- In cardiac arrest, undiluted antivenom administered as a rapid IV push is indicated in addition to standard cardiopulmonary resuscitation.
- Clinical evidence of neurotoxicity is an indication for antivenom. Early taipan antivenom may decrease the risk of progressive paralysis requiring intubation and ventilation.
- For life-threatening haemorrhage, clotting factor replacement with fresh frozen plasma (FFP) is required once adequate antivenom has been given.
- In the absence of life-threatening haemorrhage, administration of FFP, particularly within 6 hours of envenoming, may worsen coagulopathy and is not routinely indicated.

Antivenom
- The majority of taipan envenomings can safely be treated with 1 ampoule of taipan antivenom. However, in patients with severe envenoming syndromes or rapidly progressive complications, a second ampoule of taipan antivenom can be considered.
- If taipan monovalent antivenom is not immediately available, 1 ampoule of polyvalent antivenom is indicated.
- Monovalent antivenom is the preferred treatment for envenoming. However, in areas where taipan, brown and tiger snakes co-exist, patients with VICC are treated with 1 ampoule of polyvalent antivenom to cover all possibilities.

INVESTIGATIONS
- The diagnosis of envenoming is based on the correlation of history, clinical features and laboratory data.
- Routine laboratory investigations following snakebite include: FBC, EUC, CK and coagulation profile (INR, aPTT, fibrinogen, D-dimer) at presentation and at intervals thereafter (see **Chapter 5.1: Approach to snakebite**).

- Complete VICC is defined as:
  - elevated INR (at least >3 but usually unrecordable)
  - undetectable fibrinogen
  - markedly elevated D-dimer.
- Partial VICC is defined as:
  - INR abnormal but <3
  - low but detectable fibrinogen
  - elevated D-dimer.
- Recovery from VICC (INR returning to <2) usually occurs between 10 and 20 hours after the bite.
- Watch for deteriorating renal function and evidence of MAHA, indicated by raised lactate dehydrogenase (LDH) and fragmented red blood cells on blood film.

DIFFERENTIAL DIAGNOSIS
- Brown snake envenoming causes VICC, but neurotoxicity and myotoxicity are rare.
- Snakes from the tiger snake group co-exist with taipans in southern Queensland and northern New South Wales. The clinical features of envenoming by this group are indistinguishable from taipan envenoming. Polyvalent antivenom is indicated to cover both possibilities.
- Black snake envenoming is associated with myotoxicity and a mild anticoagulant coagulopathy with normal fibrinogen levels.
- Death adder envenoming causes a symmetrical descending flaccid paralysis but is not associated with coagulopathy.

DISPOSITION AND FOLLOW-UP
- All patients must be assessed in a hospital capable of providing definitive care (see **Chapter 5.1: Approach to snakebite**).
- Envenoming is excluded if patients are clinically well with no features of neurotoxicity and normal laboratory parameters at least 12 hours after the bite (and preferably 12 hours after the PBI removal). Discharge should not occur at night.
- Envenomed patients can be discharged following antivenom administration if they are clinically well with complete reversal of paralysis and the relevant laboratory parameters are improving on serial measurements:
  - INR <2
  - decreasing CK
  - no evidence of thrombotic microangiopathy (haemoglobin, platelets, creatinine).
- Patients who develop thrombotic microangiopathy require a more prolonged admission for management of acute renal failure and MAHA. Dialysis may be required for standard indications.

HANDY TIPS
- Taipan envenoming should be considered in the differential diagnosis of patients in tropical Australia who present with collapse, paralysis or a defibrinating coagulopathy.
- Point-of-care INR and D-dimer testing should never be used in suspected snakebite cases as the tests are inaccurate and unvalidated.

- Failure to consider that snakebite has occurred.
- Failure to follow the recommended approach for evaluation of snakebite.

CONTROVERSIES
- Administration of clotting factors (FFP or cryoprecipitate) after antivenom administration can result in earlier recovery from VICC but there is no evidence of benefit for clinical outcomes.
- The efficacy, safety and indications for clotting factor replacement after venom neutralisation in VICC are not yet well defined.

References
Isbister GK, Buckley NA, Page CB et al. A randomized controlled trial of fresh frozen plasma for treating venom-induced consumption coagulopathy in cases of Australian snakebite (ASP-18). Journal of Thrombosis and Haemostasis 2013; 11:1310–1318.

Sutherland SK, Tibballs J. Australian animal toxins: the creatures, their toxins and care of the poisoned patient. South Melbourne: Oxford University Press; 2001.

Trevett AJ, Lalloo DG, Nwokolo NC et al. The efficacy of antivenom in the treatment of bites by the Papuan taipan (*Oxyuranus scutellatus canni*). Transactions of the Royal Society of Tropical Medicine and Hygiene 1995; 89:322–325.

Williams D, Bal B. Papuan Taipan (*Oxyuranus scutellatus canni*) envenomation in rural Papua New Guinea. Annals of Australasian College of Tropical Medicine 2003; 4(1):6–9.

5.7 SEA SNAKES

Distribution of sea snakes

At least 30 species of sea snakes are found in coastal waters around Australia, predominantly in warmer northern waters. All sea snakes (family Hydrophiidae) are venomous and are closely related to the terrestrial Australian elapids. They are inquisitive but not aggressive and rarely bite unless they are handled or provoked.

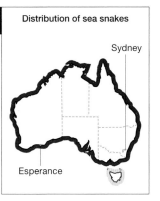

Sydney

Esperance

TOXINS

Sea snake venom is poorly characterised but contains neurotoxins and myotoxins.

CLINICAL PRESENTATION AND COURSE
- Most bites are small, superficial, relatively painless and not associated with local swelling or lymphadenitis.
- Non-specific features of envenoming include headache, nausea, vomiting and abdominal pain.
- Systemic features of neurotoxicity and myotoxicity become clinically apparent after a delay of several hours.
  - Neurotoxicity is characterised by symmetrical descending flaccid paralysis. Early signs include ptosis, blurred vision,

diplopia and difficulty swallowing. If left untreated, it may progress to generalised paralysis and respiratory failure.
— Myotoxicity may dominate the clinical picture and manifests as diffuse myalgias and myoglobinuria, and may progress to renal failure.

MANAGEMENT
See **Chapter 5.1: Approach to snakebite** for a guide to the principles of snakebite management.

Pre-hospital
- Apply a pressure bandage with immobilisation (PBI).
- Maintenance of an airway and ventilatory support may be life-saving in the pre-hospital setting.
- Transport to a hospital capable of providing definitive care.

Hospital
Resuscitation and supportive care
- Sea snake envenoming is a time-critical life-threatening emergency and patients are managed in an area capable of cardiorespiratory monitoring and resuscitation.
- Early life-threats that require immediate intervention include:
— descending flaccid paralysis with respiratory failure.
- If respiratory failure occurs and antivenom is not available, intubation and ventilation are life-saving.

Antivenom
- Sea snake antivenom (see **Chapter 6.6**) is the specific treatment of envenoming. Systemic envenoming, as evidenced by objective evidence of paralysis or myotoxicity, is treated with an initial dose of 1 ampoule.

INVESTIGATIONS
- The diagnosis of envenoming is based on the correlation of history, clinical features and laboratory data.
- Serial laboratory investigations following snakebite include: FBC, EUC, CK and coagulation profile (INR, aPTT, fibrinogen, D-dimer) at presentation and at intervals thereafter (see **Chapter 5.1: Approach to snakebite**).
- The CK rise in myotoxicity is variable and may be prolonged over several days. Severe envenomings can lead to CK levels >100 000 resulting in renal impairment.

DIFFERENTIAL DIAGNOSIS
- Other marine envenomings, although most tend to cause painful stings.
- Tiger snake and taipan envenoming also cause paralysis and myotoxicity. However, they are also associated with VICC, which does not occur in sea snake envenoming.
- Black snake envenoming is associated with myotoxicity. A mild anticoagulant coagulopathy with normal fibrinogen is also commonly seen, which does not occur in sea snake envenoming.
- Death adder envenoming causes a similar symmetrical descending flaccid paralysis, and myotoxicity (usually mild) can also occur.

DISPOSITION AND FOLLOW-UP

- All patients must be assessed in a hospital capable of providing definitive care (see **Chapter 5.1: Approach to snakebite**).
- Envenoming is excluded if patients are clinically well with no features of neurotoxicity and normal laboratory parameters at least 12 hours after the bite (and preferably 12 hours after the PBI removal). Discharge should not occur at night.
- Envenomed patients may be discharged following antivenom administration if they are clinically well with complete reversal of paralysis and the relevant laboratory parameters are improving on serial measurements:
  - decreasing CK.

HANDY TIPS

- Snakebite at sea, on the beach or in estuarine waters may be from a terrestrial snake.
- Polyvalent or other monovalent terrestrial antivenoms do not contain sea snake antivenom and are not recommended as alternatives.

PITFALLS

- Failure to consider that snakebite has occurred.
- Failure to follow the recommended approach for evaluation of snakebite.

CONTROVERSY

- Experience with sea snake envenoming is limited and the response to antivenom is poorly characterised.

Reference
White J. A clinician's guide to Australian venomous bites and stings: incorporating the updated CSL antivenom handbook. Melbourne: CSL Ltd; 2012.

5.8 AUSTRALIAN SCORPIONS

- Bothriuridae
- Buthidae
- Urodacidae

Little is known about scorpion stings in Australia, but evidence suggests that symptoms are usually limited to temporary pain at the sting site and mild non-specific systemic symptoms. This is in contrast to some scorpion stings elsewhere in the world, which are associated with life-threatening envenoming.

TOXINS
Venom contains excitatory neurotoxins.

CLINICAL PRESENTATION AND COURSE

- Symptoms are usually confined to the site of the sting.
- Severe local pain is common and usually lasts 6–12 hours, but may persist for up to 24 hours. Additional local symptoms

include erythema, tenderness, mild swelling, numbness and paraesthesia.
- Systemic effects occur in a minority of patients (10%). They are mild and self-limiting and include nausea, malaise, headache and hypertension.

MANAGEMENT
Pre-hospital
- Reassure the patient, apply an ice pack and give effective oral analgesia.
- Do not apply a pressure bandage with immobilisation (PBI).
- Patients do not require referral to hospital unless symptoms are refractory to first aid measures.

Hospital
Resuscitation and supportive care
- Scorpion stings are not life-threatening and resuscitation is not required.
- Pain refractory to simple first aid and oral analgesia can be treated with IV opioid analgesia.

Antivenom
- None available.

INVESTIGATIONS
- There are no confirmatory laboratory studies.

DIFFERENTIAL DIAGNOSIS
- Redback spider envenoming is characteristically associated with local pain, sweating and piloerection. Systemic features include pain at proximal sites, generalised sweating and dysphoria.
- Funnel-web spider envenoming is potentially lethal. It is associated with a painful bite, sweating, agitation, piloerection, cardiovascular abnormalities and neurological changes.
- Non-specific spider bites can also cause bite site pain and mild systemic symptoms, such as nausea, headache, malaise or vomiting.
- Hymenoptera (bees, wasps, ants) also cause a painful sting.
- Centipedes cause a painful bite.

DISPOSITION AND FOLLOW-UP
- Patients do not require hospital assessment unless pain is not controlled with simple analgesia or systemic symptoms develop.

HANDY TIP
- The smallest scorpions cause the most painful stings.

Reference
Isbister GK, Volschenk ES, Balit CR et al. Australian scorpion stings: a prospective study of definitive stings. Toxicon 2003; 41:877–883.

5.9 BLUEBOTTLE JELLYFISH (*PHYSALIA* SPECIES)

The bluebottle 'jellyfish' is ubiquitous in Australian coastal waters and stings occur frequently. The 'jellyfish' is a colony of multiple individual organisms functioning as a single animal. Local symptoms predominate, unlike *Physalia* stings in other parts of the world which can cause systemic envenoming. Hot water immersion provides effective symptomatic relief.

TOXINS

The toxins are contained within nematocysts (stinging organelles) on the tentacles and released on contact. A complex mixture of glycoproteins, they are yet to be well characterised.

CLINICAL PRESENTATION AND COURSE
- Stings are associated with immediate burning pain, typically lasting up to 2 hours, and linear or elliptical erythematous welts.
- Non-specific systemic symptoms, such as nausea, headache or malaise, may occur.

MANAGEMENT
- Stings are mild, self-limiting and respond to first aid measures.
- Reassure the patient.
- Place the patient under a hot shower for 20 minutes (ideal temperature 40–45°C). The shower should be hot but not scalding or uncomfortable.
- Administer effective oral analgesics.
- Do not apply a pressure bandage with immobilisation (PBI) or vinegar as this may worsen local symptoms.
- Transport to hospital is not usually required.

Antivenom
- None available.

INVESTIGATIONS
- The diagnosis is clinical, based on a high index of suspicion and correlation of history and characteristic features.

DIFFERENTIAL DIAGNOSIS
- Pain associated with Irukandji syndrome is usually delayed, severe and generalised. Significant linear dermal markings or welts are not seen.
- Envenoming by the box jellyfish (*Chironex fleckeri*) is associated with immediate pain and obvious dermal markings (large welts). Tentacles may be seen adhering to the skin.

DISPOSITION AND FOLLOW-UP
- Most patients do not require any care beyond first aid.

CONTROVERSY
- Appropriate first aid is not clearly defined. Ice packs were previously recommended as first aid for stings. The superiority of

hot water immersion has now been conclusively demonstrated. The use of vinegar remains controversial – laboratory studies suggest that it decreases the discharge rate of unactivated nematocysts but can significantly increase venom release from partially discharged nematocysts.

References
Loten C, Stokes B, Worsley D et al. A randomised controlled trial of hot water (45°C) immersion versus ice packs for pain relief in bluebottle stings. Medical Journal of Australia 2006; 184(7):329–333.

Tibballs J. Australian venomous jellyfish, envenomation syndromes, toxins and therapy. Toxicon 2006; 48:830–859.

5.10 STONEFISH

Distribution of stonefish species

- *Synanceia horrida*
- *Synanceia verrucosa*

Stonefish are extremely well-camouflaged reef fish found in the waters of northern Australia. Their dorsal spines contain venom, which is injected when external pressure is applied.

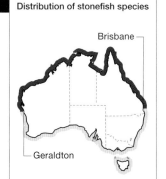

Brisbane

Geraldton

TOXINS
The venom contains pre- and post-synaptic neurotoxins, vascular permeability factors, tissue necrosis factors (hyaluronidase) and a vasodilator (stonustoxin).

CLINICAL PRESENTATION AND COURSE
- Immediate severe pain at the sting site.
- Local swelling, bruising and puncture marks. Remnants of the spine(s) may be left in the wound.
- Systemic envenoming is rare and there are no reports of deaths in Australia.
- Non-specific features of envenoming include nausea, vomiting, dizziness and dyspnoea.
- Cardiovascular signs, such as hypotension, bradycardia, collapse and pulmonary oedema, are rarely reported.

MANAGEMENT
Pre-hospital
- Reassure the patient and give simple oral analgesia.
- Immerse both limbs in hot water. The unaffected limb is also immersed to ensure the water temperature is tolerable and so prevent burns.
- Do not apply a pressure bandage with immobilisation (PBI).
- Transport all patients with significant pain refractory to first aid, or with systemic symptoms, to a medical facility.

Hospital

Resuscitation and supportive care
- Stonefish envenoming is very painful, but rarely life-threatening.
- Treatment is essentially supportive.
- Continue hot water immersion.
- Give IV opioid analgesia, repeated every 10 minutes until patient is comfortable.
- Consider regional anaesthesia with a long-acting local anaesthetic agent (e.g. ropivacaine).
- Wound care and tetanus prophylaxis as appropriate.

Antivenom
- Stonefish antivenom (see **Chapter 6.8**) is used in the treatment of severe pain refractory to hot water immersion, IV opioid analgesia or regional nerve block.
- Give 1 ampoule for every two spine puncture wounds (to a maximum of 3 ampoules).

INVESTIGATIONS
- Plain X-ray or ultrasound examination may assist detection of retained foreign bodies.

DIFFERENTIAL DIAGNOSIS
- Numerous other marine or estuarine spiny fish can cause a similar clinical presentation. Hot water immersion is the standard initial treatment for all such presentations.
- Stingray barb injury can also cause severe local pain responsive to hot water immersion.

DISPOSITION AND FOLLOW-UP
- Patients treated with opioid analgesia or antivenom may be discharged when symptoms are controlled after a period of observation.

HANDY TIPS
- Beware of retained foreign bodies and the risk of marine infection.
- Hot water should not be used following local anaesthetic infiltration because of the risk of thermal burn.

CONTROVERSY
- It is not known whether stonefish antivenom is effective for envenoming from other spiny fish.

References
Lee JYL, Teoh LC, Leo SPM. Stonefish envenomation of the hand – a local marine hazard. A series of 8 cases and review of the literature. Annals of the Academy of Medicine Singapore 2004; 33:515–520.

Little M. Stonefish (*Synanceia* species) sting. Emergency Medicine 1990; 2(4):5.

Ngo SYA, Ong SHJ, Ponampalam R. Stonefish envenomation presenting to a Singapore hospital. Singapore Medical Journal 2009; 50:506–509.

White J. A clinician's guide to Australian venomous bites and stings: incorporating the updated CSL antivenom handbook. Melbourne: CSL Ltd; 2012.

5.11 BOX JELLYFISH

● *Chironex fleckeri*

Chironex fleckeri is a large cubozoan ('box') jellyfish found in tropical Australian waters. Most stings are benign and require only symptomatic treatment. Severe envenoming can cause death within minutes of the sting, secondary to cardiac toxicity. Immediate cardiopulmonary resuscitation provides the best chance of survival, and the additional benefit of antivenom is not proven.

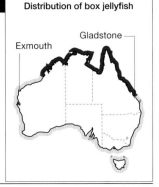

TOXINS

The toxins are contained within nematocysts (stinging organelles) on the tentacles and released on contact. The specific venom components have not been fully characterised. They are thought to affect sodium and calcium channels leading to abnormal membrane ion transport, resulting in intracellular calcium accumulation (particularly in myocardial cells) and sustained tetanic contraction ('cardiac arrest in systole'). Animal studies have also identified haemolytic and dermonecrotic venom components.

CLINICAL PRESENTATION AND COURSE

● Stings are associated with immediate severe pain, typically lasting up to 8 hours.
● Linear welts are characteristic, typically occurring in a cross-hatched pattern.
● In 30% of cases, the jellyfish tentacles are still adherent.
● Systemic envenoming is heralded by collapse or sudden death within a few minutes of the sting.
● Cardiovascular effects include hypertension, tachycardia, impaired cardiac contraction and dysrhythmias. Subsequent hypotension leads to cardiovascular collapse and cardiac arrest.
● Delayed hypersensitivity reactions occur in at least 50% of patients and manifest as pruritic erythema at the original sting site 7–14 days after the sting.

MANAGEMENT

Pre-hospital

● Patients in cardiac arrest require immediate cardiopulmonary resuscitation. Dramatic recovery has been reported following prolonged CPR performed on the beach.
● If vinegar is available, apply it liberally to all visible sting sites to inactivate undischarged nematocysts.
● Following application of vinegar, adherent tentacles should be removed as carefully as possible.

- Wash the sting sites with sea water (as fresh water can promote nematocyst discharge).
- Ice packs are recommended for pain management.
- Do not apply pressure bandaging with immobilisation (PBI) as this may increase nematocyst discharge and promote systemic envenoming.
- Patients with progressive or persistent symptoms should be assessed in hospital.

Hospital
Resuscitation and supportive care
- Box jellyfish envenoming is a potentially life-threatening emergency. However, all deaths occur within minutes of the sting, and patients who survive to reach hospital have a good prognosis.
- Patients should be managed in an area equipped for cardiorespiratory monitoring and resuscitation.
- Early life-threats that require immediate intervention include:
  - cardiac arrest
  - cardiovascular instability.
- Effective cardiopulmonary resuscitation can be life-saving and should be continued as long as possible. Dramatic recovery has been reported following prolonged CPR performed on the beach.
- If a patient remains in cardiac arrest or has significant haemodynamic compromise on arrival in hospital, resuscitation is continued and antivenom is indicated.
- Give titrated opioid analgesia to patients with pain unresponsive to first aid.

Antivenom
- The dose of box jellyfish antivenom required is not clearly defined and the effectiveness is unknown (see **Chapter 6.9**).
- Recommended doses are 1–3 ampoules over 5–10 minutes in cardiorespiratory arrest or cardiogenic shock.
- Antivenom is not recommended for the management of refractory pain.

INVESTIGATIONS
- Box jellyfish envenoming is a clinical diagnosis and no specific diagnostic investigations are indicated.
- ECG, troponin, CXR and echocardiogram are performed in patients with cardiotoxicity.

DIFFERENTIAL DIAGNOSIS
- Bluebottle stings (*Physalia* spp.) are also associated with immediate pain and dermal markings. Pain usually resolves within 1 hour and systemic symptoms are rare.
- Pain associated with Irukandji syndrome is usually delayed, severe and generalised. Significant linear dermal markings or welts are not seen.
- Decompression illness may lead to severe pain and collapse shortly after a diver has surfaced. Local pain and welts are not seen.

DISPOSITION AND FOLLOW-UP
- Patients without clinical features of systemic envenoming or local pain at 2 hours do not require further medical observation.
- Patients who require opioid analgesia or antivenom are discharged after being asymptomatic for 6 hours.

HANDY TIPS
- Reassurance is important. Despite its fearsome reputation, the vast majority of box jellyfish stings require only first aid and simple analgesia.
- Survival from cardiac arrest on the beach due to box jellyfish envenoming has been reported following prompt and prolonged CPR.
- Steroids or antihistamines may provide symptomatic relief if a delayed hypersensitivity rash occurs. Patients should be advised that skin scarring can be persistent.
- Immediate pain after a jellyfish sting, occurring in tropical waters between November and April, associated with linear welts with a cross-hatched pattern, is pathognomonic of *Chironex fleckeri* sting.

PITFALLS
- Failure to commence immediate CPR when cardiac arrest occurs on the beach.
- Administration of antivenom when not indicated.

CONTROVERSIES
- Efficacy and role of box jellyfish antivenom.
- Appropriate first aid is not clearly defined. Ice is currently recommended as appropriate topical treatment for box jellyfish stings, but it is possible that heat is more effective.

Similarly, the use of vinegar is controversial – laboratory studies suggest that it decreases the discharge rate of unactivated nematocyst stinging organelles but can significantly increase venom release from partially discharged nematocysts.

References

Currie BJ. Marine antivenoms. Journal of Toxicology – Clinical Toxicology 2003; 41:301–308.

Currie BJ, Jacups S. Prospective study of *Chironex fleckeri* and other box jellyfish stings in the 'Top End' of Australia's Northern Territory. Medical Journal of Australia 2005; 183:161–166.

Isbister GK, Palmer DJ, Weir RL et al. Hot water immersion *v* icepacks for treating the pain of *Chironex fleckeri* sting: a randomised control trial. Medical Journal of Australia 2017; 206(6):258–261. doi:10.5694/mja16.00990.

Tibballs J. Australian venomous jellyfish, envenomation syndromes, toxins and therapy. Toxicon 2006; 48:830–859.

Welfare P, Little M, Pereira P et al. An in-vitro examination of the effect of vinegar on discharged nematocysts of Chironex fleckeri. Diving and Hyperbaric Medicine 2014; 44(1):30–34.

5.12 IRUKANDJI SYNDROME

Irukandji syndrome is a potentially lethal envenoming caused by the sting of *Carukia barnesi* (and other similar) jellyfish found in coastal waters of tropical Australia. It is also reported in Hawaii, the Caribbean and South-east Asia. The defining clinical features are a severe pain syndrome, and life-threatening hypertension and pulmonary oedema may develop. Management is symptomatic and supportive.

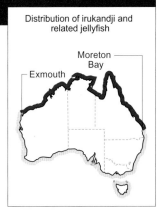

Distribution of irukandji and related jellyfish

Moreton Bay

Exmouth

TOXINS

Carukia barnsei is a small, transparent cubozoan jellyfish, with a 1–2 cm diameter cubic bell (or box) and four tentacles up to 1 m long. Pressure-sensitive nematocysts (stinging organelles) located in the tentacles and bell inject the potent venom, whose composition and mechanism of action have not been fully characterised. It is thought to act as a pre-synaptic sodium channel agonist, inducing massive catecholamine release.

CLINICAL PRESENTATION AND COURSE

- The initial sting is usually not felt and there is a delay to the onset of systemic symptoms. Local signs, such as welts or dermal markings, are minimal or absent.
- Multiple systemic symptoms develop from 30 to 120 minutes after the sting. These include a sense of impending doom, agitation, dysphoria, vomiting, generalised sweating and severe pain in the back, limbs or abdomen. Hypertension and tachycardia are common.
- Symptoms usually resolve within 12 hours.
- Severe envenoming is characterised by significant ongoing pain with high analgesic requirements. These patients are at risk of developing acute catecholamine-induced cardiomyopathy, cardiogenic shock and pulmonary oedema and may require intubation and ventilation.

MANAGEMENT

Pre-hospital

- First aid is not generally an effective option because the sting is not usually felt, symptoms are delayed in onset and a sting site is not apparent.
- Patients with significant symptoms should be assessed in hospital.

Hospital

Resuscitation and supportive care

- Irukandji syndrome is a potentially life-threatening emergency. Patients should be managed in an area equipped for cardiorespiratory monitoring and resuscitation.

- Early life-threats that require immediate intervention include:
  - severe hypertension
  - pulmonary oedema.
- Administer IV fentanyl until adequate analgesia is achieved. Large doses may be required.
  - Note: IV fentanyl is considered the opioid analgesic of choice due to a potential additional analgesic effect mediated by sodium channel antagonism.
- Severe hypertension refractory to intravenous opioid analgesia requires additional management. The initial choice is IV glyceryl trinitrate titrated to achieve a systolic blood pressure <160 mmHg. Alternative agents include nitroprusside or labetalol.
- Pulmonary oedema can develop acutely or be delayed many hours. Standard therapy with non-invasive ventilation or intubation is determined on clinical grounds.
- Development of hypotension is a significant feature that suggests cardiogenic shock from acute catecholamine-induced cardiomyopathy, requiring inotropic support (see **Chapter 2.2: Hypotension**).
- Nausea and vomiting can be difficult to control. Promethazine is an anti-emetic with additional sodium-channel-blocking effects, but can cause hypotension when given by the intravenous route. Other treatment options are droperidol or benzodiazepines.
- Ongoing severe pain is a difficult management issue and expert advice should be sought. Numerous approaches are suggested:
  - patient-controlled analgesia (PCA) infusions (including fentanyl and ketamine)
  - IV clonidine
  - Note: The use of IV magnesium is recommended by some authorities but is not clearly supported by published literature.

Antivenom
- None available.

INVESTIGATIONS
- Investigations are indicated to exclude alternative diagnoses and to assess complications in those patients who present with significant clinical features:
  - ECG, serial troponins, CXR and echocardiogram.

DIFFERENTIAL DIAGNOSIS
- Envenoming by the box jellyfish (*Chironex fleckeri*) is associated with immediate pain and obvious dermal markings (large welts). Tentacles may be seen adherent to the skin.
- Bluebottle stings (*Physalia* spp.) are associated with immediate pain and dermal markings. The pain usually resolves within 1 hour and systemic symptoms are extremely rare.
- Decompression illness may lead to generalised pain or collapse shortly after a diver has surfaced. Welts are not seen.

DISPOSITION AND FOLLOW-UP
- Patients with severe pain who require opioid analgesia may be discharged when they are clinically well and have been pain-free for a period of 6 hours.

- Prolonged symptoms can occur and delayed deterioration (>24 hours) with onset of pulmonary oedema requiring intubation and ventilation has been reported.

HANDY TIPS
- Clinical features of envenoming occur after the patient has left the water, so they may be unaware they have been stung.
- Irukandji syndrome should be considered in any patient presenting with characteristic clinical features during or shortly after swimming in tropical coastal Australian waters.
- Clinical features of dysphoria, severe generalised pain, sweating, hypertension and pulmonary oedema, in the absence of major dermal findings, are pathognomonic of Irukandji syndrome.
- Benzodiazepines, by decreasing the effects of catecholamine release, may be a useful treatment option.

PITFALL
- Failure to appreciate the risk of severe cardiotoxicity.

CONTROVERSY
- Magnesium IV has been advocated for Irukandji syndrome. There is no published evidence to support its use and it is not recommended.

References
Barnes JH. Cause and effect in Irukandji stingings. Medical Journal of Australia 1964; 1:897–904.
Huynh TT, Seymour J, Pereira P et al. Severity of Irukandji syndrome and nematocyst identification from skin scrapings. Medical Journal of Australia 2003; 178:38–41.
Little M, Mulcahy RF. A year's experience of 'Irukandji' jellyfish envenomation in far north Queensland. Medical Journal of Australia 1998; 169:638–641.
Little M, Pereira P, Carrette T et al. Jellyfish responsible for irukandji syndrome. Quarterly Journal of Medicine 2006; 99:425–427.
Macrocanis CJ, Hall NJ, Mein JK. Irukandji syndrome in northern Western Australia: an emerging health problem. Medical Journal of Australia 2004; 181(11/12):699–702.
McCullagh N, Pereira P, Cullen P et al. Randomised trial of magnesium in the treatment of Irukandji syndrome. Emergency Medicine Australasia 2012; 24(5):560–565.
Nickson CP, Waugh EB, Jacups SP et al. Irukandji syndrome case series from Australia's tropical Northern Territory. Annals of Emergency Medicine 2009; 54(3):395–403.

5.13 BLUE-RINGED OCTOPUS

- *Hapalochlaena lunulata*: northern or greater blue-ringed octopus
- *Hapalochlaena maculosa*: southern or lesser blue-ringed octopus

This small octopus is found in shallow coastal waters around Australia. It is not aggressive and bites usually occur when humans handle the animal. Envenoming causes rapid paralysis. Timely support of airway and ventilation ensures a good outcome.

TOXINS

Tetrodotoxin (maculotoxin in *Hapalochlaena maculosa*) is a potent sodium-channel-blocking neurotoxin. Venom is produced by bacteria in the salivary glands and introduced from the beak under the body of the octopus, not from the tentacles.

CLINICAL PRESENTATION AND COURSE

- The bite may not be painful.
- Local symptoms are minimal or absent.
- Systemic envenoming is characterised by a rapidly progressive symmetrical descending flaccid paralysis, which usually manifests within minutes.
- Early signs include ptosis, blurred vision, diplopia and difficulty swallowing. In severe cases, generalised paralysis, respiratory failure and secondary hypoxic cardiac arrest ensue.
- With appropriate airway support, paralysis resolves spontaneously within 1–2 days.

MANAGEMENT

Pre-hospital

- Apply a pressure bandage with immobilisation (PBI).
- Commence CPR if required.
- Transport to a hospital capable of providing definitive care.

Hospital

Resuscitation and supportive care

- Blue-ringed octopus envenoming is potentially life-threatening. Patients should be managed in an area equipped for cardiorespiratory monitoring and resuscitation.
- Early life-threats that require immediate intervention include:
  - descending flaccid paralysis with respiratory failure.
- If respiratory failure is present, intubation and ventilation are life-saving.

Antivenom

- None available.

INVESTIGATIONS

- Investigations are indicated to exclude alternative diagnoses and assess complications.
- Spirometry or peak flow measurements are useful to monitor respiratory function.

DIFFERENTIAL DIAGNOSIS

- Envenoming by the box jellyfish (*Chironex fleckeri*) is associated with collapse on the beach and sudden death following a sting. However, there is immediate severe pain and obvious dermal markings (large welts). Tentacles may be seen adherent to the skin.
- Puffer fish also contain tetrodotoxin and ingestion of these fish can lead to flaccid paralysis. The history usually permits this diagnosis to be easily distinguished from blue-ringed octopus bite.

DISPOSITION AND FOLLOW-UP

- Patients without evidence of neurotoxicity 6 hours after the bite can be discharged.
- Envenomed patients with paralysis require ventilatory support in intensive care.

- Patients remain conscious after paralysis has occurred and appropriate sedation must be given.

PITFALLS
- Failure to appreciate the possibility of rapid onset of paralysis.
- Failure to appreciate that the paralysed patient is fully aware unless sedated.

References
Cavazzoni E, Lister B, Sargent P et al. Blue-ringed octopus (*Hapalochlaena* sp.) envenomation of a 4-year-old boy: a case report. Clinical Toxicology 2008; 46:760–761.

Sutherland SK, Lane WR. Toxins and mode of envenomation of the common ringed or blue-banded octopus. Medical Journal of Australia 1969; 1:893–898.

Sutherland SK, Tibballs J. Australian animal toxins: the creatures, their toxins and care of the poisoned patient. South Melbourne: Oxford University Press; 2001.

5.14 REDBACK SPIDER

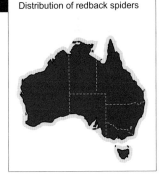

Distribution of redback spiders

- *Latrodectus hasselti*: redback spider (Australia)
- *Latrodectus katipo*: katipo spider (New Zealand)

Redback spider bite is a common envenoming in Australia. Clinical features can be distressing and refractory to symptomatic treatment but are not life-threatening. The katipo spider does not cause medically significant envenoming. The katipo spider does not cause medically significant envenoming.

TOXINS
Venom of the *Latrodectus* genus contains alpha-latrotoxin. This toxin acts pre-synaptically to open ion channels and stimulate the release of multiple neurotransmitters.

CLINICAL PRESENTATION AND COURSE
- Redback spider bites are not immediately painful.
- Intense local pain develops 5–10 minutes after the bite and is followed by sweating and piloerection within an hour. Puncture marks are not always evident and erythema, if present, is usually mild.
- Systemic envenoming (latrodectism) occurs in a significant minority of patients. Pain typically radiates proximally from the bite site to become regional, then generalised (chest, abdominal, back pain). Autonomic features include severe sweating (which may be regional [e.g. both legs] or generalised), mild hypertension and tachycardia.

- Non-specific features of envenoming include headache, nausea, vomiting and dysphoria.
- Untreated, systemic envenoming typically resolves over 1–4 days.

MANAGEMENT
Pre-hospital
- Reassure the patient, apply an ice pack and give oral analgesia such as paracetamol and anti-inflammatories.
- Do not apply a pressure bandage with immobilisation (PBI).
- Refer to hospital if the patient has local symptoms refractory to simple analgesia or clinical features of systemic envenoming.

Hospital
Resuscitation and supportive care
- Redback spider envenoming is not life-threatening and resuscitation is not required.

Antivenom
- Redback spider antivenom (see **Chapter 6.10**) has for many years been regarded as the specific treatment for refractory pain or systemic symptoms of lactrodectism; however, its clinical effectiveness has recently been questioned (see **Controversies** below).
- The standard approach is 2 ampoules given intravenously.

INVESTIGATIONS
- Laboratory investigations do not assist in diagnosis or management.
- Investigations are indicated to exclude alternative diagnoses based on clinical assessment.

DIFFERENTIAL DIAGNOSIS
- Funnel-web spider envenoming is potentially lethal. It is associated with immediate bite site pain, visible fang marks and the abrupt onset, within minutes, of a severe clinical syndrome characterised by sweating, agitation, piloerection, cardiovascular and neurological changes.
- Envenoming by *Steatoda* species (cupboard spider or brown house spider) closely resembles redback spider envenoming.
- Non-specific spider bites are associated with bite site pain and mild systemic symptoms, such as nausea, headache, malaise or vomiting. The features of latrodectism do not occur.
- Latrodectism has been mistaken for conditions such as acute surgical abdomen, acute myocardial infarction and thoracic aortic dissection.

DISPOSITION AND FOLLOW-UP
- Patients without clinical features of systemic envenoming or local pain do not require referral for medical evaluation.
- Envenomed patients may be discharged when symptoms have been controlled. Some patients re-present because of persistent symptoms.

HANDY TIPS
- The triad of local pain, sweating and piloerection increasing over the first hour is pathognomonic of redback spider bite.
- Profuse sweating and pain in both lower limbs is the characteristic clinical presentation of latrodectism.
- Consider the diagnosis in any child with abrupt onset of inconsolable crying, abdominal pain or priapism, particularly if there is evidence of localised skin erythema or sweating as a well represented clue.

PITFALL
- Failure to consider the diagnosis in the appropriate clinical setting.

CONTROVERSIES
- The clinical value of antivenom administration in the management of latrodectism has been questioned by a randomised controlled study in adults (RAVE II), showing no statistically significant clinical benefit above that of standard analgesia in control of the pain and systemic symptoms of redback envenoming.
  - However, redback antivenom out-performed the standard oral analgesic regimen (paracetamol, ibuprofen and oxycodone) for both primary and secondary end points in the study, but did not reach the pre-determined thresholds of significance.
- The decision to withhold antivenom based on the study information limits use of a potential treatment, and no alternative analgesic agent is as yet proven to be effective (including intravenous opioids or agents such as clonidine, ketamine or other neuromodulators).
- Clinical experience suggests that individual patients may benefit from antivenom – particularly paediatric patients, who were not well represented in the study.

References
Cocks J, Page CB, Chu S, Gamage I et al. Redback spider bites in children in South Australia: a 10-year review of antivenom effectiveness [published online ahead of print]. Emergency Medicine Australasia 2021. doi:10.1111/1742-6723.13869.

Isbister GK, Brown SGA, Miller M et al. A randomised controlled trial of intramuscular versus intravenous antivenom for latrodectism – the RAVE study. Quarterly Journal of Medicine 2008; 101:557–565.

Isbister GK, Gray MR. Latrodectism: a prospective cohort study of bites by formally identified redback spiders. Medical Journal of Australia 2003; 179:88–91.

Isbister GK, O'Leary MA, Miller M et al. A comparison of serum antivenom concentrations after intravenous and intramuscular administration of redback (widow) spider antivenom. British Journal of Clinical Pharmacology 2008; 65:138–143.

Isbister GK, Page CB, Buckley NA et al. Randomized controlled trial of intravenous antivenom versus placebo for latrodectism: the second Redback Antivenom Evaluation (RAVE-II) study. Annals of Emergency Medicine 2014; 64(6):620–628. doi:10.1016/j.annemergmed.2014.06.006.

Isbister GK, Sibbritt D. Developing a decision tree algorithm for the diagnosis of suspected spider bites. Emergency Medicine Australia 2006; 16:161–166.

5.15 FUNNEL-WEB (BIG BLACK) SPIDER

Distribution of funnel-web spiders

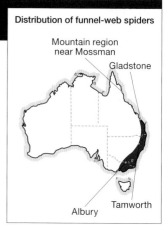

Mountain region near Mossman
Gladstone
Tamworth
Albury

Funnel-web spiders (FWSs) comprise 40 species in two genera (*Atrax* and *Hadronyche*). These potentially lethal spiders look very similar to other less medically significant big black spiders, including the trapdoor spiders (families Idiopidae and Nemesiidae) and mouse spiders (Actinopididae). For this reason, it is important to have a clinical approach to big black spider bites within the distribution of the funnel-web species.

- *Atrax robustus*: Sydney funnel-web spider
- *Hadronyche cerberea*: southern tree funnel-web spider
- *Hadronyche formidabilis*: northern tree funnel-web spider
- *Hadronyche infensa*: Toowoomba or Darling Downs funnel-web spider
- *Hadronyche macquariensis*: Port Macquarie funnel-web spider
- *Hadronyche versuta*: Blue Mountains funnel-web spider

TOXINS

Both genera of FWS produce venom that contains potent neurotoxins. Robustoxin (*Atrax* spp.) and versutoxin (*Hadronyche* spp.) prevent inactivation of sodium channels, leading to a massive increase in cholinergic and adrenergic activity.

CLINICAL PRESENTATION AND COURSE

- The patient usually gives a history of witnessed painful bite by a big black spider with large fangs.
- Local pain at the bite site is severe and fang marks are often visible.
- Local erythema and swelling are not features of FWS bite.
- Severe systemic envenoming occurs rapidly, usually within 30 minutes and almost always within 2 hours. Clinical features are a result of cholinergic and adrenergic stimulation and include:
  — general – agitation, vomiting, abdominal pain, headache and altered consciousness
  — autonomic – sweating, salivation, piloerection and lacrimation
  — cardiovascular – hypertension, tachycardia or bradycardia, acute cardiomyopathy and pulmonary oedema
  — neuromuscular – muscle fasciculations and spasms, oral paraesthesias.
- In children, the first indication of envenoming may be sudden severe illness with inconsolable crying, salivation, vomiting or collapse.

Pre-hospital
- Apply a pressure bandage with immobilisation (PBI).
- Transport to a hospital capable of providing definitive care (antivenom, resuscitation facilities and medical staff).

Hospital
Resuscitation and supportive care
- Funnel-web spider envenoming is potentially life-threatening. Patients are managed in an area equipped for cardiorespiratory monitoring and resuscitation.
- Early life-threats that require immediate intervention include:
  - cardiac arrest or cardiogenic shock
  - pulmonary oedema
  - coma.
- In cardiac arrest, 4 ampoules of undiluted antivenom administered as a rapid IV push is indicated in addition to standard cardiopulmonary resuscitation.
- Atropine may decrease respiratory secretions.

Antivenom
- Funnel-web spider antivenom (see **Chapter 6.11**) is the specific treatment of FWS envenoming.
- An initial dose of 2 ampoules is indicated for patients with systemic envenoming as evidenced by neurological, autonomic or cardiovascular features.
- The patient is observed for response to treatment. Ongoing features of envenoming prompt administration of a further dose of 2 ampoules of antivenom.
- An initial dose of 4 ampoules may be indicated in the severely envenomed patient.

INVESTIGATIONS
- Investigations are indicated to exclude alternative diagnoses and to assess complications in severe envenoming.

DIFFERENTIAL DIAGNOSIS
- Redback spider envenoming is characterised by a triad of local pain, sweating and piloerection. Systemic features include generalised pain, sweating and dysphoria. Lethal envenoming with coma, muscle fasciculations or pulmonary oedema does not occur.
- Bites by the other big black spiders (trapdoor and mouse spiders) may be associated with significant bite site pain but only mild systemic symptoms, such as nausea, headache, malaise or vomiting. Significant cardiovascular, autonomic or neurological features do not occur.
- Scorpion stings cause local pain and paraesthesia without evidence of systemic envenoming.

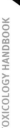

ENVENOMINGS

509

TOXICOLOGY HANDBOOK

- Patients without clinical features of systemic envenoming at 4 hours do not require further medical management.
- Envenomed patients treated with antivenom are discharged if clinically well for 12 hours. Do not discharge at night.

HANDY TIPS
- Big black spider bite in New South Wales or southern Queensland is assumed to be by a FWS and treated as such.
- Removal of the PBI only occurs when the patient is in an area equipped for cardiorespiratory resuscitation with adequate supplies of FWS antivenom.
- Tongue fasciculations are a clinical clue for systemic envenoming.
- A painful bite by a big black spider with abrupt onset of sweating, agitation, piloerection, coma and fasciculations is pathognomonic of FWS envenoming.

PITFALLS
- Failure to consider the diagnosis when spider bite is not witnessed.
- Failure to anticipate the abrupt onset of life-threatening envenoming and that delayed envenoming may occur following the release of PBI.
- Removal of PBI prior to availability of antivenom and resuscitation facilities.

References

Gray RM. A revision of the Australian funnel-web spiders (Hexathelidae: Atracinae). Records of the Australian Museum 2010; 62:285–392.

Isbister GK, Gray MR, Balit CR et al. Funnel-web spider bite: a systematic review of recorded clinical cases. Medical Journal of Australia 2005; 182:407–411.

Isbister GK, Sibbritt D. Developing a decision tree algorithm for the diagnosis of suspected spider bites. Emergency Medicine Australasia 2006; 16:161–166.

Nicholson GM, Graudins A, Wilson HI et al. Arachnid toxinology in Australia: from clinical toxicology to potential applications. Toxicon 2006; 48:872–898.

Rosengren D, White J, Raven R et al. First report of a funnel-web spider envenoming syndrome in Brisbane. Emergency Medicine Australasia 2008; 20:164–166.

5.16 WHITE-TAILED SPIDER

- *Lampona cylindrata*
- *Lampona murina*

White-tailed spiders are ubiquitous throughout Australia and previously believed to cause necrotising arachnidism, a syndrome of progressive cutaneous injury from spider venom. Published data indicate that these spiders are unlikely to cause significant dermal lesions.

TOXINS

The venom of *Lampona cylindrata* has been extensively studied and cytotoxic effects have not been noted. In contrast, venom of the brown recluse spider (*Loxosceles* spp.) native to the Americas has confirmed dermonecrotic toxins (sphingomyelinases) and in some cases is associated with the development of significant skin ulceration.

CLINICAL PRESENTATION AND COURSE
- Witnessed, painful bite.
- Three patterns of clinical effects have been identified in a prospective study of 130 *Lampona* bites where the spider was caught and formally identified by an arachnologist:
  - severe local pain of <2 hours duration
  - local pain and a red mark lasting <24 hours
  - a persistent and painful red lesion, which does not break down or ulcerate, and may last 5–12 days.
- No ulcers, necrotic lesions or infections were identified in this series.
- Mild, non-specific features of envenoming include nausea, vomiting, malaise and headache.
- Delayed pruritus occurs in up to 20% of cases.
- In many cases, a detailed history clarifies that a spider bite was not witnessed, only suspected, or that the species of spider was not formally identified.

MANAGEMENT
- Reassure the patient, apply an ice pack and give simple oral analgesia.
- Do not apply a pressure bandage with immobilisation (PBI).
- Referral to hospital is not indicated.

INVESTIGATIONS
- Investigations (including skin biopsy and microbiological cultures) may be required to determine the aetiology of skin lesions attributed to *Lampona* bites.

DIFFERENTIAL DIAGNOSIS
- If a necrotic cutaneous lesion is present, a causal association with a spider bite is a diagnosis of exclusion.
- The differential diagnoses of a chronic skin ulcer include:
  - infections (staphylococcal, streptococcal, herpes simplex, herpes zoster, gonococcal, mycobacterial, fungal)
  - diabetic ulcers
  - pyoderma gangrenosum
  - squamous cell carcinoma
  - erythema nodosum
  - chemical burn
  - lymphomatoid papulosis
  - localised vasculitis
  - factitious injury
  - traumatic.

DISPOSITION AND FOLLOW-UP
- Patients with a cutaneous ulcer may be discharged to the care of their general practitioner for further investigation or referred to a dermatologist as appropriate.

- Attribution of causation of a chronic ulcer to spider bite in Australia without extensive investigation to exclude alternative diagnosis.

References

Isbister GK, Gray MR. White-tailed spider bite: a prospective series of 130 definite bites by the *Lampona* species. Medical Journal of Australia 2003; 179:199–202.

Swanson DL, Vetter RS. Bites of the brown recluse spiders and suspected necrotic arachnidism. New England Journal of Medicine 2005; 352:700–707.

5.17 TICKS

Distribution of *Ixodes holocyclus*

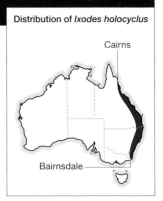

- *Ixodes cornuatus*
- *Ixodes hirsti*
- *Ixodes holocyclus*

Ticks are arachnids that attach to animal hosts to obtain blood meals in the larval, nymph and adult stages of their life cycle. There are 70 tick species found in Australia, but only the three *Ixodes* species listed above cause paralysis. Tick paralysis in humans is almost exclusively associated with *Ixodes holocyclus*, distributed in a narrow eastern coastal strip extending from far north Queensland to Victoria.

TOXINS

Ticks are found on vegetation and attach to animal hosts as they brush past. They make a small incision in the skin using mouth appendages (chelicerae) and insert a barbed feeding tube (hypostome) to begin feeding. Some species also secrete a cement-like substance from the salivary glands to enhance attachment. The toxic salivary secretions include multiple anaesthetic, anticoagulant and vasodilatory agents which facilitate feeding. These include, in the case of the adult female *Ixodes holocyclus*, a protein neurotoxin known as holocyclotoxin. It is thought to act at the pre-synaptic region of the neuromuscular junction and inhibit release of acetylcholine.

CLINICAL PRESENTATION AND COURSE

- Tick paralysis, although rare, is the most significant complication of tick bite in Australia. It usually occurs in children under 3 years of age, but has been reported in adults.
- Tick paralysis presents as a non-specific prodrome that includes drowsiness and unsteadiness of gait. This may be followed by a progressive ascending symmetrical flaccid paralysis that can take days to develop. Cranial nerves are frequently involved leading to the development of ptosis and other neurotoxic effects (oculomotor, facial and bulbar paralysis).
- Paralysis may progress for up to 48 hours after the tick is removed or falls off.

- Untreated respiratory paralysis can result in respiratory failure and death.
- Recovery in survivors is slow and it may take several weeks before strength returns to normal.
- Non-paralytic complications of tick bite include allergic reactions to salivary components ranging from local itching and inflammation to anaphylaxis, or hypersensitivity reactions and local granuloma formation due to retention of mouth parts.
- A number of human infections are transmitted by ticks, but these are outside the scope of this book.

MANAGEMENT

Pre-hospital
- The diagnosis of tick paralysis is rarely considered in the pre-hospital phase. Ventilation should be supported if necessary.

Hospital
Resuscitation and supportive care
- Tick paralysis is potentially life-threatening, the major threat being respiratory failure.
- Patients should be managed in an area equipped for cardiorespiratory monitoring and resuscitation.
- If respiratory failure develops, provision of an airway and mechanical ventilation is life-saving.
- If mechanical ventilation is required, it is likely to be required for days to weeks.

Tick removal
- The tick should be located and removed as soon as practicable.
- When the diagnosis of tick paralysis is considered, a thorough search for ticks should include the scalp, ears (including auditory canal), nose, perineum and natal cleft.
- When located, the tick is carefully removed with every attempt made to remove all of the tick mouth parts attached to the skin. The tick should be grasped as close to the skin as possible using fine forceps, veterinary tick removers or a loop of dental floss or suture material. Once grasped, the tick is then removed by applying gentle outward traction.

Antivenom
- None available for human use.

INVESTIGATIONS
- Tick paralysis is a clinical diagnosis. Investigations are directed at excluding alternative diagnoses.
- Nerve conduction studies, if performed, are abnormal with reduced amplitude of compound motor action potentials but normal conduction velocities. Sensory nerve studies are normal.

DIFFERENTIAL DIAGNOSIS
- The history of tick bite is frequently not available. The major differential diagnosis of ascending flaccid paralysis is Guillain–Barré syndrome. Location of an engorged paralysis tick by careful

searching will confirm the diagnosis of tick paralysis. Ocular signs are less frequently seen in Guillain–Barré syndrome.
- Infant botulism produces a similar clinical picture.
- Paralysis also occurs after snake and blue-ringed octopus envenoming.

DISPOSITION AND FOLLOW-UP
- All patients must be admitted for close, sequential neurological observation.
- Discharge should not occur until sustained neurological improvement is documented.
- Patients requiring ventilatory support should be managed in an intensive care unit. Several days to 1 week of ventilation followed by several weeks of convalescence can be anticipated.

HANDY TIPS
- Consider the diagnosis of tick paralysis in any young child who develops weakness or difficulty walking and resides on or has recently visited the east coast of Australia.
- Consideration of the diagnosis should always prompt a careful search for an attached tick.
- The attached tick will usually be located on the head, frequently in the scalp above the hairline or behind the ears.
- More than one tick may be attached.
- Weakness can be expected to progress for up to 48 hours after removal of the tick, and admission to hospital for close observation is recommended.

PITFALL
- Failure to admit the symptomatic child to hospital for continued observation after removal of the tick.

CONTROVERSY
- It has been suggested that forcible removal of a live tick will cause release of further toxin. It has been advocated that the tick should be killed using a pyrethrin-based insecticide or other proprietary products prior to removal but the additional value of this approach is unclear.

References
Australasian Society of Clinical Immunology and Allergy. Tick allergy 2019. Available at www.allergy.org.au/patients/insect-allergy-bites-and-stings/tick-allergy.

Diaz JH. A comparative meta-analysis of tick paralysis in the United States and Australia. Clinical Toxicology 2015; 53(9):874–883.

Edlow JA, McGillicuddy DC. Tick paralysis. Infectious Disease Clinics of North America 2008; 22:397–413.

Grattan-Smith PJ, Morris JG, Johnston HM et al. Clinical and neurophysiological features of tick paralysis. Brain 1997; 120:1975–1987.

Taylor BW, Ratchford A, van Nunen S et al. Tick killing in situ before removal to prevent allergic and anaphylactic reactions in humans: a cross-sectional study. Asia Pacific Allergy 2019; 9(2):e15. https://doi.org/10.5415/apallergy.2019.9.e15.

CHAPTER 6
ANTIVENOMS

6.1 BLACK SNAKE ANTIVENOM

This equine IgG Fab is the specific treatment of envenoming by black snakes in Australia and Papua New Guinea. The most common indications include the mulga snake (*Pseudechis australis*) and Papuan black snake (*Pseudechis papuanus*).

PRESENTATION
    18 000 unit (43–50 mL) ampoules

INDICATIONS
- Clinical evidence of systemic envenoming (see **Chapter 5.2: Black snake**)
- Laboratory evidence of anticoagulant coagulopathy
- Laboratory evidence of myotoxicity (CK >1000 IU/L)
  - Note: The recommended treatment for envenoming from red-bellied black snakes is tiger antivenom (see **Chapter 5.2: Black snake**)

CONTRAINDICATIONS
- No absolute contraindications
- Increased risk of anaphylaxis in patients who have been previously treated with antivenom or who have a known or suspected equine sera allergy

ADMINISTRATION
- Patients are managed in a monitored area where equipment, drugs and personnel are available to treat an allergic reaction.
- Administer 1 ampoule diluted in 500 mL of normal saline IV over 20 minutes.
- Pre-medication with adrenaline is unnecessary.
- Re-check the coagulation profile and CK 12 hours after antivenom administration.
  - Note: Antivenom is given as a rapid IV push if the patient is in cardiac arrest.

THERAPEUTIC END POINTS
- Resolution of systemic features of envenoming, including non-specific symptoms such as headache, abdominal pain and vomiting
- Improving laboratory values that indicate a resolving coagulopathy and falling CK

ADVERSE DRUG REACTIONS AND MANAGEMENT
Acute allergic or anaphylactic reaction
- There are limited data on the incidence of hypersensitivity reactions, but it is thought to be around 10%.
- Usually mild and manifested by erythema or urticaria. Severe cases develop hypotension.
- Immediately cease antivenom infusion.
- Give oxygen, IV fluids and administer IM adrenaline 0.01 mg/kg (max 0.5 mg) to lateral thigh (see **Chapter 6.12: Allergic reactions to antivenom** for full management description).

- Recommence antivenom infusion cautiously when clinical manifestations of anaphylaxis have improved.
  - Note: Rarely, a titrated infusion of adrenaline may be necessary to complete antivenom administration.

Serum sickness
- This relatively benign and self-limiting hypersensitivity reaction may occur 5–10 days after antivenom.
- Manifestations include fever, rash, arthralgia and myalgia.
- Oral steroids (e.g. prednisolone 25–50 mg/day in adults or 1 mg/kg/day in children) for 5 days ameliorate symptoms.
  - Note: All patients should be warned about this potential complication prior to discharge.

SPECIFIC CONSIDERATIONS
    Pregnancy: no restriction on use.
    Lactation: no restriction on use.
    Paediatric: give standard adult dose in 10 mL/kg of normal saline.

HANDY TIP
- If black snake antivenom is not readily available, 1 ampoule of polyvalent antivenom may be substituted.

PITFALLS
- Withholding antivenom from the envenomed child or pregnant woman because of concerns about the potential adverse reactions.
- Administration of antivenom to a patient who has not been envenomed.

CONTROVERSY
- Tiger snake antivenom is recommended as the preferred treatment for envenoming by the red-bellied or blue-bellied black snake. It appears to be equally effective and has the advantages of being widely available, cheaper and of smaller volume.

References

Churchman A, O'Leary MA, Buckley NA et al. Clinical effects of red-bellied black snake (*Pseudechis porphyriacus*) envenoming and correlation with venom concentrations: Australian Snakebite Project (ASP-11). Medical Journal of Australia 2010; 193:696–700.

Isbister GK, Brown SG, MacDonald E et al. Current use of Australian snake antivenoms and frequency of immediate-type hypersensitivity reactions and anaphylaxis. Medical Journal of Australia 2008; 188(8):473–476. doi:10.5694/j.1326-5377.2008.tb01721.x.

Johnston CI, Brown SGA, O'Leary MA et al. Mulga snake (*Pseudechis australis*) envenoming: a spectrum of myotoxicity, anticoagulant coagulopathy, haemolysis and the role of early antivenom therapy – Australian Snakebite Project (ASP-19). Clinical Toxicology 2013; 51:417–424.

6.2 BROWN SNAKE ANTIVENOM

This equine IgG Fab is the specific treatment of envenoming by brown snakes in Australia. These include the eastern brown snake (*Pseudonaja*

textilis), **western brown snake or gwardar (*Pseudonaja mengdeni*), dugite (*Pseudonaja affinis*) and other *Pseudonaja* species.**

PRESENTATION
1000 unit (4.5–9 mL) ampoules

INDICATIONS
- Clinical evidence of systemic envenoming (see **Chapter 5.3: Brown snake**)
- Laboratory evidence of complete or partial venom-induced consumptive coagulopathy (VICC)

CONTRAINDICATIONS
- No absolute contraindications
- Increased risk of anaphylaxis in patients who have been previously treated with antivenom or who have a known or suspected equine sera allergy

ADMINISTRATION
- Patients are managed in a monitored area where equipment, drugs and personnel are available to treat an allergic reaction.
- Administer 1 ampoule diluted in 500 mL of normal saline IV over 20 minutes.
- Pre-medication with adrenaline is unnecessary.
  - Note: Antivenom is given as a rapid IV push if the patient is in cardiac arrest.

THERAPEUTIC END POINTS
- Resolution of systemic features of envenoming

ADVERSE DRUG REACTIONS AND MANAGEMENT
Acute allergic or anaphylactic reaction
- There are limited data on the incidence of hypersensitivity reactions, but it is thought to be around 10%.
- Usually mild and manifested by erythema or urticaria. Severe cases develop hypotension.
- Immediately cease antivenom infusion.
- Give oxygen, IV fluids and administer IM adrenaline 0.01 mg/kg (max 0.5 mg) to lateral thigh (see **Chapter 6.12: Allergic reactions to antivenom** for full management description).
- Recommence antivenom infusion cautiously when clinical manifestations of anaphylaxis have improved.
  - Note: Rarely, a titrated infusion of adrenaline may be necessary to complete antivenom administration.
Serum sickness
- This relatively benign and self-limiting hypersensitivity reaction may occur 5–10 days after antivenom.
- Manifestations include fever, rash, arthralgia and myalgia.
- Oral steroids (e.g. prednisolone 25–50 mg/day or 1 mg/kg/day in children) for 5 days ameliorate symptoms.
  - Note: All patients should be warned about this potential complication prior to discharge.

Pregnancy: no restriction on use.
Lactation: no restriction on use.
Paediatric: give standard adult dose in 10 mL/kg of normal saline.

PITFALLS
- Withholding antivenom from the envenomed child or pregnant woman because of concerns about the potential adverse reactions.
- Administration of antivenom to a patient who has not been envenomed.

CONTROVERSIES
- The majority of brown snake envenomings can safely be treated with 1 ampoule of brown snake antivenom. However, in patients with severe envenoming syndromes or rapidly progressive complications, a second ampoule of brown antivenom may be considered.
- Published data indicate that administration of antivenom does not hasten recovery from VICC. It may, however, reverse or prevent other manifestations of envenoming.
- Administration of clotting factors (fresh frozen plasma or cryoprecipitate) after antivenom administration is associated with earlier recovery from VICC but not with earlier discharge from hospital.
- The efficacy, safety and indications for clotting factor replacement after venom neutralisation in VICC are not yet well defined.

References
Allen GE, Brown SCA, Buckley NA et al. Clinical effects and antivenom dosing in brown snake (*Pseudonaja* spp.) envenoming – Australian Snakebite Project (ASP-14). PLoS ONE 2012; 7(12):e53188. doi:10.1371/journal.pone.0053188.

Brown SGA, Caruso N, Borland M et al. Clotting factor replacement and recovery from snake venom-induced consumptive coagulopathy. Intensive Care Medicine 2009; 35(9):1532–1538.

Isbister GK, Brown SG, MacDonald E et al. Current use of Australian snake antivenoms and frequency of immediate-type hypersensitivity reactions and anaphylaxis. Medical Journal of Australia 2008; 188:473–476.

Isbister GK, Buckley NA, Page CB et al. A randomized controlled trial of fresh frozen plasma for treating venom-induced consumption coagulopathy in cases of Australian snakebite (ASP-18). Journal of Thrombosis and Haemostasis 2013; 11:1310–1318.

Isbister GK, Duffull SB, Brown SGA. Failure of antivenom to improve recovery in Australian snakebite coagulopathy. Quarterly Journal of Medicine 2009; 102(8):563–568.

6.3 DEATH ADDER ANTIVENOM

This equine IgG Fab is the specific treatment of envenoming by the death adder (*Acanthophis* spp.) in Australia and Papua New Guinea.

PRESENTATION
6000 unit (25 mL) ampoules

INDICATIONS
- Clinical evidence of systemic envenoming, characterised by progressive paralysis and the absence of coagulopathy (see **Chapter 5.4: Death adder**)

CONTRAINDICATIONS
- No absolute contraindications
- Increased risk of anaphylaxis in patients who have been previously treated with antivenom or who have a known or suspected equine sera allergy

ADMINISTRATION
- Patients are managed in a monitored area where equipment, drugs and personnel are available to treat an allergic reaction.
- Administer 1 ampoule diluted in 500 mL of normal saline IV over 20 minutes.
- Pre-medication with adrenaline is unnecessary.
- Observe the patient clinically and monitor serial spirometry/peak flow measurements.
  - Note: Antivenom is given as a rapid IV push if the patient is in cardiac arrest.

THERAPEUTIC END POINTS
- Resolution of systemic features of envenoming

ADVERSE DRUG REACTIONS AND MANAGEMENT
Acute allergic or anaphylactic reaction
- There are limited data on the incidence of hypersensitivity reactions, but it may be up to 40%.
- Usually mild and manifested by erythema or urticaria. Severe cases develop hypotension.
- Immediately cease antivenom infusion.
- Give oxygen, IV fluids and administer IM adrenaline 0.01 mg/kg (max 0.5 mg) to lateral thigh (see **Chapter 6.12: Allergic reactions to antivenom** for full management description).
- Recommence antivenom infusion cautiously when clinical manifestations of anaphylaxis have improved.
  - Note: Rarely, a titrated infusion of adrenaline may be necessary to complete antivenom administration.

Serum sickness
- This relatively benign and self-limiting hypersensitivity reaction may occur 5–10 days after antivenom.
- Manifestations include fever, rash, arthralgia and myalgia.
- Oral steroids (e.g. prednisolone 25–50 mg/day or 1 mg/kg/day in children) for 5 days ameliorate symptoms.
  - Note: All patients should be warned about this potential complication prior to discharge.

SPECIFIC CONSIDERATIONS
Pregnancy: no restriction on use.
Lactation: no restriction on use.
Paediatric: give standard adult dose in 10 mL/kg of normal saline.

- If death adder antivenom is not available, 1 ampoule of polyvalent antivenom may be substituted.
- If no antivenom is available, intubation and ventilation will ensure survival from respiratory failure until the features of neurotoxicity resolve over several days.

PITFALLS
- Withholding antivenom from the envenomed child or pregnant woman because of concerns about the potential adverse reactions.
- Administration of antivenom to a patient who has not been envenomed.

References

Isbister GK, Brown SG, MacDonald E et al. Current use of Australian snake antivenoms and frequency of immediate-type hypersensitivity reactions and anaphylaxis. Medical Journal of Australia 2008; 188:473–476.

Johnston CI, O'Leary MA, Brown SCA et al. Death adder envenoming causes neurotoxicity not reversed by antivenom – Australian Snakebite Project (ASP-16). PLoS Neglected Tropical Diseases 2012; 6(9):e1841.

6.4 TIGER SNAKE ANTIVENOM

This equine IgG Fab is the specific treatment for envenoming by a variety of terrestrial snakes in Australia. These include tiger snakes (*Notechis scutatus*), copperhead snakes (*Austrelaps* spp.), pale-headed and broad-headed snakes (*Hoplocephalus* spp.) and the rough-scaled snake (*Tropidechis carinatus*). It is also the preferred antivenom to treat envenoming by the red-bellied black snake *Pseudechis porphyriacus* (see Chapter 5.2: Black snake).

PRESENTATION
   3000 unit (9–12 mL) ampoules

INDICATIONS
- Clinical or laboratory evidence of systemic envenoming (see **Chapter 5.5: Tiger snake group**)
  - complete or partial venom-induced consumptive coagulopathy (VICC), neurotoxicity and myotoxicity

CONTRAINDICATIONS
- No absolute contraindications
- There is an increased risk of anaphylaxis in patients who have previously been treated with antivenom or have a known allergy to equine sera. In these settings, antivenom should be given after consideration of the risk–benefit analysis.

ADMINISTRATION
- Patients are managed in a monitored area where equipment, drugs and personnel are available to treat an allergic reaction.

- Administer 1 ampoule diluted in 500 mL of normal saline IV over 20 minutes.
- Pre-medication with adrenaline is not routinely indicated.
  - Note: Antivenom is given as a rapid IV push if the patient is in cardiac arrest.

THERAPEUTIC END POINTS
- Resolution of systemic features of envenoming
  - Note: Although tiger snake antivenom halts the progression of paralysis, established neurotoxicity is not reversed by antivenom.

ADVERSE DRUG REACTIONS AND MANAGEMENT
Acute allergic or anaphylactic reaction
- There are limited data on the incidence of hypersensitivity reactions, but it may be up to 40%.
- Usually mild and manifested by erythema or urticaria. Severe cases manifest with hypotension.
- Immediately cease antivenom infusion.
- Give oxygen, IV fluids and administer IM adrenaline 0.01 mg/kg (max 0.5 mg) to lateral thigh (see **Chapter 6.12: Allergic reactions to antivenom** for full management description).
- Recommence antivenom infusion cautiously when clinical manifestations of anaphylaxis are controlled.
  - Note: Rarely, a titrated infusion of adrenaline may be necessary to complete antivenom administration.

Serum sickness
- This relatively benign and self-limiting hypersensitivity reaction may occur 5–10 days after antivenom.
- Manifestations include fever, rash, arthralgia and myalgia.
- Oral steroids (e.g. prednisolone 25–50 mg/day or 1 mg/kg/day in children) for 5 days ameliorate symptoms.
  - Note: All patients should be warned about this potential complication prior to discharge.

SPECIFIC CONSIDERATIONS
Pregnancy: no restriction on use.
Lactation: no restriction on use.
Paediatric: give standard adult dose in 10 mL/kg of normal saline.

HANDY TIPS
- In geographical regions where brown and tiger snakes co-exist, patients who present with VICC are treated with 1 ampoule of brown and 1 ampoule of tiger antivenom.
- In areas where tiger, brown and taipan co-exist, patients are treated with 1 ampoule of polyvalent antivenom.

PITFALL
- Withholding antivenom from the envenomed child or pregnant woman because of concerns about the potential adverse reactions.

CONTROVERSIES

- Published data indicate that administration of antivenom does not hasten recovery from VICC. However, it may reverse or prevent other manifestations of envenoming – neurotoxicity, myotoxicity and thrombotic microangiopathy.
- The definitive dose of antivenom required to treat all tiger snake envenomings is not clearly established. The majority of tiger snake envenomings can safely be treated with 1 ampoule of tiger snake antivenom. However, in patients with severe envenoming syndromes or rapidly progressive complications, a second ampoule of tiger antivenom is indicated.
- Administration of clotting factors (fresh frozen plasma or cryoprecipitate) after antivenom administration can result in earlier recovery from VICC but there is no evidence of benefit for clinical outcomes.
- The efficacy, safety and indications for clotting factor replacement after venom neutralisation in VICC are not yet well defined.

References

Brown SGA, Caruso N, Borland M et al. Clotting factor replacement and recovery from snake venom-induced consumptive coagulopathy. Intensive Care Medicine 2009; 35(9):1532–1538.

Isbister GK, Brown SG, MacDonald E et al. Current use of Australian snake antivenoms and frequency of immediate-type hypersensitivity reactions and anaphylaxis. Medical Journal of Australia 2008; 188:473–476.

Isbister GK, Buckley NA, Page CB et al. A randomized controlled trial of fresh frozen plasma for treating venom-induced consumption coagulopathy in cases of Australian snakebite (ASP-18). Journal of Thrombosis and Haemostasis 2013; 11:1310–1318.

Isbister GK, Duffull SB, Brown SGA. Failure of antivenom to improve recovery in Australian snakebite coagulopathy. Quarterly Journal of Medicine 2009; 102(8):563–568.

Isbister GK, O'Leary MA, Eliott M et al. Tiger snake (*Notechis* spp.) envenoming: Australian Snakebite Project (ASP-13). Medical Journal of Australia 2012; 197(3):173–177.

Isbister GK, White J, Currie BJ et al. Clinical effects and treatment of envenoming by *Hoplocephalus* spp. snakes in Australia: Australian Snakebite Project (ASP-12). Toxicon 2011; 58:634–640.

6.5 TAIPAN ANTIVENOM

This equine IgG Fab is the specific treatment of envenoming by taipans in Australia and Papua New Guinea. These include the coastal taipan (*Oxyuranus scutellatus*), the Papuan taipan (*Oxyuranus scutellatus canni*) and the small-scaled or fierce snake (*Oxyuranus microlepidotus*).

PRESENTATION

12 000 unit (43–50 mL) ampoules

INDICATIONS

- History, clinical features and laboratory evidence of envenoming (see **Chapter 5.6: Taipan**)
  - neurotoxicity, venom-induced consumptive coagulopathy (VICC) and myotoxicity

CONTRAINDICATIONS
- No absolute contraindications
- Increased risk of anaphylaxis in patients who have been previously treated with antivenom or who have a known or suspected equine sera allergy

ADMINISTRATION
- Patients are managed in a monitored area where equipment, drugs and personnel are available to treat an allergic reaction.
- Administer 1 ampoule diluted in 500 mL of normal saline IV over 20 minutes.
- Pre-medication with adrenaline is unnecessary.
  - Note: Antivenom is given as a rapid IV push if the patient is in cardiac arrest.

THERAPEUTIC END POINTS
- Resolution of systemic features of envenoming
  - Note: Taipan antivenom halts the progression of paralysis. Established neurotoxicity is not reversed by antivenom.

ADVERSE DRUG REACTIONS AND MANAGEMENT
Acute allergic or anaphylactic reaction
- There are limited data on the incidence of hypersensitivity reactions, but it is thought to be around 20%.
- Usually mild and manifested by erythema or urticaria. Severe cases manifest with hypotension.
- Immediately cease antivenom infusion.
- Give oxygen, IV fluids and administer IM adrenaline 0.01 mg/kg (max 0.5 mg) to lateral thigh (see **Chapter 6.12: Allergic reactions to antivenom** for full management description).
- Recommence antivenom infusion cautiously when clinical manifestations of anaphylaxis have improved.
  - Note: Rarely, a titrated infusion of adrenaline may be necessary to complete antivenom administration.

Serum sickness
- This relatively benign and self-limiting hypersensitivity reaction may occur 5–10 days after antivenom.
- Manifestations include fever, rash, arthralgia and myalgia.
- Oral steroids (e.g. prednisolone 25–50 mg/day or 1 mg/kg/day in children) for 5 days ameliorate symptoms.
  - Note: All patients should be warned about this potential complication prior to discharge.

SPECIFIC CONSIDERATIONS
Pregnancy: no restriction on use.
Lactation: no restriction on use.
Paediatric: give standard adult dose in 10 mL/kg of normal saline.

HANDY TIPS
- Taipan antivenom does not reverse established paralysis. Instead, it halts the progression of paralysis.
- If taipan antivenom is not available, 1 ampoule of polyvalent antivenom may be substituted.

- Withholding antivenom from the envenomed child or pregnant woman because of concerns about the potential adverse reactions.
- Administration of antivenom to a patient who has not been envenomed.

CONTROVERSIES
- Published data indicate that administration of antivenom does not hasten recovery from VICC. However, it may reverse or prevent other manifestations of envenoming – neurotoxicity, myotoxicity and thrombotic microangiopathy.
- Administration of clotting factors (fresh frozen plasma or cryoprecipitate) after antivenom administration is associated with earlier recovery from VICC but not with earlier discharge from hospital.
- The efficacy, safety and indications for clotting factor replacement after venom neutralisation in VICC are not yet well defined.

References
Brown SGA, Caruso N, Borland M et al. Clotting factor replacement and recovery from snake venom-induced consumptive coagulopathy. Intensive Care Medicine 2009; 35(9):1532–1538.

Isbister GK, Brown SG, MacDonald E et al. Current use of Australian snake antivenoms and frequency of immediate-type hypersensitivity reactions and anaphylaxis. Medical Journal of Australia 2008; 188:473–476.

Isbister GK, Buckley NA, Page CB et al. A randomized controlled trial of fresh frozen plasma for treating venom-induced consumption coagulopathy in cases of Australian snakebite (ASP-18). Journal of Thrombosis and Haemostasis 2013; 11:1310–1318.

Isbister GK, Duffull SB, Brown SGA. Failure of antivenom to improve recovery in Australian snakebite coagulopathy. Quarterly Journal of Medicine 2009; 102:563–568.

6.6 SEA SNAKE ANTIVENOM

This equine IgG Fab is the specific treatment of envenoming by all species of sea snake (family Hydrophiidae) found in Australian waters.

PRESENTATION
1000 unit (15–35 mL) ampoules

INDICATIONS
- Clinical evidence of systemic envenoming with development of neurotoxicity (paralysis and respiratory failure – see **Chapter 5.7: Sea snakes**)
- Laboratory evidence of myotoxicity.

CONTRAINDICATIONS
- No absolute contraindications
- Increased risk of anaphylaxis in patients who have been previously treated with antivenom or who have a known or suspected equine sera allergy

ADMINISTRATION
- Patients are managed in a monitored area where equipment, drugs and personnel are available to treat an allergic reaction.
- Administer 1 ampoule diluted in 500 mL of normal saline IV over 20 minutes.
- Pre-medication with adrenaline is unnecessary.
- A single dose is sufficient to halt progression of paralysis in most cases. Following the initial dose, the patient is observed clinically and spirometry/peak flow measurements monitored.
  - Note: Antivenom is given as a rapid IV push if the patient is in cardiac arrest.

THERAPEUTIC END POINTS
- Resolution of systemic features of envenoming

ADVERSE DRUG REACTIONS AND MANAGEMENT
Acute allergic or anaphylactic reaction
- Usually mild and manifested by erythema or urticaria. Severe cases develop hypotension.
- Immediately cease antivenom infusion.
- Give oxygen, IV fluids and administer IM adrenaline 0.01 mg/kg (max 0.5 mg) to lateral thigh (see **Chapter 6.12: Allergic reactions to antivenom** for full management description).
- Recommence antivenom infusion cautiously when clinical manifestations of anaphylaxis are controlled.
  - Note: Rarely, a titrated infusion of adrenaline may be necessary to complete antivenom administration.

Serum sickness
- This relatively benign and self-limiting hypersensitivity reaction may occur 5–10 days after antivenom.
- Manifestations include fever, rash, arthralgia and myalgia.
- Oral steroids (e.g. prednisolone 25–50 mg/day or 1 mg/kg/day in children) for 5 days ameliorate symptoms.
  - Note: All patients should be warned about this potential complication prior to discharge.

SPECIFIC CONSIDERATIONS
Pregnancy: no restriction on use.
Lactation: no restriction on use.
Paediatric: give standard adult dose in 10 mL/kg of normal saline.

PITFALLS
- Withholding antivenom from the envenomed child or pregnant woman because of concerns about the potential adverse reactions.
- Administration of antivenom to a patient who has not been envenomed.

CONTROVERSY
- Historically, other antivenoms (tiger or polyvalent) have been recommended as alternatives where sea snake antivenom is unavailable. Current data do not support this recommendation.

Reference

White J. A clinician's guide to Australian venomous bites and stings: incorporating the updated CSL antivenom handbook. Melbourne: CSL Ltd; 2012.

6.7 POLYVALENT SNAKE ANTIVENOM

This equine IgG Fab is used in the treatment of envenoming by snakes in Australia and Papua New Guinea. It contains antibodies to the venom of the eastern brown snake (*Pseudonaja textilis*), mulga snake (*Pseudechis australis*), common tiger snake (*Notechis scutatus*), common death adder (*Acanthophis antarcticus*) and the coastal taipan (*Oxyuranus scutellatus*).

PRESENTATIONS

40 000 unit (~50 mL) ampoules containing:
- 1000 units brown snake antivenom
- 3000 units tiger snake antivenom
- 6000 units death adder antivenom
- 12 000 units taipan antivenom
- 18 000 units black snake antivenom

INDICATIONS
- Clinical or laboratory evidence of snake envenoming in Australia or Papua New Guinea when the appropriate monovalent antivenom is not available
- Snake envenoming presentations with VICC in areas where brown, tiger and taipan snakes co-exist (e.g. southern Queensland or northern New South Wales)
  - Note: Polyvalent antivenom is not required in Tasmania (tiger snake antivenom is recommended) or in Victoria and south-west Western Australia (a combination of brown snake antivenom and tiger snake antivenom is recommended).

CONTRAINDICATIONS
- No absolute contraindications
- Not indicated for the treatment of sea snake envenoming
- Increased risk of anaphylaxis in patients who have been previously treated with antivenom or who have a known or suspected equine sera allergy

ADMINISTRATION
- Patients are managed in a monitored area where equipment, drugs and personnel are available to treat an allergic reaction.
- Administer 1 ampoule diluted in 500 mL of normal saline IV over 20 minutes.
- Pre-medication with adrenaline is unnecessary.
  - Note: Antivenom is given as a rapid IV push if the patient is in cardiac arrest.

THERAPEUTIC END POINT
- Resolution of systemic features of envenoming

ADVERSE DRUG REACTIONS AND MANAGEMENT
Acute allergic or anaphylactic reaction
- Incidence is approximately 40%.
- Usually mild and manifested by erythema or urticaria. Severe cases manifest with hypotension.
- Immediately cease antivenom infusion.
- Give oxygen, IV fluids and administer IM adrenaline 0.01 mg/kg (max 0.5 mg) to lateral thigh (see **Chapter 6.12: Allergic reactions to antivenom** for full management description).
- Recommence antivenom infusion cautiously when clinical manifestations of anaphylaxis are controlled.
  - Note: Rarely, a titrated infusion of adrenaline may be necessary to complete antivenom administration.

Serum sickness
- This relatively benign and self-limiting hypersensitivity reaction may occur 5–10 days after antivenom.
- Manifestations include fever, rash, arthralgia and myalgia.
- Oral steroids (e.g. prednisolone 25–50 mg/day or 1 mg/kg/day in children) for 5 days ameliorate symptoms.
  - Note: All patients should be warned about this potential complication prior to discharge.

SPECIFIC CONSIDERATIONS
Pregnancy: no restriction on use.
Lactation: no restriction on use.
Paediatric: give standard adult dose in 10 mL/kg of normal saline.

HANDY TIPS
- A patient envenomed by an unknown snake may usually be appropriately treated with 1 or 2 monovalent antivenoms dependent on geography, clinical features and laboratory investigations. This is less expensive and carries a lower risk of adverse reaction than use of polyvalent antivenom.
- Polyvalent antivenom can be used as a substitute therapy for patients envenomed by taipan, black or death adder snakes if the appropriate monovalent antivenom is not available (see **Chapter 5.1: Approach to snakebite**).

PITFALLS
- Withholding antivenom from the envenomed child or pregnant woman because of concerns about the potential adverse reactions.
- Administration of antivenom to a patient who has not been envenomed.

Reference
Isbister GK, Brown SG, MacDonald E et al. Current use of Australian snake antivenoms and frequency of immediate-type hypersensitivity reactions and anaphylaxis. Medical Journal of Australia 2008; 188:473–476.

6.8 STONEFISH ANTIVENOM

This equine IgG Fab is the specific treatment of envenoming by stonefish (*Synanceia horrida* and *Synanceia verrucosa*) from Australian waters. It may also have a role in the treatment of bullrout (*Notesthes robusta*), lionfish (*Pterois volitans*) and cobbler (*Gymnapistes marmoratus*) stings.

PRESENTATION
2000 unit (1.5–3 mL) ampoules

INDICATIONS
- Severe localised pain unrelieved by intravenous opioids
- Clinical evidence of systemic envenoming

CONTRAINDICATIONS
- No absolute contraindications
- Increased risk of anaphylaxis in patients who have been previously treated with antivenom or who have a known or suspected equine sera allergy

ADMINISTRATION
- Patients are managed in a monitored area where equipment, drugs and personnel are available to treat an allergic reaction.
- Administer 1 ampoule for every two spine puncture wounds (to a maximum of 3 ampoules) undiluted by IM injection.
- Alternatively, the antivenom may be diluted in 100 mL normal saline and administered intravenously over 20 minutes.
- Pre-medication with adrenaline is unnecessary.
- Repeat doses of 1 ampoule are given until therapeutic end point is achieved (see below).

THERAPEUTIC END POINT
- Resolution of local and systemic features of envenoming

ADVERSE DRUG REACTIONS AND MANAGEMENT
Acute allergic or anaphylactic reaction
- Usually mild and manifested by erythema or urticaria. Severe cases develop hypotension.
- Immediately cease antivenom infusion.
- Give oxygen, IV fluids and administer IM adrenaline 0.01 mg/kg (max 0.5 mg) to lateral thigh (see **Chapter 6.12: Allergic reactions to antivenom** for full management description).
- Recommence antivenom infusion cautiously when clinical manifestations of anaphylaxis are controlled.
  - Note: Rarely, a titrated infusion of adrenaline may be necessary to complete antivenom administration.

Serum sickness
- This relatively benign and self-limiting hypersensitivity reaction may occur 5–10 days after antivenom.
- Manifestations include fever, rash, arthralgia and myalgia.
- Oral steroids (e.g. prednisolone 25–50 mg/day or 1 mg/kg/day in children) for 5 days ameliorate symptoms.
  - Note: All patients should be warned about this potential complication prior to discharge.

Pregnancy: pregnancy is not a contraindication to antivenom.
Lactation: no restriction on use.
Paediatric: give standard adult dose (in 10 mL/kg of normal saline if IV).

PITFALLS

- Failure to give repeat doses of antivenom following an absent, incomplete or transient response to the initial dose.
- Withholding antivenom from the envenomed child or pregnant woman because of concerns about the potential adverse reactions.
- Administration of antivenom to a patient who has not been envenomed.

CONTROVERSY

- Relative efficacy of IM versus IV route of administration.

Reference

Currie BJ. Marine antivenoms. Journal of Toxicology – Clinical Toxicology 2003; 41:301–308.

6.9 BOX JELLYFISH ANTIVENOM

This ovine IgG Fab is available for treatment of envenoming by box jellyfish (*Chironex fleckeri*) found in Australian waters. Its clinical utility is questionable.

PRESENTATION

20 000 unit (1.5–4 mL) ampoule

INDICATIONS

- Clinical features of systemic envenoming, such as cardiovascular instability and cardiac arrest (see **Chapter 5.11: Box jellyfish**)
  - Note: Significantly envenomed patients develop cardiotoxicity rapidly and require cardiopulmonary resuscitation at the beach. Routine administration of box jellyfish antivenom is not recommended for stable patients who have responded to pre-hospital resuscitation.

CONTRAINDICATIONS

- No absolute contraindications
- Increased risk of anaphylaxis in patients who have been previously treated with antivenom or who have a known or suspected ovine sera allergy

ADMINISTRATION

- Patients are managed in a monitored area where equipment, drugs and personnel are available to treat an allergic reaction.
- Pre-medication with adrenaline is unnecessary.
- Administer 1–3 ampoules diluted in 100 mL of normal saline IV over 20 minutes in patients with haemodynamic compromise.
  - Note: Six ampoules may be given as a rapid IV push if the patient is in cardiac arrest.

- Resolution of systemic features of envenoming

ADVERSE DRUG REACTIONS AND MANAGEMENT
Acute allergic or anaphylactic reaction
- Usually mild and manifested by erythema or urticaria. Severe cases develop hypotension.
- Immediately cease antivenom infusion.
- Give oxygen, IV fluids and administer IM adrenaline 0.01 mg/kg (max 0.5 mg) to lateral thigh (see **Chapter 6.12: Allergic reactions to antivenom** for full management description).
- Recommence antivenom infusion cautiously when clinical manifestations of anaphylaxis have improved.
  - Note: Rarely, a titrated infusion of adrenaline may be necessary to complete antivenom administration.

Serum sickness
- This relatively benign and self-limiting hypersensitivity reaction may occur 5–10 days after antivenom.
- Manifestations include fever, rash, arthralgia and myalgia.
- Oral steroids (e.g. prednisolone 25–50 mg/day or 1 mg/kg/day in children) for 5 days ameliorate symptoms.
  - Note: All patients should be warned about this potential complication prior to discharge.

SPECIFIC CONSIDERATIONS
Pregnancy: no restriction on use.
Lactation: no restriction on use.
Paediatric: give standard adult dose in 10 mL/kg of normal saline.

HANDY TIPS
- Most patients suffering local envenoming by box jellyfish do not develop systemic features. Local pain usually settles with ice and simple analgesia and antivenom is not indicated.
- Box jellyfish antivenom is not effective in Irukandji syndrome or for stings by other jellyfish.

PITFALL
- Administration of antivenom to patients without clinical features of systemic envenoming.

CONTROVERSIES
- Although antivenom is demonstrated to bind well to venom in vitro, it does not appear to prevent venom-induced cardiovascular collapse in vivo. This suggests that the venom acts very rapidly on the cardiovascular system and before it can be bound by antivenom. If correct, this means that antivenom is of limited clinical value.
- Although commonly advocated in patients with severe pain, there is only anecdotal evidence to support the use of antivenom for analgesia.
- Antivenom is sometimes administered by the IM route, but this route is almost certainly ineffective.

References

Currie BJ. Marine antivenoms. Journal of Toxicology – Clinical Toxicology 2003; 41:301–308.

Winter KL, Isbister GK, Jacoby T et al. An *in vivo* comparison of the efficacy of CSL box jellyfish antivenom with antibodies raised against nematocyst-derived *Chironex fleckeri* venom. Toxicology Letters 2009; 187:94–98.

6.10 REDBACK SPIDER ANTIVENOM

This equine IgG Fab is used in the treatment of envenoming by the Australian redback spider (*Latrodectus hasselti*).

PRESENTATION
> 500 unit (1–1.5 mL) ampoules

INDICATIONS
- Local pain refractory to analgesia
- Clinical features of systemic envenoming (latrodectism) (see **Chapter 5.14: Redback spider**)

CONTRAINDICATIONS
- No absolute contraindications
- Increased risk of allergic reaction in patients who have been previously treated with antivenom or who have a known or suspected equine sera allergy

ADMINISTRATION
- Patients are managed in a monitored area where equipment, drugs and personnel are available to treat an allergic reaction.
- Administer 2 ampoules diluted in 100 mL of normal saline IV over 20 minutes.
- Pre-medication with adrenaline is unnecessary.

THERAPEUTIC END POINT
- Resolution of local and systemic features of envenoming

ADVERSE DRUG REACTIONS AND MANAGEMENT
Acute allergic or anaphylactic reaction
- Acute hypersensitivity reactions occur in less than 5% of cases following IV administration of diluted antivenom and generally are of mild severity (e.g. skin rash).
- Immediately cease antivenom infusion.
- Give oxygen, IV fluids and consider administration of IM adrenaline 0.01 mg/kg (max 0.5 mg) to lateral thigh (see **Chapter 6.12: Allergic reactions to antivenom** for full management description).
- Recommence antivenom infusion cautiously when clinical manifestations of anaphylaxis are controlled.
Serum sickness
- This relatively benign and self-limiting hypersensitivity reaction occurs 5–10 days after antivenom in about 10% of cases.

- Manifestations include fever, rash, arthralgia and myalgia.
- Oral steroids (e.g. prednisolone 25–50 mg/day in adults or 1 mg/kg/day in children) for 5 days ameliorate symptoms.
  - Note: All patients should be warned about this potential complication prior to discharge.

SPECIFIC CONSIDERATIONS

Pregnancy: pregnancy is not a contraindication for antivenom treatment. Antivenom administration may have successfully reversed premature labour caused by redback spider envenoming.
Lactation: no restrictions on use.
Paediatric: give standard adult dose in 10 mL/kg of normal saline.

PITFALLS

- Withholding antivenom from the envenomed child or pregnant woman due to concerns about the potential adverse reactions. Children receive the same dose of antivenom as adults, but dilution may need to be adjusted to a suitable volume.
- Administration of antivenom to a non-envenomed patient.

CONTROVERSIES

- The clinical value of antivenom administration in the management of latrodectism has been questioned by a randomised controlled study in adults (RAVE II), showing no statistically significant clinical benefit above that of standard analgesia in control of the pain and systemic symptoms of redback envenoming.
  - However, redback antivenom out-performed the standard oral analgesic regimen (paracetamol, ibuprofen and oxycodone) for both primary and secondary end points in the study, but did not reach the pre-determined thresholds of significance.
- The decision to withhold antivenom based on the study information limits use of a potential treatment, and no alternative analgesic agent is as yet proven to be effective (including intravenous opioids or agents such as clonidine, ketamine or other neuromodulators).
- Clinical experience suggests that individual patients may benefit from antivenom – particularly paediatric patients, who were not well represented in the study.

ANTIVENOMS

533

TOXICOLOGY HANDBOOK

References

Cocks J, Chu S, Gamage L et al. Redback spider bites in children in South Australia: A 10-year review of antivenom effectiveness [published online ahead of print]. Emergency Medicine Australasia 2021. doi:10.1111/1742-6723.13869.

Isbister GK. Safety of IV administration of redback spider antivenom. Internal Medicine Journal 2007; 37:820–822.

Isbister GK, Brown SGA, Miller M et al. A randomised controlled trial of intramuscular versus intravenous antivenom for latrodectism – the RAVE study. Quarterly Journal of Medicine 2008; 101:557–565.

Isbister GK, O'Leary MA, Miller M et al. A comparison of serum antivenom concentrations after intravenous and intramuscular administration of redback (widow) spider antivenom. British Journal of Clinical Pharmacology 2008; 65:138–143.

Isbister GK, Page CB, Buckley NA et al. Randomized controlled trial of intravenous antivenom versus placebo for latrodectism: the second Redback Antivenom Evaluation (RAVE-II) study. Annals of Emergency Medicine 2014; 64(6):620–628.e2. doi:10.1016/j.annemergmed.2014.06.006.

This lapine IgG Fab is the specific treatment of envenoming by funnel-web spiders (*Atrax* spp. and *Hadronyche* spp.). It may also be useful in treating envenoming by mouse spiders (*Missulena bradleyi*).

PRESENTATION

125 units per ampoule of freeze-dried antivenom

INDICATIONS
- Clinical features of systemic envenoming (see **Chapter 5.15: Funnel-web (big black) spider**).

CONTRAINDICATIONS
- No specific contraindications
- Increased risk of anaphylaxis in patients who have been previously treated with antivenom or who have a known or suspected lapine sera allergy

---

ADMINISTRATION
- Patients are managed in a monitored area where equipment, drugs and personnel are available to manage an allergic reaction.
- Reconstitute the freeze-dried antivenom in 10 mL of sterile water.
- Administer 2 ampoules diluted in 100 mL of normal saline IV over 20 minutes.
- In the severely envenomed patient, the recommended initial dose is 4 ampoules.
- Pre-medication with adrenaline is unnecessary.
- Repeat doses of 2 ampoules are given every 2 hours until clinical features of envenoming resolve.
  - Note: Antivenom is given as a rapid IV push if the patient is in cardiac arrest.

THERAPEUTIC END POINT
- Resolution of local and systemic features of envenoming

ADVERSE DRUG REACTIONS AND MANAGEMENT
Acute allergic or anaphylactic reaction
- The risk of severe hypersensitivity reactions is low.
- Immediately cease antivenom infusion.
- Give oxygen, IV fluids and administer IM adrenaline 0.01 mg/kg (max 0.5 mg) to lateral thigh (see **Chapter 6.12: Allergic reactions to antivenom** for full management description).
- Recommence antivenom infusion cautiously when clinical manifestations of anaphylaxis are controlled.
  - Note: Rarely, a titrated infusion of adrenaline may be necessary to complete antivenom administration.

Serum sickness
- This relatively benign and self-limiting hypersensitivity reaction may occur 5–10 days after antivenom.
- Manifestations include fever, rash, arthralgia and myalgia.

- Oral steroids (e.g. prednisolone 25–50 mg/day or 1 mg/kg/day in children) for 5 days ameliorate symptoms.
  - Note: All patients should be warned about this potential complication prior to discharge.

SPECIFIC CONSIDERATIONS
Pregnancy: no restriction on use.
Lactation: no restriction on use.
Paediatric: give standard adult dose in 10 mL/kg of normal saline.

PITFALLS
- Failure to give repeat doses of antivenom following an absent, incomplete or transient response to the initial dose.
- Inadequate initial dose with life-threatening envenoming.
- Withholding antivenom from the envenomed child or pregnant woman due to concerns about the potential adverse reactions.
- Administration of antivenom to a patient who has not been envenomed.

Reference
Isbister GI, Gray MR, Balit CR et al. Funnel-web spider bite: a systematic review of recorded clinical cases. Medical Journal of Australia 2005; 182(8):407–411.

6.12 ALLERGIC REACTIONS TO ANTIVENOM

ANAPHYLAXIS
Immediate management
- Immediately cease antivenom infusion.
- Call for assistance.
- Administer adrenaline IM (lateral thigh) 0.01 mg/kg up to 0.5 mg.
- Lay patient supine if tolerated.
- Administer high-flow oxygen, airway/ventilation support if needed.
- Administer intravenous normal saline bolus 20 mL/kg.
  - Repeat IM adrenaline 0.01 mg/kg up to 0.5 mg every 3–5 minutes as needed.

Inadequate response or further deterioration
- Commence an IV adrenaline infusion according to institutional protocols:
  - A safe and effective approach is to add 1 mg of adrenaline 1:1000 to 1 L normal saline and titrate the infusion to clinical response.
  - Alternatively, add 1 mg of adrenaline 1:1000 to 100 mL normal saline and commence at 0.5–1 mL/kg/hour, titrated to response.
- If hypotension persists, repeat normal saline boluses 10–20 mL/kg as indicated.
- For bronchospasm, nebulised salbutamol and hydrocortisone IV 5 mg/kg up to 200 mg can be used as additional therapy.
  - Note: Oral antihistamines (e.g. loratadine 10 mg) are indicated for relief of urticaria and itching, but not for cardiorespiratory symptoms. Intravenous antihistamines are NOT recommended.

Infusion of antivenom can be re-started as soon as clinical manifestations of anaphylaxis are controlled. Rarely, ongoing administration of adrenaline by titrated infusion may be necessary to complete antivenom administration.

SERUM SICKNESS

This immune-mediated reaction to antivenom is a self-limiting condition, characterised by rash, fever and arthralgias. A short course of oral steroids is indicated for severe symptoms (e.g. prednisolone 25–50 mg/day in adults or 1 mg/kg/day in children for 5 days).

References

Australasian Society of Clinical Immunology and Allergy (ASCIA) Guidelines 2021. Acute Management of Anaphylaxis. Available at https://www.allergy.org.au/hp/papers/acute-management-of-anaphylaxis-guidelines.

Brown SG, Mullins RJ, Gold MS. Anaphylaxis diagnosis and management. Medical Journal of Australia 2006; 185(5):283–289.

APPENDICES

APPENDIX 1: POISONS INFORMATION TELEPHONE NUMBERS

Australia	13 11 26
New Zealand	0800 764 766 (0800 POISON)
United Kingdom	0870 6006266
United States of America	1 800 2221222

- To convert from conventional units to SI units, multiply by conversion factor.
- To convert from SI units to conventional units, divide by conversion factor.

Drug	Conventional Therapeutic range	Conventional Units	Conversion factor	SI Therapeutic range	SI Units
Carbamazepine	4–12	mg/L	4.25	17–51	micromol/L
Digoxin	0.8–2.0	ng/mL	1.281	1.1–2.6	nmol/L
Ethanol	N/A	mg/dL	0.217	N/A	mmol/L
Ethylene glycol	N/A	mg/L	16.11	N/A	micromol/L
Iron	80–180	microgram/dL	0.179	14–32	micromol/L
Lead	<10	microgram/dL	0.0483	<0.48	micromol/L
Paracetamol	10–30	microgram/mL	6.62	66–199	micromol/L
Phenobarbitone	15–40	mg/L	4.31	65–172	micromol/L
Phenytoin	10–20	microgram/mL	3.96	40–79	micromol/L
Salicylate	15–30	mg/dL	0.0724	1.1–2.2	mmol/L
Theophylline	5–15	microgram/mL	5.55	28–83	micromol/L
Valproic acid	50–120	mg/L	6.94	347–833	micromol/L

APPENDIX 3: N-ACETYLCYSTEINE (NAC) IV INFUSION FOR PARACETAMOL POISONING

Patient weight: _____ kg

Patient's weight* (kg)	INFUSION 1 200 mg/kg NAC added to 500 mL 5% glucose given over 4 hours		INFUSION 2 100 mg/kg NAC added to 1000 mL 5% glucose given over 16 hours	
	Dose of NAC (grams)	Volume of NAC (mL of 200 mg/mL NAC solution)	Dose of NAC (grams)	Volume of NAC (mL of 200 mg/mL NAC solution)
40 kg	8 g	40 mL	4 g	20 mL
50 kg	10 g	50 mL	5 g	25 mL
60 kg	12 g	60 mL	6 g	30 mL
70 kg	14 g	70 mL	7 g	35 mL
80 kg	16 g	80 mL	8 g	40 mL
90 kg	18 g	90 mL	9 g	45 mL
100 kg	20 g	100 mL	10 g	50 mL
110 kg	22 g	110 mL	11 g	55 mL

*Calculate NAC dose based on weight rounded up to nearest 10 kg. If weight >110 kg, calculate dose based on 110 kg.
Infusion 1: 200 mg/kg NAC in 500 mL 5% glucose given IV over 4 hours.
Infusion 2: 100 mg/kg NAC in 1000 mL 5% glucose given IV over 16 hours.

Clinical Institute Withdrawal Assessment of Alcohol Scale – Revised (CIWA-Ar)

NAUSEA AND VOMITING – Ask "Do you feel sick to your stomach? Have you vomited?"

0 no nausea and no vomiting
1 mild nausea with no vomiting
2
3
4 intermittent nausea with dry heaves
5
6
7 constant nausea, frequent dry heaves and vomiting

TACTILE DISTURBANCES – Ask "Have you any itching, pins and needles sensations, any burning, any numbness, or do you feel bugs crawling on or under your skin?"

0 none
1 very mild itching, pins and needles, burning or numbness
2 mild itching, pins and needles, burning or numbness
3 moderate itching, pins and needles, burning or numbness
4 moderately severe hallucinations
5 severe hallucinations
6 extremely severe hallucinations
7 continuous hallucinations

TREMOR – Arms extended and fingers spread apart

0 no tremor
1 not visible, but can be felt fingertip to fingertip
2
3
4 moderate, with patient's arms extended
5
6
7 severe, even with arms not extended

PAROXYSMAL SWEATS

0 no sweat visible
1 barely perceptible sweating, palms moist
2
3
4 beads of sweat obvious on forehead
5
6
7 drenching sweats

AGITATION

0 normal activity
1 somewhat more than normal activity
2
3
4 moderately fidgety and restless
5
6
7 paces back and forth during most of the interview, or constantly thrashes about

ORIENTATION AND CLOUDING OF SENSORIUM – Ask "What day is this? Where are you? Who am I?"

0 orientated and can perform serial additions
1 cannot do serial additions or is uncertain about date
2 disorientated for date by no more than 2 calendar days
3 disorientated for date by more than 2 calendar days
4 disorientated for place/or person

ANXIETY – Ask "Do you feel nervous?"

0 no anxiety, at ease
1 mildly anxious
2
3
4 moderately anxious, or guarded, so anxiety is inferred
5
6
7 equivalent to acute panic states as seen in severe delirium or acute schizophrenic reactions

HEADACHE, FULLNESS IN HEAD – Ask "Does your head feel different? Does it feel like there is a band around your head?" Do not rate for dizziness or light headedness

0 not present
1 very mild
2 mild
3 moderate
4 moderately severe
5 severe
6 very severe
7 extremely severe

Continued

Clinical Institute Withdrawal Assessment of Alcohol Scale – Revised (CIWA-Ar)—cont'd	
AUDITORY DISTURBANCES – Ask "Are you more aware of sounds around you? Are they harsh? Do they frighten you? Are you hearing anything that is disturbing to you? Are you hearing things that you know are not there?" 0 not present 1 very mild harshness or ability to frighten 2 mild harshness or ability to frighten 3 moderate harshness or ability to frighten 4 moderately severe hallucinations 5 severe hallucinations 6 extremely severe hallucinations 7 continuous hallucinations	**VISUAL DISTURBANCES** – Ask "Does the light appear to be too bright? Is its colour different? Does it hurt your eyes? Are you seeing anything that is disturbing to you? Are you seeing things you know are not there?" 0 not present 1 very mild sensitivity 2 mild sensitivity 3 moderate sensitivity 4 moderately severe hallucinations 5 severe hallucinations 6 extremely severe hallucinations 7 continuous hallucinations

The CIWA-Ar measures 10 symptoms. Scores of less than 8 indicate minimal withdrawal. Scores of 9-14 indicate moderate withdrawal. Scores of 15 or more indicate severe withdrawal (impending delirium tremens)

References:

Sullivan JT, Sykora K, Schneiderman J et al. Assessment of alcohol withdrawal: the revised clinical institute withdrawal assessment for alcohol scale (CIWA-Ar). British Journal of Addiction 1989; 84(11):1353-1357. doi:10.1111/j.1360-0443.1989.tb00737.x

Haber P, Lintzeris N, Proud E et al. Guidelines for the treatment of Alcohol Problems. Australian Government Department of Health and Ageing 2009.

Quigley A, Connolly C, Palmer B et al. A brief guide to the assessment and treatment of alcohol dependence. Perth, Western Australia: Drug and Alcohol Office 2015.

Dosing Guide				
Symptoms	**CIWA-Ar Score**	**Dose**		**CIWA-Ar Frequency**
		Diazepam	Lorazepam	
Mild	0-8	NIL	NIL	Record CIWA-Ar and repeat in FOUR hours
Moderate	9-14	5-15 mg	1-3 mg	Record CIWA-Ar and repeat in TWO hours
Severe	≥15	20 mg	4 mg	Record CIWA-Ar and repeat in ONE hour If no improvement in score discuss with Medical Officer
Maximum dose per 24 hours		120 mg	24 mg	Seek medical review if maximum dose reached

Adapted from: Alcohol and other drugs withdrawal management practice and pathways 2021; WA Health.

Pathways of Alcohol Metabolism

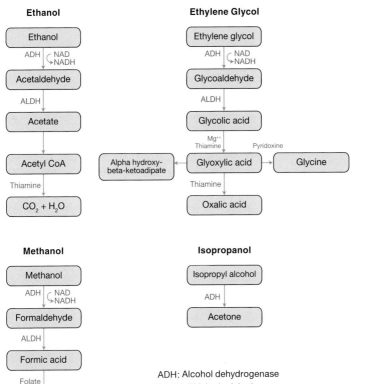

Ethanol

Ethanol
ADH ⟍ NAD
      ⤷ NADH
Acetaldehyde
ALDH
Acetate
Acetyl CoA
Thiamine
$CO_2 + H_2O$

Ethylene Glycol

Ethylene glycol
ADH ⟍ NAD
      ⤷ NADH
Glycoaldehyde
ALDH
Glycolic acid
Mg^{++} Thiamine   Pyridoxine
Alpha hydroxy-beta-ketoadipate ← Glyoxylic acid → Glycine
Thiamine
Oxalic acid

Methanol

Methanol
ADH ⟍ NAD
      ⤷ NADH
Formaldehyde
ALDH
Formic acid
Folate
$CO_2 + H_2O$

Isopropanol

Isopropyl alcohol
ADH
Acetone

ADH: Alcohol dehydrogenase
ALDH: Aldehyde dehydrogenase

APPENDICES

543

TOXICOLOGY HANDBOOK

TOXICOLOGY HANDBOOK
INDEX

Page numbers followed by '*f*' indicate figures, '*t*' indicate tables and '*b*' indicate boxes.

L

Lactation, poisoning during, 123
Lamotrigine, 282–285
LAST *see* Local anaesthetic systemic toxicity (LAST)
Lead, 285–289
Lead encephalopathy, 460
Lead poisoning, without encephalopathy, 461
Lercanidipine *see* Calcium channel blockers
Leucovorin, 426, *see also* Folinic acid
Levetiracetam *see* Anticonvulsants: Newer agents
Levobupivacaine *see* Local anaesthetics
Levocetirizine *see* Antihistamines
Lidocaine *see* Local anaesthetics
Lindane *see* Organochlorines
Lisinopril *see* Angiotensin-converting enzyme inhibitors
Lithium: acute overdose, 289–291
Lithium: chronic poisoning, 292–294
Local anaesthetics, 294–297
Local anaesthetic systemic toxicity (LAST), 294–297
Loratadine *see* Antihistamines

M

MALA *see* Metformin-associated lactic acidosis (MALA)
Malathion *see* Organophosphates
MAOIs *see* Monoamine oxidase inhibitors (MAOIs)
Marijuana *see* Cannabinoids
Mefenamic acid *see* Non-steroidal anti-inflammatory drugs (NSAIDs)
Meloxicam *see* Non-steroidal anti-inflammatory drugs (NSAIDs)
Mepivacaine *see* Local anaesthetics
Mercury, 297–303
Metabolic acidosis, non-anion-gap, 98*t*
Metabolic alkalosis, causes of, 99*t*

Metformin, 303–306
Metformin-associated lactic acidosis (MALA), 303
Methadone, 80, *see also* Opioids
Methamphetamines *see* Amphetamines
Methanol (methyl alcohol), 146–151
Methotrexate, 306–310
Methoxychlor *see* Organochlorines
Methyl alcohol *see* Methanol
Methylene blue, 439–441
Methylene chloride *see* Hydrocarbons
3,4-Methylenedioxyamphetamine (MDA) *see* Amphetamines
3,4-Methylenedioxymethamphetamine (MDMA/ecstasy) *see* Amphetamines
Methylphenidate *see* Amphetamines
Methyl salicylate *see* Salicylates
Metoprolol *see* Beta-blockers
Midazolam, 49, *see also* Benzodiazepines
Mirtazapine, 310–311
Moclobemide *see* Monoamine oxidase inhibitors
Monoamine oxidase inhibitors (MAOIs), 311–314, *see also* *specific drugs*
Morphine *see* Opioids
Mulga snake, 475–477
Mushroom poisoning, 109–117
  clinical syndromes of, 110, 111*t*–114*t*
Myocardial ischaemia, 105

N

N-acetylcysteine (NAC), 16, 441–444
N-Acetyl-p-aminophenol (APAP) *see* Paracetamol
NAI *see* Non-accidental injury (NAI)
Naloxone, 92, 444–446
Naproxen *see* Non-steroidal anti-inflammatory drugs (NSAIDs)
Neuroleptic malignant syndrome (NMS), 62–67